Clinical and Laboratory Evaluation of Human Autoimmune Diseases

Authors

RICHARD A. BRONSON, MD
Professor of Obstetrics and Gynecology
Dept. of Obstetrics and Gynecology
State University of New York at Stony Brook
Stony Brook, NY

C. LYNNE BUREK, PHD, ABMLI
Dept. of Immunology & Infectious Diseases
Johns Hopkins University
Hygiene and Public Health
615 N. Wolfe Street
Baltimore, MD 21205

DAVID J. BYLUND, MD
Scripps Reference Laboratory (SV1)
11107 Roselle Street
San Diego, CA 92121

DAVID F. CARNEY, PHD
Scripps Reference Laboratory (SV1)
11107 Roselle Street
San Diego, CA 92121

HENRY N. CLAMAN, MD
Professor of Medicine
Div. of Clinical Immunology, B-164
University of Colorado Health Science Center
4200 E. Ninth Avenue
Denver, CO 80262-0001

ROBERT I. FOX, MD, PHD
Div. of Rheumatology (MS113)
Scripps Clinic
10666 N. Torrey Pines Road
La Jolla, CA 92037

FRANCESCO M. FUSI, MD
Fondazione Centro S. Raffaele del Monte Tabor
Divisione di Ostetricia e Ginecologia
Clinica Ostetrico Ginecologica
Universita Degli Studi di Milano
Via Olgettina 60
20132 Milano, Italy

LEMING HANG, MD (deceased)
Dept. of Pathology (211C)
Scripps Clinic
10666 N. Torrey Pines Road
La Jolla, CA 92037

HENRY A. HOMBURGER, MD
Clinical Immunology Lab
Mayo Clinic
920 Hilton Bldg.
Rochester, MN 55905

GENE T. IZUNO, MD (retired)
Division of Dermatology
Scripps Clinic
10666 N. Torrey Pines Road
La Jolla, CA 92037

DAVID F. KEREN, MD
Warde Medical Laboratory
5025 Venture Drive
Ann Arbor, MI 48108

REX M. MCCALLUM, MD
Associate Clinical Professor of Medicine
Division of Rheumatology, Allergy, and Clinical Immunology
Duke University School of Medicine
Durham, NC 27710

JOHN G. MCHUTCHISON, MD
Division of Gastroenterology and Liver Diseases
Scripps Clinic
10666 N. Torrey Pines Road
La Jolla, CA 92037

JONATHAN L. MYLES, MD
Dept. of Pathology
Cleveland Clinic Foundation
9500 Euclid Avenue
Cleveland, OH 44195

ROBERT M. NAKAMURA, MD
Scripps Clinic—Department of Pathology
10666 N. Torrey Pines Road
La Jolla, CA 92037 and
Scripps Reference Laboratory
11107 Roselle Street
San Diego, CA 92121

HELENE M.A. PAXTON, PHD, MS, MT
101 Lance Court
Elkton, MD 21921

DOUGLAS A. TRIPLETT, MD
3500 E. CR350 South
Muncie, IN 47302

RAYMOND R. TUBBS, DO
Section Head, Immunopathology
Cleveland Clinic Hospital
9500 Euclid Avenue
Cleveland, OH 44195

S. KENNETH TUNG, MD
Professor, Department of Pathology
University of Virginia Health Sciences Center, Box 214
Charlottesville, VA 22908-0001

CARLOS A. VON MÜHLEN, MD, PHD
Professor of Medicine
Pontíficia Universidade Católica
Faculdade de Medicina—Hospital Sao Lucas
Av. Ipiranga 6690 conj. 325
Porto Alegre, RS, CEP 90610-000, Brazil

WILLIAM E. WINTER, MD
Professor, Pathology and Pediatrics
Dept. of Pathology
University of Florida School of Medicine
Box 100275, JHMHC
1 Miller Health Center
Gainesville, FL 32610-0275

JAMES T. WU, PHD
Professor of Pathology
Dept. of Pathology
University of Utah School of Medicine
ARUP, Inc.
500 Chipeta Way
Salt Lake City, UT 84108

Clinical and Laboratory Evaluation of Human Autoimmune Diseases

Editors

Robert M. Nakamura, MD
Chairman Emeritus
Department of Pathology
Scripps Clinic
La Jolla, California

David F. Keren, MD
Warde Medical Laboratories
Ann Arbor, Michigan

David J. Bylund, MD
The Scripps Research Institute
La Jolla, California
Scripps Reference Laboratory
San Diego, California

ASCP PRESS

American Society for Clinical Pathology
Chicago

Publishing Team
Terri Horning, Brian Franklin (production)
Alan Makinen (imaging)
Christy Prahl (editorial)
Joshua Weikersheimer (publishing direction)

Printed in Hong Kong

05 04 03 02 5 4 3 2 1

Contents

Preface

There are many immunology books today that discuss the theory and experimental progress on autoimmune diseases. The majority of these publications, by necessity, address animal experiments along with data on human diseases.

The primary purpose of this book is to present current and practical state-of-the-art information for most diagnostic clinical immunology laboratories to use in coordinating their evaluation of common human autoimmune diseases. The book tries to help clinical laboratory scientists in their day-to-day problems and consultative interaction with clinicians. It is intended for pathologists, laboratory scientists, and clinicians who are interested in the limitations and usefulness of various clinical laboratory tests for the diagnosis and evaluation of human autoimmune diseases. There is also emphasis on the correlation of clinical data with clinical laboratory tests for the diagnosis and management of human diseases.

The authors wish to acknowledge the help of many colleagues and paraprofessionals who made this book possible. However, the primary person to whom this book is dedicated is LeMing Hang, MD, who contributed so much and passed away April 22, 1997, from a complex combination of autoimmune diseases. Dr. Hang was born in Saigon, Vietnam, and received her college education in the United States, graduating from the Case Western Reserve University School of Medicine. She received her pathology residency training at Mercy Hospital in San Diego, California. Her postdoctoral training and staff work was performed at The Scripps Research Institute under the mentorship of Dr. Frank J. Dixon. She practiced pathology and immunology for several years before she passed away. She will be remembered as a complete physician; pathologist; practicing immunopathologist; and research scientist with integrity, compassion, dedication, commitment, and tenacity.

Best wishes and good luck to all of you.

Editors

SECTION I

Concepts of Autoimmunity and Related Topics

CHAPTER 1

Current and Future Role of the Diagnostic Immunology Laboratory

Robert M. Nakamura, MD

Background and Definitions

This book is primarily focused on the laboratory and clinical evaluation of human autoimmune diseases. However, autoimmune tests in the clinical laboratory are usually performed in the clinical laboratory section of diagnostic immunology laboratories. This chapter discusses the current and future directions of the diagnostic immunology laboratory that will impact lab tests for autoimmune diseases.

What Is Clinical Immunology?

In 1992, a report[1] prepared during a joint meeting of the World Health Organization (WHO; Microbiology and Immunology Support Services), the International Union of Immunological Societies (IUIS), and the International Association of Allergology and Clinical Immunology (IAACI) defined clinical immunology as follows:

> *Clinical immunology is a clinical and laboratory discipline dealing with the study, diagnosis, and care of patients with diseases or disease processes resulting from disordered immunologic mechanisms, and conditions in which immunologic manipulations form an important part of therapy and/or prevention.*

The discipline of clinical immunology also includes[1,2]

- Acquired immunodeficiency syndrome (AIDS)
- Lymphoreticular malignancies
- Infections and immunity from bacteria, viruses, and other microorganisms
- Immunogenetics
- Immune-based therapies in clinical practice

Diagnostic Immunology Laboratory

The diagnostic immunology laboratory is primarily concerned with laboratory tests to evaluate diseases mediated by primary and secondary immune mechanisms. The major categories of such diseases are[3]

- Immunodeficiency diseases
- Autoimmune disorders
- Allergies
- Transplantation immunology
- Neoplastic diseases

There has been extensive progress in the field of immunology and related areas during the last 15 years. Briefly, the areas of immunology that overlap and are related to diagnostic clinical immunology are[4–6]

- Immunobiology, which deals with the origin, inducement, and mechanisms of the immune response.
- Immunochemistry, which is concerned with the physiochemical structure and molecular actions of antigens and antibodies in vivo and in vitro. It is concerned with the many immunologic tests for serum protein abnormalities and other analytes and includes competitive binding nonisotopic assays and radioimmunoassay procedures.
- Immunopathology, which can be defined broadly as the study of diseases induced by or resulting from immune mechanisms. It is primarily concerned with unfavorable consequences in immunologic responses.
- Serology, which has classically dealt with antibodies and their reactions with antigens outside the host.
- Immunohematology, which encompasses immunology and immunochemistry of certain constituents of the blood. Tests are performed for blood group and leukocyte antigens and antibodies and for hemolytic blood disorders.
- Microbiology, which comprises the many immunologic and molecular tests related to infectious diseases.
- Immunotoxicology, which is concerned with the effects of foreign substances on host immune mechanisms. Foreign substances can induce enhanced susceptibility to infections and tumors in the host.
- Immunopharmacology, which is concerned with various humoral mediators involved in immune recognition and end-stage immunologic response.[6]

In the past several years, the diagnostic immunology laboratory has been very involved with the newer molecular deoxyribonucleic acid (DNA) and ribonucleic acid (RNA) assays, which are useful for diagnosis, evaluation, prognostic predictions, and monitoring of therapy of the many diseases mediated by immune mechanisms.[7,8]

Role of the Laboratory Scientist

Laboratory scientists and technologists need to be familiar with the many pitfalls and deficiencies in the specificity and sensitivity of various immunologic tests. In addition, test results should be correlated with newer immunologic concepts and clinical data to give the clinician meaningful information.[9]

Antibody reactions are (1) primary—the antigen and antibody react by combining with each other, ie, immunoenzymatic or immunofluorescence assays; (2) secondary—the antigen and antibody initiate a secondary reaction, such as precipitation, agglutination, or complement fixation; and (3) tertiary—the antigen-antibody reaction initiates a biochemical reaction, such as the immunoglobulin E- and antigen-mediated histamine release from mast cells seen with skin lesions.

Primary, secondary, and tertiary antibody reactions vary in their relative sensitivities.[5] The agar gel diffusion test may be considered a precipitin test with a sensitivity of 1. The electroimmunodiffusion (ED) method may increase the sensitivity 10 times,[10] and an enzyme immunoassay (EIA) or radioimmunoassay (RIA) may increase the sensitivity 10,000 times compared with the immunodiffusion assay. With the new rapid, ultrasensitive nonisotopic immunoassays, analytes can be detected in picomole and subattomole concentrations.[11] The words *zeptomole* and *yoctomole* (corresponding to 10^{-21} and 10^{-24} mol, respectively) have been introduced into the vocabulary of clinical laboratorians.[11]

Uses and Characteristics of Clinical Laboratory Tests

The various uses of laboratory tests are listed in **Table 1-1**. The most frequently performed tests are those requested by physicians to make decisions in therapy and monitor the course of diseases. Therefore, high-volume clinical laboratory tests are defined as those that are necessary for medical care and are used in therapeutic decisions or routine screening, have a rapid assay time and turnaround, and are adaptable to automation.[12]

The usefulness of a new clinical laboratory test is determined by how well it correctly differentiates diseased persons and unaffected persons.[9,13]

Table 1-1. Uses of Clinical Laboratory Tests

Diagnosis of diseases
Early detection and screening of diseases
Genetic classification of diseases
Prognostic markers
Therapeutic decisions
Monitoring and evaluation of therapy

Diagnostic Versus Evaluative Tests

Diagnostic tests are concerned with the current status of the patient. A good diagnostic test answers the question: Does this person have a disease now? The diagnostic test should also give results that are reproducible over time.[13]

On the other hand, evaluation tests are concerned with measuring changes in clinical status or disease activity. A good evaluative test helps determine whether a patient's disease status has improved or worsened over time. The evaluative test should be sensitive to change.[9,13]

For example, the indirect immunofluorescent microscopy (IFM) test for nuclear and cytoplasmic antibodies is a useful diagnostic test for systemic lupus erythematosus (SLE) or for ruling out the possibility of SLE in the differential diagnosis. However, the IFM test for nuclear cytoplasmic antibodies is a poor evaluative test to monitor disease activity of SLE, because changes in IFM test titer over time correlate poorly with other measures of disease activity.

A laboratory test that may not be important or necessary today may become important in the future when a new therapeutic drug or modality is discovered. For example, oncogene mutation assays, which are often used for clinical investigations, will become useful and important when therapeutic agents that interfere with the activation of oncogenes and prevent tumors become available.[3]

Major Factors Influencing the Use of Laboratory Tests

The major factors that influence the development of future laboratory tests, as well as changes in laboratory structure and personnel, are as follows[3]:

- Government regulations
- Health care economics
- Advances in technology
- Advances in therapeutic agents for various diseases

Government Regulations and Health Care Reform

The rapidly evolving changes in health care are being driven by the need to reduce costs. During the

Table 1-2. Criteria for Test Categories in Immunology[15]

Moderate Complexity	High Complexity
Manual procedures with limited steps	Manual procedures with multiple steps
Automated procedures that do not require operator intervention during the analytic process	Immunoassay methods requiring microscopic evaluation
	Radioimmunoassays
	Gel-based immunochemical procedures
	Electrophoresis
	Nucleotide amplification

1970s and 1980s, the rate of health care cost increases contributed to large increases in the cost of living.

Changes in the health care industry have largely been driven by technologic and therapeutic advances and demographic shifts. State and federal governments are seeking to impose a complex regulatory structure on the health care industry and service delivery system. The new proposals are initiatives to limit cost. Currently, laboratory charges comprise approximately 5% of health care bills, and managed care providers wish to reduce this number to 1%.[14]

Numerous government regulations are attempting to reduce costs and still impose strict guidelines that maintain quality control and performance standards. The clinical laboratory is one of the most regulated areas of patient care. The passage of Medicare legislation in 1965 and the implementation of the Clinical Laboratory Improvement Act (CLIA) of 1967 stimulated the development of interlaboratory proficiency survey programs and formal inspection programs by state and federal agencies as well as private organizations such as the College of American Pathologists. Under CLIA '88, regulation has been expanded to physicians' office laboratories and all other sites involving laboratory testing for humans. The personnel requirements for various test categories have been defined, and the specific responsibilities of the laboratory director and supervisor have been delineated.

Under CLIA '88, many of the analytes in immunology are classified in both the moderate- and high-complexity categories. The characteristics used to classify the test procedures for these analytes are listed in **Table 1-2**.[15] The new regulations and changing health care environment will decrease the demand for per-patient use of highly complex and esoteric immunology laboratory tests.

Health Care Economics

The high cost of health care is constantly addressed today by government agencies, health care providers, and third-party payers. To help with the current problems, many managed care programs have been developed. The payment for health care has shifted from fee-for-service to prepaid capitation per case and per diem payment for inpatient hospital services.[3,16]

What Is Managed Care?

Peterson and Hilborne[16] have defined managed care as anything that alters or interferes with the traditional autonomous decisions made by a patient and a physician regarding the patient's care. The scenario of the physician functioning as the patient's advocate has changed to one in which the patient's needs and desires are balanced against the need for cost control. A health maintenance organization (HMO) is a government-qualified prepaid health plan organization and is the model for a managed health care delivery system.

What Is Managed Competition?

Under this health care reform system, the government sets the rules for the minimum benefits package and criteria for competition, with the goal of a market-based approach that improves access and contains costs. Managed competition is expected to encourage health care providers and third-party payers to form alliances, joint ventures, and partnerships to expand and improve current HMOs. The new health care organizations are expected to provide employers with health plans carrying a fixed premium and will compete by contract on price, quality, patient outcomes, and patient satisfaction.[17]

Role of the Clinical Laboratory in Managed Care

Clinical laboratorians must understand the financial arrangement between clinicians and hospitals and work with the clinicians to increase efficiency and productivity and to reduce inappropriate testing. Under the new managed care plans, the clinical laboratory becomes a cost center, and resources must be managed carefully. Any test performed is a net expenditure; there is no increase in incremental revenue from ordering additional "esoteric" tests because there is no payment per test.

Much of the reimbursement for clinical laboratory tests in the future will be made on a contract basis. Thus, for many hospital laboratories, the charge for a particular test will be reimbursed at a fixed specific amount regardless of the actual cost involved in producing a particular test result.[18]

Clinical laboratory professionals must redefine their role in managed care and become integral players in the management of patient care. The clinical laboratory provides important clinical information for an effective mandated care program.[18]

Types of Immunology Laboratories

There are different types of immunology laboratories: acute care (hospital laboratories), primary reference laboratories, and secondary reference laboratories. Each is geared toward providing different tests, depending on turnaround time requirements for diagnostic and therapeutic evaluation. The highly complex tests that do not require a rapid turnaround time are decentralized and performed in reference laboratories. Centralization of tests offers the advantages of cost effectiveness and higher volume. A secondary reference laboratory may perform the more specialized low-volume tests.

Advances in Technology

The new technologic advances that are likely to bring about many changes in the immunology laboratory are shown in **Table 1-3**.

Recombinant DNA Technology

Recombinant DNA technology has led to the development of many new applications in clinical immunology and medicine. Many nucleotide probe assays have been developed for the diagnosis and monitoring of infectious diseases, genetic diseases, immune-mediated diseases, and cancer. The Human Genome Project has been completed and already gene therapy is a reality.[1] Many new laboratory tests will be needed to evaluate and monitor immune diseases treated with gene therapy.[19,20]

Synthetic Peptide Technology

With the advances in recombinant DNA technology, DNA can be cloned and sequenced easily, rapidly, and accurately. The translation of nucleotide sequences into amino acid sequences has become commonplace. Because the amino acid sequences of many proteins are in computer programs, one can obtain the unique specific peptide structures of a virus, protein, hormone, etc. A peptide can be selected for its hydrophilic, hydrophobic, and antigenic properties, and a specific monoclonal antibody to it can be produced.

Numerous peptides have been identified as neurotransmitters and brain hormones. Besides medical therapeutic uses, synthetic peptides are useful for developing specific diagnostic assay kits for use in infectious and many other diseases. Synthetic peptide immunoassays have been developed to detect human immuno-deficiency virus (HIV) and especially to identify specific infections caused by HIV-1 and HIV-2 subspecies.[21]

Table 1-3. Technologic Advances Influencing the Future of Immunology Laboratories[3,13]

Antibody design (combined monoclonal and recombinant DNA technology)
Rapid, automated solid-phase and homogeneous immunochemical assay instruments
DNA/RNA probe tests and amplification systems, such as polymerase chain reaction
Synthetic peptides
Biosensors
Supercomputers with image storage and retrieval
Cellular immune assays, cytokines, and adhesion molecules

Biosensors

Biosensors are synergistic devices combining biochemistry and microelectronics that simplify biochemical and chemical analysis on a microscopic or macroscopic scale.[22,23] Some biosensors, such as gas sensory electrodes, do not contain an immobilized biologic material and are more robust and reliable.

There are 4 main types of biosensors[22]:

- Small, handheld devices
- Bench-type analyzers or multisample automated analyzers
- Flow devices (bioreactors) for on-line monitoring of continuous processes
- Continuous in vivo or implanted monitors

The current trend is toward miniaturization of biosensors. In the future, data from small biosensors used at the point of care will be sent to central laboratory computers by wireless means.

Supercomputers

Computers of the future will report laboratory data using graphics, and will be able to retrieve previous data on the same patient. Thus, the clinician can easily see trends and changes in a specific analyte. Future reports will be in a consultative format with interpretive information, and many immunology laboratory tests will help monitor the innovative complex forms of therapy and will require reporting of information beyond the level of the specific analyte.

Besides interpretive profiling of laboratory tests, the technology will allow extensive image storage and retrieval and the transmission of pictures and data. This will have an impact in the area of anatomic pathology, especially with regard to image analysis and immunohistochemical analysis.

Cellular Immune Assays, Cytokines, and Adhesion Molecules

Technologic instruments will be developed so cellular marker assays will be routine in most hospital laboratories. These cellular markers and receptor assays will be necessary for evaluating diseases and monitoring future therapeutic modalities. Flow cytometry and image analyzers will be common instruments in the immunology laboratory.[3]

Considerable advances in cellular immunology have been achieved through various in vitro studies of isolated lymphocytes or macrophages under defined conditions. These studies have shown that all stages of development, growth, proliferation, and activation are regulated and influenced by the intracellular elaboration of numerous cytokines. Cytokines are signaling molecules involved in communication between cells. They are polypeptide products of activated cells that influence the states of activation, proliferation, and differentiation.[3]

Cytokines are released during the effector phase of cellular stimulation and are important in translating immune recognition. A particular cytokine produced by one cell type may affect the production of cytokines by other cell types. Cytokines are involved in immunoregulation and hematopoietic blood development. Several have been cloned and are used for therapeutic purposes.

Criteria for Evaluation of Diagnostic Technology

Most new diagnostic technologies have not been assessed adequately to determine whether their application improves health.[24] Guyatt et al[25] have presented guidelines for the evaluation of diagnostic techniques to determine their range of possible uses, diagnostic accuracy, impact on the health care provider, therapeutic impact, and impact on patient outcomes. The criteria are listed in **Table 1-4**.

Advances in Therapy

As stated previously, many laboratory tests are unimportant for diagnosis or evaluation until a special drug or specific treatment modality becomes available. Such tests then become necessary for treatment decisions. There have been many advances in the therapy of immunologically mediated diseases. Some of the important advances are[3]

- Therapeutic immunosuppression in autoimmune diseases and transplantation
- Cytokines, growth factors, and cytokine receptor analogs and antagonists
- Cell adhesion molecules and therapeutic modalities
- Interferon therapy
- Gene therapy of immune diseases
- Cancer gene therapy
- Immunotherapy of cancer

Therapeutic Immunosuppression in Autoimmune Diseases and Transplantation

Autoimmunity is a concept that explains "normal" regulatory physiologic mechanisms as well as the pathogenesis of a number of diseases. Autoimmunity can be pathologic and induce immunologic injury to the host, as is the case with diseases such as autoimmune thyroiditis and systemic lupus erythematosus. Autoimmunity may also play a role in a wide range of clinical states, including physiologic clearance of dead cells and cell components, aging, response to rival and microbial infections, and generalized immunologic diseases.[26]

In the nonspecific immunosuppressive treatment of autoimmune disease, there are different levels of treatment[27,28]:

- Corticosteroids, which suppress autoimmune reactions and reduce inflammation
- Chemical immunosuppressive drugs such as cyclophosphamide
- Cyclosporine and FK506 (immunosuppressive drugs for transplantation)

The newer therapeutic modalities and those under development involve[3]

- T-cell vaccination
- Monoclonal antibodies to CD3, CD4, T-cell receptors, and class II major histocompatibility complex (MHC) molecules
- Peptide therapy for blocking antigens to MHC molecules

The above 3 specific targets involve the recognition and antigen processing of the immune system.

Conclusion and Future Expectations

In the future, the immunology laboratory will provide tests on a disease-oriented basis rather than by assay methodology. The laboratorian will perform the humoral and cellular immune tests as well as the nucleotide tests needed for the evaluation and monitoring of immune-mediated diseases. The laboratorian will also perform complex assays to help monitor the new therapeutic options. The laboratory scientist will work closely with clinicians and provide consultative information.

There will be a trend toward

- Centralization of complex immunologic and nucleotide probe assays, which may require a turnaround time of 1 day or more.
- Decentralization of tests that are important for monitoring critical patients in intensive care, coronary care, or transplantation surgery.
- Decentralization of high-volume tests to alternative sites such as the patient's bedside and the physician's office. The tests that are urgently needed for medical treatment decisions will be transferred rapidly to these sites when biosensors become available.

Most pathologists agree that the major factors that will influence the future of the immunology laboratory are government regulations, health care economics, technology, and advances in therapy. New diagnostic technologies should be used to provide a better understanding of disease processes, with the prospect of more effective treatments. However, many ethical issues regarding genetic testing and screening exist.[29] The insurance

Table 1-4. Criteria for the Evaluation of Diagnostic Technology[25]

Technologic capability	The ability of the technology to perform to specifications in a laboratory setting has been demonstrated.
Range of possible uses	The technology promises to provide important diagnostic information in a number of clinical situations.
Diagnostic accuracy	The technology provides information that allows health care workers to make more accurate assessments regarding the presence and severity of disease.
Impact on health care providers	The technology allows health care workers to be more confident of their diagnoses and thereby decreases their anxiety and increases their comfort.
Therapeutic impact	The therapeutic decisions made by health care providers are altered as a result of applying the technology.
Patient outcome	Application of the technology results in a benefit to the patient.

providers may identify patients at risk and not provide insurance or increase premiums.

A negative aspect of new technologic developments is that some health care providers may be tempted to use new diagnostic tests to serve their own economic and administrative purposes. However, new diagnostic techniques also can be used to predict late-onset genetic diseases and behavioral disorders, thus reflecting the strategies of health care providers to reduce costs, minimize the risk of malpractice suits, and plan for the efficient use of health care resources.[30]

In the future, a renewed focus on preventive medicine will place emphasis on predictive tests to screen for data that identify important population phenotypes that represent risk factors.[9] Tests may soon be used to identify genes in patients who are predisposed to autoimmune diseases.

Autoimmune diseases are usually revealed at a late stage of their natural history, and immunointervention is used only when all other treatments have failed. This should change in the future with the early prediction of disease onset using genetic tests and immunologic markers. Early identification of at-risk patients will allow selective intervention with autoantigen-specific therapy. Experimental models of spontaneous autoimmune diseases show that at these early stages,[31] the autoimmune response is much more sensitive to immunointervention than in later stages.[31] It is also obvious that such early intervention prevents the occurrence of the irreversible lesions that characterize advanced autoimmune diseases.[9,31]

The discovery of immunologic tests that allow prediction, early diagnosis, or prognosis of autoimmune diseases is the subject of intensive research. The most spectacular progress has been achieved in insulin-dependent diabetes,[32] in which islet cell autoantibodies can be found several years before the onset of clinical disease (as defined by insulin requirement). The quality of prediction is sufficient to enable recognition of future diabetics with a reliability approaching 80%. It remains true, however, that some diabetics never show the presence of islet cell antibodies (KA31: GAD, IA2, ICA-69 antibodies) regardless of the antibody assay used, and that some ICA-positive subjects fortunately never become diabetic. One may assume that the inclusion of a T-cell assay would improve the quality of prediction, because the disease is apparently exclusively mediated by a cellular immune reaction.

References

1. Lambert PH, Metzger H, Miyamoto T. Clinical immunology: Guidelines for its organization, training and certification—relationship with allergology and other medical disciplines. A WHO/IUIS/IAACI report. *Clin Immunol Immunopathol.* 1993;69:234–243.
2. Bloch KJ. What is a clinical immunologist? *Pediatr Clin North Am.* 1994;41:591–596.
3. Nakamura RM, Bylund DJ. Factors influencing changes in the clinical immunology laboratory. *Clin Chem.* 1994;40:2193–2204.
4. Kwapinski JBG. A concept of modern immunology. In: Kwapinski JBG, ed. *Research in Immunochemistry and Immunobiology.* Vol. 2. Baltimore, MD: University Park Press; 1972:vii.
5. Nakamura RM. *Immunopathology: Clinical Laboratory Concepts and Methods.* Boston, MA: Little Brown & Co; 1974:3–9.
6. Burrell R, Flaherty DK, Sauers LJ. *Toxicology of the Immune System: A Human Approach.* New York, NY: Van Nostrand Reinhold; 1992:1–9.
7. Nakamura RM. College of American Pathologists Conference XXIV on Molecular Pathology: Introduction. *Arch Pathol Lab Med.* 1993;117:455–456.
8. Nelson DL, Kurman CC. Molecular genetic analysis of the primary immunodeficiency disorders. *Pediatr Clin North Am.* 1994;41:657–663.
9. Osterland CK. Laboratory diagnosis and monitoring in chronic systemic autoimmune diseases. *Clin Chem.* 1994;40:2146–2153.
10. Purves LR, Geddes EW. A more sensitive test for alpha fetoprotein. *Lancet.* 1972;I:47.
11. Kricka LJ. Selected strategies for improving sensitivity and reliability of immunoassays. *Clin Chem.* 1994;40:347–357.
12. Nakamura RM, Bylund DJ. New developments in clinical laboratory molecular assays. *J Clin Lab Anal.* 1992;6:73–83.
13. Ward MM. Evaluative laboratory testing assessing tests that assess disease activity. *Arthritis Rheum.* 1995;38:1555–1563.
14. Young DS, Bruns DE, Doumas BT, et al. The future of clinical chemistry and its role in healthcare: A report of the Athena Society. *Clin Chem.* 1996;42:96–101.
15. Abbott DB, Homburger HA. HHS categorization of CLIA tests systems in laboratory immunology. *Clin Immunol Newsletter.* 1993;13:9–11.
16. Peterson P, Hilborne LH. Facing managed care's challenge to pathology. *Am J Clin Pathol.* 1993;99(suppl):S3–S6.
17. Cohen C. View from Washington—reimbursement and regulatory trends. *Am J Clin Pathol.* 1993;99(suppl):S17–S21.
18. Skootsky SA, Oye RK. The changing relationship between clinicians and the laboratory medicine specialist in the managed care era. *Am J Clin Pathol.* 1993;99(suppl):S7–S11.

19. Anderson WF. Human gene therapy. *Science.* 1992;256:808–813.
20. Mulligan RD. The basic science of gene therapy. *Science*. 1993;260:926–932.
21. Smith RS, Parks DE. Synthetic peptide assays to detect human immunodeficiency virus types 1 and 2 in seropositive individuals. *Arch Pathol Lab Med*. 1990;114:254–258.
22. Nakamura RM, Kasahara Y, Rechnitz GA. *Immunochemical Assays and Biosensor Technology for the 1990s*. Washington, DC: American Society of Microbiologists; 1992.
23. Gronow M. Biosensors. *Trends Biochem Sci.* 1984;9:336–340.
24. Berger ML, Hillman HL, Bryan R, et al. Economic analysis of health care technology. A report on principles. *Ann Intern Med.* 1995;122:61–70.
25. Guyatt GH, Tugwell PX, Feeny DH, et al. A framework for clinical evaluation of diagnostic technologies. *Can Med Assoc J.* 1986;134:587–594.
26. Nakamura MC, Nakamura RM. Contemporary concepts of autoimmunity and autoimmune diseases. *J Clin Lab Anal*. 1992;6:275–289.
27. Bach JF. *Monoclonal Antibodies and Peptide Therapy in Autoimmune Diseases*. New York, NY: Marcel Dekker; 1993.
28. Hoffman ES. Immunosuppressive therapy for autoimmune diseases. *Ann Allergy*. 1993;70:263–274.
29. Durfey SJ. Ethics and the human genome project. *Arch Pathol Lab Med.* 1993;117:466–469.
30. Nelken D, Taneredi L. *Dangerous Diagnostics—The Social Power of Biological Information.* New York, NY: Basic Books; 1989:207.
31. Bach JF. Predictive medicine in autoimmune diseases: From the identification of genetic predisposition and environmental influence to precocious immunotherapy. *Clin Immunol Immunopathol*. 1994;72:156–161.
32. Palmer JD. Predicting IDDM (insulin dependent diabetes mellitus). Use of humoral markers. *Diabetes Res*. 1993;1:104–115.

CHAPTER 2

Concepts of Autoimmunity and Autoimmune Diseases

Robert M. Nakamura, MD

Normally, each person is endowed with an immune system that develops and can distinguish "self" from "nonself," or foreign. Generally, the host immune system is capable of responding to any invading foreign molecule and usually avoids adverse reactions against antigens of the host (self-antigens).[1,2]

However, many pathways and alterations of self-recognition control mechanisms can initiate an autoimmune response. *Autoimmunity* has been defined broadly as the failure of an organism to recognize its own healthy tissue as self and includes any immune response to the host's own tissue, whether it is humoral (eg, circulating autoantibodies) or cellular (eg, delayed hypersensitivity). Autoimmunity is also defined by the presence of autoantibodies and/or T cells that react against self-antigens.[2]

The normal response to self-antigens has 3 stages[3]:

- *Autorecognition* can be defined as the normal regulatory interaction in cells of the immune system for the autorecognition of membrane idiotype receptors and major histocompatibility complex (MHC) molecules to maintain tolerance, handling, and elimination of metabolic and catabolic substances, regardless of origin (self or nonself).
- *Autoimmunity* is characterized by enhanced autoreactions concomitant to nonself reactions due to disturbances such as infections and trauma with an intact immunologic network.
- In *autoimmune diseases*, the autoimmune responses and severe derangements of the immunologic network lead to pathologic injury.

Natural Autoimmune Response Versus Autoimmune Diseases

In 1900, Erlich and Morgenroth[4] postulated the concept of *horror autotoxicus*, which said that the body does not normally mount immune responses against itself. It was also believed that if an autoimmune response did occur, it was harmful to the host. During the 1990s, numerous research advancements in immunology, molecular biology, and immunogenetics influenced a change in thinking regarding the autoimmune response and autoimmune disease.

Today, we know that autoimmune responses are not rare and self-antigens may elicit a "natural" autoimmunity of the host without an accompanying autoimmune disease. Newer evidence and research have indicated that autoimmune responses may be normal and important in regulating the immune system.[5–7] Therefore, not all autoimmune responses are harmful or "forbidden." Certain responses, such as the recognition of cell surface antigens encoded by the MHC and anti-idiotypic responses against self-idiotypes, are important for the diversification and normal functioning of an intact immune system.[3,8]

Some benign or normal autoimmune responses may serve a regulatory function within the immune network. Autoimmune responses may be important for normal regulatory mechanisms, such as physiologic clearance of dead cells or cell components involved in aging. Autoantibodies that react with tissue antigens of the host may not cause tissue injury or produce disease.[1–9]

However, autoimmunity can be pathologic and induce immunologic injury to the host by leading to accompanying diseases such as autoimmune thyroiditis and systemic lupus erythematosus (SLE). In organ-specific diseases such as autoimmune thyroiditis, the autoimmune response is the major factor in initiating the tissue injury. However, there are other diseases in which the immunologic response is secondary to the initial tissue injury. The term "autoimmune disease" has generally been assigned to those conditions in which an autoimmune mechanism or injury has contributed to the pathogenesis of the disease.

In summary, autoimmunity is a concept that may explain the pathogenesis of a number of diseases with an immune etiology, but also may help explain "normal" physiological and immunologic regulatory mechanisms in a wide range of clinical states, including the physiologic clearance of dead cells and components, aging, and response to viral and microbial infections.

The Role of the Major Histocompatibility Complex in Self- and Nonself-Recognition

The MHC is involved in determining responsiveness or nonresponsiveness to self- and nonself-immunogens.[8]

Normal Immune System

The normal immune system recognizes foreign antigens by 3 different types of recognition structures:

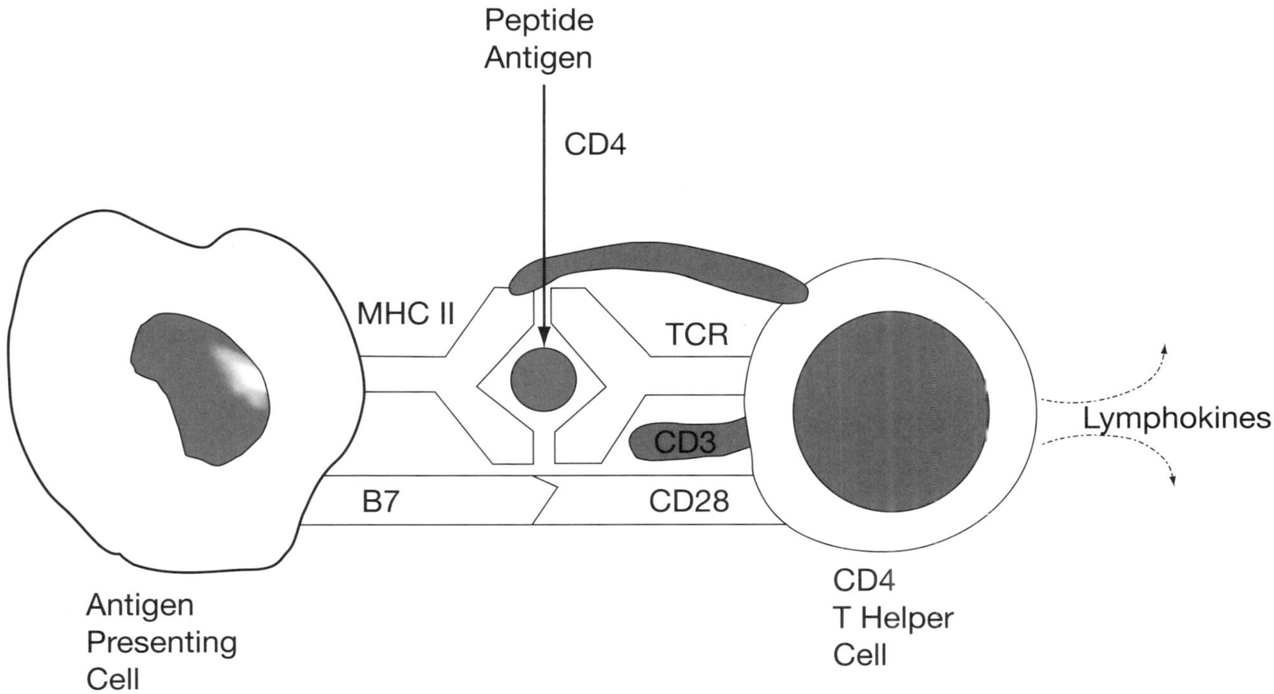

Figure 2-1. The ternary complex. Schematic representation of the trimolecular interaction between the MHC class II molecule, peptide antigen, and the T-cell receptor (TCR) involved in the induction of a normal immune response. Two signals are necessary to activate lymphocytes: (1) A CD4+ helper T cell with TCR recognizes a processed peptide antigen presented by an MHC class II molecule; and (2) A costimulatory signal, which activates CD4+ T cells to produce cytokines, is provided by the interaction between CD28 and B7. B7 is produced by the antigen-presenting cell only when it is activated.

- Immunoglobulins (Igs), or antibodies, which are expressed or secreted by an activated B cell or plasma cell
- T-cell receptors (TCRs), which are responsible for mediating T-cell recognition of antigens presented by histocompatibility antigens
- Glycoprotein products of the MHC

The first 2 types of structures are found only on lymphocytes, whereas MHC glycoproteins are present on the surface of all nucleated cells in the body. Each of the fully developed lymphocytes expresses a specific and unique Ig or TCR, and all of the cells of the same host express the same MHC gene products.[7]

The MHC molecules are highly polymorphic. Class I molecules are expressed on most cell types and are recognized by the CD8+ subset of mature T cells. Class II molecules (HLA-DR, HLA-DP, HLA-DQ) are found largely on cells with antigen-presenting cell function and are recognized by DC4+ T cells.[8,10,11]

Certain antigens such as intracellular viral antigens are preferentially presented by class I molecules to CD8+ T cells. The CD8– T cells are directed to destroy cells invaded by viruses, producing abnormal antigens. Class II molecules are directed toward presentation of external or alloantigens processed through the cytosomal system to CD4+ T cells.

In the initiation of a CD4+ T-cell response, a T cell with the α-β receptors must recognize a self-peptide or foreign peptide within the peptide-binding groove of a self class II MHC molecule[8,10,12] (**Figure 2-1**). T cells are bound to intact self-antigen molecules, and the antigen must be processed and cleaved into peptide fragments and presented on the surface of antigen-presenting cells with class II or class I MHC molecules that serve as targets for CD4+ and CD8+ T cells, respectively.[8,12,13]

The immunoglobulin receptors of B cells are capable of binding native antigen, which is not processed. B cells can bind self-components, and low levels of nonpathologic "natural" autoantibodies are found in the normal state.[14,15] Autoantibodies may be an epiphenomenon (appearing as a result of, rather than being responsible for, the primary autoimmune process).

The 3 main functions of T cells are (1) to help B cells, (2) to induce inflammatory reactions, and (3) to induce killing. These functions are acquired only after T-cell activation and are influenced by both the environment and the cytokines produced by cell-to-cell interaction.[16]

Natural Killer Cells and Major Histocompatibility Complex Class I Molecules

Natural killer (NK) cells constitute a distinct population of lymphocytes.[17,18] These cells are involved in helping the host mechanisms to eliminate neoplasms. However, they also play a major role in immune response to invading microorganisms such as viruses and (particularly) intracellular pathogens.

The expression of MHC class I molecules protects cells against lysis by NK cells. Natural killer cells are believed to recognize self-MHC class I molecules; the combination of self-peptide and MHC class I molecules blocks NK cell–mediated lysis.[17,19]

T-Cell Involvement in Self and Nonself Recognition

The control of self-nonself discrimination is the primary responsibility of the T cell. Discrimination of self- from nonself-antigens and MHC molecules is achieved by negative and positive selection of T cells in the thymus. Harmful T cells with receptors that bind to self-molecules are deleted before they can mount immune responses.[12]

Thus, the 2 requirements for the initiation of autoimmune disease are

1. Incomplete elimination of self-reactive T cells
2. Presentation of self-antigens as an MHC II/self-antigen complex

T-Cell Activation

Native T cells are first stimulated by the interaction of T-cell α-β receptors and specific peptides presented by the MHC (first signal). However, for the T cell to acquire full effector function, it needs a costimulatory signal that is antigen-nonspecific (second signal). This is delivered by CD28 molecules, which interact with B7 on antigen-presenting cells (see Figure 2-1), although other possibilities for the secondary signal exist. Activation of helper T cells by this mechanism is followed by the production of cytokines and immune response amplification. Signal 1 in the absence of the signal 2 results in T-cell inactivation or anergy, which is associated with a blocking of interleukin gene transcription.[20] This mechanism also prevents self-antigens from initiating an autoimmune response. It is believed that only certain cells—such as macrophages, dendritic cells, and possibly activated B cells—can deliver both the first and second signals.[21,22]

γ-δ T Cells

In contrast to conventional α–β T cells, which are specific for antigenic peptides presented by the MHC, the γ-δ T cells can directly recognize proteins and nonproteinaceous phospholigands.[9,23] Therefore, the role of γ-δ T cells in immune response to microbial infections has been clearly documented.

γ–δ T lymphocytes may play a role in autoimmunity through the production of cytokines that induce heat shock proteins (hsps).[24] γ–δ cells recognize epitopes of stress proteins.

Cytokines and Helper T Cells

Cytokines are important molecules that mediate interactions within the immune system. The cytokines include the various interleukins, interferons, and related molecules. Certain cytokines are effectors that promote autoimmune reactions, whereas others serve to suppress the development of autoimmunity. The factors that regulate cytokine production are complex.

There are 2 types of helper T cells: Th_1 and Th_2. Activated T cells under the influence of surrounding cytokines may differentiate into Th_1 or Th_2.[16,25] The Th_1 cells produce interleukin-2 (IL-2) and interferon gamma (IFN-γ), induce inflammatory responses, and help produce opsonizing antibodies that bind to Fc receptors and phagocytes. Th_1-dominated responses may be involved in the pathogenesis of organ-specific autoimmune disorders, acute allograft rejection, and contact dermatitis. In contrast, Th_2 responses may be responsible for certain systemic autoimmune diseases and atopic disorders.

Subsets of CD4+ T cells have been defined as Th_1 and Th_2 based on the profile of cytokines they produce.[16,25] In addition to IL-2 and IFN-γ, Th_1 cells produce tumor necrosis factor-α and lymphotoxin-α, which can promote or inhibit Th_2 cells. The Th_1 cells generally promote T-cell inflammatory immune reactions.

In contrast, the Th_2 cells promote humoral immunity and produce IL-4, IL-10, and IL-5 and inhibit delayed hypersensitivity responses as well as Th_1-cell functions. Autoimmune responses may arise from defects in abnormal regulation of the Th_2 cells or infection stimuli with polyclonal activation of a Th_1 response.

Relationship of Tolerance and Autoimmunity

Weigle[26–28] defined autoimmunity as a termination of natural unresponsiveness or tolerance to self. *Immunologic unresponsiveness* is the inability to initiate a detectable immune response to an antigenic challenge; *tolerance* is commonly used in transplantation immunology to include factors besides immunologic events, such as drug resistance. Tolerance and unresponsiveness are used interchangeably in this chapter, because only the immune system is discussed.

Immunologic tolerance is an active physiologic process, and 2 types of tolerance have been described[28,29]:

Central tolerance. No antibody is produced because response immune cells are missing (due to clonal deletion of specific autoreactive T cells).

Peripheral tolerance. An antibody may be produced initially, but is then suppressed and controlled by other components of the immune system (suppressor T cells, antibodies), anti-idiotypes, and immune complexes. Autoimmune disease may result from a failure in peripheral tolerance. The peripheral tolerance is dynamic rather than static and operates at many different sites of interactions from TCRs, MHC molecules, differential signaling, and cytokines.[30]

Mechanisms of Induction of Self-Tolerance

Self-tolerance is not genetically predetermined in the germline, but is acquired somatically by mechanisms that delete or inactivate autoreactive clones during the embryonic development of the immune system. The mechanisms of tolerance are important in the pathogenesis of autoimmune diseases. Current concepts in the mechanisms of self-tolerance include clonal deletion, clonal anergy, and active suppression.

Clonal Deletion

The host individual acquires the ability to distinguish self and nonself during fetal life with the development of the immune system. The natural unresponsive state develops as a result of direct contact between self constituents and receptor sites on the surface of lymphocytes reactive to these antigens. This is a phenomenon predicted by Burnet,[31,32] who developed the *clonal selection theory,* which proposed that the contact of antibody-forming cells with their respective antigens during fetal or early postnatal life leads to destruction or inactivation of the corresponding clones. Thus, Burnet's hypothesis was that the thymus deletes clones of lymphocytes with receptors for self-antigens.

The maturation of lymphocytes occurs continuously, and the autoantigen must be present to induce tolerance in the newly arising lymphocytes. If the particular autoantigen is not present and in contact with the new lymphocytes, termination and breakdown of tolerance may occur, with initiation of an autoimmune reaction.[26–28]

One of the primary mechanisms for inducing and maintaining self-tolerance is the clonal deletion of autoreactive T cells within the thymus. Clonal deletion results from a specific biochemical process, *programmed cell death* or *apoptosis,* which causes lysis of the cell nucleus and enzymatic degradation of its DNA contents. Clonal T-cell deletion occurs in the thymus under direct genetic control.[33,34] Clonal deletion occurs at the CD4+/CD8+ double-positive or single-positive stage of T-cell development in the thymus and involves participation of CD8 or CD4 molecules in the recognition of MHC class I or class II molecules.[8,35,36]

Evidence to support the concept of clonal deletion came from Owen's classic study of chimeric cattle,[37] which showed that animals sharing a placenta demonstrate tolerance to the incompatible blood cells of their sibling for their lifetime. Additionally, the experimental production of tolerance by Billingham et al[38] demonstrated that unresponsiveness is acquired during fetal or early postnatal life and is inherited genetically.

Clonal Anergy

Clonal deletion does not remove all autoreactive T cells, especially for tissue-specific sequestered antigens, such as lens proteins, sperm antigens, and brain tissue antigens.[35] In the case of brain antigens, there may be a lack of expression of class I or class II molecules in the target organ during presentation of the antigen with resulting tolerance.

Clonal anergy is the term used when the autoreactive T cells with low affinity are not deleted in the thymus gland but are functionally inactivated.[7,29] There may be a downregulation or suppression of autoreactive T cells in the thymus. In the periphery of the immune system, the autoreactive T cells may encounter antigen in the absence of MHC molecules or another signal from antigen-presenting cells, leading to functional inactivation and an inability to produce IL-2.

Normally, T and B lymphocytes capable of binding self-antigens are present. However, in a healthy individual, the lymphocytes are incapable of proliferation in response to self-antigens. Nossal and Pike[29] have shown experimentally that B lymphocytes capable of binding tolerated self-antigens are not deleted. These B lymphocytes are not reactive and normally do not proliferate or produce autoantibody because of a lack of helper T-cell signal.

Active Suppression

Autoreactive lymphocytes (T cells and B cells) may be actively suppressed by regulatory or suppressor T cells that inactivate or lyse autoreactive cells.[33,35,36] Three factors are potentially capable of suppressing autoimmune or self-directed immune responses:

- Non–antigen-specific suppressor T cells.
- Antigen-specific suppressor T cells. These suppressor cells are referred to as "anti-idiotypic" and react with the variable portion of TCRs. Their role is inactivation of a specific population of T cells. Two types of suppressor cells, idiotypic and anti-idiotypic, also can be present.
- Anti-idiotypic antibodies. In the network theory of immune response regulation proposed by Jerne,[39] the immune system is regarded as a web of variable domains based on interactions between idiotypes. The collection of idiotypes is found on any individual immunoglobulin molecule. Under this theory, antigen elicits the production of antibodies bearing idiotypic determinants (antibody 1) that are able to induce synthesis of anti-idiotypic determinants by anti-idiotypic antibodies (antibody 2). The idiotypic determinants of the anti-idiotypic antibodies can themselves elicit the production of other anti-idiotypic antibodies. The immune response is regulated by the suppressive action of the anti-idiotypic antibodies on both B and T cells.[39–42]

How T Cells Are Rendered Tolerant to Self-Antigens

T cells undergo a maturation process in the thymus. Two steps are involved[13,38]:

1. Negative selection with deletion of autoreactive precursor T cells (T cells that bind avidly to self-MHC antigens).
2. Positive selection in which there is preferential maturation of T cells that can recognize foreign antigenic peptides in association with self-MHC molecules.

The T cells are rendered tolerant to self-antigens as follows:

1. Self-reactive T cells may be killed and clonally deleted. About 99% of developing T cells die during thymic maturation, and those that emerge show marked depletion of autoreactive specificities.
2. T cells reactive with self-antigens that "leak out" and emerge from the thymus are often rendered nonfunctional or anergic. Clonal anergy, as discussed earlier, describes a condition in which T cells may be nonfunctional due to a lack of accessory signals even though the thymic receptor interacts with the antigen.
3. Autoreactive T cells capable of activation may be suppressed by other components of the immune system, such as suppressor cells.

Differences Between T Cells and B Cells in the Induction of Tolerance

T cells and B cells interact in the production of autoantibodies. The mechanism of induction of the unresponsive state to self antigens at the cellular level differs between the 2 types of cells.[27–29,43]

On the cellular level, macrophages or antigen-presenting cells, in conjunction with MHC molecules, B cells, and T cells, are involved in tolerance or unresponsiveness. The direct cooperation of T- and B-lymphocytes in this process is well confirmed.[27–29]

Both T cells and B cells can become tolerant. However, the kinetics of induction of tolerance differ greatly between the 2 lymphocyte populations. Many autoantigens such as thyroglobulin, protein hormones, and solubilized membrane antigens circulate in limited concentrations in body fluid. Given the limited concentrations of these self-components, the unresponsive state is maintained only by the T cells and not the B cells. The natural unresponsive state is maintained to antigens such as native thyroglobulin because of the lack of helper T-cell signal; thus, autoantibody production is not initiated.

High doses of antigen are required to induce tolerance in both T and B lymphocytes. This was demonstrated experimentally with induction of tolerance to human γ-globulin in mice. The thymocytes of the mouse become tolerant to human γ-globulin within 24 hours of exposure, and this tolerance lasts for 100 days. By contrast, B-cell tolerance requires an induction period of 15 to 21 days. The long latent period between exposure and tolerance to human γ-globulin in mice may indicate that the bone marrow cells are relatively resistant to tolerance or that thymic cell–bone marrow interaction is required before tolerance can be induced. Even with high doses of antigen, the unresponsive state of B lymphocytes is often incomplete, and a low-affinity antibody can be formed.[28]

In the case of thyroglobulin and its involvement in thyroiditis, only T lymphocytes may be tolerant, leaving B lymphocytes able to respond to autoantigens suitably presented to them with T-lymphocyte help. Mechanisms allowing the requirement for specific T lymphocytes responding to autoantigens to be bypassed will be discussed later in this chapter. Tolerance of autoantigen on the basis of the selective unresponsiveness of T lymphocytes can easily be bypassed by various viral or microbial infections and other events.[1,2]

In contrast to their unresponsiveness to thyroglobulin, neither T cells nor B cells appear to be unresponsive to basic protein, and specific antigen-binding cells to basic protein have been detected in both T- and B-cell populations. By deleting either the T cells or B cells, it has been demonstrated that T cells and not antibodies are responsible for induction of experimental allergic encephalitis.

Principal Factors in the Etiology of Autoimmune Diseases

No single theory or mechanism can explain all features of autoimmune diseases,[44] most of which are multifactorial in etiology. Autoimmunity arises when there is an abnormal interaction of T cells and B cells with autoantigen. Autoimmune diseases are frequently associated with genetic and viral factors that interact with the immune system and influence regulation. Genetically determined lymphocyte membrane antigens in humans determine the magnitude of mixed lymphocyte reactions and may be closely associated with the development of autoimmunity. Although the exact mechanisms relating genetic factors and autoimmunity are unclear, it is likely that immune response genes, lymphocytic surface antigens, and possible receptors for specific viruses are often involved in multiple mechanisms or pathways.

Genetic Factors

Susceptibility to autoimmune diseases is multifactorial and polygenic. Multiple genes contribute to the induction of pathogenic autoimmunity, and no single genetic abnormality is sufficient to produce a specific autoimmune disease.[45]

Most autoimmune diseases are not inherited in a simple mendelian segregation. Study of monozygotic twins shows that concordance for autoimmune diseases is much less than 100%, and varies from less than 5% for multiple sclerosis to 30% for type 1 diabetes.[46] Even with a proven susceptible genotype, not all individuals will develop autoimmunity.

The autoimmune diseases are strongly influenced by genes involved within the MHC, particularly class I (HLA-A, HLA-B, HLA-C) and class II (Ia, HLA-D, HLA-DR) antigens.[47] There is a well-documented association between many autoimmune diseases and HLA antigens.[8,11,47] The association of such antigens has been striking in cases of ankylosing spondylitis, in which as many as 90% of patients are found to possess HLA-B27 antigens. This association does not imply that the disease is directly caused by possession of the HLA-B27 antigen. Certain autoimmune diseases, particularly organ-specific disorders such as idiopathic Addison's disease, Graves' disease, type 1 (insulin-dependent) diabetes, chronic active hepatitis, and Sjögren's syndrome, occur more frequently in individuals who have the HLA-B8 antigen. Other diseases, such as multiple sclerosis and rheumatoid arthritis, appear to be associated with lymphocyte-defined genetic loci whose products on the cell membranes are responsible for mixed lymphocyte reactivity.

The presence of certain cell surface molecules encoded by the HLA-D region shows a strong association with some autoimmune diseases. Examples of diseases with strong HLA-DR associations include dermatitis herpetiformis and celiac disease with HLA-DR3, pemphigus and rheumatoid arthritis with HLA-DR4, type 1 diabetes with HLA-DR3 or HLA-DR4, SLE with HLA-DR2 and HLA-DR3, Sjögren's syndrome with HLA-DR2 and/or HLA-DR3, Graves' disease (hyperthyroidism) with HLA-DR3, and myasthenia gravis with HLA-DR3 and HLA-DR2.[8,11,47]

One current hypothesis proposes the existence of a primary autoimmune gene that is not a part of the MHC on the sixth chromosome but is located in another yet unknown region.[48] This hypothesis proposes that the HLA genes function as secondary genes to allow expression of specific autoantibodies. Therefore, both MHC alleles and non-MHC genes are involved in autoimmune disease susceptibility.

Sex and Hormonal Factors

Women are more frequently affected by autoimmune diseases than are men.[3,33,49,50] Female-male ratios of greater than 5:1 have been reported in scleroderma, SLE, Sjögren's syndrome, Hashimoto's disease, and primary biliary cirrhosis.[49,50]

Do sex hormone levels explain the female predominance of autoimmunity? If so, one would expect peak age incidence of autoimmune diseases to occur when sex hormone levels are highest. For example, the peak incidence of SLE at 25 to 34 years of age in black women is consistent with this expectation.[51]

However, the pattern of highest incidence when female hormone levels are highest is not observed in the following diseases:

- Rheumatoid arthritis. The incidence of this disease continues to rise with age into the eighth decade of life. Some investigators feel that the incidence pattern in rheumatoid arthritis is consistent with decreased levels of serum adrenal anabolic steroids. They have observed a significantly lower mean serum level of dihydroepiandrosterone sulfate but not of cortisol among younger premenopausal women before the onset of rheumatoid arthritis.[52]
- Hashimoto's disease. The peak incidence occurs in the postmenopausal years, at 50 to 59 years of age.[53]

Hormonal factors play a definite role in autoimmunity. However, differences in sex hormone levels do not result in corresponding modulation of or susceptibility to the development of a specific autoimmune disease, such as SLE or rheumatoid arthritis. For example, pregnancy often induces a remission of rheumatoid arthritis, but not of SLE.[52] Similarly, women who have given birth are at reduced risk of developing rheumatoid arthritis but not SLE.

Sex hormones play an important role in the regulation of the immune system and modulate the autoimmune response.[50] Estrogens are known to influence suppressor T-cell activity and indirectly increase helper T cells; they also influence cytokine production and potentiate *IL-1* concentrations. Estradiol-17β inhibits expression of the human *IL-6* gene through an indirect estrogen receptor–mediated effect on the promoter transcription activity.[54]

Environmental Factors

Infections with bacteria, viruses, and other pathogens play an important role in the initiation of autoimmune responses. Infection does not always induce autoimmunity, even in genetically susceptible hosts. The context of the infection is very important. Only the direct analysis of patients and their environment can reveal the pathogenetic mechanism of postinfectious autoimmunity.[55]

Infectious agents may activate self-reactive and inflammatory disease in acute, chronic, or latent infections. Drugs and toxins also have been shown to initiate autoimmune disease, as is the case with procainamide and drug-induced SLE.[1,56] The association of many autoimmune diseases with preceding infection may support the concept of molecular mimicry, in which the initial autoimmune response can be triggered by a cross-reacting environmental pathogen.[57–60]

Infection and Autoimmunity

Several human infections demonstrate significant features of autoimmunity. Examples of such infections include bacterial endocarditis, streptococcal pharyngitis, Lyme disease, trypanosomiasis, and human immunodeficiency virus (HIV).

A second group of diseases, listed in **Table 2-1**, is autoimmune in nature, and there is a good possibility of an infection involved in the etiology and pathogenesis of each disease. Examples include type 1 diabetes, rheumatoid arthritis, SLE, and ankylosing spondylitis.[57]

Infectious agents may cause autoimmune diseases through normal antigen-processing pathways: antigenic peptides derived from the various infectious agents are presented to T lymphocytes as part of the HLA–antigenic peptide complex.

Table 2-1. Autoimmune Diseases With Possible Evidence of Infection Involved in the Pathogenesis[57,60-63]

Disease	Possible Infectious Agents
Insulin-dependent diabetes	Coxsackievirus
	Rubella virus
	Cytomegalovirus
Rheumatoid arthritis	Epstein-Barr virus
	Parvovirus
	Mycobacteria, mycoplasms
Systemic lupus erythematosus	Type C retroviruses
	Epstein-Barr virus
Ankylosing spondylitis	*Klebsiella* species

Table 2-2. Viruses and Autoimmune Diseases

Autoimmune Disease	Virus(es) Possibly Involved
Autoimmune hepatitis	Hepatitis viruses
Cryoglobulinemia	Hepatitis C virus
Type 1 diabetes mellitus	Coxsackievirus
	Chickenpox virus
Myocarditis, cardiomyopathy	Coxsackievirus
Rheumatoid arthritis	Retrovirus
	Epstein-Barr virus
Sjögren's syndrome	Herpes simplex virus
	Epstein-Barr virus
Systemic lupus erythematosus	Retroviruses
	Epstein-Barr virus

Modified from Aichele et al.[61]

Hypotheses to explain the association of autoimmune disease with infectious agents involve molecular mimicry and sequestered antigens.[57-60]

Molecular Mimicry—Under this hypothesis, a self molecule and a molecule on the infectious agent share a similar epitope (antigenic determinant). Two scenarios may be possible:

1. The immunologic similarity of the epitopes means the host regards the infectious agent as self and not foreign. No immune response is initiated and the agent can produce an autoimmune disease by some unknown mechanism.
2. The epitope on the infectious agent is recognized as foreign, causing initiation of an immune response. The immune response then recognizes the "self-epitope" as foreign and initiates an "autoimmune response," producing the autoimmune disease.

Sequestered-Antigen Hypothesis—During an infection, a normally sequestered self-antigen is exposed and initiates an "autoimmune response." Therefore, molecular mimicry may involve human target organs and specific components of the infectious organism, and host HLA cell surface molecules may share antigens with presumed bacterial and viral initiators of disease.

Viruses and Autoimmunity

It has been proposed that viruses are involved in several diseases with autoimmune pathogeneses.[60–65] Some of these viruses are listed in **Table 2-2**. Viral involvement with autoimmune reactions may be caused by molecular mimicry and/or superantigen activation of autoreactive T cells.

For example, Epstein-Barr virus (EBV) latently infects essentially the entire adult population and expresses a number of antigens genetically related to human proteins.[62,66] The virus has been implicated in the pathogenesis of Sjögren's syndrome, rheumatoid arthritis, and other diseases.[62,66] It has been shown to induce differing autoantibodies in certain autoimmune diseases.

The main factor linking EBV to the onset of autoimmune disorders is the appearance of numerous autoantibodies of varied specificity during the acute phase of infectious mononucleosis. Some of the autoantibodies noted in these infections are to the following antigens[66]:

- Smooth muscle (tubulin)
- Intermediate filaments

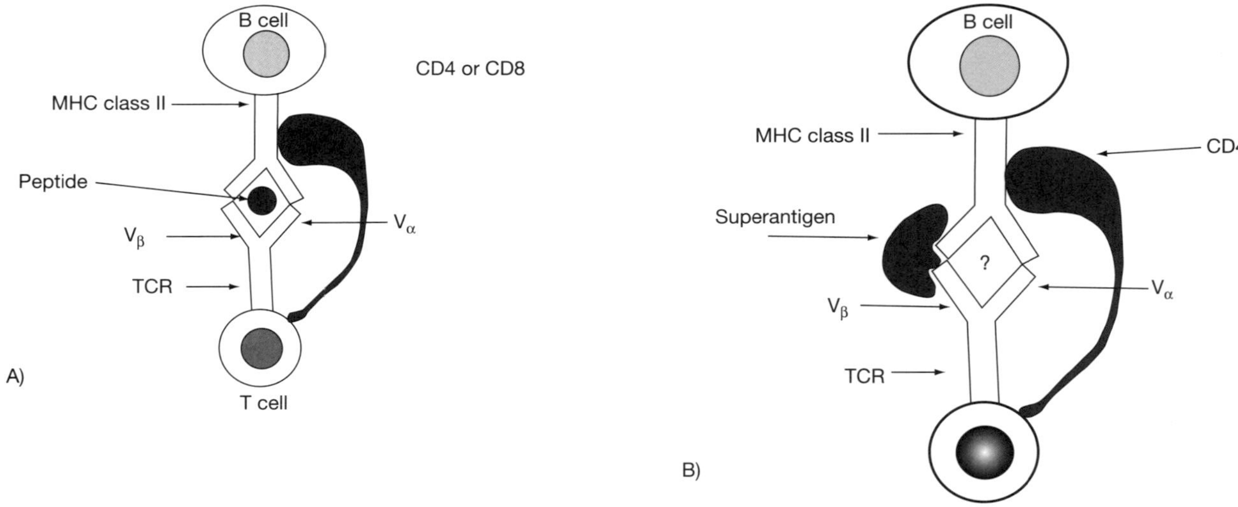

Figure 2-2. Classic peptide and superantigen recognition. **A.** In classical antigen recognition, a processed peptide is presented by an MHC class I or class II molecule to a T-cell receptor (TCR). **B.** In superantigen recognition, the superantigen cross-links the TCR Vb chain with the MHC class II molecule. It is not known whether antigenic peptides are bound to MHC.

- Cardiolipins
- Histones
- T lymphocytes (membrane antigens)
- Other nuclear antigens

Unequivocal evidence that implicates viruses in type 1 diabetes has not been established. However, circumstantial evidence does not exclude the possibility that viral infection of the B cells of pancreatic islets can initiate autoimmune destruction of B cells.

The Role of Superantigens—Superantigens are bacterial, viral, or retroviral proteins that can activate a large proportion of T cells.[67–70] In contrast to the classic peptide-antigen immunologic recognition scenario (**Figure 2-2A**), superantigen recognition has the following features:

- Superantigens do not require processing to small peptides and can act as complete or partially processed proteins (**Figure 2-2B**).
- Superantigens can bind to MHC class II molecules and stimulate T cells through the TCR V_β chain. The other parts of the TCR necessary for classic antigen recognition are not necessary with superantigen activation.
- Superantigens can activate a large portion of the immune system shortly after infection. The activated cells may have a wide variety of antigen specificities. These superantigens are able to initiate T-cell and polyclonal B-cell responses.
- The polyclonal expansion of activated T cells may result in the production of large quantities of cytokines with activation of autoreactive lymphocyte populations.

Superantigens have been found in a wide variety of infectious agents, such as staphylococci, streptococci, mycoplasma, *Yersinia*, retroviruses, HIV, and other viruses.[67–70] Recent evidence suggests that superantigens may be relevant to the pathogenesis of autoimmune and immunodeficiency disorders. Superantigens have been implicated in the induction of rheumatoid arthritis and multiple sclerosis because of the expansion of particular autoreactive V_β-bearing T cells in affected patients.[67–70]

Inductive Mechanisms of Autoimmunity

In the initiation of an autoimmune response, one or both of the following events may be involved[5,7,71]:

- Autologous antigen may be presented abnormally to a normal immune system. This may result from hyperexpression of MHC class II gene products.
- There may be an alteration of the immune system itself caused by a defective suppressor

Table 2-3. Inductive Mechanisms of Autoimmunity[1–3,8,87]

T-cell bypass
Alternative helper T-cell signal initiation
Polyclonal B-cell activation
Sequestered antigen release
Loss of suppressor activity
Molecular mimicry
Heat shock proteins
Idiotypic antibodies
Apoptosis

mechanism, altered neuroendocrine regulation, or several abnormalities.

The immunologic imbalance may arise from an alteration in and disturbance of the activities of suppressor and helper T-cells. As stated earlier, the immunologic imbalance is modulated by genetic, hormonal, viral, and environmental factors.[3,7,71]

Several inductive mechanisms of autoimmunity are listed in **Table 2-3**. There may be some overlap of certain basic reactions, such as cross-reactivity.

T-Cell Bypass Mechanism

In a healthy individual, the T cell is tolerant and the B cell is competent. No autoantibody is formed by the absence of the helper T-cell signals (**Figure 2-3A**). However, the autoantigens can form immunogenic units with antigens that are able to initiate the helper T-cell signal to stimulate the existing immunocompetent B cell.[1,2] Any procedure that nonspecifically activates lymphocytes, such as adjuvants or a graft-versus-host reaction with allogenic cells, can stimulate production of autoantibodies by bypassing T-cell specificity (**Figure 2-3B**). A nontolerant immunocompetent B cell can be stimulated to produce autoantibody without the need for an immunocompetent-specific T cell. The B cells may be stimulated by 2 general pathways:

- The autoantigens or cross-reactive foreign antigens may form immunogenic units to initiate helper T-cell signals to stimulate immunocompetent B cells. Helper determinants may be drugs, viruses, or bacteria.
- The immunocompetent B cells may be nonspecifically stimulated by viruses, adjuvants, or allogenic cells, initiating a graft-versus-host reaction to produce autoantibodies. This phenomenon is referred to as *polyclonal activation* of B cells.[43,72] The polyclonal activation of B cells in the induction of autoimmune reaction in vivo plays a prominent role in certain spontaneous autoimmune diseases. Many bacterial antigens, such as lipopolysaccharides and viruses (eg, EBV) can initiate B-cell activation.

T-cell bypass autoimmune reaction may be seen with drug administration, virus infection, adjuvant effect, bacterial infection, degradation and alteration of autoantigens, and allogenic cells (**Table 2-4**).

Drug Administration

Binding of the drug or metabolite to host tissue may initiate a host T-lymphocyte response against the drug. The drug combined with the host tissue may also initiate a helper T-cell signal to stimulate competent B cells with autoantibody production.

There are many examples of autoimmune manifestations following drug administration. A drug-induced lupus erythematosus syndrome is not uncommon in patients treated with procainamide or hydralazine.

Adjuvant Effect and Bacterial Infections

Immunologic adjuvants are nonspecific stimulators of lymphocytes and can help initiate autoimmune responses. Lipopolysaccharides or purified protein derivatives of tuberculin are polyclonal B-cell activators, and Freund's complete adjuvant is a nonspecific T-cell stimulator.[68,73] The need for a specific T cell is bypassed (**Figure 2-4**). Bacterial infections with liberation of products of adjuvant activity, such as *Bordetella pertussis* infection, may produce polyclonal lymphocyte activation and autoimmunity.[60]

Degradation and Alteration of Autoantigens

Tissue damage with alteration of host antigens may elicit an autoimmune reaction. Partial degradation can expose antigenic determinants that are unavailable in the self molecules, and these can react with T lymphocytes to induce autoimmunity. Many bacterial, viral, and parasitic infections are associated with transient positive tests for antiglobulin of the rheumatoid factor type, and partial degradation or alteration of host antigens is among the underlying mechanisms.

Allogenic Cells

When live allogenic lymphocytes are injected into a recipient, the primary event is a graft-versus-host reaction. The donor T lymphocytes respond to the

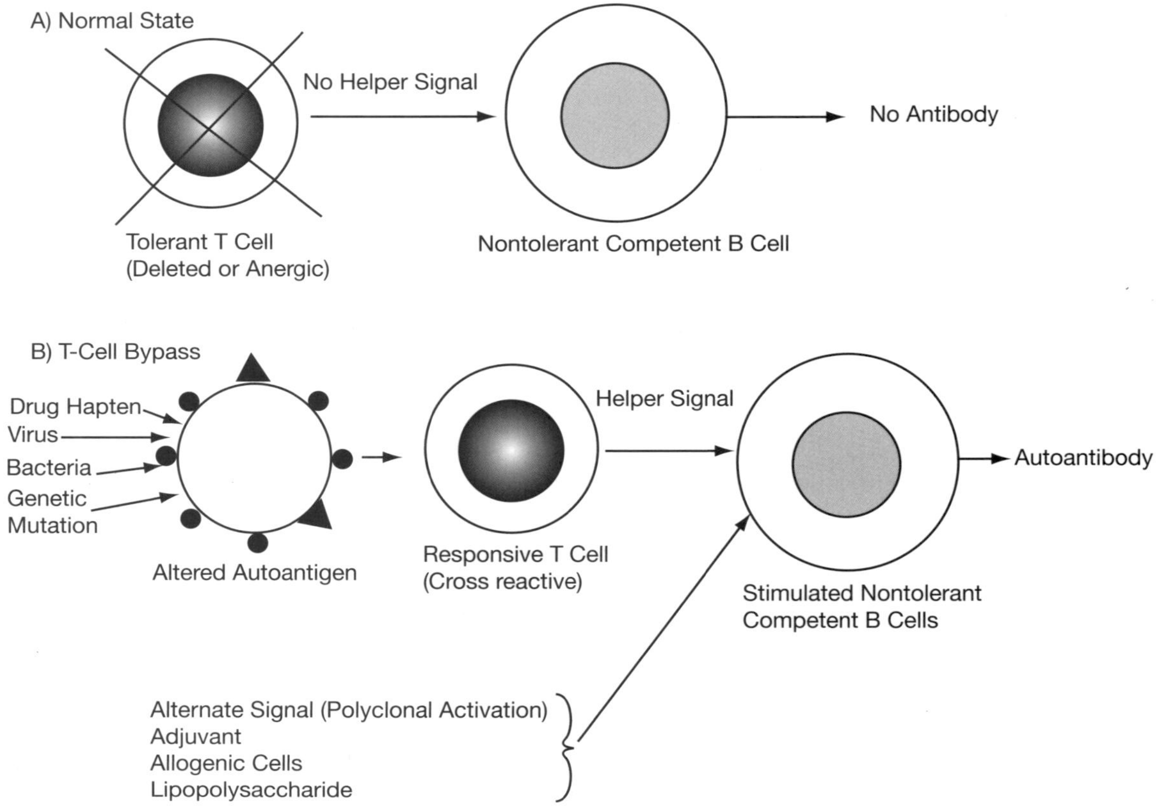

Figure 2-3. T-cell bypass mechanisms. **A.** In a normal person, the tolerant T cell has been deleted or is anergic. Thus, there is no helper T-cell signal to initiate antibody response. **B.** Various mechanisms (drug haptens, viruses, bacteria, and genetic mutations) alter the autoantigen to stimulate a responsive T cell to generate the helper signal. Also, a polyclonal B-cell activation may be initiated by direct stimulation of B cells.

Table 2-4. T-Cell Bypass Mechanisms (Alternate T-Cell Signal or Polyclonal B-Cell Stimulation)

Drug administration
Viral infection
Bacterial infection
Adjuvant effect
Degradation and alteration of autoantigen
Allogenic cells

MHC of the lymphoid and hematopoietic cells of the recipient. The stimulation of the lymphoid tissue in the recipient is manifested by profound lymphoreticular hyperplasia, with germinal center enlargement and plasmacytosis. The donor T-cell reaction initiates proliferation of the recipient B cells.

In a normal person, autoantibody formation does not occur, because T lymphocytes are unable to react to autoantigens. However, when host B cells are nonspecifically stimulated by the donor T cells, as in the graft-versus-host reaction, there is an allogenic effect leading to the production of antibodies. With this mechanism, the need for carrier-specific T lymphocytes can be bypassed. Hence, the graft-versus-host reaction results in the formation of autoantibodies.[1,2]

T-Cell Bypass Mechanism in Thyroiditis (Example of an Organ-Specific Autoimmune Disease)

Most autoantigens, such as thyroglobulin, protein hormones, and soluble membrane antigen, circulate in very low concentrations. Prolonged exposure to these antigens normally produces selective tolerance in T lymphocytes, allowing B lymphocytes to

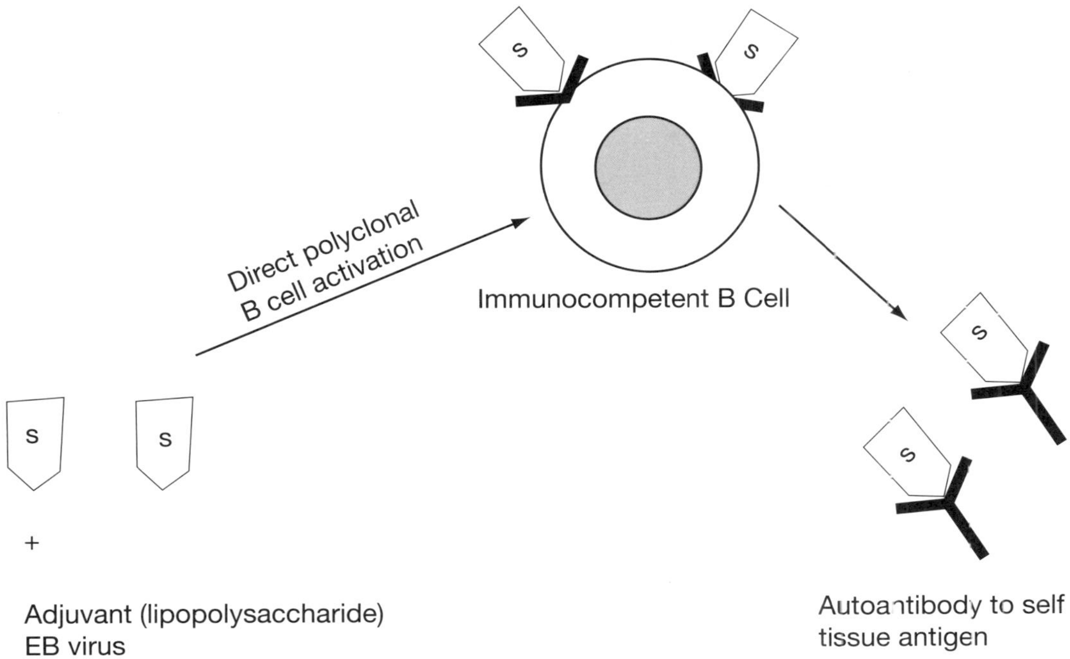

Figure 2-4. Adjuvant effect and bacterial infections. Bacterial infections may initiate an autoimmune reaction by an immunologic adjuvant effect. The adjuvants nonspecifically stimulate T cells to initiate a helper T-cell effect. In the case of lipopolysaccharides, direct activation with polyclonal stimulation of B cells can occur with the production of autoantibodies.

bind and be stimulated by autoantigens presented to them with appropriate T-lymphocyte help.[1,2,28,73] Under such circumstances, the requirements for T lymphocytes responding to autoantigenic determinants can be bypassed.

The classic example of the mechanism of T-cell specificity bypass is in experimental thyroiditis (**Figure 2-5**). Overwhelming evidence from studies of experimental animal thyroiditis as well as human thyroiditis has shown that the major factor in initiating tissue injury is the humoral autoantibody response.

It was previously thought that thyroglobulin was a sequestered antigen. However, it has been shown that thyroglobulin antigen is actually present in the circulation in very small amounts after birth and can equilibrate between the intravascular and extravascular compartments. In organs that are frequently associated with autoimmune disease, it is thought that extremely low concentrations of self-antigen, such as thyroglobulin, are in the circulation. These concentrations are sufficient to maintain tolerance at the T-cell level, but not at the level of B cells or bone marrow cells. This is not a completely healthy condition, because unresponsiveness at the thymus level is adequate to inhibit antibody response. Problems can arise if a situation such as viral transformation or genetic mutation is superimposed. This permits the thymus cells to react with the altered portion of the gene and the self-antigen. Interaction then takes place with the immunocompetent bone marrow cells, and the autoimmune process is initiated.

The same mechanism involved in thyroiditis may operate in other organ-specific diseases, such as primary adrenal gland atrophy, parathyroid hypoplasia, and primary ovarian atrophy. The organs involved release extremely small concentrations of self-antigens during the development of the natural unresponsive state. Tolerance is then developed at the T-cell level and not at the B-cell level.

Sequestered-Antigen Release Reaction

This reaction involves the stimulation of competent T cells and/or B cells by sequestered self-antigens.[1,2,28,35] Sequestered antigens such as sperm antigens and lens proteins are not available or accessible to the normal immune cells. Therefore, no self-tolerance to these antigens develops. Such antigens may induce

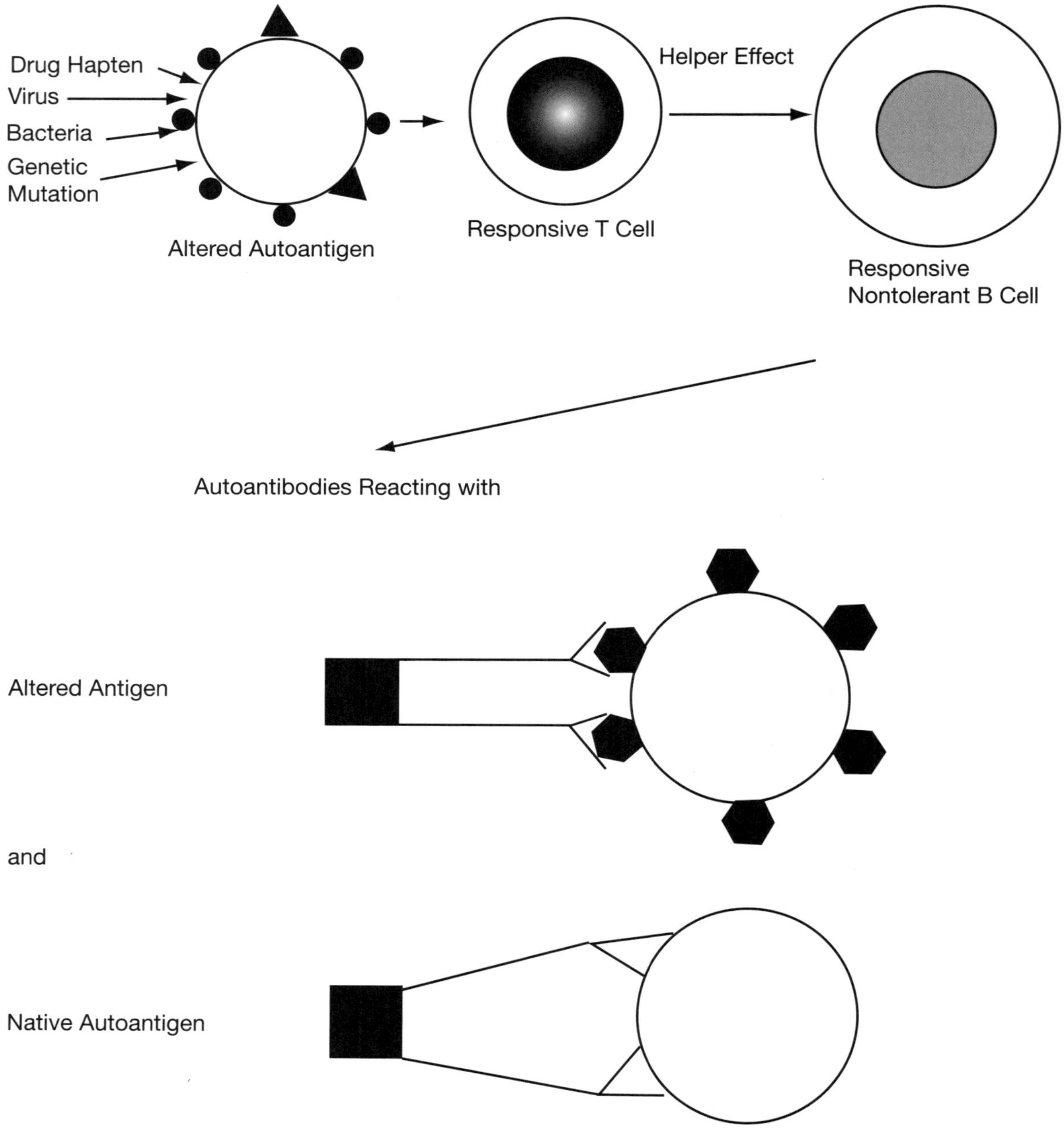

Figure 2-5. T-cell specificity bypass. In thyroiditis and certain other organ-specific autoimmune diseases, T-cell specificity is bypassed by various means to initiate a helper T-cell signal that stimulates B cells to produce autoantibodies. The responsive T cell may be cross-reactive with the self-antigen, such as thyroglobulin.

an autoimmune reaction when they are released into the immune system by tissue injury. When the sequestered antigen is released, the host T cells recognize it as foreign, initiate a helper T-cell signal, and stimulate the B cell to proliferate and divide.

Myelin basic protein, a brain antigen, has been considered a sequestered antigen, lying as it does behind anatomic barriers. In contrast to T-cell unresponsiveness to thyroglobulin, immunocompetent T cells and B cells to myelin basic protein exist normally

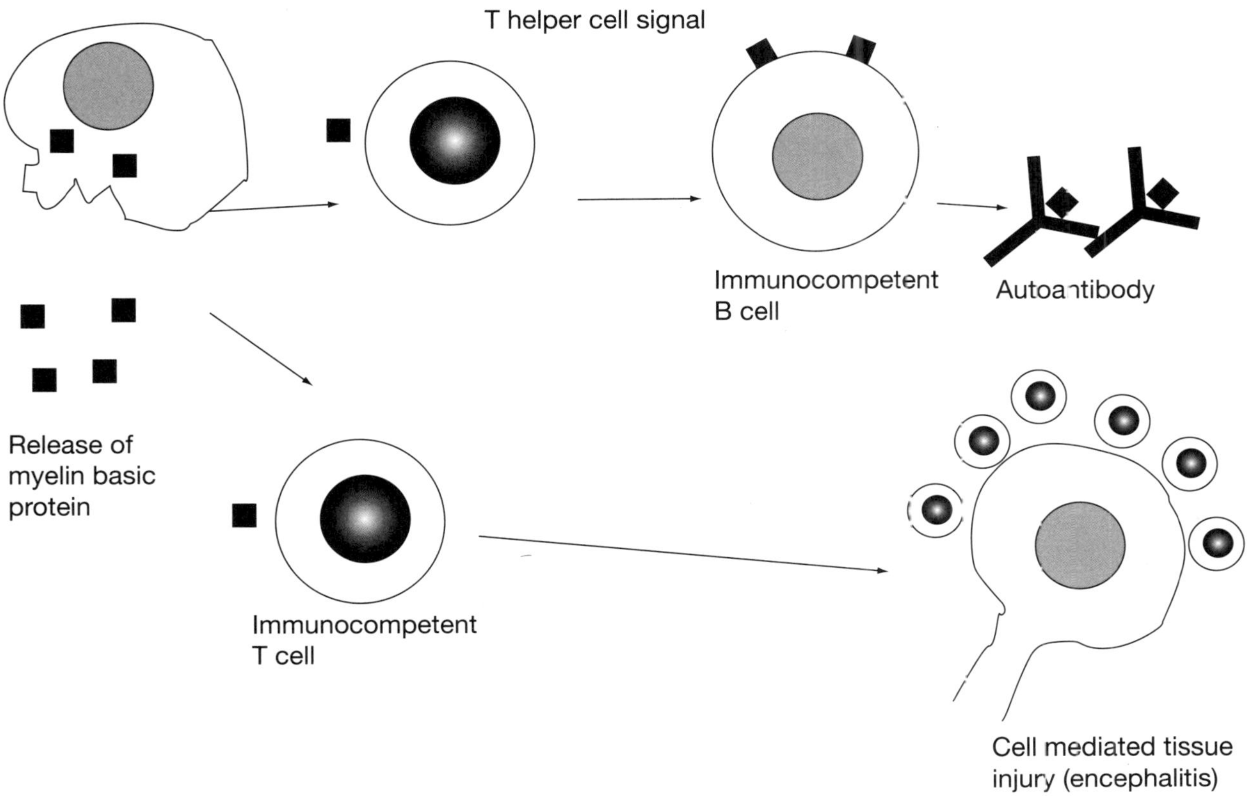

Figure 2-6. Sequestered antigen release mechanisms of autoimmunity in experimental and postinfectious encephalitis. The sequestered antigen is myelin basic protein. When released by various means, such as viral inflammation, it stimulates both immunocompetent T cells and B cells. The primary mechanism of injury in experimental and postviral encephalitis is a cell-mediated injury.

(**Figure 2-6**). The normal unresponsive state to myelin basic protein may be ascribed to the sequestered nature of the antigen or to the lack of expression of MHC class I or class II molecules in the target organ.[35] It has been demonstrated experimentally that the T cells are primarily responsible for induction of experimental allergic encephalitis immunization with myelin basic protein.[28]

Loss of Suppressor Activity

Normally, the presence of a suppressor T cell may block a self-antigen from triggering a helper T-cell signal[3,7,36] (**Figure 2-7A**). The suppressor T cells may also block and inhibit modification of the competent B cells to produce autoantibody (**Figure 2-7B**). As discussed previously, both antigen-specific and non–antigenic-specific suppressor T cells play a regulatory role in a cytotoxic reaction.

Molecular Mimicry

As described earlier, molecular mimicry is a sharing of epitopes in linear or 3-dimensional presentation by disparate proteins from entirely different sources. A good example is the relationship of group A streptococcal membranes and human cardiac myosin, which is implicated in cardiac rheumatic fever.

Autoimmunity provoked by molecular mimicry may occur when the microbial and host determinants are similar enough to cross-react and yet different enough to terminate or break immunologic tolerance.[60,70–75] What evidence is there that molecular mimicry causes disease? Findings regarding 2 diseases can be presented[76–79]:

- Celiac disease in humans is characterized by injury of the small intestine and gastrointestinal malabsorption. The celiac disease is activated by the protein α-gliadin, which is a component

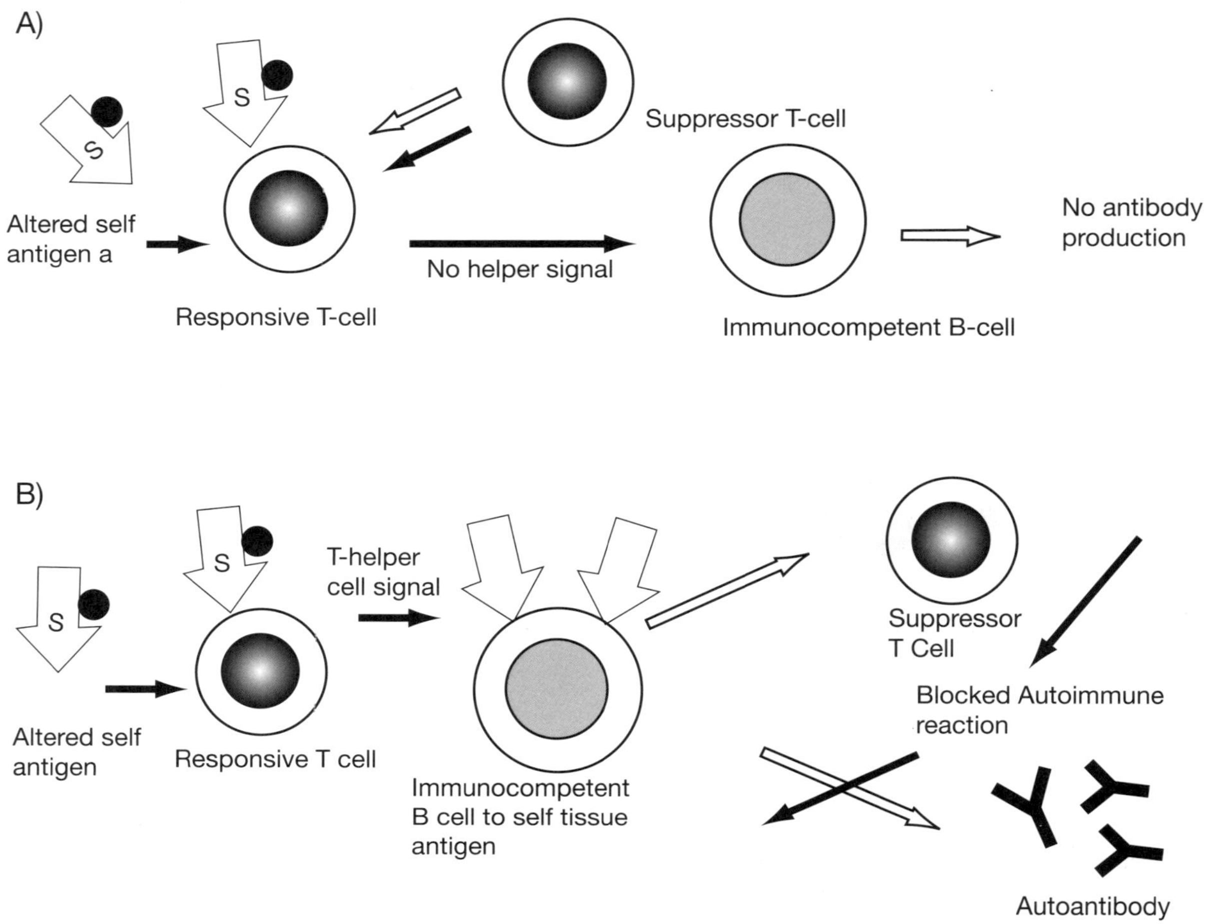

Figure 2-7. Prevention of autoimmune reaction by suppressor T cells. **A.** Suppressor T cells may inhibit helper T-cell signals to prevent autoimmune response. **B.** Suppressor T cells also may prevent autoimmune reaction by suppressing B-cell proliferation, blocking antibody production.

of wheat gluten. α-Gliadin shares 8 amino acids with a protein of human adenovirus 12 (Ad-12), which inhabits the intestinal tract. The antibodies against adenovirus 12 cross-react with gliadin. Additionally, 89% of patients with celiac disease showed evidence of infection by Ad-12 virus, versus 17% of control patients. A cross-reactive immune response against the α-gliadin initially induced by Ad-12 intestinal infection probably plays a role in the pathogenesis of celiac disease.

- Ninety-five percent of patients with ankylosing spondylitis and 80% of those with Reiter's syndrome carry the HLA-B27 allele, compared with 7% of the general population. There is a 6 amino acid homology between the hypervariable domain of HLA-B27 and *Klebsiella pneumoniae*. In patients with ankylosing spondylitis and Reiter's syndrome, the autoimmune response may be initiated by a *Klebsiella* infection and directed against HLA-B27.

Heat Shock Proteins and the Role of γ–δ T Cells

Heat shock (stress) proteins (hsps) constitute a family of proteins divided into subfamilies and named for their approximate molecular masses in kilodaltons: hsp 90, hsp 70, hsp 65, and so on.[24,80,81] They are characterized by high degrees of sequence homology. For example, the human and bacterial versions of hsp 65 are identical in approximately

50% of their amino acid residues.[80,81] The heat shock proteins are highly conserved and are essential for the survival of all cells. They are produced in augmented amounts to combat the denaturation produced by heat and other metabolic, toxic, and physical types of stress.

Immune responses to heat shock proteins have been observed in many infections, including tuberculosis, Legionnaire's disease, Lyme disease, chlamydial infections, and Chagas' disease. For example, hsp 65 is an immunodominant antigen during many infections. The T-cell cross-reactivity to hsp 65 may be a factor in the development of certain autoimmune diseases, including type 1 diabetes, rheumatoid arthritis, and multiple sclerosis.[80,81]

Bacterial heat shock proteins are major target antigens for cell-mediated immune-effector mechanisms.[82] Although highly conserved, the bacterial heat shock proteins are sufficiently different from their mammalian homologues to be immunogenic and perceived as foreign by the host immune system.

Viruses differ from bacteria in that they do not carry hsp genes and can cause enhanced expression of endogenous host heat shock proteins, which in turn may stimulate a subset of γ–δ T cells. T cells bearing the γ–δ TCR may be reactive to self hsp and are part of the immune system.[82-84] The γ–δ T cells differentiate in the thymus, possess surface markers, and mediate a variety of functions characteristic of T lymphocytes.

The exact interaction of heat shock proteins and γ–δ T cells has yet to be elucidated. Doherty et al[82] have hypothesized that, following certain viral infections, there is increased expression of host hsp 65 which is reactive with γ–δ T cells. The lymphokines and cytokines secreted by the γ–δ T cells may initiate autoimmunity if the reaction occurs in sites such as joints, where normal physiologic processes may not readily clear the inflammatory cells.

Anti-idiotype and Autoimmune Diseases

Idiotype is a term for the antigenic constitution of the variable regions (idiotypes). Anti-idiotypes are antibodies produced following idiotypic stimulation. Jerne[39] has proposed that during the normal course of immune response, "auto–anti-idiotypes" are generated. The auto–anti-idiotypes are primarily autoimmune reactions; however, they play a major role in regulation by either enhancing or suppressing idiotype inflammation.[85–87]

Shoenfeld[88] has presented evidence from clinical observations and experimental animal models that some autoimmune diseases in which the autoantigen, such as DNA cardiolipin, is not very immunogenic may follow a common infection. In the host response to the infection, the antibodies against the infecting agent carry a pathogenic idiotype of a specific antibody. In a person who is susceptible and prone to autoimmunity, the pathogenic idiotype initiates an autoimmune disease with dysregulation of the immune system. In the animal experiments conducted by Shoenfeld[89,90] and others[91] with idiotypic induction of autoimmunity, the animal counterparts of SLE, antiphospholipid syndrome, and Wegener's granulomatosis were observed.

Apoptosis

Apoptosis is an active process of cellular self-destruction. It is a physiologic process of selective cell deletion that occurs during embryogenesis, metamorphosis, tissue atrophy, and tumor regression.[92–94] In contrast, necrosis is a degenerative process.

Activation-induced apoptosis is a primary mechanism for deletion of T cells with specificities that may be harmful to the host. These include autospecific T cells. The surface molecules involved in activation-induced apoptosis are the FAS protein and FAS ligand (FASL), as well as the TCR, which modulates the expression and function of these molecules.[92-94] FAS is a cell surface molecule belonging to the tumor necrosis factor family.[92-93]

Recently, a direct link between FAS-mediated apoptosis and human SLE has been identified.[95] Decreased apoptosis in SLE is associated with increased production of a soluble form of the FAS molecule, which can inhibit apoptosis. Thus, different defects in FAS/APO1 (CD95) interaction with its ligand or in the signaling of apoptosis may contribute to autoimmune disease.[93]

Criteria for Human Autoimmune Disease

In 1957, Witebsky et al[96] established criteria for the autoimmune etiology of human disease. These criteria, modeled after Koch's postulate, were as follows:

- The autoimmune response is recognized in the form of antibody- or cell-mediated immunity.

- The corresponding autoantigen should be identified.
- An analogous autoimmune response is induced in an experimental animal.
- The immunized animal also must develop a similar disease.

More recently, in light of knowledge gained from monoclonal antibody and molecular biology technology, Rose and Bona[97] proposed that three types of evidence could be used to establish that a human disease is truly autoimmune in origin:

1. Direct evidence from transfer of pathogenic antibody or pathogenic T cells
2. Indirect evidence based on reproduction of the autoimmune disease in experimental animals
3. Circumstantial evidence from clinical clues, including
   - association with other autoimmune diseases in the same person or family
   - lymphocytic infiltration of the target organ, especially if there is a restriction in V gene usage
   - statistical association with a specific MHC haplotype or aberrant expression of MHC class II antigens on the affected organ
   - favorable response to immunosuppression

Such circumstantial evidence alone cannot define an autoimmune disease. However, it provides impetus for further investigation.

One group of antibody-mediated autoimmune diseases that fulfills the Witebsky-Rose criteria for autoimmunity includes myasthenia gravis, pemphigus vulgaris, hyperthyroidism (Graves' disease), and autoimmune thrombocytopenia. A second group of diseases generally regarded as autoimmune diseases that do not fulfill the Witebsky-Rose criteria includes SLE, primary biliary cirrhosis, polymyositis, and scleroderma. These diseases are suspected of being autoimmune on the basis of immunologic, genetic, hormonal, and environmental factors.[59] Autoantigens are implicated and identified; however, the antigens are intracellular molecules or ubiquitous compounds. Immunizing experimental animals with the autoantigens does not cause disease. Moreover, the passive transfer of the specific autoantibodies usually cause immune injury or overt clinical manifestations.

The human disease counterparts induced in the mice were SLE, antiphospholipid syndrome, primary biliary cirrhosis, and Wegener's granulomatosis.[80,90] Thus, Shoenfeld[88] postulates a relationship between infection and autoimmunity. The infection with a common pathogen triggers production of idiotypes of autoantibodies. In healthy individuals, the idiotypic cascade ends with Ab_2 (anti-Id). In genetically susceptible subjects, the Ab_3 (autoantibodies) develop with accompanying clinical manifestations. For example, high titers of 16/6 Id pathogenic idiotypes of anti-DNA have been found in patients infected with *Mycobacteria tuberculosis, Klebsiella*, and other gram-negative bacteria.[98]

In light of this evidence, Shoenfeld[88] has postulated a new classification of autoimmune diseases in which idiotypic dysregulation may play a significant role in pathogenesis. In different animal experiments, Shoenfeld[89,90] and others[91] have presented evidence of inducing autoimmune conditions following immunization of healthy mice with specific autoantibody emulsified in Freund's adjuvant. Following immunization with Ab_1 (Id) and production of Ab_2 (anti-Id), the mice can develop Ab_3 (anti–anti-Id). These idiotypic antibodies have autoantibody characteristics and are associated with the serologic and clinical manifestations of the disease.

Effector Mechanism in Autoimmune Diseases

The activation of self-reactive T cells by a specific mechanism sets in motion the events leading to autoimmune tissue injury. In systemic autoimmune diseases, as demonstrated by SLE and related connective tissue disorders, the following features are noted[99,100]:

- The major autoantigens, including components of nuclei and cell surfaces, are widely distributed in different tissues of the body.
- The formation of multiple autoantibodies is characteristic.
- The effectors of systemic diseases are generally humoral, involving autoantibody itself or immune complexes.

In organ-specific autoimmune diseases, the principal antigens are unique to the target organ. The effector mechanisms may be either humoral or cellular primarily depending on the nature and disposition of the antigen. In practice, most autoimmune diseases are probably produced by a combination of these pathogenetic mechanisms, including T cells and B cells, cytokines, and various other mediators.

Classification of Autoimmune Diseases

Human autoimmune diseases can be classified in several ways. Traditionally, they have been divided between organ-specific and non–organ-specific (or systemic) autoimmune diseases, depending on whether the response is primarily against antigens localized to particular organs or widespread antigens. The common target organs in organ-specific diseases include the thyroid, adrenals, stomach, and pancreas. The systemic autoimmune diseases include SLE and the various systemic rheumatic diseases. There is considerable overlap, and Roitt[101] proposed the concept of a spectrum of autoimmune diseases.

Autoimmune Diseases by Major Histocompatibility Complex Classes I and II

Susceptibility to many autoimmune diseases is strongly influenced by genes encoded in the MHC, particularly class I (HLA-A, HLA-B, HLA-C) and class II (Ia, HLA-D, HLA-DR) molecules.[8,10] Major histocompatibility complex class I autoimmune diseases fall into two main categories[8]:

- HLA-B27–related spondyloarthropathies, which include ankylosing spondylitis, Reiter's syndrome, and reactive arthropathy
- Psoriasis vulgaris, which is associated with HLA-B12, HLA-B16, and HLA-B17

These diseases show a male predominance, which is noted in ankylosing spondylitis and Reiter's syndrome.

In MHC class II–associated diseases, there are also two main groups:

- Organ-specific autoimmune diseases
- Systemic autoimmune diseases

Generally, MHC class II–associated autoimmune diseases show a female predominance, most marked in SLE and hyperthyroidism.[8]

Autoimmune Diseases by Final Effector Mechanisms

Autoimmune diseases also can be classified according to the predominant final effector mechanism of immunologic tissue injury.[6,102] Examples of such mechanisms are

- Antibody mediated—seen in Goodpasture's syndrome with glomerulonephritis due to basement membrane autoantibodies; antireceptor autoantibodies (eg, tumor-specific antigen and acetylcholine receptors in hyperthyroidism and myasthenia gravis, respectively)
- Immune complex mediated—seen in SLE, polyarteritis nodosa, immune complex glomerulonephritis
- T-cell mediated—seen in type 1 diabetes, autoimmune chronic hepatitis, and multiple sclerosis

Mackay-Rose Classification of Autoimmune Diseases

Autoimmune diseases vary widely in their expression, mediation, and outcome. Mackay and Rose[103,104] have proposed a reasonable classification into the following groups.

Organ-Specific Autoimmune Diseases

Disease is focused in a single organ with demonstration of corresponding organ-specific autoantibodies and/or T cells. Multiple organ-specific autoantibodies are usually present. Examples include thyroiditis, adrenalitis, gastritis, and type 1 insulin-dependent diabetes mellitus.

"Paradoxic" Organ-Specific Autoimmune Diseases

In this group, the disease is localized mainly to a particular tissue or organ. There is a systemically distributed autoantigen and a demonstrable "marker." Autoantibody has no evident relationship to actual pathogenesis or cause of tissue injury. Examples of this group of diseases (with their corresponding antibodies) are

- Sjögren's syndrome (anti-SS-A/Ro and SS-B/La)
- Polymyositis (anti-Jo-1)
- Primary biliary cirrhosis (antimitochondrial antibody)
- Vasculitis (antibodies to neutrophil cytoplasmic enzymes)

Cell-Specific Autoimmune Diseases

These diseases primarily involve a discrete cellular element or product that may be dispersed throughout the body. There is a well-defined antibody to a cell-specific antigen or receptor. Examples include myasthenia gravis and Goodpasture's syndrome.

Multisystem Autoimmune Diseases

These diseases demonstrate multiple antibodies to widely distributed cell surface or intracellular antigens. The pathogenic consequences and mechanism of injury are due mostly to deposited immune complexes. Examples are SLE and progressive systemic sclerosis.

In this book, human diseases have been categorized by the traditional organ system involvement. Therefore, the following classification is used to group autoimmune disorders into 4 major categories (see Chapter 8).

- Endocrine organ-specific autoimmune diseases
- Systemic autoimmune diseases, including SLE and other systemic rheumatic diseases
- Autoimmune diseases grouped by primary organ system involvement, including autoimmune diseases of the skin, kidney, and nervous system
- Other autoimmune diseases

Summary

Autoimmunity can be defined by the presence of autoantibodies and/or T cells that react against self-antigens. Not all autoimmune responses are harmful or "forbidden." Considerable research has indicated that autoimmune responses may be normal and important in the regulation of the immune system. Autoimmunity plays a role in a wide range of clinical states (including physiologic clearance of dead cells) and cell components, aging, response to viral and microbial infections, and generalized immunologic diseases.

Autoimmunity can be pathologic and induce immunologic injury to the host with disease. The term "autoimmune disease" has been generally assigned to conditions in which an autoimmune mechanism or injury has contributed to the pathogenesis.

Susceptibility to autoimmune diseases is multifactorial and polygenic. There is a definite association between autoimmune diseases and MHC alleles. Non-MHC genes also are involved in disease susceptibility.

No single theory or mechanism can explain the phenomenon of autoimmunity or autoimmune disease. There are many etiologic factors involved in autoimmunity, including genetic, hormonal, immunologic, and environmental factors. Numerous mechanisms of autoimmunity have been discussed. There may be an alteration with dysregulation of the immune system with defective generation of normal suppressor mechanisms or an altered neuroendocrine regulation. The altered immune system makes the host more susceptible to autoimmune disease, but autoimmune reactions can occur in a host with a normal immune system. The complex interactions of the various components of the immune system, including the MHC molecule, TCRs, and effector molecules in the induction of tolerance and autoimmunity also have been examined.

References

1. Nakamura RM, Binder WL. Current concepts and diagnostic evaluation of autoimmune disease. *Arch Pathol Lab Med.* 1988;112:869–877.
2. Nakamura MC, Nakamura RM. Contemporary concepts of autoimmunity and autoimmune diseases. *J Clin Lab Anal.* 1992;6:275–289.
3. Talal N. In: Talal N, ed. *Autoimmunity: Genetic Immunologic, Virologic, and Clinical Aspects.* New York, NY: Academic Press; 1977.
4. Ehrlich P, Morgenroth J. In: Himmelweit F, ed. *The Collected Papers of Paul Ehrlich—1990.* Oxford, England: Pergamon Press; 1956:205–215.
5. Theofilopoulos AN, Dixon FJ. Autoimmune diseases, immunopathology and etiopathogenesis. *Am J Pathol.* 1982;108:321–365.
6. Rose NR. Current concepts of autoimmune disease. *Transplant Proc.* 1988;20:3–10.
7. Rose NR. The concept of autoimmunity and autoimmune disease. In: Krawitt EL, Wiesner RH, eds. *Autoimmune Liver Diseases.* New York, NY: Raven Press, Ltd; 1991:1–20.
8. Sinha AA, Lopez MT, McDevitt HO. Autoimmune diseases: The failure of self tolerance. *Science.* 1990;248:1380–1388.
9. Nakamura RM. *Immunopathology: Clinical Laboratory Concepts and Methods.* Boston, MA: Little Brown and Co; 1974.
10. Bach FH. The major histocompatibility complex and its relationship to autoimmune disease. In: Talal N, ed. *Autoimmunity: Genetic Immunologic, Virologic, and Clinical Aspects.* New York, NY: Academic Press; 1977:3–32.
11. Braun WE, Zachary A. The HLA histocompatibility system in autoimmune states. In: Deodhar SD, ed. *Autoimmune Diseases: Clinics in Laboratory Medicine.* Vol. 8. Philadelphia, PA: WB Saunders Co; 1988:351–372.
12. Von Boehmer H, Kisielow P. Self-nonself discrimination by T-cells. *Science.* 1990;248:1369–1373.
13. Sprent J, Gao EK, Webb SR. T-cell reactivity to MHC molecules: Immunity versus tolerance. *Science.* 1990;248:1357–1363.
14. Möller G, ed. *Immunological Reviews: Autoimmunity* No. 94. Copenhagen, Denmark: Munksgaard; 1986.

15. Cohen IR. Regulation of autoimmune disease: physiological and therapeutic. *Immunol Rev.* 1986;94:5–21.

16. Romagnani S. TH_1 and TH_2 in human disease. *Clin Immunol Immunopathol.* 1996;80:225–235.

17. Yokoyama WM. Natural killer cell receptors specific for major histocompatibility complex class I molecules. *Proc Natl Acad Sci U S A.* 1995;92:3081–3085.

18. Moretta L, Mingari MC, Pende D, et al. The molecular basis of natural killer (NK) cell recognition and function. *J Clin Immunol.* 1996;16:243–253.

19. Versterg R. NK cells and T-cells: Mirror images? *Immunol Today.* 1992;13:244–247.

20. Lanzavecchia A. Identifying strategies for immune intervention. *Science.* 1993;260:937–944.

21. Marrock P, Kappler JW. How the immune system recognizes the body. *Sci Am.* 1993;269:81–89.

22. Harlan DM, Abe R, Led KP, et al. Potential roles of the B7 and CD28 receptor families in autoimmunity and immune evasion. *Clin Immunol Immunopathol.* 1995;75:99–111.

23. Kaufmann SHE. γ/δ and other unconventional T lymphocytes: What do they see and what do they do? *Proc Natl Acad Sci U S A.* 1996;93:2272–2279.

24. Schultz DR, Arnold PI. Heat shock (stress) proteins and autoimmunity in rheumatic diseases. *Semin Arthritis Rheum.* 1993;22:357–374.

25. Romagnani S. Biology of human TH1 and TH2 cells. *J Clin Immunol.* 1995;15:121–129.

26. Weigle WO. Recent observations and concepts in immunological unresponsiveness and autoimmunity. *Clin Exp Immunol.* 1971;9:437–447.

27. Weigle WO. Immunological tolerance and immunopathology. *Hosp Pract.* 1977;12:71.

28. Weigle WO. Analysis of autoimmunity through experimental models of thyroiditis and allergic encephalomyelitis. *Adv Immunol.* 1980;30:159–273.

29. Nossal GJV, Pike BL. Clonal anergy: Persistence in tolerance mice of antigen-binding B lymphocytes incapable of responding to antigen or mitogen. *Proc Natl Acad Sci U S A.* 1980;77:1602–1606.

30. Ottenhoff THM. Selective modulation of T-cell responses in autoimmunity and cancer. *Immunol Today.* 1996;17:54–55.

31. Burnet FM. *The Clonal Selection Theory of Acquired Immunity.* Cambridge, England: Cambridge University Press; 1959.

32. Burnet FM. In Burnet FM, ed. *Autoimmunity and Autoimmune Disease.* Philadelphia, PA: FA Davis & Co; 1972.

33. Schwartz RS, Rose NR. Autoimmunity: Experimental and clinical aspects. *Ann N Y Acad Sci.* 1986;475:1–427.

34. Heath VL, Saoudi A, Seddon BP. The role of the thymus in the control of autoimmunity. *J Autoimmun.* 1996;9:241–246.

35. Miller A, Hafler DA, Weiner HL. Tolerance and suppressor mechanisms in experimental autoimmune encephalomyelitis: Implications for immunotherapy of human autoimmune diseases. *FASEB J.* 1991; 5:2560–2566.

36. Miller KB, Schwartz RS. Autoimmunity and suppressor T lymphocytes. *Adv Intern Med.* 1982;27:281–313.

37. Owen RD. Immunogenetic consequences of vascular anastomosis between bovine twins. *Science.* 1945;102:400–401.

38. Billingham RE, Brent L, Medauar PB. Actively acquired tolerance of foreign cells. *Nature.* 1953;172:603–606.

39. Jerne NK. The natural selection theory of antibody formation. *Proc Natl Acad Sci U S A.* 1955;41:849–859.

40. Bona C, Kohler H. Immune networks. *Ann N Y Acad Sci.* 1983;418:1–230.

41. Geha RS. Current concepts in immunology: Regulation of the immune response by idiotypic antiidiotypic interactions. *N Engl J Med.* 1981;305:25–28.

42. Male DK. Idiotypes and autoimmunity. *Clin Exp Immunol.* 1986;65:1–9.

43. Goodman ME, Weigle WO. Role of polyclonal B-cell activities in self/nonself discrimination. *Immunol Today.* 1981;2:54–57.

44. Shoenfeld Y, Isenberg D. The mosaic of autoimmunity. *Immunol Today.* 1989;10:123–126.

45. Theofilopoulos AN. The basis of autoimmunity: Part II: Genetic predisposition. *Immunol Today.* 1995;16:150–159.

46. Rotter JI, Landau EM. Measuring the genetic contribution of a single locus to a multilocus disease. *Clin Genet.* 1984;26:529–542.

47. Rose NR, Mackay IR. Genetic predisposition to autoimmune diseases. In: Rose NR, Mackay IR, eds. *The Autoimmune Disease.* Orlando, FL: Academic Press; 1985:1–25.

48. Bias WB, Reveille JD, Beaty TH, et al. Evidence that autoimmunity in man is a Mendelian dominant trait. *Am J Hum Genet.* 1986;39:584–602.

49. Nelson JL. Maternal-fetal immunology and autoimmune disease. Is some autoimmune disease autoalloimmune or allo-autoimmune? *Arthritis Rheum.* 1996;39:191–194.

50. Cutolo M, Sulli A, Seriolo B, et al. Estrogens and the immune response and autoimmunity. *Clin Exp. Rheumatol.* 1995;13:217–226.

51. Hochberg MC. The incidence of systemic lupus erythematosus in Baltimore, Maryland, 1970–1977. *Arthritis Rheum.* 1985;28:80–86.

52. Masi AT. Sex hormones and rheumatoid arthritis: Cause or effect relationships in a complex pathophysiology? *Clin Exp Rheumatol.* 1995;13:227–240.

53. Furszfir J, Kurland L, Woolner L, et al. Hashimoto's thyroiditis in Olmsted County, Minnesota, 1935–1967. *Mayo Clin Proc*. 1970;45:586–596.

54. Pottratz ST, Bellido T, Mocharia H, et al. 17B-estradiol inhibits expression of human interleukin-6 promoter-reporter constructs by a receptor-dependent mechanism. *J Clin Invest*. 1994;93:944–950.

55. Kotb M. Infection and autoimmunity: A story of the host, the pathogen, and the copathogen. *Clin Immunol Immunopathol*. 1995;74:10–22.

56. Hokama Y, Nakamura RM. *Immunology and Immunopathology: Basic Concepts*. Boston, MA: Little Brown and Co; 1982.

57. Nygard NR, Schwartz BD. Infection and autoimmunity. *Adv Intern Med*. 1993;38:337–359.

58. Tomer Y, Davies TF. Infection, thyroid disease and autoimmunity. *Endocr Rev*. 1993;14:107–120.

59. Shoenfeld Y. Common infections, idiotypic dysregulation, autoantibody spread and induction of autoimmune diseases. *J Autoimmun*. 1996;6:235–239.

60. Friedman H, Rose NR, Bendinelli M, eds. *Microorganisms and Autoimmune Diseases*. New York, NY: Plenum Press; 1996.

61. Aichele P, Bachmann MF, Hengartner H, et al. Immunopathology or organ–specific autoimmunity as a consequence of virus infection. *Immunol Rev*. 1996;152:21–45.

62. Vaughan JH. The Epstein-Barr virus in autoimmunity. *Springer Semin Immunopathol*. 1995;17:203–230.

63. Kalden JR, Gay S. Retrovirus and autoimmune rheumatic diseases. *Clin Exp Immunol*. 1994;98:1–5.

64. Manns MP. Viruses and autoimmune liver diseases. *Intervirology*. 1993;35:108–115.

65. Dyrberg T, Mackay P, Michelsen B, et al. Viruses and diabetes mellitus. In: Friedman H, Rose NR, Bendinelli M, eds. *Microorganisms and Autoimmune Diseases*. New York, NY: Plenum Press; 1996:105–127.

66. Garzelli C. Epstein-Barr virus and autoimmunity. In: Friedman H, Rose NR, Bendinelli M, eds. *Microorganisms and Autoimmune Diseases*. New York, NY: Plenum Press; 1996:197–218.

67. Drake CE, Kotzin BL. Superantigens: Biology, immunology, and potential role in disease. *J Clin Immunol*. 1992;12:149–162.

68. Friedman SM, Posnett DN, Tumang JR, et al. A potential role for microbial superantigens in the pathogenesis of systemic autoimmune disease. *Arthritis Rheum*. 1991;34:468–480.

69. Acha-Orbea H. Bacterial and viral superantigens: Roles in autoimmunity? *Ann Rheum Dis*. 1993;52:S6–S16.

70. Johnson HM, Torres BA, Soos JM. Superantigens: Structure and relevance to human diseases. *Proc Soc Exp Biol Med*. 1996;212:99–109.

71. Rose NR. Pathogenic mechanisms in autoimmune diseases. *Clin Immunol Immunopathol*. 1989;53:S7–S16.

72. Dziarski R. Autoimmunity: Polyclonal activation or antigen induction. *Immunol Today*. 1988;9:340–342.

73. DeGroot LJ, Quintans J. The causes of autoimmune thyroid disease. *Endocr Rev*. 1989;10:537–562.

74. Cunningham MW. Streptococci and rheumatic fever. In: Friedman H, Rose NR, Bendinelli M, eds. *Microorganisms and Autoimmune Diseases*. New York, NY: Plenum Press; 1996:13–66.

75. Fujinami RS, Oldstone MBA. Amino acid homology between the encephalitogenic site of myelin basic protein and virus: Mechanism for autoimmunity. *Science*. 1985;230:1043–1045.

76. Oldstone MA. Molecular mimicry and autoimmune disease. *Cell*. 1987:50:819–820.

77. Schwimmbeck PL, Yu DTY, Oldstone MBA. Autoantibodies to HLA-B27 in the sera of HLA-B27 patients with ankylosing spondylitis and Reiter's syndrome. *J Exp Med*. 1987;166:173–181.

78. Oldstone MBA. Molecular mimicry as a mechanism for the cause and as a probe uncovering etiologic agent(s) of autoimmune disease. *Curr Top Microbiol Immunol*. 1989;45:127–135.

79. Tsuchiya N, Williams RC. Molecular mimicry—hypothesis or reality? *West J Med*. 1992;157:133–138.

80. Winfield JB, Jarjour WN. Stress proteins, autoimmunity, and autoimmune disease. *Curr Top Microbiol Immunol*. 1991;167:161–189.

81. Res P, Thole J, de Vries R. Heat-shock proteins and autoimmunity in humans. *Springer Semin Immunopathol*. 1991;13:81–98.

82. Doherty PC, Allan W, Eichelberger M, et al. Heat-shock proteins and the gamma-delta T-cell response in virus infections: Implications for autoimmunity. *Springer Semin Immunopathol*. 1991;13:11–14.

83. Janeway CA Jr, Jones B, Hayday A. Specificity and function of T-cells bearing gamma delta receptors. *Immunol Today*. 1988;9:73–76.

84. O'Brien RL, Born W. Specificity of mycobacterial/self reactive gamma delta cells. *Curr Top Microbiol Immunol*. 1990;173:143–150.

85. Plotz PH. Autoantibodies are anti-idiotypic antibodies to antiviral antibodies. *Lancet*. 1983;2:824–826.

86. Cooke A, Lydyard PM, Roitt IM. Autoimmunity and idiotypes. *Lancet*. 1984;2:723–725.

87. Bauman GP, Hurtubise P. Anti-idiotypes and autoimmune disease. In: Deodhar SD, ed. *Auto-immune Diseases. Clinics in Laboratory Medicine*. Vol. 8. Philadelphia, PA: WB Saunders Co; 1988:399–407.

88. Shoenfeld Y. Idiotype induction of autoimmunity: A new classification of autoimmune disease. *Isr J Med Sci*. 1994:11–14.

89. Shoenfeld Y. Idiotypic induction of autoimmunity: Do we need an autoantigen? *Clin Exp Rheumatol.* 1994;12(suppl 11): S37–S40.

90. Shoenfeld Y. Idiotypic induction of autoimmunity: A new aspect of the idiotypic network. *FASEB J.* 1994;8:1296–1301.

91. Shoenfeld Y, Amital H, Ferrone S, et al. Anti-idiotypes and their application under autoimmune, neoplastic and infectious conditions. *Int Arch Allergy Immunol.* 1994;105:211–223.

92. Mountz JD, Zhou T, Su X, et al. The role of programmed cell death as an emerging new concept for the pathogenesis of autoimmune diseases. *Clin Immunol Immunopathol.* 1996;80:S2–S14.

93. Mountz JD, Wu J, Cheng J, et al. Autoimmune disease—a problem of defective apoptosis. *Arthritis Rheum.* 1994;37:1415–1420.

94. Ogawa N, Dang H, Talal N. Apoptosis and autoimmunity. *J Autoimmun.* 1995;8:1–19.

95. Cheng J, Zhou T, Liu C, et al. Identification of a soluble form of the fas molecule that protects cells from fas-mediated apoptosis. *Science.* 1994;263:1759–1761.

96. Witebsky E, Rose NR, Terplan K, et al. Chronic thyroiditis and autoimmunization. *JAMA.* 1957;164:1439–1447.

97. Rose NR, Bona C. Defining criteria for autoimmune diseases (Witebsky's postulates revisited). *Immunol Today.* 1993;14:426–430.

98. Sela O, El-Roeiy A, Isenberg DA, et al. A common DNA antibody idiotype in sera of patients with active pulmonary tuberculosis. *Arthritis Rheum.* 1987;30:50–55.

99. Nakamura RM, Bylund DJ. Contemporary concepts for the clinical and laboratory evaluation of systemic lupus erythematosus and "lupus-like" syndromes. *J Clin Lab Anal.* 1994;8:347–359.

100. Lahita RG. *Systemic Lupus Erythematosus.* 2d ed. New York, NY: Churchill Livingstone; 1992.

101. Roitt IM. Autoimmunity and autoimmune diseases. In: Roitt IM, Brostoff J, Male DK, eds. *Immunology.* 3d ed. St. Louis, MO: Mosby; 1993:24.1–24.

102. Druet P. Diagnosis of autoimmune diseases. *J Immunol Methods.* 1992;150:177–184.

103. Mackay IR. Autoimmunity: Paradigms of Burnet and complexities of today. *Immunol Cell Biol.* 1992;70:159–171.

104. Mackay IR, Rose NR. Autoimmunity: Horizons. In: Rose NR, Mackay IR, eds. *The Autoimmune Disease II.* San Diego, CA: Academic Press; 1992:409–430.

CHAPTER 3

Human Natural Autoantibodies: Definition, Laboratory Testing, and Clinical Significance

LeMing Hang, MD, and Robert M. Nakamura, MD

Background and Definitions

In 1966, Boyden[1] reported the presence of "natural autoantibodies" (NAAs) in healthy individuals without autoimmune disorders or other disease symptoms. He proposed that these NAAs might be related to previously unknown antigenic triggers or subclinical infections. However, subsequent studies showed that production of NAAs did not require or depend on specific antigenic stimulation.[2] Currently, NAAs are regarded as essential constituents of physiologic autoimmunity, reactive with and capable of binding to various cellular components such as nuclear, cytoskeletal, and membrane proteins, as well as circulating immunoglobulins, cytokines, clotting factors, and hormonal polypeptides. There is no evidence of familial tendency in NAA occurrence.[2–5]

Epidemiologic Surveys of Natural Autoantibodies

Natural autoantibodies can be detected in healthy individuals of any age, including neonates. Incidence of NAA occurrence tends to increase with age. Less than 10% of sera from children and young adults contain NAAs, whereas 20% to 30% of sera from adults and the elderly test positive for NAAs. Moreover, in the elderly, NAAs may comprise over 20% of total immunoglobulins.[5] Combined surveys of over 10,000 healthy adult and elderly subjects[2–5] showed a varying incidence of different types of NAAs: 16% of cases were antimicrosomal; 13% were antiactin (smooth muscle); 10% were antithyroglobulin; 8% were antinuclear; 5% were anti-immunoglobulin (anti-Ig) G, or rheumatoid factor; 2.5% were antimitochondrial; 3% were antilymphocyte; and 0.5% were anti–Sjögren's syndrome A/Ro (SSA-Ro). A smaller survey[2–4] of 269 sera from healthy children also found various types of NAAs, such as antinuclear, antimitochondrial, antiactin, and anti-IgG, with incidence rates ranging from 0.6% to 3% (**Table 3-1**).

Laboratory Assay Methods for Natural Autoantibodies

Detection and quantitation of NAAs can be performed by direct assay methods, such as enzyme-linked immunosorbent assay (ELISA), immunofluorescence (IF), radioimmunoassay (RIA), immunoblot (IB), or flow cytometry. Alternative methods to demonstrate NAA production are in vitro stimulation and expansion of immunoglobulins secreting B cells isolated from the peripheral blood of test subjects, using polyclonal B-cell activators, such as pokeweed mitogen and Epstein-Barr virus. Somatic cell hybridization and cell fusion with myeloma techniques also are available, and these assays offer higher sensitivity as well as specificity.[6–8]

Physical Properties and Characteristics of Natural Autoantibodies

The majority of NAAs are polyreactive low-affinity IgMs, but IgG and IgA NAAs also can be detected, although they are usually masked by polyreactive IgM NAAs (**Table 3-2**). All three isotype NAAs have antiself and anti-idiotypic activities, capable of binding to multiple self- and non-self-antigens. The antigenic binding ability of

Table 3-1. Incidence of Natural Autoantibodies in Sera of Healthy Populations[3]

Natural Autoantibody	Number of Sera Tested	Positive Results (%)
Antinuclear	3,784	8
Antimitochondrial	2,500	2.5
Anti–SSA-Ro	2,500	0.5
Anti-IgG (rheumatoid factor)	245	5
Antithyroglobulin	215	10
Antimicrosomal	197	16
Antilymphocyte	93	3
Antiactin (smooth muscle)	65	13

Abbreviations: SSA-Ro = Sjögren's syndrome A/Ro; IgG = immunoglobulin G.

Table 3-2. Physical Properties and Characteristics of Natural Autoantibodies[3]

May be immunoglobulin M, G, or A isotypes
May be low affinity or high avidity
May be polyreactive or monospecific, reacting with self- and nonself-antigens
Have antigenic repertoires similar to those of autoimmune diseases
Are usually nonpathogenic
Are important in immunologic homeostasis
Are part of regulatory and idiotypic networks
May inhibit natural killer cells and interferon activity

NAAs depends on local concentrations of antigens and antibodies, as well as the density of major histocompatibility complex (MHC) class II molecules expressed by immune cells. The avidities of polyreactive IgM NAAs for their respective autoantigens range from 10^{-5} to 10^{-10} mol. The monoreactive IgA and IgG NAAs show more variable avidities, ranging from 10^{-3} to 10^{-11} mol in magnitude. These avidity ranges are apparently comparable to those of T-cell receptors.[9–11]

As stated previously, NAAs show reactivity with a wide panel of autoantigens that have been highly conserved during evolution. Examples of such autoantigens are histone, DNA, RNA, actin, myosin, and myelin, as well as circulating cytokines, cellular enzymes, phospholipids, polypeptide hormones, and neural glycosides. Although the NAA antigenic repertoire bears some resemblance to that seen in autoimmune diseases, NAAs usually are not associated with pathologic tissue lesions and are subjected to autoregulation by the idiotype–anti-idiotype network.[5,12–14]

Sources of Natural Autoantibodies

Placental cord blood cells, CD5+ B cells, and fetal liver cells are the main sources of NAAs. The size of the CD5+ B-cell pool in a given individual is genetically determined and regulated. In neonates, CD5+ B cells are found in the omentum and liver. In adults, CD5+ pre-B cells reside in the bone marrow, while the more mature CD5+ B cells populate the lymph nodes, tonsils, peripheral blood, and spleen.[15,16] These mature cells have receptors for immunostimulatory cytokines, such as interleukin-2 (IL-2) and interleukin-5 (IL-5), but the cells themselves can produce inhibitory cytokines, such as interleukin-10 (IL-10), to regulate helper T-cell activities.[15,17] The total CD5+ B-cell population is higher in early neonatal life and in patients with infections, autoimmune diseases, monoclonal lymphoproliferative disorders, and tumors.[18–22] Synthesis of NAAs by CD5+ B cells is encoded by unmutated, highly conserved germline genes.[23] In addition to producing NAAs, CD5+ B cells are capable of initiating cytotoxic activities, directing the autoregulatory idiotype network, processing antigens for presentation to T cells, and inducing immunologic tolerance.[24–26]

With repeated exposure of autoantigens, CD5+ B cells can undergo affinity maturation. This creates the potential of the cells generating somatically mutated, antigen-specific, high-affinity IgG and IgA "pathogenic" autoantibodies similar to those detected in autoimmune diseases.[27,28]

Natural Autoantibodies and the Idiotype Network

Idiotypes are antigenic epitopes located in the antigen-binding regions of antibody molecules. Jerne[29] postulated that the immune response to an antigen can lead to the formation of idiotype, anti-idiotype, and anti–anti-idiotype networks. The tertiary structure of an anti-idiotype can be similar or identical to that of the initial antigen. Thus, the idiotype network can promote formations of various types of antigen-antibody complexes for more effective modulation and regulation of immune responses.[30]

Cross-reactive NAAs with idiotypic properties are present in neonates, healthy adults, autoimmune disease patients, and their primary relatives.[31,32] The immunologic response of a given individual can be enhanced or suppressed by NAAs and their idiotypic networks. For example, sera from patients with cold agglutinin disease who test positive for anti-DNA expressing 16/6 idiotype can induce a disease similar to systemic lupus erythematosus (SLE) in mice recipients; on the other hand, the disease symptoms of certain lupus patients can be ameliorated by infusion of anti-idiotypic antibodies with anti-DNA activity.[33,34]

The determining factors for these apparently divergent idiotypic responses seem to be (1) the antigen-antibody ratio; (2) the affinity, avidity, isotypes, and tertiary conformations of the involved antibodies; (3) the density and types of MHC molecules expressed by the effector and target cells; and (4) the individual's genetic background.[11–14,29,30,35]

The Physiologic Roles of Natural Autoantibodies

During fetal development, NAAs participate in morphogenesis and organogenesis. Throughout an individual's life, NAAs perform various immunoregulatory and physiologic functions to maintain homeostasis. The polyreactivity of NAAs allows them to bind with multiple autoantigens as well as nonself-antigens and perform several important and necessary tasks. These tasks are[9,36,37]

- To serve as the first line of defense against invading agents by enhancing phagocytosis and complement-mediated lysis of these agents
- To complex with various types of altered host tissue or microbial antigens thus preventing the induction of inappropriate or pathologic autoimmunity
- To facilitate the removal of immunogenic metabolic and catabolic wastes from the host body, thus averting sustained immunostimulatory and autoimmune events

The following observations strongly support that NAAs are essential for maintenance of physiologic autoimmunity, homeostasis, and immunoregulation:

- Natural autoantibody titers increase during viral, bacterial, and parasitic infections. Some of these NAAs exhibit rheumatoid factor–like activity, serving to downregulate any heightened immune response and to prevent potential pathogenic autoimmunity.[38,39]
- Natural autoantibodies can bind to pathogenic immune complexes to enhance removal of these complexes from host tissue and circulation.[11,36]
- Natural autoantibodies with antiactin reactivities can facilitate binding of nonself-antigens to negatively charged cell membrane to initiate helper, suppressor, or cytotoxic T-cell activities.[3,11,24]
- Natural autoantibodies with proteolytic properties for vasoactive intestinal polypeptides may be involved in metabolism of these intestinal peptides.[40]
- Natural autoantibodies with idiotypic properties can mediate acute rejection in transplant recipients.[41]
- Natural autoantibodies with antiphospholipid activity may play a physiologic role in eliminating senescent erythrocytes by binding to their surface lipids.[37,42]
- Natural autoantibodies with anti-IgE activity can regulate and modulate allergic disease states. Such NAAs are found in 35% of nonatopic individuals and 71% of atopic individuals.[43]
- Natural autoantibodies with anti–factor VIII activity are present in healthy individuals without coagulopathy. These NAAs can inhibit factor VIII activity in pooled normal plasma but not in autologous plasma. At present, the clinical significance of this "inhibitory" effect is unclear.[44]

The Pathogenic Potential of Natural Autoantibodies

The determining factors for induction of physiologic versus pathologic autoimmune responses are (1) the duration of the antigenic stimuli; (2) the titer, isotype, affinity, and avidity of the antibodies produced; and (3) the types of effector T cells and cytokines generated.[12] The consequences of interactions among these factors can either restore "orderly connectivity" of immune networks, ensuring physiologic homeostasis, or disrupt such connectivity, resulting in pathogenic autoimmune tissue injury.[12–14] Several NAAs and their pathogenic potentials are listed in **Table 3-3**.

Several studies[11,14,18,25] have shown that NAAs coexist with their pathogenic "counterparts" and that

CD5+ B cells can, under certain conditions, produce "pathogenic" NAAs. The investigators proposed that CD5+ B-cell hyperactivity with increased synthesis of NAAs occurs during the early phase of physiologic autoimmune responses to pathogens and other environmental insults. These initial NAAs serve to eliminate potential immunogens and to prevent sustained autoimmune events. However, individuals who are genetically susceptible to autoimmune disease may have CD5+ B-cell clones that may expand, mature, and somatically mutate to higher affinity-avidity NAAs when they are subjected to persistent or repeated antigenic stimuli. These high-avidity NAAs can cause immune complex–mediated tissue injury under conditions that promote local inflammatory cytokine activities.[26–30]

Thus, CD5+ B cells can be the source of both physiologic and pathogenic NAAs. The following observations offer supporting evidence that NAAs coexist with their pathogenic counterparts and contribute to autoimmune tissue injuries:

- Polyreactive anti-DNA autoantibodies in SLE patients bear idiotopes similar to those of NAAs in healthy individuals; both types cross-react with phospholipids.[31,42]
- Immune complexes eluted from kidney and skin lesions of SLE patients contain monospecific, high-avidity anti-DNA autoantibodies, as well as IgM and IgG NAAs. Two types of anti-DNA autoantibodies can be found in SLE patients: polyreactive low-affinity types and monoreactive high-avidity types.[36,46–48]
- Many of the autoantibodies produced by human hybridomas derived from SLE patients are polyreactive IgMs with physical properties similar to those of NAAs.[49]
- Immunoglobulin gene expression and site-directed mutagenesis studies have shown that CD5+ B cells in SLE and rheumatoid arthritis patients are the main source for both IgM NAAs and pathogenic IgG anti-DNA autoantibodies and rheumatoid factors.[50–52]
- Some of the NAAs found in patients with reactive, inflammatory monoclonal gammopathies or lymphoproliferative malignancies can cause autoimmune hemolytic anemia, vasculitis, cryoglobulinemia, arthropathy, and peripheral neuropathy.[53–58]

Natural Autoantibodies and Monoclonal Gammopathies

Monoclonal gammopathies in patients with reactive or neoplastic lymphoproliferation may be composed of monoclonal NAAs. Up to 10% of monoclonal NAAs have cross-reactive and anti-idiotypic properties.[59] The types and relative frequencies of these monoclonal NAAs are as follows: anti–SSA-Ro (23%), anti-Smith antigen (anti-Sm) (16%), antihistone (14%), anti-DNA(6%), and rheumatoid factors (5%). Monoclonal NAAs that react with neural glycolipids and blood group antigens also have been identified. Although most monoclonal NAAs are germline encoded and usually not associated with clinical autoimmune disease, some have been shown to be pathogenic, apparently causing vasculitis, serositis,

Table 3-3. Natural Autoantibodies with Pathogenic Potential[45]

Type of Natural Autoantibody*	Associated Clinical Symptoms
Anti-IgG	Cryoglobulinemia, vasculitis
Anti–SSA-Ro	Vasculitis, symptoms of sicca syndrome
Antiactin (smooth muscle)	Symptoms of polymyositis
Antiphospholipid	Lupus anticoagulant activity
Anti–factors V, VII, VIII, and X	Presence of coagulation inhibitors
Anti–DNA 16/6 idiotype	Induced SLE-type disease
Anti-Ii RBC antigen	Hemolytic anemia, presence of cold agglutinins
Antithyroglobulin (in myeloma)	Hypothyroidism
Antimyelin (in monoclonal gammopathies)	Peripheral neuropathy

Abbreviations: IgG = immunoglobulin G; SSA-Ro = Sjögren's syndrome A/Ro; RBC = red blood cell.
**Most entries are natural autoantibodies of monoclonal gammopathies.*

rheumatoid arthritis, peripheral neuropathy, hemolytic anemia, and coagulopathy (see Table 3-3).[53,56–62]

Natural Autoantibodies and Tumor Development

Tumor development is a prolonged process sometimes lasting half of an individual's lifetime.[63] Tumor progression depends on host humoral and cellular factors. In vitro, NAAs are capable of tumor immunomodulation by interacting with the various types of receptors found on tumor cells. These are receptors for T cells, immunoglobulins, lymphokines, and cytokines. In vivo, the NAAs found in cancer patients apparently display antitumor, anti-IgG, anti-interferon, anti-interleukin, and antilymphocyte reactivities. Whether these NAAs are present to control tumor progression or promote tumor growth has not been clarified. Natural autoantibodies may have the potential to promote or prohibit tumor growth.[64]

Patients with lymphoid and epithelial malignancies have increased CD5+ B cells and NAA titers but decreased capacity to mount appropriate immune responses. The CD5+ B cells are thought to be responsible for their immunosuppressive state.[65] At present, the exact roles of NAAs in tumor development and growth are unclear, but various types of investigative studies are in progress.[66–68]

Therapeutic Roles of Natural Autoantibodies

Patients with certain types of autoimmune diseases, most notably those who are autoantibody mediated, may respond to high-dose intravenous immunoglobulin (IVIG) infusion. The polyreactive NAAs present in the pooled normal plasma used for IVIG are thought to be responsible for the improvement of disease symptoms by inducing anti-idiotypic immunosuppression.[69–71] Autoimmune diseases exhibiting such therapeutic responses include immune leukocytopenia, chronic idiopathic thrombocytopenia, myasthenia gravis, Guillain-Barré syndrome, anti-neutrophilic cytoplasmic antibody (ANCA)–related vasculitis, posttransfusion purpura, autoimmune thyroiditis, bullous pemphigoid, and lupus anticoagulant–related spontaneous abortions.[72–79] The following are some of the proposed mechanisms by which NAAs can modulate and ameliorate these autoimmune diseases:

- Inhibition of monocyte activation by blocking surface Fc receptors of phagocytic cells[79]
- Regulation of activities of T cells, natural killer cells, and autoantibody-producing B cells[80]
- Prevention of complement and immune complex binding to target cell membranes[81]
- Aversion of immune complex tissue injury by acting as anti-idiotypic antibodies that bind and occupy the F(ab)2 sites of pathogenic autoantibodies[82]
- Enhancement of the removal of pathogenic immune complexes by promoting their solubility[83]
- Initiation of idiotypic suppression by activating CD8+ suppressor T cells[84,85]

One or more of these mechanisms may operate simultaneously to achieve the optimal therapeutic effects. Examples of autoimmune diseases that respond to NAA-induced anti-idiotypic immunosuppression are those in which anti-idiotypic antibodies against pathogenic autoantibodies can be detected in "remission sera." The list of such diseases includes SLE, Guillain-Barré syndrome, anti–factor VIII coagulopathy, myasthenia gravis, and systemic vasculitis.[69,85] As studies of interrelationships among autoimmune diseases, NAAs, and the idiotype network continue, more diseases may be added to this list.

Summary

Natural autoantibodies are present in sera from healthy individuals of all ages, including neonates. These autoantibodies are synthesized by CD5+ B cells. They are mostly polyreactive low-avidity IgMs, but also may be monoreactive high-avidity IgG and IgA isotypes. Natural autoantibodies can bind to nuclear, cytoplasmic, and cell surface membrane proteins, as well as to circulating polypeptides, hormones, cytokines, and phospholipids. The incidence and types of NAAs found in healthy populations range from 0.5% for anti–SSA-Ro, 5% for rheumatoid factor, and 8% for antinuclear to over 10% for antiactin, antimicrosomal, or other cytoskeletal proteins. Natural autoantibodies usually are not associated with clinical autoimmune disease and are considered essential components of physiologic autoimmunity, necessary for immunoregulation and maintenance of immunologic homeostasis.

The clinically significant physiologic functions and unique properties of NAAs are as follows:

- The antigenic repertoire of NAAs bears some resemblance to that seen in autoimmune diseases, but NAAs usually are not pathogenic.
- Natural autoantibodies serve as precursors of antibodies to exogenous antigen and the first line of defense against invading pathogens. Their titers are higher in individuals with viral, bacterial, or parasitic infections.
- Natural autoantibodies show extensive cross-reactivity with bacterial antigens and organic haptens, promoting the removal of these agents from the circulation.
- Natural autoantibodies can bind with damaged and senescent cell components to facilitate elimination of these catabolic wastes, averting molecular mimicry and potential autosensitization of T cells or B cells.
- Natural autoantibodies contribute to cytotoxic, natural killer, phagocytic, stimulatory, and inhibitory immunologic activities. Some NAAs have proteolytic activity for vasoactive intestinal polypeptides.
- Natural autoantibodies are part of the idiotypic network for maintenance of self-tolerance and immunoregulation. The therapeutic effects of IVIG in some autoimmune diseases have been attributed to the idiotypic properties of NAAs.
- A number of monoclonal gammopathies (10% to 30%) may have NAA properties, and some of these may be pathogenic.
- When subjected to repeated or persistent antigenic stimuli, the CD5+ B cells—which are the major sources of polyreactive low-avidity NAAs—can proliferate and undergo somatic mutation
- To synthesize monoreactive high-avidity NAAs with pathogenic potential.

References

1. Boyden SV. Natural antibodies and the immune response. *Adv Immunol.* 1966;5:1–27.
2. Avrameas S. Natural autoantibodies: Self-recognition and physiological autoimmunity. In: Shoenfeld Y, Isenberg DA, eds. *Natural Autoantibodies. Their Physiological Role and Regulatory Significance.* Boca Raton, FL: CRC Press Inc; 1993:1–14.
3. Abu-Shakra M, Shoenfeld Y. What are natural autoantibodies? In: Shoenfeld Y, Isenberg DA, eds. *Natural Autoantibodies: Their Physiological Role and Regulatory Significance.* Boca Raton, FL: CRC Press Inc; 1993:15–33.
4. Varela F, Anderson A, Dietrich G, et al. Population dynamics of natural antibodies in normal and autoimmune individuals. *Proc Natl Acad Sci U S A.* 1991;88:5917–5921.
5. Dighiero G, Lymberi P, Guilbert B, et al. Natural autoantibodies constitute a substantial part of normal circulating immunoglobulins. *Ann N Y Acad Sci.* 1986;475:135–145.
6. Kalsi J, Isenberg DA. Measurement of natural autoantibodies. In: Shoenfeld Y, Isenberg DA, eds. *Natural Autoantibodies: Their Physiological Role and Regulatory Significance.* Boca Raton, FL: CRC Press Inc; 1993:35–57.
7. Lydyard PM. Flow cytometry developments, use of monoclonal antibodies and cell purification. *Curr Opin Immunol.* 1990:2:923–926.
8. Seigneurin M, Guilbert B, Bourgeat MJ, et al. Polyspecific natural antibodies and autoantibodies secreted by human lymphocytes immortalized with EBV. *Blood.* 1988;71:581–585.
9. Monestier M, Bonna C. Antibodies possessing multiple antigen specificities and exhibiting extensive idiotypic cross-reactivity. *Int Rev Immunol.* 1988;3:59–70.
10. Schwartz RS. Autoimmunity and autoimmune diseases. In: Paul WE, ed. *Fundamental Immunology.* 3rd ed. NewYork, NY: Raven Press; 1993:1034–1095.
11. Avrameas S. Natural autoantibodies: From "horror autotoxicus" to "gnothi seauton." *Immunol Today.* 1991;12:154–158.
12. Varela FJ, Coutinho A. Second generation immune network. *Immunol Today.* 1991;12:159–166.
13. Cooke A, Lydyard PM, Roitt IM. Mechanism of autoimmunity: A role for cross-reactive idiotypes. *Immunol Today.* 1987;8:170–172.
14. Cohen IR, Cooke A. Natural autoantibodies might prevent autoimmune disease. *Immunol Today.* 1986;7:363–364.
15. Buskila D, Mackenzie LE, Shoenfeld Y, et al. The biology of CD5+ B cells. In: Shoenfeld Y, Isenberg DA, eds. *Natural Autoantibodies: Their Physiological Role and Regulatory Significance.* Boca Raton, FL: CRC Press Inc; 1993:125–142.
16. Kipps TJ. The CD5 B cell. *Adv Immunol.* 1989;47:117–185.
17. Fiorentino DF, Zlotnik A, Vieira P, et al. IL-10 acts on the antigen presenting cell to inhibit cytokine production by TH1 cells. *J Immunol.* 1991;146:3444–3451.
18. Youinou D, Buskila D, MacKenzie LE, et al . CD5 positive B cells and disease. In: Shoenfeld Y, Isenberg DA, eds. *Natural Autoantibodies: Their Physiological Role and Regulatory Significance.* Boca Raton, FL: CRC Press Inc; 1993:143–165.

19. Becker H, Weber C, Storch S, et al. Relationship between CD5+ B cells and systemic autoimmunity. *Clin Immunol Immunopathol*. 1990;56:219–225.

20. Hayakawa K, Hardy RR. Normal, autoimmune, and malignant CD5 B cells: The Ly-1 B lineage? *Annu Rev Immunol*. 1988;6:197–218.

21. Kazbay K, Osterland CK. The frequency of CD5+ B cells in autoantibody positive and negative autoimmune disease and in neonatal cord blood. *Clin Exp Rheumatol*. 1990;8:231–235.

22. Stein R, Witz IP, Ovadia J, et al. CD5+ cells and natural autoantibodies in patients with cancer. *Clin Exp Immunol*. 1991;65:418–422.

23. Siminovitch KA, Misner V, Kwong PC, et al. A natural autoantibody is encoded by germline heavy and lambda light chain variable region genes without somatic mutation. *J Clin Invest*. 1989;84:1675–1678.

24. Raveche ES. Possible immunoregulatory role for CD5+ B cells. *Clin Immunol Immunopathol*. 1990;56:135–150.

25. Roosnek E, Lanzvecchia A. Efficient and selective presentation of antigen-antibody complexes by rheumatoid factor B cells. *J Exp Med*. 1991;173:487–489.

26. Coutinho A. Beyond clonal selection and network. *Immunol Today*. 1989;11:63–88.

27. Ikematsu H, Harindranath N, Casali P. Somatic mutations in the VH genes of high affinity antibodies to self and foreign antigens produced by human CD5+ and CD5– B cells. *Ann N Y Acad Sci*. 1992;651:319.

28. Kocks C, Rajewsky K. Stepwise intraclonal maturation of antibody affinity through somatic hypermutation. *Proc Natl Acad Sci U S A*. 1988;85:8206–8210.

29. Jerne NK. The generative grammar of the immune system. *Science*. 1985;229:1057–1064.

30. Male DK. Idiotypes and autoimmunity. *Clin Exp Immunol*. 1986;65:1–9.

31. Isenberg DA, Shoenfeld Y, Walport M, et al. Detection of cross-reactive anti-DNA antibody isotype in the serum of SLE patients and of their relatives. *Arthritis Rheum*. 1985;28:999–1007.

32. Youinou P, MacKenzie L, Katsikis P, et al. The relationship between CD5 expressing B lymphocytes and serological abnormalities in RA patients and their relatives. *Arthritis Rheum*. 1990;33:339–348.

33. Shoenfeld Y, Mozes E. Pathogenic idiotypes of autoantobodies in autoimmunity: Lessons from new experimental models of SLE. *FASEB J*. 1990;4:2646–2651.

34. Zouali M, Diamond B. Idiotype-mediated intervention in systemic lupus erythematosus. *J Autoiummun*. 1990;3:381–385.

35. Ammital-Teplizki H, Lymbery P, Tomer Y, et al. The idiotypic network, autoimmunity, and natural autoantibodies. In: Shoenfeld Y, Isenberg DA, eds. *Natural Autoantibodies: Their Physiological Role and Regulatory Significance*. Boca Raton, FL: CRC Press Inc; 1993:175–204.

36. Louzir H, Tenynck T, Gorgi Y, et al. Enzyme immunoassay analysis of antibody specificities present in the circulating immune complexes of selected pathological sera. *J Immunol Methods*. 1988;128:1695–1699.

37. Wiener E, Wickramasinghe SN. Natural autoantibodies may play a role in ineffective erythropoiesis during megaloblastic haemopoiesis. *Clin Exp Immunol*. 1991;83:121–125.

38. Nakamura M, Burastero SE, Notkins AL, et al. Human monoclonal rheumatoid factor-like antibodies from CD5 B cells are polyreactive. *J Immunol*. 1988;140:4180–4186.

39. Lydyard PM, Quarety-Papafio R, Broker B, et al. The repertoire of early human B cells: High frequency of autoreactivity and polyreactivity. *Scand J Immunol*. 1990;31:33–43.

40. Paul S, Volle DJ, Mei S. Affinity chromatography of catalytic autoantibody to vasoactive intestinal peptide. *J Immunol*. 1990;145:1196–1199.

41. Turman MA, Casali P, Notkins AL, et al. Polyreactivity and antigen specificity of human xenoreactive monoclonal and serum natural antibodies. *Transplantation*. 1991;52:710-717.

42. Alarcon-Segovia D. Antiphospholipids as natural autoantibodies. In: Shoenfeld Y, Isenberg DA, eds. *Natural Autoantibodies: Their Physiological Role and Regulatory Significance*. Boca Raton, FL: CRC Press Inc; 1993:261–265.

43. Williams R, Griffiths RW, Emmons JD. Naturally occurring human antiglobulins with specificity for IgE. *J Clin Invest*. 1972;51:955–963.

44. Algiman M, Dietrich G, Nydegger UE, et al. Natural antibodies to factor VIII (anti-hemophilic factor) in healthy individuals. *Proc Natl Acad Sci U S A*. 1992;89:3795–3799.

45. Papadopoulos NM, Costello R, Ceroni M, et al. Identification of HIV-specific oligoclonal immunoglobulins in the serum of carriers of HIV antibody. *Clin Chem*. 1988;34:937–935.

46. Van Es JH, Frits HJ, Gmelig M, et al. Somatic mutation in the variable region of a human IgG anti-dsDNA autoantibody suggests a role for antigen in the induction SLE. *J Exp Med*. 1991;173:461–470.

47. Suzuki N, Sakane T, Engleman EG. Anti-DNA antibodies production by CD5+ and CD5– cells of patients with SLE. *J Clin Invest*. 1990;85:238–247.

48. Madaio MP, Carlson J, Catoldo J, et al. Murine monoclonal anti-DNA antibodies bind directly to glomerular antigens and form immune complexes. *J Immunol*. 1987;138:2883–2889.

49. Shoenfeld Y, Rauch J, Massicotte H, et al. Polyspecificity of monoclonal lupus antibodies produced by human-human hybridoma. *N Engl J Med*. 1983;308:414–420.

50. Burastero SE, Casali P, Wilder RL, et al. Monoreactive high affinity and polyreactive low affinity rheumatoid factors are produced by CD5+ B cells from patients with rheumatoid arthritis. *J Exp Med*. 1988;168:1979–1992.

51. Casali P, Burastero SE, Nakamura M, et al. Human lymphocytes making rheumatoid factor and antibody to ssDNA belong to Leu1+ B cell subset. *Science*. 1987;236:77–81.

52. Zouali M. From the preimmune repertoire to pathogenic autoantibodies. In: Shoenfeld Y, Isenberg DA, eds. *Natural Autoantibodies: Their Physiological Role and Regulatory Significance*. Boca Raton, FL: CRC Press Inc; 1993:237–246.

53. Grunebaum E, Buskila D, Shoenfeld Y. Serum human immunoglobulins (monoclonal gammopathies) as natural autoantibodies. In: Shoenfeld Y, Isenberg DA, eds. *Natural Autoantibodies. Their Physiological Role and Regulatory Significance*. Boca Raton, FL: CRC Press Inc; 1993:81–107.

54. Shoenfeld Y, Vilner Y, Coates AR, et al. Monoclonal anti-tuberculosis antibodies react with DNA and monoclonal anti-DNA autoantibodies react with *Mycobacterium tuberculosis. Clin Exp Immunol*. 1986;66:255–261.

55. Rubin L, Urowitz MB, Pruzanski W. Systemic lupus erythematosus with paraproteinemia. *Arthritis Rheum*. 1984;27:638–644.

56. Duhrsen U, Augener W, Zwingers T, et al. Spectrum and frequency of autoimmune derangements in lymphoproliferative disorders. Analysis of 637 cases and comparison with myeloproliferative diseases. *Br J Haematol*. 1987;67:235–239.

57. Borche L, Lim A, Binet JL, et al. Evidence that chronic lymphocytic leukemia B lymphocytes are frequently committed to production of natural autoantibodies. *Blood*. 1990;76:562–569.

58. Kyle RA. Monoclonal gammopathy of undetermined significance(MGUS): A review. *Clin Haematol*. 1982; 11:123–150.

59. Kunkel HG, Agnello V, Joslin FG, et al. Cross-idiotypic specificity among monoclonal IgM proteins with anti-globulin activity. *J Exp Med*. 1973;137:331–342.

60. Sestak AL, Harley JB, Yoshida S, et al. Lupus/Sjögren's autoantibody specificities in sera with paraproteins. *J Clin Invest*. 1987;80:138–144.

61. Hamblin TJ, Oscier DJ, Young BJ. Autoimmunity in chronic lymphocytic leukemia. *J Clin Pathol*. 1986;39: 713–716.

62. Freddo L, Ariga T, Saito M. The neuropathy of plasma cell dyscrasia: Binding of IgM M-protein to peripheral nerve glycolipids. *Neurology*. 1985;35:1420.

63. Farber E, Rubin H. Cellular adaptation in the origin and development of cancer cells. *Cancer Res*. 1991;51:2751–2761.

64. Witz IP. Naturally occurring antibodies and tumor development and progression. In: Shoenfeld Y, Isenberg DA, eds. *Natural Autoantibodies: Their Physiological Role and Regulatory Significance*. Boca Raton, FL: CRC Press Inc; 1993:247–258.

65. Paglieroni T, Caggiano V, Mackenzie M. CD5+ immunoregulatory B cell subsets. *Am J Hematol*. 1988;28:276–280.

66. Witz IP. Tumor-bound immunoglobulins: In situ expression of humoral immunity. *Adv Cancer Res*. 1977;25:95–158.

67. Cahalon L, Korem S, Gonen B, et al. Autoantibody-mediated regulation of tumor growth. *Ann N Y Acad Sci*. 1992;651:393–408.

68. Witz IP, Agaasy-Cahalon L. Do naturally occurring antibodies play a role in the progression and proliferation of tumor cells? *Int Rev Immunol*. 1988;3:133–145.

69. Nydegger URSE. Hypothetic and established action mechanism of therapy with immunoglobulins. In: Imbach P, ed. *Immunotherapy with IVIG*. New York, NY: Academic Press; 1991:27–36.

70. Rossi F, Kazatchkine MD. Anti-idiotypes against autoantibodies in pooled normal human polyspecific immunoglobulins. *J Immunol*. 1989;143:4104–4109.

71. Buskila D, Shoenfeld Y. From the practical viewpoint—immunomodulation with natural auto-anti-idiotypic antibodies: The role of treatment with IVIG. In: Shoenfeld Y, Isenberg DA, eds. *Natural Autoantibodies: Their Physiological Role and Regulatory Significance*. Boca Raton, FL: CRC Press Inc; 1993:303–336.

72. Becton DL, Kinney TR, Chaffee S, et al. High dose IVIG for severe platelet alloimmunization. *Pediatrics*. 1984;74:1120–1122.

73. Barbui T, Bassan R, Viero P, et al. Pure white cell aplasia treated with high dose IVIG. *Br J Haematol*. 1984;58:556–562.

74. Van Doorn PA, Brand A, Rossi F, et al. On the mechanism of high dose IVIG treatment of patients with chronic inflammatory demyelinating polyneuropathy. *J Neuroimmunol*. 1990;29:57–64.

75. Rossi F, Jayne DR, Lockwood CM, et al. Anti-idiotypes against anti-neutrophil cytoplasmic antigen autoantibodies in normal human polyspecific IgG for therapeutic use and in the remission sera of patients with systemic vasculitis. *Clin Exp Immunol*. 1991;83: 298–303.

76. Becker T, Panzer S, Maas D, et al. High dose IVIG for post-transfusion purpura. *Br J Haematol*. 1985;61: 149–155.

77. Roubaty C, Bedin C, Charreire J. Prevention of experimental autoimmune thyroiditis through the anti-idiotypic network. *J Immunol*. 1989;144:2167–2174.

78. Godard W, Roujeau JC, Guillot B, et al. Bullous pemphigoid and IVIG. *Ann Intern Med*. 1985;103:965.

79. Coulman C, Peters A, McIntyre J, et al. The use of IVIG for the treatment of recurrent spontaneous abortion. In: Imbach P, ed. *Immunotherapy with IVIG*. New York, NY: Academic Press; 1991:395–400.

80. Mannhalter JW, Ahmad R, Wolf HM, et al. Effect of polymeric IgG on human monocyte function. *Int Arch Allergy Appl Immunol*. 1987;82:159–167.

81. Engelhard D, Warner JL, Kapoor N, et al. Effect of IVIG on natural killer cell activity: Possible association with autoimmune neutropenia and ITP. *J Pediatr*. 1986;108:77–81.

82. Lockwood CM. Therapeutic opportunities in systemic vasculitis. In: Imbach P, ed. *Immunotherapy with IVIG*. New York, NY: Academic Press; 1991:297–306.

83. Sato M, Kojima H, Koshikawa S. Modification of immune complexes deposited in glomeruli in tissue section treated with sulfonized gammaglobulins. *Clin Exp Immunol*. 1986;64:623–628.

84. Delfraissy JK, Techernia G, Laurian Y, et al. Suppressor cell function after IVIG treatment in adult chronic ITP. *Br J Haematol*. 1985;60:315–322.

85. Macey MG, Newland AC. CD4 and CD8 subpopulation changes during high dose IVIG treatment. *Br J Haematol*. 1990;76:513–520.

CHAPTER 4

Interrelationships of Immunodeficiency, Autoimmunity, and Malignancies

LeMing Hang, MD, and Robert M. Nakamura, MD

Since the 1950s, numerous clinical studies have noted the increased incidence of malignancies in patients diagnosed with autoimmune or immunodeficiency diseases. However, the reported extent of increased malignancy risk varied widely, from twice to several hundred times over that of age-matched controls.[1–9] The causes of such large variations observed by the investigators in these retrospective clinical and epidemiologic surveys have been attributed to differences in data collection methodologies, the extent of patient collaboration, the lack of uniform sample size, criteria for selection of positive versus control patient groups and the types of tumors, and the presence of certain inherent biases in statistical analysis.[5–9]

The limitations imposed by methodologic differences and statistical bias have made confirmation of previous reports and studies regarding malignancy risk in autoimmune and immunodeficient patients challenging and difficult. Nevertheless, the goals of this chapter are to (1) review these studies and reexamine the data and evidence presented; (2) indicate the malignancy risk in patients with and without an immunologic disease diagnosis; (3) identify the common factors linking immunodeficiency, autoimmunity, and malignancy; (4) provide clinical and laboratory guidelines to help in evaluating immunodeficiency states; and (5) discuss examples of lymphoid and epithelial malignancies that can mimic autoimmune disease, or "autoimmune paraneoplastic syndromes."

Malignancies in Autoimmune and Immunodeficiency Diseases

In general, malignancies associated with autoimmune and immunodeficiency diseases can be categorized into 4 groups:

- Malignancies developing in patients with autoimmune diseases
- Malignancies developing in patients with immunodeficiency diseases
- Lymphoid malignancies mimicking "systemic autoimmune diseases"
- Epithelial malignancies mimicking "systemic autoimmune diseases"

In earlier epidemiologic studies, patients in the latter 2 groups may have had autoimmune paraneoplastic syndromes but were misclassified as "autoimmune disease patients developing malignancies."

Incidence and Types of Malignancies in Patients With Autoimmune Disease

Autoimmune events cause persistent tissue damage. The compensatory repair and regenerative processes in the targeted organs may progress from cellular atypia to dysplasia and neoplasia. Close correlations between mucosal epithelial dysplasia and subsequent colorectal carcinoma have been demonstrated in patients with long-standing autoimmune ulcerative and Crohn's colitis. Studies from the 1950s reported the risks of adenocarcinoma to be 20 to 40 times higher for patients with autoimmune diseases when compared with age-matched controls.[2] More recent surveys of ulcerative colitis patients with long-term clinical and endoscopic follow-ups indicate that 10% to 20% of nonpolyposis colitis patients develop adenocarcinoma; colitis patients with familial polyposis are at much higher risk, with 50% to 90% possibly harboring multifocal and recurrent adenocarcinoma.[10–12] Additional examples of autoimmune injury–related malignancies (**Table 4-1**) are bronchoalveolar adenocarcinomas developing in 5% to 9% of scleroderma patients and thyroid lymphoma being found in 10% of autoimmune thyroiditis patients 2 to 25 years after the onset of autoimmune disease.[13–16,28–30] Approximately 10% of Sjögren's syndrome and rheumatoid arthritis patients develop malignant B-cell or T-cell lymphomas.[17–19]

Incidence and Types of Malignancies in Patients With Immunodeficiency Disease

Immunodeficiency diseases may be congenital or acquired, the former occurring mostly in children and the latter in adults. The various types of immunodeficiency diseases are listed in **Table 4-2**. Congenital immunodeficiency diseases are consequences of different types of genetically predetermined developmental and/or functional defects in cells of the immune system. The deficient cells may be T, B, phagocytic, or granulocytic. Not all congenital immunodeficiency diseases have been associated with increased frequencies of malignancies. Patients with congenital immunoglobulin (Ig) A deficiency, ataxia-telangiectasia, Wiskott-Aldrich syndrome, X-linked agammaglobulinemia, and common variable immunodeficiency (CVI) show definite increased incidences (5% to 11%) of malignancy, usually lymphoma or leukemia.[9,20,21,31,34,35]

Table 4-1. Incidence of Malignancy in Autoimmune and Immunodeficiency Diseases[6,9,13-27]

	Incidence of Malignancy (%)	No. of Possible Patients/ Total No. of Patients
Autoimmune diseases		
Rheumatoid arthritis	10	19/1,294
Systemic lupus erythematosus	< 3	1/36
Sjögren's syndrome	10	46/485
Polymyositis/dermatomyositis (2 studies)	7, 24	9/590, 5/27
Scleroderma	9	20/262
Mixed connective tissue disease	10	4/40
"Unclassified" autoimmune syndromes	23	25/108
Ulcerative colitis	5-30	*
Lymphocytic thyroiditis	10	*
Congenital immunodeficiency diseases		
X-linked agammaglobulinemia	5	*
Ataxia-telangiectasia	9	9/102
Wiskott-Aldrich syndrome	12	36/301
Common variable immunodeficiency	11	11/98
Acquired immunodeficiency diseases		
Bone marrow transplant	Up to 3	54/2,150
HIV infection (AIDS)	3-14	*

**Actual number of patients not given; percentages stated.*

Of additional significance is that concurrent or subsequent gastrointestinal tract adenocarcinomas tend to occur more frequently in patients with CVI, congenital IgA deficiency, and ataxia-telangiectasia.[35] This unique predisposition to gastrointestinal tract adenocarcinoma has prompted more extensive clinical analysis and studies. The additional studies noted more severe gastrointestinal tract lymphoid hyperplasia and recurrent flares of inflammatory bowel disease in the malignancy-prone patient group. Adenocarcinoma is found during the fifth and sixth decades of the patient's life. Defective immune surveillance and malignant degeneration of chronically irritated colonic mucosa have been implicated as the most likely causes of carcinogenesis in these patients.[11,35]

Acquired immunodeficiency diseases occur in bone marrow and various organ allograft recipients treated with antilymphocyte agents, patients with excessive immunoglobulin loss, those with certain chronic viral infections, and individuals with immune paralysis from other causes. The incidence of epithelial and lymphoid malignancies in this group of patients ranges from 3% to 12%. The types of malignancy that develop are diverse, including squamous cell carcinoma, human papillomavirus–related carcinoma, hepatocellular carcinoma, Kaposi's sarcoma, and high-grade B-cell or T-cell lymphomas.[22–24,36] T-cell depletion, defective immune surveillance, and abnormal oncogene activation have all been implicated as contributing factors to the induction of neoplasm in patients with acquired immunodeficiency diseases. Evidence of viral-induced oncogenesis has been noted by several epidemiologic studies with laboratory demonstration of viral DNA in tumor cells.[25,26,37]

Factors Linking Immunodeficiency, Autoimmunity, and Malignancy

Although the immunologic hypoactivity of immunodeficiency diseases seems to be in distinct contrast to the immunologic hyperactivity of autoimmune diseases, certain studies suggest that patients

Table 4-2. Classification of Immunodeficiency Diseases[31–33]

- Congenital Immunodeficiency Diseases
  - B-cell antibody production defects* (50%)
    - X-linked infantile agammaglobulinemia
    - Transient hypogammaglobulinemia
    - X-linked immunodeficiency with hyper-IgM
    - Selective or salivary IgA deficiency
    - Dysgammaglobulinemia with normal or increased immunoglobulins
  - Combined T-cell and B-cell defects (20%)
    - Swiss type agammaglobulinemia
    - Wiskott-Aldrich syndrome (immunodeficiency with thrombocytopenia and eczema)
    - Ataxia-telangiectasia
    - Common variable immunodeficiency
    - Immunodeficiency with thymoma
    - Immunodeficiency with short-limb dwarfism
    - Immunodeficiency with generalized hematopoietic hypoplasia
    - Hyper-IgE syndrome
    - Adenosine deaminase deficiency
  - Phagocytic deficiencies with recurrent deep skin abscesses (18%)
  - T-cell defects (10%)
    - Thymic dysplasia/hypoplasia (DiGeorge syndrome)
    - Episodic lymphopenia with lymphocytotoxin
    - Chronic mucocutaneous candidiasis
    - Nucleoside phosphorylase deficiency with red cell aplasia
  - Hereditary complement component deficiencies (2%)
- Acquired Immunodeficiency Diseases
  - Human immunodeficiency virus or chronic Epstein-Barr virus
  - Bone marrow transplantation
  - Prolonged immunosuppressive therapy
  - Excessive immunoglobulin loss due to nephrotic syndrome or gastrointestinal telangiectasia
  - Systemic autoimmune diseases, including sarcoidosis
  - Lymphoid or epithelial malignancies
  - Nutritional deficiencies: biotin, zinc, selenium (may be associated with hyperalimentation)
  - Uremia or various systemic toxic conditions, including sepsis

**Other defects mimicking antibody deficiency may include intercellular adhesion molecule or cytokine defects (recurrent periodontitis and sepsis).*

with either autoimmune or immunodeficiency disorders who develop malignancies may share certain immunoregulatory and immunogenetic abnormalities. These abnormalities may be (1) T-cell dysfunctions; (2) aberrant major histocompatibility complex (MHC) expressions; and (3) cellular oncogene dysregulation, usually related to chromosome breakage and other structural defects. The carcinogenic potentials of these immunoregulatory and genetic abnormalities are discussed in this section.

T-Cell Dysfunctions

Defective T-cell functions have been implicated in the induction of immunodeficiency, autoimmune, and neoplastic diseases.[6,8,9,37] Defective CD4+ T-cell production of cytokines, such as interleukin-2 (IL-2), causing B-cell maturation failure, has been proposed as the cause of CVI, and treatment with IL-2 improves patients' immune status.[38] Patients with various types of autoimmune diseases have suppressor T- or helper T-cell dysfunctions. Despite excessive B-cell hyperactivity and circulating autoantibodies, these patients have defective cellular and humoral immunity.[4,6] Moreover, 10% to 20% of patients with congenital or acquired immunodeficiency diseases have concurrent autoimmune hemolytic anemia, pernicious anemia, or autoimmune thrombocytopenia.[39–41] B-cell hyperactivity, increased autoantibodies, lupus anticoagulants, and autoimmune-mediated cytopenias are often found in individuals infected with human immunodeficiency virus (HIV) and depleted T-cell counts.[42,43] Thus, T-cell defects and dysfunctions occur in patients with either immunodeficiency or autoimmune diseases, predisposing them to the development of malignancies.

Aberrant Major Histocompatibility Complex Expression

Major histocompatibility complex expressions by cells of the immune-recognition system determine an individual's immunocompetence. Aberrant MHC overexpression can initiate autoimmune tissue destruction, whereas MHC underexpression can lead to defective immune surveillance and unregulated clonal and/or neoplastic cellular proliferation.[37,44] Certain MHC haplotypes are noted more frequently in autoimmune, immunodeficiency, and neoplastic diseases. For example, HLA-DR3 and B8 are associated with rheumatoid arthritis, Sjögren's syndrome, congenital IgA deficiency, aggressive forms of HIV infections, CVI, familial Waldenström's macroglobulinemia, and chronic lymphocytic leukemia.[45–48] The MHC haplotypes shared by patients with autoimmune, immunodeficiency, and neoplastic diseases may be indicators of related underlying genetic susceptibility to aberrant MHC expression and other immunoregulatory defects. In vitro evidence of spurious aberrant MHC class II expression has been demonstrated in tumor cells from malignancies developing in patients with either autoimmune or immunodeficiency diseases.[27,37]

Cellular Oncogene Dysregulation With Chromosome Breakage/Structural Defects

Human cellular oncogenes and proto-oncogenes are recombinants of viral and host DNA sequences incorporated as part of the normal human genome. In healthy states, these cellular oncogenes are "normal functional" genes that help control cell proliferation and differentiation. Examples of functional human cellular oncogenes are c-*myc*, which serves as growth factor to promote cellular proliferation; c-*ras*, which regulates cell cycles by initiating and controlling microtubule and cytoskeletal formation; and *Bcl*-2, which can induce or inhibit apoptosis. These oncogenes are capable of enhancing and regulating each other's replication and functions.[49–52]

Cellular oncogene displacement and dysregulation occur with chromosome breakage or defective structural alterations of chromosomes (ie, translocations and mutations). Such oncogene dysregulations can lead to abnormal activation, causing excessive genome multiplication. These displaced, dysregulated, and abnormally activated oncogenes can cause immunologic disarray and neoplastic transformation of the affected cells. The following are examples of oncogene dysregulation observed in (or associated with) patients with autoimmune, neoplastic, or immunodeficiency diseases:

- Increased *Bcl*-2 and c-*ras* oncogene mRNAs were detected in fibroblastoid cells of rheumatoid synovia; increased expression of c-*myc* and c-*ras* oncogenes were detected in lymphocytes of patients with systemic lupus erythematosus (SLE) and other autoimmune diseases.[51–53]
- Abnormal c-*myc* expression has been implicated in the induction of lung carcinomas.[54]
- c-*myc* dysregulation has been postulated as the triggering factor that converts benign indolent monoclonal gammopathies to aggressive myelomas.[55]
- c-*myc* and c-*ras* dysregulation have been observed in malignancies developing in patients with HIV-related immunodeficiency diseases.[56,57]
- Displacements of the c-*myc* oncogene to the proximity of the immunoglobulin heavy chain were found.
- Chromosome breakage point translocation t(14;8)(q24;q32) occurs in both HIV-related and sporadic Burkitt's lymphoblastic lymphomas.[58]
- Displacement of the *Bcl*-2 oncogene to the proximity of the immunoglobulin heavy chain were found; chromosome breakage point translocation t(14;18)(q32;q21) is identified in up to 89% of follicular center B-cell malignant lymphomas.[59,60]
- TCL1 oncogene activation and chromosome breakage translocations at points t(14;14)(q11;q32) and t(7;14)(q35;q32) are noted in preleukemic T cells from the peripheral blood of patients with ataxia-telangiectasia.[61]
- Nijmegen breakage syndrome, a variant of ataxia-telangiectasia congenital immunodeficiency disease, is characterized by

chromosome fragility, hypersensitivity to radiographs, and multiple breakages on chromosomes 7 and 14, with increased frequency of translocations involving 7q12, 7q35, 14q12, and 14q32 break points.[62]

In addition to the common factors linking patients with autoimmune, immunodeficiency, and neoplastic diseases (defective T-cell immune surveillance, aberrant MHC expression, and cellular oncogene dysregulation), environmental factors, such as repeated exposure to oncogenic viruses, physical and chemical carcinogens, irradiation, and biologic toxins, can trigger or enhance underlying immunoregulatory and immunogenetic susceptibilities.

Clinical and Laboratory Guidelines for Evaluating Immunodeficiency Disorders

In contrast to autoimmune diseases in which evidence of circulating autoantibodies and immune tissue injury are present at the time of presentation, the clinical warning signs of immunodeficiency disorders are more subtle and may even be "absent." Moreover, immunodeficient patients may present with autoimmune or "rheumatic" disease symptoms. For example, patients with IgA or complement deficiency may have clinical signs of SLE, Sjögren's syndrome, polymyositis, or vasculitis. Patients with acquired immunodeficiency syndrome and coinfected with Epstein-Barr virus (EBV) and cytomegalovirus may have generalized lymphadenopathy; lymphocytosis; hypergammaglobulinemia with multiple types of circulating autoantibodies, including lupus anticoagulants; vasculitis; and myositis. Patients with phagocytic and/or CD8+ T-cell disorders may present with clinical findings of psoriasis, arthritis, uveitis, urethritis, or spondyloarthropathy syndromes.[63]

Congenital immunodeficiency diseases are infrequent, the incidence being approximately 1 in 10,000. Acquired immunodeficiency diseases are more common and usually associated with poor nutrition (diets lacking zinc, biotin, and/or selenium), malabsorption, excessive renal or gastrointestinal immunoglobulin loss, and certain chronic viral infections. Thorough review of the patient's environmental, drug, nutritional, and family histories should be an integral part of the assessment. The following clinical and laboratory guidelines[31–33,63,64] can be helpful for patient evaluation.

Clinical Warning Signs

These signs should suggest the presence of immunodeficiency states and diseases (**Table 4-3**):

- T-cell defects should be suspected when patients develop severe systemic illness following common viral infection or vaccines, persistent oral *Candida* lasting 6 months despite treatment, mucocutaneous candidiasis with granulomatous skin lesions, or graft-versus-host disease after blood transfusions.
- B-cell–antibody production defects should be suspected when patients have recurrent pyogenic infection at multiple sites, frequent and persistent diarrhea, or early childhood "inflammatory bowel disease" symptoms.
- Combined T-cell and B-cell defects should be suspected when patients have unexplained anemia or thrombocytopenia, telangiectasia of the sclera or ear, persistent/recurrent eczema or skin infections, and other signs already listed.
- Deficiencies of leukocyte enzyme, complement components, and cytokines may mimic B-cell defects. Patients with these deficiencies may have recurrent periodontitis, deep subcutis abscesses, chronic osteomyelitis, and septic episodes. Myeloperoxidase defects show very few symptoms.

Initial Laboratory Screening Test Panel

The initial screening tests should include (1) complete blood cell count with differential; (2) serum protein electrophoresis and immunoglobulins; (3) HIV and EBV profiles, if indicated by the patient's history; (4) skin tests with at least 3 different antigens; and (5) screens for complements C3, C4, and CH50. Over 95% of suspected immunodeficiency cases can be ruled out by this test panel (**Table 4-4**). However, it should be emphasized that "normal values" at a certain point for the patient's age do not absolutely exclude certain immunodeficiency diseases. Detection of B-cell and/or antibody production defects with late disease onset may require repeated screening.

Disease-Specific Laboratory Test Panel

If the results from the initial screening tests and family/clinical history review are compatible or strongly suggestive of immunodeficiency, further

Table 4-3. Clinical Warning Signs of Immunodeficiency Diseases[31–33,63,64]

B-cell–antibody production defects	Recurrent pyogenic infection at multiple sites Recurrent/persistent diarrhea or early onset "childhood" inflammatory bowel disease (Deep skin abscesses or chronic osteomyelitis may be signs of primary leukocyte defect.) (Recurrent neisserial infection may be signs of congenital complement deficiency.)
T-cell defects	Severe systemic illness produced by common viral infection or vaccine Anergy by skin test Persistent oral *Candida* lasting 6 months despite treatment Mucocutaneous candidiasis with granulomatous skin lesions Graft-versus-host disease after blood transfusion
T-cell and B-cell defects	Absent HLA-associated immune response (cannot be tissue typed) Unexplained anemia or thrombocytopenia Telangiectasia of the sclera or ear Skin lesions (eczema or infections) Other signs of T-cell and B-cell defects
Adult immunodeficiency diseases with rheumatic warning signs	
IgA or complement deficiency	Systemic autoimmune disease symptoms such as SLE, Sjögren's syndrome, polymyositis, and vasculitis Recurrent neisserial infections with sepsis
HIV coinfection with EBV and CMV	Generalized lymphadenopathy Hypergammaglobulinemia B-cell hyperactivity Anticardiolipin autoantibodies Diffuse infiltrative lymphocytosis syndrome Dysregulated cytokine production/activity Vasculitis, polymyositis
Macrophage/CD8 T-cell disorders	Psoriatic arthritis Reiter's disease Spondyloarthropathy syndromes
Direct CD4 T-cell depletion	Osteomyelitis Pyomyositis Infectious arthritis

Abbreviations: HLA = human leukocyte antigen; IgA = immunoglobulin A; SLE = systemic lupus erythematosus; HIV = human immunodeficiency virus; EBV = Epstein-Barr virus; CMV = cytomegalovirus.

disease-specific testing may be indicated (see Table 4-4). These additional tests may include

- Immunoglobulin isotypes and/or IgG subclasses
- Flow cytometry for T-cell and B-cell immunophenotyping
- Cell cycle/DNA analysis of T-cell and B-cell proliferative responses
- Immunoassay or bioassay for cytokines and leukocyte adhesion molecules
- Bioassays for neutrophil chemotaxis, microbicidal activity, and superoxide production
- Functional assays for complement activation
- Measurement of adenosine deaminase or nucleoside phosphorylase activity
- In situ hybridization or reverse transcriptase polymerase chain reaction for detection of genetic (chromosome) defect markers

It cannot be overemphasized that timely, accurate, and effective communications among the pathologist, technologist, and clinician are of the utmost importance in patient evaluation and management.

Table 4-4. Laboratory Tests to Evaluate Immunodeficiency[31–33,63,64]

Initial screening test panel	Complete blood cell count with differential Serum protein and immunoglobulins HIV and EBV profiles, if indicated by history Skin tests with at least 3 different antigens Complement C3, C4, and CH50 tests
Disease-specific test panel (if indicated by history and results of initial screening tests)	Immunoglobulin isotypes and/or IgG subclasses (ELISA) T-cell and B-cell immunophenotyping (flow cytometry) T-cell and B-cell proliferative responses (cell cycle/DNA analysis) Cytokine profile of T cells and macrophage/monocytes (immunoassay or bioassay) Leukocyte adhesion molecule profile (ELISA) Neutrophil chemotaxis, microbicidal activity, superoxide production (bioassays) Complement activation complex and complement functional assays Enzyme assays: adenosine deaminase or nucleoside phosphorylase Genetic defect markers (in situ hybridization or RT-PCR)

Abbreviations: HIV = human immunodeficiency virus; EBV = Epstein-Barr virus; ELISA = enzyme-linked immunosorbent assay; RT-PCR = reverse transcriptase polymerase chain reaction.

Guidelines for Recognizing Malignancies That Mimic Autoimmune Diseases

Autoimmune Diseases Mimicked by Lymphoid Malignancies

Patients with lymphoproliferative disorders often present with various types of autoimmune disease symptoms, depending on the titers and antigenic specificities of the associated monoclonal autoantibodies and the tissue sites of lymphoid infiltration.[65–67] The most frequent symptoms are those mimicking rheumatoid arthritis, vasculitis, and SLE.

Constant bone and arthritic pain that worsen at night may be signs of multiple myeloma. Myelomas often involve the vertebrae, and 48% of patients have compression fractures. Patients with Waldenström's macroglobulinemia often have multilocular cyst–like bone lesions on radiograph. Plasma cell dyscrasia with amyloidosis also can mimic Sjögren's syndrome, and affected patients may have joint stiffness, polymyalgia, and carpal tunnel or Raynaud's-type syndromes. Synovial biopsies may show monotonous lymphoid infiltrates or amyloid deposits. Idiopathic fasciitis or amyloidosis also can be the presenting clinical symptoms of adult T-cell malignant lymphoma, Hodgkin's disease, and (less likely) carcinoma.[67,68]

Urticarial vasculitis with osteosclerotic bone lesions can be symptoms of IgM myeloma; other lesions associated with IgM myelomas include palpable purpura, distal limb necrosis, Raynaud's syndrome, and membranous glomerulonephritis.[66–69] Granulomatous angiitis of the central nervous system or "mass effect" may be presenting symptoms of T-cell lymphomas. Giant cell arteritis and polymyalgia rheumatica may be presenting symptoms of B-cell lymphomas.[66,67]

Systemic lupus erythematosus symptoms occur in patients with myeloma or lymphoma when their clinical courses are complicated by fever, serositis with effusions, and microangiopathic glomerulonephritis. These patients may have either low-titer nonspecific antinuclear antibodies (ANAs) or antigen-specific monoclonal autoantibodies, such as anti-DNA, anti-Sm, or anti-Sjögren's syndrome A/Ro.[6,68] Monoclonal gammopathies developing in patients with SLE, rheumatoid arthritis, or Sjögren's syndrome can be warning signs of incipient malignant B-cell lymphoma.[16,66,67,70]

Autoimmune Diseases Mimicked by Epithelial Malignancies

Patients with occult carcinomas may present with neuromyopathic, rheumatoid-type arthritic, vasculitic, or dermatopathic pemphigoid symptoms.

These are manifestations of "autoimmune paraneoplastic syndromes," defined as distinct disease entities in which the clinical symptoms involve other organs separate from the sites of neoplasm growth. Various rheumatic disease–like autoimmune paraneoplastic syndromes have been reported in patients with carcinomas of the lung (27%), gynecologic and/or müllerian type (14%), prostate (12%), colon (10%), and breast (7%).[71–73]

Immune mechanisms apparently mediate many of these autoimmune paraneoplastic syndromes, because patients with carcinomas are exposed to continuous antigenemia originating from tumor and surrounding damaged host tissue.[71,74] Numerous studies have provided evidence of "shared-antigenic epitope" between tumor and host tissue as the cause of these autoimmune responses. Some of these progress to "pathogenic autoimmunity" with consequent immune complex tissue damage and clinical manifestations of autoimmune rheumatic diseases. The following are examples of the various types of autoimmune paraneoplastic syndromes:

- Polymyositis symptoms can occur in patients with carcinomas of the lung, prostate, colon, ovary, and vagina. Circulating autoantibodies that cross-react with tumor antigen and "normal" muscle cells can be detected in some but not all patients.[75–77]
- Rheumatoid-type arthritis may be the presenting symptom in patients with carcinomas of the lung, breast, prostate, kidney, or head and neck.[78–82]
- Pemphigoid skin lesions associated with autoantibodies to epidermal intercellular and basement membrane are found in patients with either lymphoma or carcinoma.[83,84]

Also of clinical significance are antinucleolar and anticentromere autoantibodies found in patients with malignancies but without clinical autoimmune disease or autoimmune paraneoplastic syndromes. Antinucleolar autoantibodies have been detected in 31% of patients with hepatocellular carcinoma and 13% of cirrhotic patients with chronic liver disease. These autoantibodies show immunologic specificity for nucleolar antigens NOR-90 and fibrillarin, which are essential proteins for ribosomal synthesis.[85]

Anticentromere autoantibodies can be found in up to 30% of patients with carcinoma of the breast, lung, gastrointestinal tract, ovary, or prostate. These autoantibodies show immunologic specificity for mitotic cell cycle–dependent centromere proteins p33od/CENP-F, which are not detected in sera from patients with scleroderma.[86]

Antinuclear autoantibodies with nucleolar and/or cytoplasmic antigenic specificities can be detected in over 70% of patients with melanomas. At present, there is no obvious explanation for these "clinically silent" ANAs. They appear to be produced in response to specific intranuclear cell cycle antigens of proliferating cells.[85,87]

Summary

Review of past and current clinical studies confirms a definite increased risk of malignancy in patients with autoimmune and immunodeficiency diseases. Malignancies develop in 3% to 10% of patients with autoimmune diseases and 5% to 12% of patients with certain congenital and acquired immunodeficiency diseases, compared with less than 0.4% in aged-matched controls without immunologic diseases (see Table 4-1). T-cell dysfunction, aberrant MHC expression, and cellular oncogene dysregulation associated with chromosome breakages and/or mutations have been demonstrated in a significant number of patients. These are the most likely common factors linking immunodeficiency, autoimmunity, and malignancy. Various environmental (biologic and chemical) agents can trigger, promote, and accelerate the growth of these tumors. The interrelationships of immunodeficiency, autoimmunity, and malignancy are summarized in **Table 4-5**.

Furthermore, up to 27% of patients with lymphoid or epithelial malignancies may have rheumatic-type autoimmune paraneoplastic syndromes (**Table 4-6**). When evaluating patients with clinical symptoms of immunologic diseases, the following points are worth noting:

- Idiopathic myositis symptoms may be signs of occult lung, colon, or prostate carcinoma.
- Carpal tunnel syndrome, fasciitis, and or amyloidosis may be presenting symptoms of plasma cell malignancies, lymphoma, and (less likely) carcinoma.
- Raynaud's-type ischemia, distal limb necrosis, or vasculitis can be warning signs of either occult malignant lymphoma or carcinoma.
- Monoclonal gammopathies developing in patients with SLE, rheumatoid arthritis, or Sjögren's syndrome are suggestive of incipient or occult malignant lymphoma.

Table 4-5. Interrelationship of Immunodeficiency, Autoimmunity, and Malignancy[6,8,9,16,17,25,27,37,39,48–62,88]

Common immunologic and genetic factors	Defective T-cell immune surveillance Aberrant MHC expression Cellular oncogene dysregulation associated with chromosome translocation/mutations
Environmental agents exacerbating immunologic and genetic defects	Persistent or recurrent viral infections Prolonged exposure to biologic or chemical cytotoxins Irradiation
Systemic autoimmune disease symptoms	May be the clinical manifestation in 23% of patients with malignancies
Autoimmune paraneoplastic syndromes	With neuromyopathic, arthritic, vasculitic, or pemphigoid symptoms, may occur in up to 27% of patients with carcinomas. Associated autoantibodies are directed against shared antigenic epitopes of the patient's tumor cells and normal cells. One third of patients may respond to treatment with remissions.

Abbreviation: MHC = major histocompatibility complex.

Table 4-6. Incidence of Autoimmune Paraneoplastic Symptoms in Various Carcinomas[6,68-84, 88-90]

Site of Carcinoma	No. of Patients With Autoimmune Symptoms/ Total No. of Patients	Percentage
Lung	23/84	27.4
Prostate	7/56	12.5
Colon	11/105	10.5
Uterus	3/36	8.3
Breast	18/250	7.2
Ovary	2/29	6.9

- Unclassified autoimmune SLE or rheumatoid arthritis symptoms with low-titer nonspecific ANAs may be associated with carcinomas of the lung, breast, or gastrointestinal tract.
- Immune complex–mediated membranous glomerulopathy may be a presenting symptom of occult lymphoma or carcinoma.

Finally, although cancer patients with autoimmune paraneoplastic syndromes were previously associated with poor prognoses, more recent studies have shown that with early diagnosis and appropriate therapy, 30% to 50% of these patients respond to treatment with remissions of both tumor and autoimmune symptoms.[6,7] Thus, knowledge and alertness of the plethora of autoimmune, immunodeficiency, and paraneoplastic disease manifestations that can occur in patients harboring malignant neoplasms allow timely institution of antitumor therapy that can improve their quality of life and may even save their lives.

References

1. Lindsay S, Dailey ME, Friedlander J, et al. Chronic thyroiditis: A clinical and pathological study of 354 patients. *J Clin Endocrinol Metab.* 1952;12:1578–1586.
2. Weckesser EC, Chinn AB. Carcinoma of the colon complicating chronic ulcerative colitis. *JAMA.* 1953;152:905–908.
3. Hitchcock CR, Maclean LD, Sullivan WA. The secretory and clinical aspect of achlorhydria and gastric atrophy as precursors of gastric cancer. *J Natl Cancer Inst.* 1957;18:795–799.

4. Nakamura RM. Autoimmunity, unresponsiveness, and interrelationships: Human cancer and autoimmunity. In: Nakamura RM, ed. *Immunopathology: Clinical Laboratory Concepts and Methods*. Boston, MA: Little, Brown and Co; 1974:201–224.
5. Oleinick A. Leukemia or lymphoma occurring subsequent to an autoimmune disease. *Blood*. 1967;29:144–153.
6. McCarty GA. Autoimmunity and malignancy. *Med Clin North Am*. 1985;69:599–615.
7. Sela O, Shoenfeld Y. Cancer in autoimmune diseases. *Semin Arthritis Rheum*. 1988;18:77–87.
8. Fudenburg HH. Genetically determined immune deficiency as the predisposing cause of "autoimmunity" and lymphoid neoplasia. *Am J Med*. 1971;51:295–298.
9. Gatti RA, Good RA. Occurrence of malignancy in immunodeficiency diseases: A literature review. *Cancer*. 1971:28:89–94.
10. Collins RH Jr, Feldman M, Fordtran JS. Colon cancer, dysplasia, and surveillance in patients with ulcerative colitis. *N Engl J Med*. 1987;316:1654–1658.
11. Riddell RH, Goldman H, Ransohoff DF, et al. Dysplasia in inflammatory bowel disease: Standardized classification with provisional applications. *Hum Pathol*. 1983;11:931–968.
12. Haggitt RC, Reid BJ. Hereditary gastrointestinal polyposis syndromes. *Am J Surg Pathol*. 1986;10:871–887.
13. Peters-Golden M, Wise RA, Hochberg M, et al. Incidence of lung cancer in systemic sclerosis. *J Rheumatol*. 1985;12:113–117.
14. Holm LE, Blomgren H, Lowhagen T. Cancer risk in patients with chronic lymphocytic thyroiditis. *N Engl J Med*. 1985;312:601–604.
15. Hamburger JL, Miller JM, Kini SR. Lymphoma of the thyroid. *Ann Intern Med*. 1983;99:685–693.
16. Compagno J, Oertel JE. Malignant lymphoma and other lymphoproliferative disorders of the thyroid gland. A clinicopathologic study of 245 cases. *Am J Clin Pathol*. 1980;74:1–11.
17. Symmons DPM, Ahern M, Bacon PA, et al. Lymphoproliferative malignancy in rheumatoid arthritis: A study of 20 cases. *Ann Rheum Dis*. 1984;43:132–135.
18. Isenberg DA, Griffith MH, Rusis M, et al. T cell lymphoma in a patient with longstanding rheumatoid arthritis and Sjögren's syndrome. *Arthritis Rheum*. 1987;30:115–117.
19. Anaya JM, McGuff HS, Banks PM, et al. Clinicopathological factors relating malignant lymphoma with Sjögren's syndrome. *Semin Arthritis Rheum*. 1996;25:337–346.
20. Spector BD, Perry GS, Kersey JH. Genetically determined immunodeficiency diseases and malignancy. *Clin Immunol Immunopathol*. 1978;11:12–29.
21. Rosenblatt HM, Shearer WT. Immune deficiency and cancer. In: Finegold M, Bennington JL, eds. *Pathology of Neoplasia in Children and Adolescents*. Philadelphia, PA: WB Saunders Co; 1986:31–45.
22. Cunningham-Rundles C, Siegel FP, Cunningham-Rundles S, et al. Incidence of cancer in 98 patients with common varied immunodeficiency. *J Clin Immunol*. 1987;7:294–299.
23. Penn I. Tumor incidence in human allograft recipients. *Transplant Proc*. 1979;11:1047–1051.
24. Bhatia B, Ramsay NK, Steinbuch M, et al. Malignant neoplasm following bone marrow transplantation. *Blood*. 1996;87:3633–3639.
25. Penn I. Depressed immunity and the development of cancer. *Cancer Detect Prev*. 1994;18:241–252.
26. Patil P, Elem B, Zumla A. Pattern of adult malignancies in Zambia (1980–1989) in light of the HIV epidemic. *J Trop Med Hyg*. 1995;98:281–283.
27. Kinlen LJ. Malignancy in autoimmune diseases. *J Autoimmun*. 1992;5(suppl A):363–371.
28. Haddad R, Massaro D. Idiopathic diffuse interstitial fibrosis, atypical epithelial proliferation, and lung cancer. *Am J Med*. 1968;45:211–219.
29. Jones AW. Alveolar cell carcinoma occurring in idiopathic interstitial pulmonary fibrosis. *Br J Dis Chest*. 1970;64:78–84.
30. Fraire AE, Greenberg SD. Carcinoma and diffuse interstitial fibrosis of lung. *Cancer*. 1973;31:1078–1086.
31. Hong Richard. Problems in host defense. In: Henry JB, ed. *Clinical Diagnosis and Management by Laboratory Methods*. 19th ed. Philadelphia, PA: WB Saunders Co; 1996:1003–1012.
32. Pacheco SE, Shearer WT. Laboratory aspects of immunology. *Pediatr Clin North Am*. 1994;4:623–655.
33. Paxton H, Cunningham-Rundles S, O'Gorman MRG. Laboratory evaluation of the cellular immune system. In: Henry JB, ed. *Clinical Diagnosis and Management by Laboratory Methods*. 19th ed. Philadelphia, PA: WB Saunders Co; 1996:877–912.
34. Nakamura RM. The immune system and immune deficiency diseases. In: Nakamura RM, ed. *Immunopathology: Clinical Laboratory Concepts and Methods*. Boston, MA: Little, Brown and Co; 1974:3–42.
35. Swift M, Sholman L, Perry M, et al. Malignant neoplasm in the families of patients with ataxia-telangiectasia. *Cancer Res*. 1976;36:209–215.
36. Hermaszewski RA, Webster ADB. Primary hypogammaglobulinemia: A survey of clinical manifestations and complications. *Q J Med*. 1993;86:31–42.
37. Guardiola J, Maffei A. Control of MHC class II gene expression in autoimmune, infectious, and neoplastic diseases. *Crit Rev Immunol*. 1993;13:247–268.

38. Cunningham-Rundles C, Mayer L, Sapira E, et al. Restoration of Ig secretion in vitro in CVI by in vivo treatment with polyethylene glycol-conjugated human recombinant IL2. *Clin Immunol Immunopathol*. 1992;64:46–56.

39. Friedman JM, Fialkow PJ, Davis SD, et al. Autoimmunity in the relatives of patients with immunodeficiency diseases. *Clin Exp Immunol*. 1977;28:375–388.

40. Stephen RS, Gershwin EM. The association and relationships of congenital immunodeficient states and autoimmune phenomena. *Semin Arthritis Rheum*. 1979;9:98–123.

41. Liblau RS, Bach JF. Selective IgA deficiency and autoimmunity. *Int Arch Allergy Immunol*. 1992;99:16–27.

42. Morris L, Distenfield A, Amorosi E, et al. Autoimmune thrombocytopenia purpura in homosexual men. *Ann Intern Med*. 1982;96:714–717.

43. Bloom EJ, Abrams DI. Lupus anticoagulants in the acquired immunodeficiency syndrome. *JAMA*. 1986;256:491–493.

44. Redondo M, Concha A, Oldiviela R, et al. Expression of HLA class I and II antigens in bronchogenic carcinoma: Its relationship to cellular DNA content and clinical pathological parameters. *Cancer Res*. 1991;51:4948–4954.

45. Nepom GT, Erlich H. MHC class II molecules and autoimmunity. *Annu Rev Immunol*. 1991;9:493.

46. Blattner WA, Garber JE, Mann DL, et al. Waldenström's macroglobulinemia and autoimmune disease in a family. *Ann Intern Med*. 1980;93:830–834.

47. Lockard Conley C, Misiti J, Laster AJ. Genetic factors predisposing to CLL and to autoimmune disease. *Medicine*. 1980;59:323–334.

48. Schaffer FM, Palermos J, Zhu ZB, et al. Individuals with IgA deficiency and common varied deficiency share polymorphisms of MHC class III genes. *Proc Natl Acad Sci U S A*. 1989;86:8015–8019.

49. Bos JL. The *ras* gene family and human carcinogenesis. *Mutation Res*. 1988;195:255–271.

50. Hunter T. Cooperation between oncogenes. *Cell*. 1991;66:249–270.

51. Muller-Ladner U, Kriegsmann J, Gay RE, et al. Oncogenes in rheumatoid arthritis. *Rheum Dis Clin North Am*. 1995;21:675–690.

52. Boumpas DT, Tsokus GC, Mann DL, et al. Increased proto-oncogene expression in peripheral blood lymphocytes from patients with SLE and other autoimmune diseases. *Arthritis Rheum*. 1986;29:755–760.

53. Mountz JD, Steinberg AD, Klinman DM, et al. Autoimmunity and increased C-*myc* transcription. *Science*. 1984;226:1087–1089.

54. Gazdar AF. The molecular and cellular basis of lung cancer. *Anticancer Res*. 1994;4:261–267.

55. Lust JA. Roles of cytokines in the pathogenesis of monoclonal gammopathies. *Mayo Clin Proc*. 1994;69:691–704.

56. Levine AM. Epidemiology, clinical characteristics and management of AIDS-related lymphoma. *Hematol Oncol Clin North Am*. 1991;5:331–342.

57. Gaidano G, Dalla-Favera R. Biologic aspects of HIV-related lymphoma. *Curr Opin Oncol*. 1992;4:900–906.

58. Croce CM. Molecular biology of lymphomas. *Semin Oncol*. 1993;20(suppl 5):31–46.

59. Weisenburger DD, Chan WC. Lymphomas of follicles: Mantle cell and follicular center cell lymphomas. *Am J Clin Pathol*. 1993;99:409–420.

60. Fit K, Changati RS. Chromosomal aberrations in non-Hodgkin's lymphomas: Biologic and clinical correlations. *Hematol Oncol Clin North Am*. 1991;5:853–869.

61. Narducci MG, Virgilio L, Isobe M, et al. TCL1 oncogene activation in preleukemic T cells from a case of ataxia-telangiectasia. *Blood*. 1995;86:2358–2364.

62. Weemaes CM, Smeets DF, Horstink M, et al. Variants of Nijmegen breakage point syndrome and ataxia-telangiectasia. *Immunodeficiency*. 1993;4:109–111.

63. Silviu I. Adult immunodeficiency and rheumatic disease. *Rheum Dis Clin North Am*. 1996;22:53–73.

64. Fleisher TA. Evaluation of the potentially immunodeficient patients. *Adv Intern Med*. 1996;41:1–30.

65. Hamblin TJ, Oscier DJ, Young BJ. Autoimmunity in chronic lymphocytic leukemia. *J Clin Pathol*. 1986;39:713–716.

66. Duhrsen U, Augener W, Zwingers T, et al. Spectrum and frequency of autoimmune derangements in lymphoproliferative disorders. Analysis of 637 cases and comparison with myeloproliferative diseases. *Br J Haematol*. 1987;67:235–239.

67. Duna GF, Cash JM. Rheumatic manifestations of dysproteinemias and lymphoproliferative disorders. *Rheum Dis Clin North Am*. 1996;22:39–51.

68. DeCross AJ, Sahasrabudhe DM. Paraneoplastic Raynaud's phenomenon. *Am J Med*. 1992;92:570–572.

69. Greer JM, Longley S, Edwards NL, et al. Vasculitis associated with malignancy: Experience with 13 patients and literature review. *Medicine*. 1988;76:222–230.

70. Chan LS, Hanson CA, Cooper KD. Concurrent eosinophilic fasciitis and cutaneous T-cell lymphoma. *Arch Dermatol*. 1991;127:862–865.

71. Pfingsgraff J, Buckingham RB, Killian PJ, et al. Palmar fasciitis and arthritis with malignant neoplasms: A paraneoplastic syndrome. *Semin Arthritis Rheum*. 1986;16:118–125.

72. Naschitz JE, Yeshurun D, Abrahamson J. Arterial occlusive disease in occult cancer. *Am Heart J*. 1992;124:738–745.

73. Naschitz JE, Yeshurun D, Zuckerman E, et al. Cancer-associated fasciitis and panniculitis. *Cancer*. 1994;73: 231–235.

74. Norris SH. Paraneoplastic glomerulopathies. *Semin Nephrol*. 1993;13:258–272.

75. Callen JP. Myositis and malignancy. *Curr Opin Rheumatol*. 1994;6:590–594.

76. Hochberg MC, Feldman D, Stevens MB. Adult onset polymyositis/dermatomyositis: An analysis of clinical and laboratory features and survival in 76 patients with a review of the literature. *Semin Arthritis Rheum*. 1986;15:168–178.

77. Ueyama H, Kumamoto T, Araki S. Circulating autoantibody to muscle protein in a patient with paraneoplastic myositis and colon cancer. *Eur Neurol*. 1992;32:281–284.

78. Shenberger KN, Schned AR, Taylor TH. Rheumatoid disease and bronchogenic carcinoma: Case report and review of literature. *J Rheumatol*. 1984;11:226–228.

79. Simon RD, Ford LE. Rheumatoid-like arthritis associated with colon carcinoma. *Arch Intern Med*. 1980;140:698–700.

80. Schattner A, Shani A, Talpaz M, et al. Rheumatoid factor in the sera of patients with gastrointestinal carcinoma. *Cancer*. 1983;52:2156–2161.

81. Susal C, Maier H, Lorenz K, et al. Association of IgA-anti-Fab autoantibodies with disease stage in head-and neck cancer. *Int J Cancer*. 1994;57:47–50.

82. Caldwell DS. Carcinoma polyarthritis: Manifestation and differential diagnosis. *Med Grand Rounds*. 1982;1:378–385.

83. Moioka S, Sakuma M, Ogawa H. The incidence of internal malignancies in autoimmune blistering diseases: Pemphigus and bullous pemphigoid in Japan. *Dermatology*. 1994;189(suppl 1):82–84.

84. Helm TN, Camisa C, Valenzuela R, et al. Paraneoplastic pemphigus: A distinct autoimmune vesiculobullous disorder associated with neoplasm. *Oral Surg Oral Med Oral Pathol*. 1993;75:209–213.

85. Haruhiko I, Ochs RL, Kiyosawa K, et al. Nucleolar antigens and autoantibodies in hepatocellular carcinoma and other malignancies. *Am J Pathol*. 1992;140:859–870.

86. Casiano CA, Humbel RL, Peebles C, et al. Autoimmunity to the cell cycle-dependent centromere protein p33od/CENP-F in disorders associated with cell proliferation. *J Autoimmun*. 1995;8:575–586.

87. Thomas PJ, Kaur JS, Aitcheson CT, et al. Antinuclear, antinucleolar, and anticytoplasmic antibodies in patients with malignant melanoma. *Cancer Res*. 1983;43:1372–1380.

88. Naschitz JE, Yeshurun D, Rosner I. Rheumatic manifestations of occult cancer. *Cancer*. 1995;75:2954–2958.

89. Cupps TR, Fauci AS. Neoplasm and systemic vasculitis: A case report. *Arthritis Rheum*. 1982;25:475–477.

90. Kelly C, Baird G, Foster H, et al. Prognostic significance of paraproteinemia in rheumatoid arthritis. *Ann Rheum Dis*. 1991;50:290–294.

CHAPTER 5

Cryoglobulins, Immune Complexes, and Autoimmune Diseases

David F. Keren, MD

Twenty years ago, a plethora of assays was developed to detect circulating immune complexes. Many studies employing these assays to investigate a wide variety of conditions, autoimmune diseases prominent among them, were published at that time. Unfortunately, the assays were not useful for diagnosing any particular condition, were not the most useful method available for estimating prognosis, and were not the best way to follow patients with autoimmune disease.[1]

The presence of circulating immune complexes does not indicate that an autoimmune disease is present. Immune complexes may be found in patients with infections (minor or catastrophic), neoplasms, or autoimmune disease. Circulating immune complex assays record part of the physiologic process for removal of antigens from the body. As such, they are a snapshot of a complex, dynamic process. Obvious clinical relevance is found only in the direct demonstration of immune complexes deposited in tissues, such as in renal or skin biopsies.[1]

Therefore, for the past decade, this author has recommended that assays for circulating immune complexes not be performed on patients. These assays may be useful in large epidemiologic studies to determine trends, and specific assays for antigens in the complexes may be useful in research projects. However, they are not practical for following individual patients and are not recommended for routine patient care.

Circulating Immune Complexes

A MEDLINE review of articles with "circulating immune complexes" in the title indicates a dramatic decline in the number of papers published on the topic since the early 1980s, when these assays were at the height of their popularity (**Figure 5-1**). More recent publications concerning immune complex assays have included research papers that explore the specificity of the antibody or antigens in the complexes and the variety of techniques to detect them rather than their mere presence.[2–9] Although these assays have provided interesting biologic information about the diseases studied, they are not recommended for use in following individual patients. Information from epidemiological studies on circulating immune complexes may provide useful information for better performing some important routine testing. For instance, a recent report noted that hepatitis B surface antigen (HBsAg) may be bound to circulating immune complexes in the serum of patients who are infected with the human immunodeficiency virus (HIV).[8] To better detect the HbsAg in the sera from those patients, an acid dissociation step was needed. However, there was no need to perform the older general circulating immune complex assays for clinical purposes. With very limited resources and the availability of key assays of widely accepted prognostic significance, such as determining the HIV RNA viral load required for appropriate care of these patients, the potential benefits of research-related use of the circulating immune complex assay must be distinguished from its lack of a clinical use.

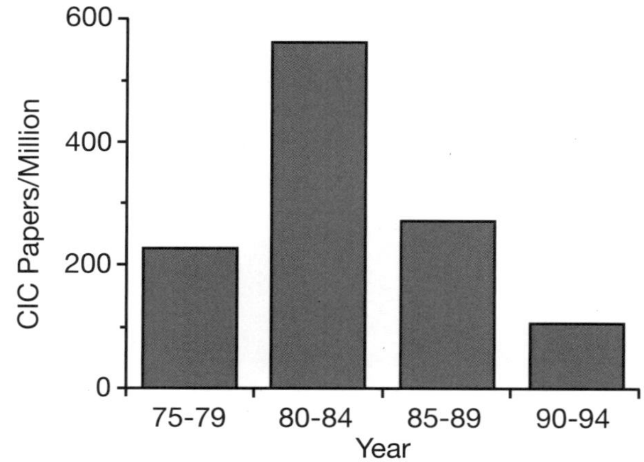

Figure 5-1. Number of papers containing the phrase "circulating immune complexes" (CIC) in the title or as key words for the indicated time periods.

However, one form of circulating immune complex is routinely assayed for patient care. Cryoglobulins are clinically important and unique molecules that must be investigated in a timely manner for the well-being of the patient. This chapter reviews the current classification of cryoglobulins, the clinical indications that should motivate a search for their presence, and the methods for detection and characterization of these molecules.

Cryoglobulin Evaluation

Definition of Cryoglobulins

Cryoglobulins are molecules that aggregate and precipitate at temperatures below 37°C. This phenomenon may occur in vivo or in vitro. Cryoglobulins are extremely heterogeneous molecules that have been classified into 3 biochemical types. Yet within each of the 3 types, there is considerable heterogeneity.

Because of this heterogeneity, the clinical presentation, detection, and characterization of patients with cryoglobulins is problematic and subjective. Although cryoglobulins aggregate and precipitate at less than 37°C, they can be difficult to detect because their precipitation may depend on assay conditions such as collection and transportation methods, ionic strength, pH, concentration of the cryoprecipitating immunoglobulin, and temperature.[10–14] Cryoglobulins are also heterogeneous with regard to the temperature at which they precipitate. Typically, large amounts of cryoglobulin create more problems clinically than do small amounts; however, quantity is not the only important factor. Those cryoglobulins that precipitate at temperatures above 25°C are uncommon, but may be particularly hazardous.[15] Because the temperature in the periphery of the body is lower than that at the center, and because vascular circulation is typically slower in the legs than in the arms, cryoglobulins often form first in the lower legs. When the cryoglobulin precipitates in blood vessels near the skin, they initiate a local vasculitis with complement activation, and when they pass through the circulation to the remainder of the body, neurologic and renal involvement may be seen.[16] Deposition of the cryoglobulin in nerves, blood vessels, and glomeruli attest to the devastation that may occur after cryoglobulins form.[17,18]

Classification of Cryoglobulins

Although the classification of cryoglobulins is evolving because of strong evidence implicating hepatitis C virus (HCV) with mixed cryoglobulins, the classification by Brouet et al[16] remains the standard that clinicians and laboratories use for categorization. The authors divided cryoglobulins into types I, II, and III.[16,19]

About 25% of cryoglobulins fall into the type I category. Typically, these cryoglobulins are the easiest to detect and identify because they are homogeneous monoclonal products that are present in relatively large quantities in serum. This does not mean they are identical from one patient to another. Even monoclonal cryoglobulins differ in their physicochemical characteristics. They are homogeneous in that they are monoclonal proteins in patients who have plasma cell and/or B-cell lymphoproliferative disorders, including multiple myeloma, Waldenström's macroglobulinemia, and lymphoma or leukemia. Typically, the monoclonal proteins in type I cryoglobulinemia are present in much greater concentrations (usually >500 mg/dL) than are the cryoproteins in type II and type III cryoglobulinemia. In some cases of type I cryoglobulinemia, the antigenic specificity of the monoclonal protein has been characterized.[20] Although this may be of interest to researchers, it is not required for the routine laboratory evaluation of cryoglobulin.

Because type II and type III cryoglobulins contain polyclonal immunoglobulins, they are called "mixed cryoglobulins." Type II cryoglobulins contain a monoclonal component, usually immunoglobulin (Ig) M, whereas type III cryoglobulins do not. In type II cryoglobulins, the monoclonal component has rheumatoid factor activity and reacts with polyclonal IgG and occasionally polyclonal IgA. It is usually present in much smaller amounts than is the monoclonal component in type I cryoglobulin.

The term *essential mixed cryoglobulin* may cause confusion. It is applied to cases of type II and type III cryoglobulinemia when no underlying condition (other than Sjögren's syndrome) is present.[21] Autoimmune diseases, especially Sjögren's syndrome, occur in about 25% of patients with mixed cryoglobulinemias.[22] Often, patients with both type II and type III cryoglobulinemia have a recognizable underlying condition such as HCV, lymphoproliferative disease, or autoimmune disease (other than Sjögren's syndrome). When type II and type III cryoglobulins are present in patients who have another condition, they are referred to as *secondary mixed cryoglobulins*. The category of essential mixed cryoglobulins was much larger before studies in the 1990s that indicated a strong association of these types of cryoglobulin with HCV.[23–27]

Immunochemically, cryoglobulins are particularly interesting molecules. One feature that points to a commonality between these heterogeneous structures is that 60% of cases of type II essential cryoglobulinemia have a specific cross-reactive rheumatoid factor idiotype (Wa). Idiotypes are specific antigens located on antigen-binding sites of immunoglobulins.[28] The presence of this idiotype suggests that it may be involved with the common characteristic of cryoprecipitation. Other idiotypes described among IgM-κ rheumatoid factors in type II cryoglobulinemias include Po and Bla. Together,

Po, Wa, and Bla account for about 80% of the rheumatoid factor activity.[29]

There are probably several mechanisms involved in cryoglobulin precipitation that vary from one patient to another. Certainly the manner in which they precipitate (gelatinous or crystalline) and the clinical symptoms of their presence differ among patients. Although it has been reported that an abundance of hydrophobic amino acids, unusual glycosylation, interchain disulfide bond cleavage, or a relatively large net negative charge may predispose a protein to cryoprecipitation, this has been a controversial view and there is no consensus about the mechanism at the present.[11,30–32]

Clinical Manifestations of Cryoglobulinemia

Cutaneous symptoms include Raynaud's phenomenon and palpable purpura (**Table 5-1**). The latter is most common in the lower extremities, although it may be seen on the arms and the buttocks, while the trunk and the face are usually spared.[33] Brouet et al[16] reported that 66% of their patients presented with either skin lesions or vasomotor attacks. Histologically, the skin lesions show a vasculitis with fibrinoid degeneration in the walls of the vessels. The lumen of the vessel may contain the cryoglobulin, which may have a hyaline appearance on routine hematoxylin-eosin sections of the tissue.[16] Neutrophils in various stages of degeneration also may be seen, and extravascular erythrocytes account for the characteristic palpable purpura. In rare instances, the skin lesions may progress to frank necrosis. The purpura may be worsened by a variety of situations, depending on the patient and the specific cryoglobulin. Exposure to cold, prolonged standing, and drugs such as penicillin or aspirin have been reported to potentiate the skin lesions in some patients.[16]

Table 5-1. Clinical Features of Essential Mixed Cryoglobulinemia[33]

Feature	Mean Age/Percent of EMC Patients With Symptoms
Average age	51 years
Purpura	95%
Arthralgia	72%
Peripheral neuropathy	25%
Renal failure	30%
Liver involvement	70%
Sjögren's syndrome	25%
Raynaud's phenomenon	25%

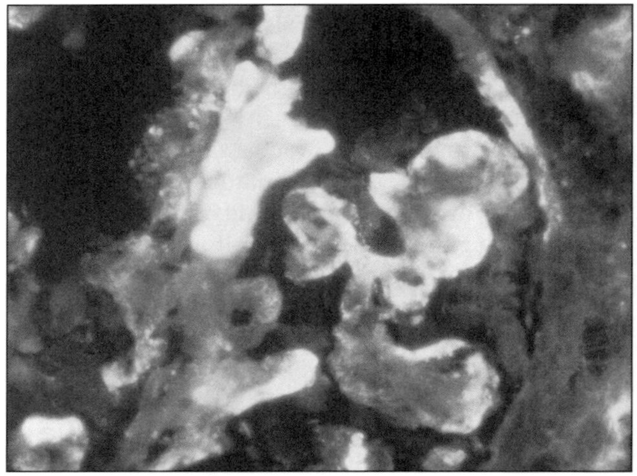

Figure 5-2. Dark-field photomicrograph of a glomerulus from a patient with type III cryoglobulinemia. The glomerulus is stained with fluorescein-conjugated antihuman IgG. Capillaries are filled with precipitated cryoglobulin.

Renal Involvement

About 20% of the patients studied by Brouet et al[16] had glomerular injury, yet other reports focusing on type II cryoglobulinemia reported renal disease in as many as 75% of their patients.[34] Renal disease usually involves the glomeruli, with a wide variety of diagnoses, including chronic glomerulonephritis, membranoproliferative glomerulonephritis, mesangiocapillary glomerulonephritis, and focal and segmental glomerulonephritis.[16,27,35] The presence of cryoglobulinemia in patients with autoimmune diseases such as systemic lupus erythematosus (SLE) significantly increases the likelihood that the individual will develop renal disease.[35] In many patients, hyaline thrombi can be found occluding glomerular capillaries. The hyaline structures in the glomerular capillaries can be identified as immunoglobulins by immunofluorescence (**Figure 5-2**). The thrombi are also often positive by periodic acid–Schiff (PAS) assay.[36]

Depending on the characteristics of the cryoglobulin, ultrastructural studies may demonstrate amorphous, homogeneous, or crystalline structures.[16,37]

Some scientists have noted an association between cryoglobulins, HCV, and membranoproliferative glomerulonephritis.[27] A multivariate analysis of the clinical outcomes of 105 patients with essential mixed cryoglobulinemia and renal involvement determined that key factors in predicting the likelihood of dialysis or death were patient age (older than 50 years of age), purpura, splenomegaly, cryocrit greater than 10%, C3 levels of less than 54 mg/dL, and serum creatinine greater than 1.5 mg/dL.[38]

Joint Involvement

Patients with cryoglobulinemia may have a variety of arthritic complaints. Although a few patients have rheumatoid arthritis, most have polyarthralgia, which may be accompanied by myalgia.[36,39,40] These polyarthralgias and myalgias have been found in patients with HCV-associated cryoglobulinemia.[40] The arthralgia is usually symmetric and the patients do not have morning stiffness.[33] Although rheumatoid factor is often positive in patients with type II or type III cryoglobulinemia, these individuals should not be classified as having rheumatoid arthritis unless they fit the clinical diagnostic criteria. Rheumatoid factor is elevated in a wide variety of inflammatory and infectious conditions and is not specific to rheumatoid arthritis. However, the level of rheumatoid factor may decline in patients treated with interferon alfa, implying a possible link between the rheumatological manifestations of type II or type III cryoglobulinemia and the treatment for HCV.[41]

Neurologic Involvement

Tingling sensations and numbness are signs of peripheral neuropathy that often accompany essential mixed cryoglobulinemias. A few patients demonstrated motor loss after a period of years, and Brouet et al[16] recorded 2 cases of patients with central neurologic involvement, one of whom experienced temporary blindness. In patients with Waldenström's macroglobulinemia, neurologic symptoms often relate to the hyperviscosity problems that are characteristic of that condition. It is uncommon for patients with type I cryoglobulins, other than those with Waldenström's macroglobulinemia, to suffer from neurologic symptoms. Patients with type II and type III cryoglobulinemia are more likely than those with type I to have peripheral neuropathy.[42,43] Immunofluorescence and ultrastructural studies demonstrated IgM cryoglobulin deposits in the peripheral nerves of a patient with cryoglobulinemia and Waldenström's macroglobulinemia.[44]

Cryoglobulins and Hepatitis C Virus

Hepatitis C and Mixed Cryoglobulinemias

Until recently, the relatively high percentage of patients with mixed cryoglobulinemia and liver involvement was somewhat surprising (see Table 5-1). Although some early studies hypothesized a relationship between hepatitis B virus and cryoglobulinemia, they were not supported by subsequent investigations.[45–47] In the 1990s, a close relationship was established between HCV infection and the development of type II and type III cryoglobulins.[23,48–50] Agnello and colleagues[24] reported that 16 of 19 patients with type II cryoglobulinemia had HCV RNA in their plasma; 8 also had positive serology to HCV. In a study of a large group of patients with HCV infection documented by biopsy, serology, and molecular demonstration of HCV RNA, Cacoub et al[47] reported that approximately 50% of patients had either type II or type III cryoglobulinemia. Interestingly, the duration of hepatitis was twice as long (14 years) in patients with type II cryoglobulinemia as in patients with type III.[47] This led to the suggestion that the disease may evolve from type III to type II due to an unknown event that permits unrestricted replication by one clone.

Because of the association between the duration of hepatitis and the apparent evolution of a type III to a type II cryoglobulinemia, other workers[51] have recorded an association between HCV and the development of monoclonal gammopathies, especially in patients with genotypes 1b and 2a/c. Indeed, HCV has been found in patients with monoclonal gammopathies not associated with cryoglobulinemia, which implies a hematopoietic tropism for this virus.[52]

Hepatitis C Virus and Cryoglobulin Therapy

The relationship between type II and type III cryoglobulinemia and HCV is of more than academic interest. It affects the type of therapy offered to affected individuals. Individuals who have type II and III cryoglobulinemia due to autoimmune disease rather than HCV infection would not benefit from antiviral therapy, whereas, those patients with HCV may. Interferon alfa has been used in several studies[53–55] and was shown to improve both the liver and renal manifestations of the disease. In a controlled study of 53 patients with HCV-related type II cryoglobulinemia, Misiani et al[56] reported that many patients who received interferon alfa-2a therapy showed significant improvement in their symptoms and a decrease in the amount of cryoglobulin present. Symptoms recurred when the therapy was discontinued.

However, interferon alfa is not a panacea. The therapy may help some patients improve, whereas others do not respond at all.[57] Zimmermann et al[58] recorded the case of a patient with type II mixed cryoglobulinemia associated with HCV and vasculitis in whom the vasculitis worsened during the interferon alfa-2a therapy. Serum aminotransferase levels improved and became normal in the patient during the therapy. Following discontinuation of the therapy, aminotransferase levels rose again, but the vasculitis and cutaneous symptoms improved. The researchers hypothesized that the different HCV subtypes may make a difference in the response to interferon therapy, but no subtype analysis was offered.

Other scientists[59] have hypothesized that the demonstrated increase in anti-GOR antibodies (antibodies that react with both viral and host antigens) in patients with HCV-associated type II cryoglobulinemia suggests that the antibodies represent the result of molecular mimicry between human and viral epitopes.

Although the relationship between type II cryoglobulinemia and HCV is strong, many cases of type II cryoglobulinemia are not associated with HCV and may occur with a wide variety of clinical lymphoproliferative or autoimmune processes.[60] Patients with Sjögren's syndrome and type II cryoglobulinemia do not usually have HCV, and the presence of type II cryoglobulin in these patients is highly associated with the development of B-cell lymphoma.[61]

Similarly, despite the strong association of many cases of mixed cryoglobulinemia with HCV, about 50% of patients with type III cryoglobulinemia experience other infectious conditions (including cytomegalovirus), autoimmune diseases, and un-known conditions, but not lymphoproliferative disorders.[35,62] Typically, the rheumatoid factor is IgM, and cryoglobulin is present in low concentration (<100 mg/dL).[16] The profile of a typical patient with autoimmune disease and type III essential mixed cryoglobulinemia is that of a 50-year-old woman.[22]

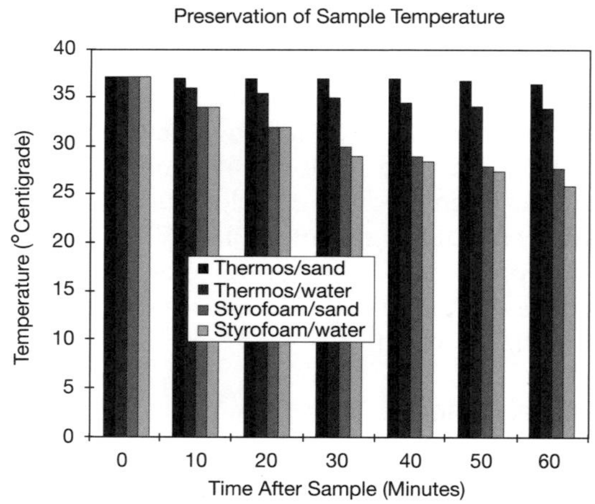

Figure 5-3. Lowering of temperature shown for 1 hour after a sample is preserved under the indicated conditions.

Laboratory Characterization of Cryoglobulins

Temperature of the Initial Sample

Maintaining sample temperature at 37°C is critically important in detecting cryoglobulins. If possible, the patient should be brought to the laboratory to minimize the possible cooling of a specimen during transportation time. In addition, the specimen should be drawn in a prewarmed tube or syringe. When it is not practical to bring the patient to the laboratory due to the condition of the patient or the location of the laboratory, sample temperature may be maintained during transportation by using a thermos filled with 37°C sand (**Figure 5-3**).[10] As a quality assurance measure, the temperature of specimens transported to the laboratory should be recorded at the time of receipt.

Clot separation also must be performed at 37°C. The serum is then split into 2 tubes, one held at 4°C and the other at 37°C.[63] Samples are examined once daily for 3 days. If a precipitate is present in the 4°C tube but not in the 37°C tube, the specimen is interpreted as positive for cryoglobulin.

The amount of cryoglobulin may be quantified by a variety of methods. A simple choice is the cryocrit assay.[63] To perform this test, the serum is separated at 37°C and placed in a hematocrit tube. After incubating at 4°C for 72 hours, the sample is centrifuged (still at 4°C) at 3,000 rpm for 30 minutes and the cryocrit is recorded.[63] The cryocrit test has the advantage of not being dependent on redissolving the cryoglobulin, and no protein is lost during the wash steps needed for protein quantification. However, not all cryoglobulins form clear-cut precipitates, and cryocrits may therefore not provide adequate information. Bloch[64] pointed out that when the cryoglobulin precipitates as a cryogel, it may adhere to the wall of the centrifuge tube rather than settling as a clear-cut precipitate. Bloch recommended that measurement of the serum monoclonal component was the most reliable means of measuring the cryoglobulin in cases where the cryoglobulin tends to gel.

In all cases of cryoglobulinemia, it is possible to quantify the total amount of protein present in the cryoglobulin. One milliliter of the serum is placed in a tube that is kept at 4°C for 72 hours. After the sample is centrifuged at 2,500 rpm for 30 minutes, the supernatant is removed. The cryoglobulin is washed 3 times in cold phosphate-buffered saline, and is then redissolved in 1 mL of 37°C buffer from the protein assay to be used. Results are expressed as cryoglobulin protein/mL of serum.

Classification of the cryoglobulinemia as type I, II, or III requires immunofixation. Immunoelectrophoresis is no longer the preferred procedure for evaluating monoclonal gammopathies.[65] After the precipitate is washed at least 3 times with cold barbital buffer, it is redissolved for analysis. The cryoglobulin usually dissolves upon heating to 37°C. If the cryoglobulin does not dissolve at 37°C, the pH or salt concentration may be adjusted. Grose[66] suggests adding 5% acetic acid to a mixture of saline and the cryoprecipitate to facilitate the process. If the cryoglobulin proves difficult to redissolve, the type of cryoglobulin can be characterized based on differences between the serum immunoglobulin and rheumatoid factor level before and after cryoprecipitation.[19] After the sample is dissolved, immunofixation is performed. A type I cryoglobulin will have only the monoclonal protein (M-protein) with one light chain and one heavy chain type. The monoclonal protein is usually present in large quantity (typically >500mg/dL). A type II cryoglobulin will have a relatively small IgM, usually κ, but occasionally λ M-protein in the serum together with polyclonal IgG (containing both κ and λ polyclonal reactions). A type III cryoglobulin will have only polyclonal immunoglobulins present by immunofixation.

Because of the strong association between HCV and type II and III cryoglobulins, it is advisable to assay all cryoglobulin-positive patients for the presence of anti-HCV using the enzyme-linked immunosorbent assay (ELISA). However, molecular characterization of the precipitate for the presence of HCV viral RNA is not routinely recommended because the serology establishes the diagnosis and HCV RNA measurement by polymerase chain reaction (PCR) in serum is the most useful way to follow the infection. Related literature should be reviewed carefully, however, because monitoring interferon alfa-2a therapy may require molecular studies on the plasma or the cryoprecipitate for the amount of HCV RNA.

Precautions

The unrecognized presence of a cryoglobulin in serum may create problems in other laboratory tests. In serum protein electrophoresis and immunofixation, the cryoglobulin may leave a precipitate at the origin (the agarose gel is cold relative to the precipitating temperature for many cryoglobulins). This produces a band at the origin that is in direct proportion to the dilution of the patient's serum used in each lane. When such an immunoprecipitate appears at the origin of all or several lanes (depending on the concentration of patient serum applied to the lane), it is useful to repeat the immunofixation, but overlay one lane with buffer only. When a precipitate is seen in the buffer-only lane, it is highly likely that a cryoglobulin is present. It is then recommended that the clinician send a fresh sample to the laboratory, obtained under the temperature-controlled circumstances detailed earlier, for formal cryoglobulin evaluation.

In addition to difficulties encountered with immunofixation, cryoglobulins may cause problems with tests of complement activation and complement consumption, because some cryoglobulins bind to C1q and begin the complement cascade.[67] Consequently, complement and C4 levels may be decreased in patients with activation of the complement pathway.[22,29] In addition, cryoprecipitates may be interpreted as leukocytes by some automated hematology analyzers, making a manual count necessary.[68,69]

Because cryoglobulin testing is not well standardized, serial evaluations are not recommended to follow disease activity.[63]

Summary

In summary, whereas epidemiological studies for the presence and content of circulating immune complexes may provide useful data about disease states, these assays are not useful for following individual patients. One type of immune complex, cryoglobulins, is critically important to detect, characterize, and measure. The key to detection of cryoglobulins is to be sure that blood samples are preserved at 37°C at the time of the initial sampling, during transportation, and in the laboratory until the serum is separated into two tubes: one kept at 37°C and the other at 4°C for up to 7 days. When a cryoglobulin is detected, it must be characterized immunochemically by washing the sample extensively (at least 3 times in cold buffer) and performing an immunofixation. The cryoglobulin may be characterized by measuring the total protein in the cryoglobulin or performing a cryocrit. Serial evaluations of cryoglobulin are not currently recommended due to the lack of standardization of cryoglobulin testing. HCV testing should be performed on sera of all patients with Type II or III cryoglobulins.

References

1. Keren DF. Assays for circulating immune complexes. In: Homburger HA, Batsakis JB, eds. *Clinical Laboratory Annual: 1985.* New York, NY: Appleton-Century-Crofts; 1985:105–142.
2. Mironova MA, Klein RL, Virella GT, et al. Anti-modified LDL antibodies, LDL-containing immune complexes, and susceptibility of LDL to in vitro oxidation in patients with type 2 diabetes. *Diabetes.* 2000;49: 1033–1041.
3. Van Hoeyveld E, Bossuyt X. Evaluationof seven commercial ELISA kits compared with the C1q solid-phase binding RIA for detection of circulating immune complexes. *Clin Chem.* 2000;46:283–285.
4. Gussin HA, Russo KL, Teodorescu M. Effect of circulating immune complexes on the binding of rheumatoid factor to histones. *Ann Rheum Dis.* 2000;59: 351–358.
5. Tsai JF, Margolis HS, Jeng JE, et al. Increased IgM class circulating immune complexes in acute hepatitis A virus infection. *Clin Immunol Immunopathol.* 1996;78:291–295.
6. Tai AW, Newkirk MM. An autoantibody targeting glycated IgG is associated with elevated serum immune complexes in rheumatoid arthritis. *Clin Exp Immunol.* 2000;120:188–193.
7. Nezlin R. A quantitative approach to the determination of antigen in immune complexes. *J Immunol Methods.* 2000;237:1–17.
8. Stanojevic M, Zerjav S, Jevtovic DJ, et al. HbsAg as the antigen component of circulating immune complexes in HIV-infected patients. *Biomed Pharmacother.* 2000;54:163–167.
9. Tsai JF, Margolis HS, Jeng JE, et al. Circulating immune complexes in chronic hepatitis related to hepatitis C and B viruses infection. *Clin Immunol Immunopathol.* 1995;75:39–44.
10. Keren DF, Di Sante AC, Mervak T, et al. Problems with transporting serum to the laboratory for cryoglobulin assay: A solution. *Clin Chem.* 1985;31: 1766–1767.
11. Lawson EQ, Brandau DT, Trautman PA, et al. Electrostatic properties of cryoimmunoglobulins. *J Immunol.* 1988;140:1218–1222.
12. McLeod BC, Sassetti RJ. "Hypocryoglobulins": Enhanced cryoprecipitation from hypotonic serum in patients with vasculitis. *Arch Intern Med.* 1984;144:1381–1385.
13. Brandau DT, Trautman PA, Steadman BL, et al. The temperature-dependent stoichiometry of mixed cryoimmunoglobulins. *J Biol Chem.* 1986;261:16385–16391.
14. Aizawa Y, Zawadzki ZA. Monoclonal IgG1 immunoglobulinaemia with strictly pH dependent cryoprecipitability. *Clin Exp Immunol.* 1979;37:265–275.
15. Letendre L, Kyle RA. Monoclonal cryoglobulinemia with high thermal insolubility. *Mayo Clin Proc.* 1982;57:629–633.
16. Brouet J, Clauvel J, Danon F, et al. Biologic and clinical significance of cryoglobulins. *Am J Med.* 1974;57:775–788.
17. Vital A, Vital C, Ragnaud J, et al. IgM cryoglobulin deposits in the peripheral nerve. *Virchows Arch A Pathol Anat Histopathol.* 1991;418:83–85.
18. Scully RE, Mark EJ, McNeely WF, et al. Case 11-1989. Case records of the Massachusetts General Hospital. Weekly clinicopathological exercises. *N Engl J Med.* 1989;320:718–728.
19. Keren DF. Conditions associated with monoclonal gammopathies. In: Keren DF. *High-Resolution Electrophoresis and Immunofixation: Techniques and Interpretation.* 2nd ed. Boston, MA: Butterworth; 1994:211–282.
20. Mills LE, Brettman LR, Jetoft JE, et al. Crystallocryoglobulinemia resulting from human monoclonal antibodies to albumin. *Ann Intern Med.* 1983;99:601–604.
21. Meltzer M, Franklin EC, Elias K, et al. Cryoglobulinemia—a clinical and laboratory study. II. Cryoglobulins with rheumatoid factor activity. *Am J Med.* 1966;40:837–856.
22. Gorevic PD, Galanakis D, Finn AF Jr. Cryoglobulins. In: Rose NR, de Nacario EC, Folds JD, et al, eds. *Manual of Clinical Laboratory Immunology.* 5th ed. Washington, DC: ASM Press;1997:217–223.
23. Ferri C, Greco F, Longombardo G, et al. Association between hepatitis C virus and mixed cryoglobulinemia. *Clin Exp Rheumatol.* 1991;9:621–624.

24. Agnello V, Chung RT, Kaplan LM. A role for hepatitis C virus infection in type II cryoglobulinemia. *N Engl J Med*. 1992;327:1490–1495.

25. Dammacco F, Sansonno D. Antibodies to hepatitis C virus in essential mixed cryoglobulinemia. *Clin Exp Immunol*. 1992;87:352–356.

26. Ferri C, Greco F, Longombardo G, et al. Antibodies to hepatitis C virus in patients with mixed cryoglobulinemia. *Arthritis Rheum*. 1991;34:1606–1610.

27. Johnson RJ, Gretch DR, Yambe H, et al. Membranoproliferative glomerulonephritis associated with hepatitis C virus infection. *N Engl J Med*. 1993;328:465–470.

28. Agnello V. Rheumatoid factor cross idiotypes. *Springer Semin Immunopathol*. 1988;10:203–214.

29. Finn AF, Gorevic PD. Pathogenic paraproteins: Gammopathies and cryoglobulinemia. *Curr Opin Rheumatol*. 1990;2:652–660.

30. Brandau DT, Lawson EQ, Middaugh CR, et al. The effect of interchain disulfide bond cleavage on the cold induced precipitation of cryoimmunoglobulins. *Immunol Invest*. 1986;15:447–462.

31. McClure SP, Hurtubise PE. Laboratory and clinical evaluation of cryoglobulinemia. *Clin Immunol News*. 1983;4:7–9.

32. Levo Y. Nature of cryoglobulinaemia. *Lancet*. 1980;1:285–286.

33. Abel G, Zhang Q-X, Agnello V. Hepatitis C virus infection in type II mixed cryoglobulinemia. *Arthritis Rheum*. 1993;36:1341–1349.

34. Frankel AH, Singer DR, Winearls CG, et al. Type II essential mixed cryoglobulinaemia: Presentation, treatment and outcome in 13 patients. *Q J Med*. 1992;82:101–124.

35. Howard TW, Iannini MJ, Burge JJ, et al. Rheumatoid factor, cryoglobulinemia, anti-DNA, and renal disease in patients with systemic lupus erythematosus. *J Rheumatol*. 1991;18:826–830.

36. Iwasaki M, Okabe H, Ochi Y. Renal and neurologic symptoms due to cryoglobulinemia complicated with rheumatoid arthritis and Sjögren's syndrome. *Rinsho Byori*. 1992;40:665–669.

37. Ishimura E, Nishizawa Y, Shoji S, et al. Heat-insoluble cryoglobulin in a patient with essential type I cryoglobulinemia and massive cryoglobulin-occlusive glomerulonephritis. *Am J Kidney Dis*. 1995;26:654–657.

38. Tarantino A, Campise M, Banfi G, et al. Long-term predictors of survival in essential mixed cryoglobulinemic glomerulonephritis. *Kidney Int*. 1995;47:618–623.

39. Bekavac J, Varas MA, Ardiles A, et al. Cryoglobulins in rheumatoid arthritis: Exhaustive detection, immunochemical findings and clinical expression. *Rev Med Chil*. 1994;122:180–185.

40. Bon E, Cantagrel A, Moulinier L, et al. Rheumatic manifestations of chronic hepatitis C and response to the treatment with interferon alpha-2b. *Rev Rhum Ed Fr*. 1994;61:497–504.

41. Sepp NT, Umlauft F, Illersperger B, et al. Necrotizing vasculitis associated with hepatitis C virus infection: Successful treatment of vasculitis with interferon-alpha despite persistence of mixed cryoglobulinemia. *Dermatology*. 1995;191:43–45.

42. Nemni R, Corbo M, Fazio R, et al. Cryoglobulinaemic neuropathy. A clinical, morphological and immunocytochemical study of 8 cases. *Brain*. 1988;111:541–552.

43. David WS, Peine C, Schlesinger P, et al. Nonsystemic vasculitic mononeuropathy multiplex, cryoglobulinemia, and hepatitis C. *Muscle Nerve*. 1996;19:1596–1602.

44. Vital A, Vital C, Ragnaud J, et al. IgM cryoglobulin deposits in the peripheral nerve. *Virchows Arch A Pathol Anat Histopathol*. 1991;418:83–85.

45. Levo Y, Gorevic PD, Hanna MD, et al. Liver involvement in the syndrome of mixed cryoglobulinemia. *Ann Intern Med*. 1977;87:287–292.

46. Galli M. Cryoglobulinemia and serological markers of hepatitis viruses. *Lancet*. 1991;338:758–759.

47. Cacoub P, Fabiani FL, Musset L, et al. Mixed cryoglobulinemia and hepatitis C virus. *Am J Med*. 1994;96:124–132.

48. Domingo JM, Romero S, Moreno JA, et al. Hepatitis C virus infection and mixed cryoglobulinemia in patients with lymphoproliferative diseases. *Haematologica*. 1999;84:94–96.

49. Misiani R, Bellavita P, Fenili D, et al. Hepatitis C virus infection in patients with essential mixed cryoglobulinemia. *Ann Intern Med*. 1992;117:573–577.

50. Levey JM, Bjornsson B, Banner B, et al. Mixed cryoglobulinemia in chronic hepatitis C infection: A clinicopathologic analysis of 10 cases and review of recent literature. *Medicine*. 1994;73:53–67.

51. Andreone P, Gramenzi A, Cursaro C, et al. Monoclonal gammopathy in patients with chronic hepatitis C virus infection. *Blood*. 1996;88:1122.

52. Mangi A, Clemente R, Musto P, et al. Hepatitis C virus infection and monoclonal gammopathies not associated with cryoglobulinemia. *Leukemia*. 1996;10:1209–1213.

53. Ferri C, Marzo E, Longombardo G, et al. Interferon-alpha in mixed cryoglobulinemia patients: A randomized, crossover-controlled trial. *Blood*. 1993;81:1132–1136.

54. Casato M, Lagana B, Antonelli G, et al. Long-term results of therapy with interferon alpha for Type II essential mixed cryoglobulinemia. *Blood*. 1991;78:3142–3147.

55. Ferri C, Marzo E, Longombardo G, et al. Interferon alfa-2b in mixed cryoglobulinaemia: A controlled crossover trial. *Gut*. 1993;34(suppl):S144–S145.

56. Misiani R, Bellavita P, Fenili D, et al. Interferon alfa-2a therapy in cryoglobulinemia associated with hepatitis C virus. *N Engl J Med*. 1994;330:751–756.

57. Arranz FR, Diaz RD, Diez LI, et al. Cryoglobulinemia vasculitis associated with hepatitis C virus infection. A report of eight cases. *Acta Derm Venereol*. 1995;75:234–236.

58. Zimmerman R, Konig V, Bauditz J, et al. Interferon alfa in leukocytoclastic vsculitis, mixed cryoglobulinaemia, and chronic hepatitis C. *Lancet*. 1993;341:561–562. [Letter]

59. Ballare M, Quaglia V, Di Natale C, et al. Anti-GOR antibodies in type II mixed cryoglobulinemia associated with hepatitis C virus infection. *Ann Ital Med Int*. 1995;10:98–101.

60. Shpilberg O, Ehrenfeld M, Berkovitz M, et al. Hairy cell leukemia with an autoimmune syndrome, paraproteinemia, and cryoglobulinemia. *South Med J*. 1989;82:1552–1554.

61. Tzioufas AG, Boumba DS, Skopouli FN, et al. Mixed monoclonal cryoglobulinemia and monoclonal rheumatoid factor cross-reactive idiotypes as predictive factors for the development of lymphoma in primary Sjögren's syndrome. *Arthritis Rheum*. 1996;39:767–772.

62. Witzke O, Kassubek J, Bonmann E, et al. Cryoglobulinemia: A complication of infectious disease. *Clin Investig*. 1994;72:1048–1050.

63. Kallemuchikkal U, Gorevic PD. Evaluation of cryoglobulins. *Arch Pathol Lab Med*. 1999;123:119–125.

64. Bloch KJ. Quoted by: Scully RE, Mark EJ, McNeely WF, et al. Case 30-1995. Case records of the Massachusetts General Hospital. Weekly clinicopathological exercises. *N Engl J Med*. 1995;333:862–868.

65. Keren DF, Alexanian R, Goeken JA, et al. Guidelines for clinical and laboratory evaluation of patients with monoclonal gammopathies. *Arch Pathol Lab Med*. 1999;123:106–107.

66. Grose MP. *Clinical Immunology Tech Sample*. No. CI-2. Chicago, IL: ASCP Press; 1988.

67. Sheehan C. Autoimmunity. In: Sheehan C, ed. *Clinical Immunology. Principles and Laboratory Diagnosis*. Philadelphia, PA: JB Lippincott; 1990:327.

68. Banfi G, Grazioli V, Dolci A, et al. Detection of a case of pseudolymphocytosis due to cryoglobulins. *J Clin Lab Anal*. 1990;4:319–323.

69. Banfi G, Bunini PA. Detection of cryoglobulins by Coulter counter model S-plus IV/D. *Clin Lab Haematol*. 1988;10:453–459.

CHAPTER 6

Complement and Autoimmune Diseases

David F. Carney, PhD

The complement system consists of a series of circulating blood proteins that participate in the body's inflammatory response and host defense mechanisms. Complement proteins play an important role as inflammatory mediators, participate in the opsinization of foreign particulate matter (including a variety of microorganisms), and cause cytolytic reactions against certain susceptible prokaryotic and eukaryotic cells and enveloped viruses.[1–3] The complement system consists of over 30 functionally diverse proteins.[3] These proteins can function as enzymes, regulatory inhibitors and inactivators, membrane-integrated receptors, and lytic pore formers.[2]

Activation of the complement system follows an activation cascade that comprises 2 separate pathways called the classical and alternative pathways[4] (**Figure 6-1**). These 2 pathways converge at the stage of C3 activation, which then leads to subsequent activation and assembly of the 5 proteins of the terminal pathway.[1–3] Activation of the classical pathway is initiated primarily through the interaction of C1q with immune complexes that contain immunoglobulin (Ig) M and some classes of IgG.[2,3] Classical pathway activation also can be triggered by such diverse substances as C-reactive protein, rheumatoid factor, certain viruses, tissue damage products, lipopolysaccharides, and serum amyloid A protein. The classical pathway uses C1q, C1r, C1s, C4, and C2, and activation of this pathway ultimately leads to activation of C3.[2] Another form of classical pathway activation uses mannose binding protein, which is structurally similar to C1q and activates the classical pathway in a manner independent of C1.[8]

Alternative pathway activation also ultimately leads to activation of C3, but uses factor B, factor D, and properdin (factor P) instead of C1, C4, and C2.[5] The alternative pathway is activated by many agents, including repeating polysaccharides, endotoxin, virally infected cells, some Ig light chains, immune complexes, C3 nephritic factor, and cobra venom factor.[6] The alternative pathway is also subject to autoactivation, which depends on features of the surfaces to which activated C3 (C3b) binds.[2] It is of significant clinical importance that complement can be activated by a number of biopolymers used in cardiopulmonary bypass, hemodialysis, and other related procedures.[9] Formation of C3b via either the classical or alternative pathway initiates activation of the terminal pathway and assembly of the terminal complex.[1–3]

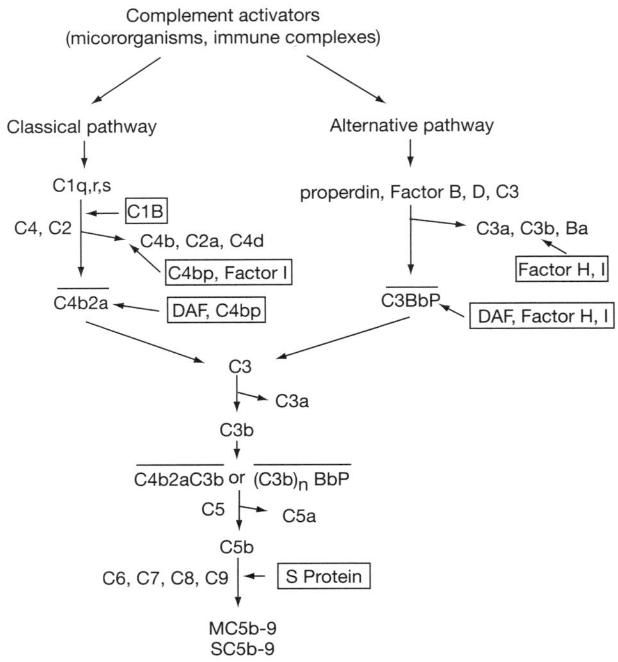

Figure 6-1. Classical and alternative pathways of the complement activation cascade.[1-3,5-7] Components followed by a, b, or d indicate proteolytic fragments of the parent component. Enzyme complexes are indicated with a bar (eg, $\overline{\text{C4b2a}}$). The $\overline{\text{C4b2a}}$ and $\overline{\text{C3bBbP}}$ enzymes convert C3 to C3a and C3b. The $\overline{\text{C4b2aC3b}}$ and $\overline{\text{(C3b)}_n\text{BbP}}$ enzymes convert C5 to C5a and C5b. Components in boxes are regulatory proteins, with arrows indicating the site of regulation. Abbreviations: DAF = decay acceleration factor; C4bp = C4 binding protein; C1EI = C1 esterase inhibitor; MC5b-9 = C5b-9 formed within a membrane lipid bilayer; SC5b-9 = C5b-9 that remains in solution due to binding to S protein (vitronectin).

The terminal complex is formed by sequential activation and assembly of C5b, C6, C7, C8, and 1 to 12 molecules of C9 into a multimeric complex.[10] Assembly of the C5b-9 terminal complex can occur either in solution or within membrane lipid bilayers.[11] The C5b-9 complex has a cylindrical structure with an inner internal pore of up to 10 nm in diameter.[10] Whereas a single C5b-9 channel within the plasma membrane of an erythrocyte is sufficient for erythrocyte lysis, multiple C5b-9 are required for nucleated cell lysis because nucleated cells rapidly remove C5b-9 from the cell surface.[10] A sublytic number of C5b-9 or the intermediates C5b-8 or C5b-7 formed in the plasma membrane of nucleated cells can cause cell activation via the generation of signals that include elevated intracellular Ca^{2+}.[10]

In addition to the complement proteins C1 through C9, many other proteins also participate in the process of complement activation, mainly as regulators and inhibitors[1,3] (see Figure 6-1). These proteins include C1 esterase inhibitor (C1EI), decay acceleration factor (DAF), C4 binding protein, factor I, factor H, S protein, CD59, and the complement receptors CR1 and CR3.[2] The proteins have diverse functions, such as protease inhibition, decay acceleration, cofactor activity, and inhibition of terminal complex assembly.[1–3] Detailed characterization of these proteins can be found in a number of reviews.[12–14]

Complement Assays: An Overview

Because complement plays a central and diverse role in the immune response, the finding of depressed or elevated circulating levels of intact complement components or their activation products in patients is usually clinically nonspecific.[15–17] The most notable exception to this generalization is patients suspected of having a genetic deficiency in any one of the complement proteins, in which case diagnosis can be confirmed by assaying for the suspected deficient component.[18] Another disease group that may be diagnosed with the aid of complement assays is the hereditary and acquired angioedemas. Complement measurements sometimes may be clinically useful for other diseases, especially when they are targeted at diagnosing or monitoring specific clinical conditions. For example, complement activation may be extensive in certain autoimmune diseases, such as systemic lupus erythematosus (SLE) or rheumatoid arthritis.[16,19] In diseases accompanied by in vivo complement activation, complement measurements may be useful for monitoring clinical activity or the patient's response to treatment.[16,19,20]

Assays of complement components can be divided broadly into those that measure levels of intact components and those that measure levels of complement activation products[3,16,17] (**Tables 6-1** and **6-2**). Measurement of intact components is often used as an indirect measure of complement activation, based on the assumption that complement activation reduces circulating levels of intact complement proteins due to consumption. In the context of this discussion, consumption refers to proteolytic conversion of intact complement proteins to activation fragments.[3] However, there are 2 inherent problems associated with correlating in vivo complement activation with measurements of intact components. First, mild-to-moderate complement activation may not reduce circulating intact components to levels below normal, considering the broad normal ranges typically observed for these proteins in most laboratories.[21] For

Table 6-1. Assays That Measure Intact Complement Proteins

Assay Types	Components Measured	Methods	Method Principle
Functional		Erythrocyte suspension	Erythrocyte lysis and hemoglobin release
CH_{50}	C1, C2, C4 (C3, C5-C9)		
		Agarose gel	Erythrocyte lysis; zone of hemolysis
AP_{50}	Factors B and D; properdin (C3, C5-C9)	Liposome	Lysis of liposome containing trapped marker
		ELISA	Measurement of SC5b-9 via in vitro complement activation
Antigenic	C1-C9; factors B, D, and H; C1EI; C4bp; properdin; protein S	Nephelometry	Rate of immune precipitate formation
		Radial immunodiffusion	Size of precipitin ring around sample well
		Immunoelectrophoresis	Immunostaining after electrophoretic separation
		ELISA	Capture and detecting antibodies required

Abbreviation: ELISA = enzyme-linked immunosorbent assay.

Table 6-2. Complement Activation Products

Classification	Product	Comments
Multimolecular activation products	C1-C1EI	Moderate sensitivity, high specificity for classical pathway activation
	C3bBbP	Short half-life in vivo
	SC5b-9	Stable in vitro, long half-life in vivo, no spontaneous formation, sufficient circulating levels of protein S required
Activation fragments	C3a	Special handling of patient samples required to minimize generation of any activation fragments by in vitro activation
	iC3b	Factors H and I required to obtain iC3b from C3
	C3c, C3dg	Circulating levels of all C3 fragments poorly defined clinically
	C3d	Stable, long half-life
	C4a	Cleared by kidneys; renal disease may cause retention in the circulation
	C4b	Circulating levels of all C4 fragments poorly defined clinically
	C4d	Conversion of C4 to C4d dependent on factor I and C4 bp
	Ba	Cleared by kidneys; renal disease may cause retention in the circulation
	Bb	Sensitive, reliable indicator of alternative pathway activation

Abbreviation: C1EI = C1 esterase inhibitor.

example, consumption of as little as 5% to 10% of available serum C3 reflects massive activation, but serum C3 levels might be well within normal limits.[19] Second, the sensitivity of these assays is further compromised by the fact that most complement proteins behave as acute phase reactants.[17,21,22] Thus, the increased synthesis of these proteins during the acute phase response could mask evidence of consumption in antigenic or functional assays.

Despite these drawbacks, assays that measure intact components may be clinically useful in specific disease management when properly used. A 1988 International Union of Immunological Societies/World Health Organization (IUIS/WHO) report pertaining to complement assays[23] stated that functional complement assays were considered "essential" in patients with suspected inherited complement deficiencies. Measurements of intact complement components were considered "helpful" in the management of a variety of autoimmune disorders, such as SLE.

Measurements of complement activation products are generally far more sensitive for detecting complement activation than are measurements of intact complement proteins or functional assays.[17,19] However, these assays must be used cautiously because the clinical utility of complement activation product assays for specific diseases is not yet firmly established, and sample handling can significantly affect assay results (as will be discussed later in this chapter). The consensus of the IUIS/WHO report[23] concluded that complement activation assays were "not essential" for the diagnosis of any condition but could be "useful" in monitoring the effects of treatment in patients whose disease process is accompanied by in vivo complement activation.

Measurement of Intact Complement Proteins

Functional Complement Assays

The CH_{50} and AP_{50} assays assess the integrity of the classical and alternative pathways, respectively[17,21] (see Table 6-1). In these assays, patient serum complement is activated by antibody-sensitized sheep erythrocytes (CH_{50}) or unsensitized rabbit or chicken erythrocytes (AP_{50}), either in suspension or in agarose gel. Complement activation and progression through an intact cascade is indicated by the formation of a functional C5b-9 terminal complex, which, when formed within erythrocyte membranes, causes cell lysis. Thus, these assays can detect abnormalities in any of the complement pathway proteins. Lysis is quantitated by using spectrophotometry to measure hemoglobin release for suspended cells or by measuring the area of hemolysis around the central well containing the patient sample in agarose gels. Patient values are usually compared with those obtained from a normal serum or serum pool. These assays are accurate and reliable when done properly but tend to be cumbersome and difficult to standardize because the results are affected by the age and concentration of the erythrocytes, ionic strength, pH, the quality of antibody sensitization, and reaction times and temperatures.[21] The agarose gel method should continue to stimulate interest with the introduction of commercially available standardized kits.

Newer-generation functional assays, which have replaced the need for erythrocytes, include indicator systems, such as marker-loaded liposomes that mimic the lipid bilayer properties of erythrocytes, and formats based on enzyme-linked immunosorbent assays (ELISAs) that measure fluid phase SC5b-9 captured on the plate by antibodies to C5, C9, or neoantigens on C5b-9.[24] Patient results are typically compared with a standard material (often obtained by pooling normal donors) to report a standard unit value relative to normal.[3] These newer assays are particularly attractive because they are amenable to automation.

Functional complement assays are generally used for assessing the integrity of the entire complement cascade, and as such may be useful as an initial screen when complement system involvement is suspected. These assays are particularly useful in screening for genetic complement deficiencies, but are also commonly used to measure complement consumption in patients with autoimmune disorders such as SLE.[16,21] They also may be (but are not commonly) used for measuring the activities of individual complement proteins.[25] The levels of individual components are usually assayed by immunochemical methods rather than by functional assays.[17,21]

Antigenic Complement Assays

The levels of intact complement components are most often determined using immunoassays with highly specific monoclonal or polyclonal antibodies directed against individual complement proteins. Although these assays are particularly useful in ruling out specific genetic complement deficiencies, they are probably more often used as an indirect measure of complement activity in vivo via a measurement of consumption.[19,21] Antigenic assays include those that measure components of both the classical and alternative pathways, the most common of which are C1q, C3 (or C3c), C4, and factor B.[3,15] C2 is often included in this group, not only because C2 deficiency is by far the most common genetic complement deficiency, but also because C2 levels may be a more sensitive indicator of complement consumption in vivo due to C2's low plasma concentration relative to the other complement proteins.[21]

Although a variety of methods are available for measuring complement proteins by antigenic assays, the 2 most commonly used methods are rate nephelometry and radial immunodiffusion (RID)[3,15] (see Table 6-1). These methods measure the rate or the extent of immunoprecipitation, respectively, which is proportional to the amount of complement protein (antigen) present under optimized experimental conditions.[15] These assays require a standard curve using standard materials, preferably in the form of serum or plasma, that contain known quantities of the complement proteins to be measured. In addition to these techniques, immunoelectrophoretic and ELISA methodologies are used in complement antigenic assays.[17,21]

Complement Activation Product Assays

Whereas levels of intact complement proteins are an indirect and insensitive measure of complement activation in vivo, assays of complement activation products are highly specific and significantly more sensitive for this purpose.[19,21,26] Complement activation products are classified both by virtue of their molecular nature—that is, multimolecular complexes versus split products (proteolytic fragments)—and by the activation pathway (classical, alternative, or terminal) from which they are derived. Multimolecular complexes include C1-C1EI (classical), C3bBbP (alternative), and SC5b-9 (terminal)[16,19] (see Table 6-2). "Sandwich" ELISAs have been designed for all 3 complexes based on trapping the complex on a solid support using a capture antibody that recognizes one of the constituents (anti-C1s, anti-properdin, and anti-C9) and then detecting the complex using an antibody to a separate component (anti-C1EI, anti-C3, and anti-S, respectively).[19,21] These complexes are highly specific indicators of complement activation and are relatively stable in vitro with long half-lives.[16] Thus these assays offer clear advantages for assessing complement activation in clinical practice.

The anaphylatoxins—especially C3a and C4a—as well as other split products, such as Ba, Bb, and C4d, are also sensitive indicators of complement activation and may be useful for assessing disease activity and for monitoring the response to treatments aimed at reducing inflammatory episodes.[16,17,21] For example, Ba, Bb, C3a, C3d, and C4d levels have been found to correlate better with disease activity than C3, C4, and CH_{50} levels.[19,27–29] However, widespread use of assays that measure complement activation fragments is still forthcoming and their clinical utility remains unknown.

Most of the newer-generation assays for split products are based on sandwich ELISAs and use monoclonal antibodies to neoantigens expressed on the activation fragment but not the intact fragment.[17,19,21] Detecting antibodies are either monoclonal antibodies against a second antigenic site or polyclonal antibodies. An *activation index*, which is defined as the ratio of the split product to the intact factor, may be useful for evaluating some diseases, including SLE, cryoglobulinemia, sepsis, and membranoproliferative glomerulonephritis type I.[27,30] The activation index is useful because it can give an estimate of the fractional catabolic rate of the intact components.[30] Examples of activation indexes include ratios for C4d/C4 and Bb/factor B.

Despite the high sensitivity and specificity of complement activation product assays, some caution is warranted before interpreting these measurements. For example, a potential disadvantage of measuring activation fragments with low molecular weights, such as C4a and Bb, is that their circulating levels may be falsely elevated in patients with impaired renal function because these fragments are normally excreted in urine.[31] Another disadvantage of these assays is the fact that patient samples that are not properly collected and processed can show significant in vitro complement activation, thus yielding falsely elevated results.[3,16] (The issue of specimen collection is addressed in more detail later in this chapter.)

C1 Esterase Inhibitor Assays

C1 esterase inhibitor assays are particularly important to aid in the diagnosis of a hereditary or acquired deficiency or dysfunction of C1EI[12] (**Table 6-3**). C1EI abnormalities are observed in hereditary angioedema (HAE), an autosomal dominant disorder characterized by recurrent subcutaneous or mucosal edema.[32] Two forms of HAE have been described.[33] The more common variety, type I HAE, accounts for 85% of affected patients and is characterized by low circulating levels of antigenic C1EI protein due to a synthetic or regulatory gene defect.[15] In addition, the C1EI in affected patients typically also has reduced functional activity. The second variety of HAE, type II HAE, similarly presents with dysfunctional C1EI. However, the antigenic levels of C1EI in affected patients may be normal or decreased.[15]

Both antigenic and functional C1EI assays are recommended for patients suspected of having HAE. C1 esterase inhibitor antigenic assays are usually performed by rate nephelometry or RID. For measurement of functional C1EI activity, both qualitative and quantitative assays have been described.[34,35] In the qualitative assay, as first described by Ziccardi and Cooper,[34] patient serum complement is first activated in vitro and then assayed by RID using anti-C1r. If functional C1EI is present, it binds to activated C1r and subsequently masks anti-C1r binding sites on C1r. Thus, no precipitin ring indicates the presence of functional C1EI and vice versa. A quantitative C1EI functional assay based on measuring residual C1s after incubation with C1EI in the patient's serum has been reported.[36] A commercially available ELISA functional C1EI assay also is available.

In addition to qualitative and quantitative defects in C1EI, autoantibodies to C1EI that presumably inhibit C1EI functional activity are sometimes found in association with a syndrome called acquired angioedema.[37] In this disease, anti-C1EI is not always present, and C1EI antigenic levels may be normal or variably decreased.[32,33] Enzyme-linked immunosorbent assay is the preferred method for detecting C1EI autoantibodies. In the standard method, C1EI autoantibodies bind to purified C1EI coated in ELISA plate wells.[37] Because IgM, IgA, and (primarily) IgG C1EI autoantibodies have been observed,[33] either a polyclonal detecting reagent or all 3 individual Ig-detecting reagents should be employed in the standard method.

Table 6-3. Clinical Utility of C1 Esterase Inhibitor Assays

Disease	C1EI Antigen	C1EI Function	C1EI Autoantibody
Type I HAE	Decreased	Decreased	Negative
Type II HAE	Normal or decreased	Decreased	Negative
Type I AAE	Normal or decreased	Decreased	Negative
Type II AAE	Normal or decreased	Decreased	Positive

Abbreviations: C1EI = C1 esterase inhibitor; HAE = hereditary angioedema; AAE = acquired angioedema.

Circulating Immune Complex Assays

Circulating immune complexes (CICs) and complement are intimately related, not only because CICs are potent complement activators but also because complement fragments that bind CICs in vivo help prevent immune precipitation, solubilize immune aggregates, and promote CIC clearance via binding to cell surface complement receptors.[38–40] Circulating immune complexes differ markedly in size and molecular character, due in part to the diverse physiochemical properties of the antigens and antibodies that comprise them.[41] Small CICs activate complement poorly and are inefficient in promoting the immune response. Large complexes are potent complement activators but are rapidly cleared from the circulation. Intermediate-sized CICs may be the most pathologic because they activate complement well but are not cleared from the circulation as efficiently as are large complexes.[41] Circulating immune complexes may contain Ig of any of the 3 classes (IgM, IgG, and IgA) and include the IgG subclasses IgG1 through IgG4.[39,41] All 3 Ig classes are clinically relevant, so appropriate considerations should be made when choosing and designing CIC assays. Circulating immune complex assays are not particularly sensitive or reliable as indices of disease activity.[41–43] According to the 1988 IUIS/WHO report,[23] detection of CICs was not considered essential in any clinical condition but may be helpful for assessing and monitoring disease activity in conditions such as rheumatoid arthritis and SLE. Circulating immune complexes have been found in a wide variety of diseases, some of which are listed in **Table 6-4**.

A large number of CIC assays vary markedly in methodology as well as in the size and type of CIC detected[17,39,41] (**Table 6-5**). With the notable exception of methods that detect CIC via binding to staphylococcal protein A or to monoclonal rheumatoid factor,[41] most assays measure CIC by quantitating complement activation fragments (eg, C1q, C3bi, C3dg) that are bound to the CIC.[17,41]

The complement-dependent CIC assays are divided into 2 groups. In the first group, CICs are detected by measuring free CICs that bind to complement fragments in vitro in the assay reaction mixture. Two assays in this group are the fluid-phase and solid-phase C1q binding assays.[46,47] The fluid-phase C1q assay is based on CICs binding to radiolabeled C1q, after which the labeled CIC-C1q multimers are quantitated after separation from the unbound label.[47] The results are often expressed in terms of percent of total labeled C1q bound to the CIC. In the solid-phase C1q assay, CICs are allowed to bind to ELISA plates coated with purified C1q.[46] Bound CICs are detected using a tagged anti-Ig. The results are typically compared with a standard curve consisting of heat-aggregated IgG. One major disadvantage of the solid-phase method is that monomeric Ig autoantibodies to C1q also are detected with this method.[48] Anti-C1q autoantibodies reportedly are not detected in the fluid-phase C1q binding assay.[49]

The second group of complement-dependent CIC assays, which includes the Raji cell assay and the conglutinating complement absorption test, are based on the measurement of CIC–complement fragment complexes preformed in vivo.[50,51] The assays already mentioned detect C3bi and/or C3dg fragments attached to CICs.[41] Newer-generation sandwich ELISAs designed for CIC measurement using purified complement fragments offer greater sensitivity, specificity, and reproducibility.[52] Other commercially available assays are based on the detection of CICs bound to C1q or C3 fragments using monoclonal antibodies against these complement fragments as capture reagents, followed by anti-Ig antibodies as detecting reagents.

Measurement of CICs has been extremely difficult to standardize for a number of reasons. Substantial variations have been observed in the amount of

Table 6-4. Examples of Diseases Associated With Circulating Immune Complexes[38,40,44,45]

Class	Disease
Autoimmune	SLE Rheumatoid arthritis Sjögren's syndrome Scleroderma Behçet's disease Mixed connective tissue disease Seronegative spondyloarthropathies Vasculitis
Infectious disease	Streptococcal infections Viral hepatitis Cytomegalovirus AIDS Mycobacterial infections Parasitic infections
Pulmonary	Cystic fibrosis Idiopathic interstitial pneumonitis
Allergy	Asthma Rhinitis
Cutaneous	Dermatitis herpetiformis Cutaneous vasculitis Psoriasis
Renal	Glomerulonephritis Nephrotic syndrome
Neurologic	Multiple sclerosis Myasthenia gravis Guillain-Barré syndrome
Endocrine	Diabetes Hashimoto's disease Graves' disease

Abbreviations: SLE = systemic lupus erythematosus; AIDS = acquired immunodeficiency syndrome.

Table 6-5. Circulating Immune Complex Assays

Complex Measured	Assays
x-CIC*	Fluid-phase C1q binding assay Solid-phase C1q binding assay
C1q-CIC, C3bi-CIC, C3dg-CIC†	Raji cell assay Conglutinin binding assay ELISA; anti-C1q or C3 activation fragments as capture antibody

Abbreviations: CIC = circulating immune complex; ELISA = enzyme-linked immunosorbent assay.

**x-CIC indicates circulating immune complexes that contain available C1q binding sites.*

†Assays for these immune complexes measure the complement activation fragment that is bound to the immune complex.

CIC detected among the various assays, probably due to assay differences in the size range of CICs detected, the Ig classes measured, and the large interassay variation noted for some assays, particularly the Raji cell assay.[53] The results of an interlaboratory comparison of 6 CIC methods performed in 9 laboratories revealed poor to modest agreement.[54] The lack of agreement was attributed in part to the reference preparation used for testing.[54] In addition, many of the assays detect aggregated IgG, so care must be taken to avoid artifactual in vitro Ig aggregation in patient samples.[41] Finally, the lack of a WHO international standard or equivalent, as well as the inherent difficulties involved in the preparation of in-house CIC standards, has contributed significantly to the lack of interlaboratory correlation.

Complement Autoantibody Assays

Two groups of autoantibodies against complement proteins have been found to be clinically relevant: anti-C1EI and "nephritic factor" autoantibodies.[55–59] Anti-C1EI, which is associated with type II acquired angioedema, was discussed earlier. Nephritic factor autoantibodies are composed of at least 3 types, which are directed against various activated complement complexes.[55-58] The term *nephritic* refers to the fact that all are found in association with glomerulonephritis, particularly membranoproliferative glomerulonephritis (MPGN). The autoantibodies referred to as NFa (more commonly known as C3 nephritic factor) are directed against activated factor B as part of the C3bBb complex. C3 nephritic factor causes prolongation of C3 cleaving activity, with resulting decreased circulating C3 levels.[57] The autoantibody NFt similarly binds to the C3bBb complex but differs in that it converts C3 more slowly, requires properdin for maximum effectiveness, and causes activation of the terminal pathway.[56] The autoantibody C4 nephritic factor (NFc) binds to a neoantigen exposed in the C4b2a complex.[55] Anti-C1q belongs to a fourth class of nephritic factor autoantibodies.[59] Anti-C1q antibodies cause disregulation of classical pathway activation, leading to a decrease in C2 and C4. [59] Serum anti-C1q is best recognized as a diagnostic marker for hypocomplementemic urticarial vasculitis syndrome.[60,61] Anti-C1q also has been found in association with autoimmune-mediated renal disease, such as MPGN, in which anti-C1q may be located within subendothelial immune deposits. In addition, anti-C1q is found in up to 46% of SLE patients.[49] In these patients, serum anti-C1q is associated with MPGN and thus may be a useful marker for monitoring the progression or activity of renal disease.[62] Diseases associated with nephritic factor autoantibodies are summarized in **Table 6-6**.

Assays for nephritic factors, particularly C3 and C4, are based on cross-immunoelectrophoresis, hemolytic, and ELISA assay formats. In cross-immunoelectrophoresis assays, C3b and C3c are measured after alternative pathway activation of reagent serum in the presence of patient serum that contains nephritic factors.[67] Hemolytic assays are based on the ability of nephritic factors in patient serum to alter the rate of decay of C3bBb or C4b2a on erythrocytes.[68] An ELISA method has been reported that quantitates nephritic factors by measuring their effect on C3bBbP complexes formed in ELISA plates using purified components.[69]

Table 6-6. Diseases Associated With Antinephritic Antibodies[20,55,63-66]

Autoantibody	Diseases
NFa	Type II MPGN; partial lipodystrophy; poststreptococcal glomerulonephritis; SLE; idiopathic rapidly progressive glomerulonephritis, occasionally associated with types I and III MPGN
NFt	Types I and III MPGN
NFc	Type I MPGN; acute postinfectious glomerulonephritis; SLE; chronic glomerulonephritis
Anti-C1q	SLE; Sjögren's syndrome; Types I, II, and III MPGN; HUVS

Abbreviations: MPGN = membranoproliferative glomerulonephritis; SLE = systemic lupus erythematosus; HUVS = hypocomplementemic urticarial vasculitis syndrome.

Clinical Conditions That Warrant the Use of Complement Assays

Recurrent Infections

Although relatively rare, genetic complement deficiencies should be considered for patients with recurrent infections, especially systemic neisserial infections such as meningococcal meningitis or meningococcemia.[3,17,18] In patients with recurrent bacterial, viral, fungal, or parasitic infections without genetic complement deficiencies, evidence of complement activation may frequently be present, especially activation of the alternative pathway.[3,70] Quantitative measurements of complement activation in these patients may or may not correlate with severity of disease.[3]

Autoimmune/Immune Complex Diseases

Many autoimmune-mediated clinical syndromes have been associated with complement activation, but the most widely studied are SLE and serum sickness.[19,71] The clinical disease activity in these syndromes has been shown in some patients to rise and fall in indirect proportion with CH_{50}, C3, and C4 levels.[17,19] However, levels of the multimolecular activation products C1-C1EI, C3bBbP, and SC5b-9, as well as the split products C3d, C4d-Ba, and Bb are reported to be better markers of disease activity than measurements of intact complement components.[16,19,27,29,30,72] This general scheme also holds true for rheumatoid arthritis and other rheumatic diseases.[16] Patients with renal disorders and associated immune complex disease may demonstrate depressed levels of intact complement components, such as C3 and C4, as well as elevations in activation fragments or complexes such as Ba, Bb, C3a, C4a, C3dg, and SC5b-9.[3,15,27,29,73] As mentioned previously, serum measurements of small activation fragments in diseases with impaired renal function should be interpreted with caution, because some of these fragments may be cleared normally by the kidney.[16]

Other Diseases

A wide variety of diseases or conditions accompanied by in vivo complement activation other than those already mentioned may also exhibit abnormal circulating complement values. Adult respiratory distress syndrome associated with sepsis or trauma can be accompanied by significant activation of both the classical and alternative pathways.[74] In hemolytic-uremic syndrome, approximately 33% of children may have hypocomplementemia in the acute phase of the disease. Persistently abnormal complement levels in this syndrome may be a poor prognostic indicator.[75] In demyelinating diseases, such as multiple sclerosis, complement activation products have been demonstrated in the cerebrospinal fluid.[76] Complement activation during hyperacute rejection may be mediated by the classical pathway via antibodies to the endothelium of the transplanted organ or the alternative pathway via direct interaction of complement with the donor endothelium.[77] Various forms of extracorporeal circulation, such as cardiopulmonary bypass, hemodialysis, and apheresis, are associated with inflammatory reactions involving complement.[8] Thus, the degree of complement activation may be an important factor in determining biocompatibility. In all of these diseases or conditions, intact complement components may be decreased and/or complement activation products may be increased, which may or may not correlate with the severity of the disease or condition.[2] Examples of various diseases associated with abnormal serum complement levels are shown in **Table 6-7**.

Sample Processing

Certain handling requirements are necessary for blood specimens used for complement component evaluation to prevent in vitro activation and to preserve functional complement activity. Specimen handling requirements are more stringent for some assays than for others, but generally it is recommended that plasma or serum be separated from cells and stored at or below –70°C as soon as possible after

Table 6-7. Diseases or Conditions That Frequently Demonstrate Abnormal Complement Circulating Levels

Disease Class	Disease or Condition	Complement Assays	References
Angioedema	HAE, AAE	C1EI antigen and functional, anti-C1EI	12,78,79
Autoimmune/ immune complex disease	C deficiencies (C1q, C1r, C1s, C2-C4)	F→A	18,71,80
	Heterologous serum sickness	M,S,F,A	19,29,47
	Rheumatoid arthritis (vasculitis)	M,S,F,A	2,15
	Essential mixed cryoglobulinemia	M,S,F,A	49
	System vasculitis	M,S,F,A	2,15
	MPGN and other forms of glomerulonephritis	M,S,F,A, nephritic factors	2,41
	Hypocomplementemic urticarial vasculitis syndrome	M,S,F,A, anti-C1q	2,73
	IgA nephropathy	M,S,F,A	49,59,61
Infectious	C deficiency (C1q; C2-C9; factors I, D, and H; properdin)	F→A	18,80
	Recurrent neisserial and meningococcal infections	M,S,F,A	81
	Poststreptococcal glomerulonephritis	M,S,F,A	41
	Septic shock	M,S,F,A	70
	Pneumococcal sepsis	M,S,F,A	41
	Gram-negative sepsis	M,S,F,A	41
	Viremias (hepatitis B, measles, dengue)	M,S,F,A	41
	Parasitemias (trypanosomiasis, malaria, babesiosis)	M,S,F,A	41
	Fungal (cryptococcal)	M,S,F,A	3
Other	PNH	DAF or CD59 by flow cytometry	2,18
	ARDS	M,S,F,A	74
	Hemolytic uremic syndrome	M,S,F,A, factor H	75
	Demyelinating diseases	M,S in CSF	76
	Allograft rejection	M,S,F,A	77
	Extracorporeal devices	M,S,F,A	9
	Preeclampsia	M,S,F,A	2

Abbreviations: C1EI = C1 esterase inhibitor; HAE = hereditary angioedema; AAE = acquired angioedema; SLE = systemic lupus erythematosus; MPGN = membranoproliferative glomerulonephritis; F = functional assay (CH_{50}, AP_{50}); M = complement fragment assay (multimolecular complex); S = complement fragment assay (split product); A = antigenic assay for intact components; PNH = paroxysmal nocturnal hemoglobinuria; ARDS = adult respiratory distress syndrome; DAF = decay acceleration factor; CSF = cerebral spinal fluid.

collection.[16,21] Serum is preferred over plasma for functional assays (unless highly diluted EDTA plasma samples are used in the assay), because ethylenediaminetetraacetic acid (EDTA) inhibits complement activation. For serum preparation, whole blood is allowed to clot at room temperature for no more than 1 hour, after which the serum is separated by centrifugation and then aliquoted and frozen. In the author's laboratory, antigenic complement assays for intact factors have not shown significantly different values for matched serum and EDTA plasma samples. For measurement of CICs, the assay results may be altered in samples subjected to repeated freeze/thaw cycles or heat inactivation of complement (56°C for at least 30 minutes) that can cause aggregation of IgG.[41]

Particular attention to sample handling is necessary for complement activation product assays.[16,17,21] Even minimal in vitro complement activation can alter patient results significantly due to the high sensitivity of these assays.[16,21] Blood samples must be collected in EDTA and stored on ice until the plasma is promptly separated and frozen. The addition of proteinase inhibitors, such as nafamostat mesylate (Futhan, Terumo Corporation, Tokyo, Japan) is helpful when sample processing is delayed.[16,21]

Summary

A wide variety of assays are currently available in the clinical laboratory for evaluating the complement system. Assays can broadly be divided into those that quantitate intact complement proteins or proteolytic activation fragments in plasma and those that detect serum autoantibodies that cause disregulation of the complement system. Assays that quantitate intact complement proteins are useful for ruling out genetic deficiencies but are less useful for evaluating the small decreases in intact components that frequently occur as a consequence of complement activation in inflammatory disorders. Complement activation fragment assays are highly sensitive and specific for monitoring complement activation, but their clinical utility is not well defined. Assays that measure C1EI using functional or antigenic methods are useful for diagnosis of hereditary angioedema. Circulating immune complex assays may be useful for assessing or monitoring disease activity in conditions such a RA or SLE, as well as a variety of other diseases. Assays that detect C3 and C4 nephritic factors, as well those that detect autoantibodies to C1EI and C1q, are helpful as an aid in the diagnosis of various autoimmune diseases. Diagnostic testing to evaluate the complement system can be useful for patients with a wide variety of immune-related diseases and conditions. However, complement assays are most beneficial for diagnosis of genetic complement deficiency, for diagnosis and monitoring of immune complex-mediated diseases, for etiologic diagnosis of chronic urticaria or recurrent angioedema, and for evaluation of patients with recurrent infections.

References

1. Lim HW. The complement system: Activation, modulation, and clinical relevance. *Dermatol Clin*. 1990;8:609–618.
2. Holers VM. Complement. In: Rich RR, Fleisher TA, Schwartz BD, et al, eds. *Clinical Immunology Principles and Practice*. St. Louis, MO: Mosby Year Book; 1996:363–391.
3. Khan WA, Wigfall DR, Frank MM. Complement and kinins: Mediators of inflammation. In: Henry JB, ed. *Clinical Diagnosis and Management by Laboratory Methods*. 19th ed. Philadelphia, PA: WB Saunders Co; 1996:928–946.
4. Lachmann PJ, Hughes-Jones NC. Initiation of complement activation. *Springer Semin Immunopathol*. 1984;7:143–162.
5. Müller-Eberhard HJ, Schreiber RD. Molecular biology and chemistry of the alternative pathway of complement. *Adv Immunol*. 1980;29:1–53.
6. Pangburn MK. Activation of complement via the alternative pathway. *Fed Proc*. 1983;42:139–143.
7. Müller-Eberhard HJ. Chemistry and function of the complement system. *Hosp Pract*. 1977;12:33–43.
8. Matsushita M, Fujita T. Activation of the classical complement pathway by mannose-binding protein in association with a novel C1s-like serine protease. *J Exp Med*. 1992;176:1497–1502.
9. Chenoweth DE. Anaphylatoxin formation in extracorporeal circuits. *Complement*. 1986;3:152–165.
10. Shin ML, Carney DF. Cytotoxic action and other metabolic consequences of terminal complement proteins. *Prog Allergy*. 1988;40:44–81.
11. Bhakdi S, Roth M. Fluid-phase SC5b-8 complex of human complement: Generation and isolation from serum. *J Immunol*. 1981;127:576–580.
12. Davis AE III. C1 inhibitor and hereditary angioneurotic edema. *Annu Rev Immunol*. 1988;6:595–628.
13. Lachmann PJ. The control of homologous lysis. *Immunol Today*. 1991;12:312–315.

14. Parker CJ. Regulation of complement by membrane proteins: An overview. *Curr Top Microbiol Immunol.* 1992;178:1–6.

15. Glovsky MM. Applications of complement determinations in human disease. *Ann Allergy.* 1994;72:477–490.

16. Ahmed AEE, Peter JB. Clinical utility of complement assessment (mini review). *Clin Diagn Lab Immunol.* 1995;2:509–517.

17. Fries LF III. Diagnostic evaluation of the complement system. In: Rich RR, Fleisher TA, Schwartz BD, et al, eds. *Clinical Immunology Principles and Practice.* St. Louis, MO: Mosby Year Book; 1996:2157–2168.

18. Winkelstein JA, Sullivan KE. Complement deficiencies. In: Rich RR, Fleisher TA, Schwartz BD, et al, eds. *Clinical Immunology Principles and Practice.* St. Louis, MO: Mosby Year Book; 1996:662–676.

19. Buyon JP, Tamerius J, Belmont HM, et al. Assessment of disease activity and impending flare in patients with systemic lupus erythematosus: Comparison of the use of complement split products and conventional measurements of complement. *Arthritis Rheum.* 1992;35:1028–1037.

20. West CD. The complement profile in clinical medicine. Inherited and acquired conditions lowering the serum concentrations of complement component and control proteins. *Complement Inflamm.* 1989;6:49–64.

21. Porcel JM, Peakman M, Senaldi G, et al. Methods for assessing complement activation in the clinical immunology laboratory (mini review). *J Immunol Methods.* 1993;157:1–9.

22. Whaley K. Measurement of complement activation in clinical practice. *Complement Inflamm.* 1989;6:96–103.

23. Bentwich Z, Beverley PCL, Hammarstrom L, et al. Laboratory investigations in clinical immunology: Methods, pitfalls, and clinical indications. A second IUIS/WHO report. IUIS/WHO working group. *Clin Immunol Immunopathol.* 1988;49:478–497.

24. Sanders ME, Schmetz MA, Hammer CH, et al. Quantification of activation of the human terminal complement pathway by ELISA. *J Immunol Methods.* 1985;85:245–256.

25. Whaley K. Measurement of complement. In: Whaley K, ed. *Methods in Complement for Clinical Immunologists.* New York, NY: Churchill-Livingstone; 1985:77–139.

26. Maillet F, Fremeaux-Bacchi V, Uhring-Lambert B, et al. Assessment of complement activation in clinical samples. *J Immunol Methods.* 1992;156:171–178.

27. Belmont HM, Hopkins P, Edelson HS, et al. Complement activation during systemic lupus erythematosus: C3a and C5a anaphylatoxins circulate during exacerbations of disease. *Arthritis Rheum.* 1986;29:1085–1089.

28. Sanders ME, Alexander EL, Koski CL, et al. Detection of activated terminal complement (C5b-9) in cerebrospinal fluid from patients with central nervous system involvement of primary Sjögren's syndrome or systemic lupus erythematosus. *J Immunol.* 1987;138:2095–2099.

29. Abramson SB, Weissmann G. Complement split products and the pathogenesis of SLE. *Hosp Pract.* 1988;23:45–56.

30. Rabson AR. Complement activation. In: Rose NR, Conway de Macario E, Folds JD, et al, eds. *Manual of Clinical Laboratory Immunology.* 5th ed. Washington, DC: ASM Press; 1997:187-191.

31. Abou-Ragheb HHA, Williams AJ, Brown CB, et al. Plasma levels and mode of excretion of the anaphylatoxins C3a and C4a in renal disease. *J Clin Lab Immunol.* 1991;35:113–119.

32. Gelfand JA, Boss GR, Conley CL, et al. Acquired C1 esterase inhibitor deficiency and angioedema: A review. *Medicine.* 1979;58:321–328.

33. Davis AE III, Cicardi M. C1 inhibitor autoantibodies. In: Peter JB, Shoenfeld Y, eds. *Autoantibodies.* Amsterdam, the Netherlands: Elsevier Science; 1996:126–131.

34. Ziccardi RJ, Cooper NR. Development of an immunological test to assess C1 inactivator function in human serum and its use for the diagnosis of hereditary angioedema. *Clin Immunol Immunopathol.* 1980;15:465–471.

35. Cicardi M, Bisiani G, Cugno M, et al. Autoimmune C1 inhibitor deficiency: Report of eight patients. *Am J Med.* 1993;95:169–175.

36. Munkvad S, Jespersen J, Gram J, et al. Effects of methylamine and heparin on a rapid chromogenic assay of C1-esterase inhibitor in plasma. *Clin Chem.* 1990;36:737–741.

37. Jackson J, Sim RB, Whelan A, et al. An IgG autoantibody which inactivates C1-inhibitor. *Nature.* 1986;323:722–724.

38. Kimberly RP. Immune complexes in the rheumatic diseases. *Rheum Dis Clin North Am.* 1987;13:583–596.

39. Phillips TM. Immune complex assays: Diagnostic and clinical application. *Crit Rev Clin Lab Sci.* 1989;27:237–264.

40. Davies KA, Schifferli JA, Walport MJ. Complement deficiency and immune complex disease. *Springer Semin Immunopathol.* 1994;15:397–416.

41. Ruddy S, Moxley G. Clinical utility of assays for immune complexes and complement. *Immunol Allergy Clin North Am.* 1994;14:387–400.

42. McCarthy D, Goddard DH, Holborrow EJ, et al. The effect of IgG aggregate size and concentration on reactivity in immune complex assays. *J Immunol Methods.* 1981;47:349–358.

43. McDougal JS, Hubbard M, Strobel PL, et al. Comparison of five assays for immune complexes in the rheumatic diseases. Performance characteristics of the assays. *J Lab Clin Med*. 1982;100:705–719.

44. Nydegger UE, Davis JS. Soluble immune complexes in human disease. *CRC Crit Rev Clin Lab Sci*. 1980;12:123–170.

45. Theofilopoulos AN, Dixon FJ. Immune complexes in human diseases. *Am J Pathol*. 1980;100:531–594.

46. Abrass CK, Nies KM, Louie JS, et al. Correlation and predictive accuracy of circulating immune complexes with disease activity in patients with systemic lupus erythematosus. *Arthritis Rheum*. 1980;23:273–282.

47. Lloyd W, Schur PH. Immune complexes, complement and anti-DNA in exacerbations of systemic lupus erythematosus (SLE). *Medicine*. 1981;60:208–217.

48. Hack CE, Belmer AJM. The IgG detected in the C1q solid-phase immune-complex assay is not always of immune-complex nature. *Clin Immunol Immunopathol*. 1986;38:120–128.

49. Wener MH, Uwatoko S, Mannik M. Antibodies to the collagen like region of C1q in sera of patients with autoimmune rheumatic diseases. *Arthritis Rheum*. 1989;32:544–551.

50. Eisenberg RA, Theofilopoulos AN, Dixon FJ. Use of bovine conglutinin for the assay of immune complexes. *J Immunol*. 1977;118:1428–1434.

51. Andrews BS, Ascher MS, Barada FA Jr, et al. The Raji cell radioimmunoassay in patients with systemic lupus erythematosus: Clinical significance and relationships to other serologic variables assessed by discriminant analysis. *J Rheumatol*. 1985;12:718–723.

52. Durand CG, Burge JJ. A new enzyme-linked immunosorbent assay (ELISA) for measuring immunoconglutinins directed against the third component of human complement: Findings in systemic lupus erythematosus. *J Immunol Methods*. 1984;73:57–66.

53. McDougal JS, Hubbard M, McDuffie FC, et al. Comparison of five assays for immune complexes in the rheumatic diseases: An assessment of their validity for rheumatoid arthritis. *Arthritis Rheum*. 1982;25:1156–1166.

54. Nydegger UE, Svehag SE. Improved standardization in the quantitative estimation of soluble immune complexes making use of an international reference preparation: Results of a collaborative multicentre study. *Clin Exp Immunol*. 1984;58:502–509.

55. Halbwachs L, Levillé M, Lesavre PH, et al. Nephritic factor of the classical pathway of complement. *J Clin Invest*. 1980;65:1249–1256.

56. Clardy CW, Forristal J, Strife CF, et al. A properdin dependent nephritic factor slowly activating C3, C5 & C9 in MPGN types I and III. *Clin Immunol Immunopathol*. 1989;50:333–347.

57. Tsokos GC, Stitzel AE, Patel AD, et al. Human polyclonal and monoclonal IgG and IgM complement 3 nephritic factors: Evidence for idiotypic commonality. *Clin Immunol Immunopathol*. 1989;53:113–122.

58. Peter JB. Nephritic factor antibodies. In: Peter JB, ed. *Use and Interpretation of Tests in Clinical Immunology*. 8th ed. Santa Monica, CA: Specialty Laboratories; 1991:169–170.

59. Wener MH, Mannik M. C1q autoantibodies. In: Peter JB, Shoenfeld Y, eds. *Autoantibodies*. Amsterdam, the Netherlands: Elsevier Science; 1996:132–138.

60. Zeiss CR, Burch FX, Marder RJ, et al. A hypocomplementemic vasculitis urticarial syndrome: Report of four new cases and definition of the disease. *Am J Med*. 1980;68:867–875.

61. Wisnieski JJ, Baer AN, Christensen J, et al. Hypocomplementemic urticarial vasculitis syndrome: Clinical and serologic findings in 18 patients. *Medicine*. 1995;74:24–41.

62. Siegert CE, Daha MR, Tseng CM, et al. Predictive value of IgG autoantibodies against C1q for nephritis in systemic lupus erythematosus. *Ann Rheum Dis*. 1993;52:851–856.

63. Gigli I, Sorrillo J, Halbwachs L, et al. Mechanism of action of the C4 nephritic factor. *J Exp Med*. 1981;154:1–12.

64. Jackson EC, McAdams AJ, Strife CF, et al. Differences between membranoproliferative glomerulonephritis types I and III in clinical presentation, glomerular morphology, and complement perturbation. *Am J Kidney Dis*. 1987;9:115–120.

65. Fujita T, Sumita T, Yoshida S, et al. C4 nephritic factor in a patient with chronic glomerulonephritis. *Clin Lab Immunol*. 1987;22:65–70.

66. Tanuma Y, Ohi H, Hatano M. Two types of C3 nephritic factor: Properdin-dependent C3NeF and properdin-independent C3NeF. *Clin Immunol Immunopathol*. 1990;56:226–238.

67. Giclas PC, Wisnieski JJ. Autoantibodies to complement components. In: Rose NR, Conway de Macario E, Folds JD, et al, eds. *Manual of Clinical Laboratory Immunology*. 5th ed. Washington, DC: ASM Press; 1997:960–967.

68. Daha MR, Fearon DT, Austin KF. C3 nephritic factor (C3NeF): Stabilization of fluid phase and cell-bound alternative pathway convertase. *J Immunol*. 1976;116:1–7.

69. Seino J, van der Wall Bake WL, van Es LA, et al. A novel ELISA assay for the detection of C3 nephritic factor. *J Immunol Methods*. 1993;159:221–227.

70. Lin RY, Astiz ME, Saxon JC, et al. Alterations in C3, C4, factor B, and related metabolites in septic shock. *Clin Immunol Immunopathol*. 1993;69:136–142.

71. Agnello V. Lupus diseases associated with hereditary and acquired deficiencies of complement. *Semin Immunopathol*. 1986;9:161–178.

72. Rother E, Lang B, Coldeway R, et al. Complement split product C3d as an indicator of disease activity in systemic lupus erythematosus. *Clin Rheumatol.* 1993;12:31–35.

73. Hebert LA, Cosio FG, Birmingham DJ. The role of the complement system in renal injury. *Semin Nephrol.* 1992;12:408–427.

74. Langlois PF, Gawryl MS. Complement activation occurs through both classical and alternative pathways prior to onset and resolution of adult respiratory distress syndrome. *Clin Immunol Immunopathol.* 1988;47:152–163.

75. Gonzalo A, Mampaso F, Gallego N, et al. Hemolytic uremic syndrome with hypocomplementemia and deposits of IgM and C3 in the involved renal tissue. *Clin Nephrol.* 1981;16:193–199.

76. Hartung H-P, Jung S, Stoll G, et al. Inflammatory mediators in demyelinating disorders of the CNS and PNS. *J Neuroimmunol.* 1992;40:197–210.

77. Dalmasso AP. The complement system in xenotransplantation. *Immunopharmacology.* 1992;24:149–160.

78. Rosen FS, Alper CA, Pensky J, et al. Genetically determined heterogeneity of the C1 esterase inhibitor in patients with hereditary angioneurotic edema. *J Clin Invest.* 1971;50:21–43.

79. Alsenz J, Bork K, Loos M. Autoantibody-mediated acquired deficiency of C1 inhibitor. *N Engl J Med.* 1987;316:1360–1366.

80. Nusinow SR, Zuraw BL, Calrd JG. The hereditary and acquired deficiencies of complement. *Med Clin North Am.* 1985;69:487–503.

81. Figueroa JE, Densen P. Infectious diseases associated with complement deficiencies. *Clin Microbiol Rev.* 1991;4:359–395.

CHAPTER 7

Human Cytokines: Classification, Clinical Significance, and Laboratory Assays

LeMing Hang, MD, and Robert M. Nakamura, MD

First discovered and described in the 1970s, cytokines are low-molecular-weight regulatory polypeptides (monomer form < 30 kd), which are distinct from immunoglobulins. They are produced and secreted primarily by activated T cells and macrophages. With their versatile hormonelike properties, cytokines serve as cell-to-cell messengers, mediating the physiologic and immunologic events in homeostasis. They communicate and coordinate complex interactions among immune effector and tissue target cells during antigenic challenges. They can exert proinflammatory, anti-inflammatory, immunostimulatory, immunosuppressive, growth promoting, inhibitory, and antitumor effects.[1–4] Over 20 different cytokines have been isolated and characterized. The cytokine family currently includes at least 13 types of interleukins (IL-1 through IL-13), several types of interferons (IFNs), tumor necrosis factors (TNFs), and cellular growth factors.[2,3]

In a healthy individual, cytokines interact to help maintain immunologic and physiologic homeostasis. Increased production and release of cytokines occur when the immune system is activated by pathogens, complement by-products, or immune complexes. The additional cytokines "network" to initiate and propagate complex synergistic, antagonistic, and at times paradoxic events. They can (1) induce or suppress their own production and synthesis of other cytokines, (2) recruit circulating immune effector cells to sites of inflammation, and (3) stimulate effector cells to produce additional immune cell growth factors.[2,4–6] Thus, unregulated or defective cytokine synthesis and release can have pathologic consequences. Cytokine dysregulation and dysfunction have been implicated in various inflammatory, autoimmune, and immunodeficiency diseases.[7–9]

This chapter reviews the current classification and functional characteristics of cytokines; their role in various inflammatory and immunologic diseases; laboratory methods for cytokine testing; and the clinical application of cytokines for disease evaluation, therapy, and prevention.

Classification of Cytokines

As indicated in **Table 7-1**, cytokines can be categorized into the following functionally different groups:

- Proinflammatory/immunostimulatory
- Anti-inflammatory
- "Pleotrophic" (having immunostimulatory, immunosuppressive, and reparative functions)
- Hematopoietic growth factors
- Interferons

Immunobiologic and Pathologic Properties of Cytokines

Interleukin-1, originally known as lymphocyte-activating factor, is produced by white blood cells, activated immune cells, and nonimmune cells (ie, astrocytes and keratinocytes). Synthesis and secretion of IL-1 are stimulated by infection, tissue injury, antigenic challenge, and endotoxins. Once secreted, IL-1 can induce T cells to produce other synergistic cytokines. The local effect of IL-1 is proinflammatory/immunostimulatory, yet IL-1 may induce leukopenia and systemic shock by enhancing production of prostaglandins and nitric oxides. Investigational studies have noted an inverse relationship between the survival of patients in septic shock and their plasma IL-1 and TNF-α levels. Corticosteroids, IL-10, TGF-β, and IL-1 receptor antagonist (ra) can suppress IL-1 synthesis and its activities.[2,10,11]

Originally called T-cell growth factor, IL-2 is produced by activated helper T (Th^1) cells. Circulating IL-2 levels are increased in states of immune activation, such as infection, tissue graft rejection, and autoimmune diseases. Interleukin-2 can activate various immune cells to express IL-2 receptors; stimulate additional Th^1-cell proliferation; and promote the release of IL-1, IL-6, TNF-α, and IFN-γ. Cyclosporine and corticosteroids inhibit IL-2 activity and receptor expression.[1–4,8]

Interleukin-3, originally known as a colony forming unit stimulator, is produced primarily by activated T cells. It stimulates production and maturation of bone marrow precursor cells, mast cells, and specific T-cell subsets.[12]

Interleukin-4, produced by helper T (Th^2) cells, has multiple diverse immunostimulatory and regulatory properties. This type of cytokine can promote immunoglobulin (Ig) E isotype switch and eosinophil-mediated cytotoxicity, inhibit monocytic superoxide production, and deactivate macrophages. Recent studies have shown that IL-4 can antagonize the pathogenic effects of IL-1 and TNF-α released by Th^1 cells. Thus, IL-4 cytokines are being considered for use as immunotherapeutic agents to treat Th^1-related autoimmune diseases.[13,14]

Table 7-1. Major Cytokines: Classification by Functional Characteristics[1-5]

Cytokine	Primary Cell Source	Principal Effect
Proinflammatory and/or immunostimulatory		
IL-1	Myelocytes, NK cells, astrocytes, keratinocytes	Inflammatory and hematopoietic; activates T and B cells; pyrogenic
IL-2	T cells, activated lymphocytes	Activates T and NK cells, expands T cells; induces B-cell maturation
IL-5	Th² cells	Promotes IgA switch and eosinophilia; increases GI tract mucosal immunity
IL-6	Th² cells, fibroblasts, other cells	Increases possibility of intrauterine infections, glomerulonephritis, and myeloma
IL-7	Bone marrow cells, thymic stromal cells	Activates cytotoxic T and NK cells
IL-8	Most immune system cells	Promotes chemotaxis and lymphocyte homing
IL-9	Activated T lymphocytes	Stimulates thymus and erythroid precursors
TNF-α	Macrophages, other cells	Promotes thrombosis and cell necrosis; mediates host response to endotoxins
Anti-inflammatory		
IL-1ra	Th¹ cell	Blocks IL-1 receptor effects (antagonist)
IL-4	Th² cell	Promotes IgE switch and eosinophil cytotoxicity; deactivates macrophages; inhibits monocytes; suppresses Th¹- and Th²-induced inflammation; inhibits IFN-γ, IL-1, and TNF-α function
IL-10	T cells, B cells, thymocytes	Suppresses lymphocyte-cytokine synthesis
TGF-β	Megakaryocytes, osteocytes	Suppresses immune-mediated tissue injuries; promotes wound repair
Hematopoietic growth factors		
IL-3	T cells	Promotes growth of early myeloid cells
IL-6	T cells, fibroblasts, other cells	Promotes B-cell growth and Ig synthesis
IL-7	Stromal cells	Induces pre-B and T-cell proliferation
IL-11	Bone marrow stromal cells	Increases megakaryocytes and platelets
GM-CSF	T cells, other cells	Induces myelopoiesis
G-CSF, M-CSF	Monocytes, other cells	Generates neutrophils and macrophages
Pleotrophic		
IL-12	Macrophages, dendritic cells, EBV-infected lymphocytes, neutrophils	Activates NK and B cells, induces synthesis of inflammatory and immunosuppressive cytokines; exerts antitumor effect
IL-13	T cells	Downgrades IL-1 and IL-6 activities; promotes B-cell proliferation
Interferons		
IFN-α	Leukocytes	Inhibits viral proliferation
IFN-β	Fibroblasts	Promotes repair and tissue fibrosis; inhibits TNF-a activity
IFN-γ	Th¹ and NK cells	Induces and enhances MHC expression by macrophages and target cells; promotes endothelial ICAM synthesis; inhibits B-cell maturation

Abbreviations: NK = natural killer; Th¹/Th² = helper T; Ig = immunoglobulin; GI = gastrointestinal; TNF = tumor necrosis factor; ra = receptor antagonist; IFN = interferon; TGF = transforming growth factor; GM-CSF = granulocyte-macrophage colony-stimulating factor; G-CSF = granulocyte colony-stimulating factor; M-CSF = macrophage colony-stimulating factor; EBV = Epstein-Barr virus; MHC = major histocompatibility complex; ICAM = intercellular adhesion molecules.

Originally known as eosinophil differentiation factor, IL-5 is produced by activated T cells. It can stimulate basophil production and enhance the immune response of gastrointestinal tract mucosa to parasitic infections.[15,16]

Produced by immune and nonimmune cells, IL-6 induces mesangial and keratinocytic cell proliferation, B-cell maturation to plasma cells, and T-cell synthesis of inflammatory cytokines. Levels of IL-6 are increased in patients with glomerulonephritis, plasmacytomas, infection, and various inflammatory states including autoimmune diseases.[17]

Interleukin-7, previously called pre-B cell growth factor, is produced mostly by stromal cells. These cytokines are potent T-cell mitogens and promoters of cytotoxic as well as activated killer cell development.[18]

Produced by immune cells, fibroblasts, and endothelial cells, IL-8 initiates and enhances chemotaxis by inducing endothelial expression of intercellular adhesion molecules (ICAMs), lymphocyte homing, and degranulation. It also can promote tumor growth and angiogenesis.[19,20]

Interleukin-9, produced by activated T cells, stimulates production of megakaryocytes and erythroid precursors. It also can promote IgE synthesis.[21]

Originally termed cytokine synthesis inhibitory factor, IL-10 is produced by activated Th[2] cells. This type of cytokine suppresses inflammation by inducing IL-1ra production and "deactivating" monocytes and macrophages.[10,11,22,23]

Interleukin-11 is produced by bone marrow stromal cells. It promotes megakaryocyte colony growth, platelet production, and hematopoiesis.[24]

Interleukin-12 and IL-13 are pleotrophic cytokines. Interleukin-12, produced by macrophages, dendritic cells, Epstein-Barr virus–infected lymphocytes, and neutrophils, has immunostimulatory, antitumor, and antiangiogenic properties. It enhances cellular and humoral immunity by inducing Th[1] and Th[2] cells to synthesize cytokines and by directly activating natural killer (NK) and B cells.[25,26] Interleukin-13, produced by activated T cells, promotes B-cell proliferation but downregulates the inflammatory activities of IL-1 and IL-6.[1–3]

Tumor necrosis factors, produced mostly by macrophages, have proinflammatory and antitumor activities. They promote tissue thrombosis and cellular necrosis. Increased levels of these factors are seen in patients with sepsis, immune activation, and autoimmune diseases.[27–29]

Transforming growth factor–beta (TGF-β), produced by megakaryocytes and osteocytes, suppresses immune-mediated tissue injury and promotes wound healing.[30–32]

Type I interferons (IFN-α and IFN-β), produced by leukocytes and fibroblasts, have antiviral "interference" properties. Type II interferons (IFN-γ) are produced by T cells and have pleotrophic immunostimulatory and inflammatory properties. They can induce T cells, macrophages, and target cells to express major histocompatibility complex (MHC), promote endothelial cell expression of ICAMs, enhance NK cell cytotoxicity, and inhibit B-cell maturation. Interferon-gamma also can stimulate monocytes and granulocytes to release IL-1 and hydrogen peroxides. It has been implicated in the pathogenesis of various types of autoimmune diseases.[33–35]

Intercellular Adhesion Molecules and Their Clinical Significance

Intercellular adhesion molecules are a family of proinflammatory glycoproteins, produced and expressed by cells of the immune system and endothelium. There are at least 6 types of ICAMs, designated as lymphocyte activating factor (LAF; IL-1), membrane attack complex–1, selectin, integrin, integrin ligands, and CD44 molecules. These glycoproteins promote and perpetuate immune-mediated target tissue damage by inducing circulating leukocytes to adhere to endothelium and transmigrate to inflammatory sites. Intercellular adhesion molecules also may enhance tumor cell dissemination and metastasis. Defective function and production of ICAMs have been noted in various immunodeficiency diseases.[1,36-38]

Regulation of Cytokine Activities and Interactions

The physiologic activities and immunopathologic effects of various cytokines are regulated and modulated by the following processes:

- Inhibition of cytokine receptor expression on target cell surfaces
- Production of cytokine receptor antagonists
- Secretion of soluble cytokine receptors to intercept cytokine activities
- Competitive binding of cytokine receptors with cytokine antibodies and nonimmune proteins

Inhibition of Cytokine Receptor Expression on Target Cell Surfaces

To initiate the intended immunologic and inflammatory events, cytokines induce synthesis and expression of their respective receptors on target cell surfaces. Cytokine receptors allow the interaction of cytokines with intracellular tyrosine kinase pathways to signal enzymatic and physiologic changes. Cytokine receptor expression by target cells may be inhibited or enhanced by other cytokines.[4,29,39]

Production of Cytokine Receptor Antagonists

Cytokine receptor antagonists, induced by IL-10, serve to inhibit binding of cytokines to their surface receptors on target cells. The IL-1 receptor antagonist has been the most extensively studied. It shares 26% amino acid homology with IL-1, and an excess of 10 to 100 times the normal level of IL-1 receptor antagonists is needed to prevent IL-1 from binding with receptors on target cells. The antagonistic effects on IL-1 function do not interfere with "physiologic immunity." Phase I trials using IL-1ra for the treatment of endotoxin shock, rheumatoid arthritis, graft-versus-host disease, myeloproliferative disorders, and asthmatic crisis have been instituted.[39–42]

Secretion of Soluble Cytokine Receptors

"Soluble" cytokine receptors are found in the blood and tissues of healthy individuals as well as patients with inflammatory and immunologic diseases. These soluble receptors are generated by either proteolysis of the extracellular domains of cell surface receptors or splicing of cDNA. They bind with cytokines to inhibit their effect but may paradoxically prolong the half-life of their respective cytokines by serving as "carrier proteins."[1,39–41]

Competitive Binding of Cytokines With Antibodies and Nonimmune Proteins

Natural autoantibodies (NAAs) that react with IL-1, TNF-α, and IL-6 cytokines can be found in up to 20% of healthy individuals.[42–45] Nonimmune proteins, such as uromodulin and α_2-microglobulins, which are synthesized in the kidney and liver, can bind to various cytokines. These NAAs and nonimmune proteins interfere with cytokine immunoassays, but their in vivo activities and clinical significance are unclear.[39,46,47]

Role of Cytokines in Immunologic Diseases

Cytokine defects, dysfunction, and dysregulation have been observed in various types of immunodeficiency and autoimmune diseases. Examples of immunodeficiency diseases associated with cytokine defects and dysfunction (**Table 7-2**) include the following:

- X-linked severe combined immunodeficiency disease is associated with IL-2-RG gene mutation and production of structurally defective IL-2 cytokines. Such IL-2 defects cause helper T-cell and B-cell incompetence.[1,8]

Table 7-2. Immunodeficiency Diseases Associated With Cytokine Defects[48-53]

Disease	Defect
X-linked SCID	IL-2-RG gene mutation, causing defects in IL-2 molecules
SCID with eosinophilia (Omenn's syndrome)	T-cell defects in cytokine production with insufficient IFN-γ and IL-2 but excessive IL-4, IL-5, and IL-10
Hyper-IgM immunodeficiency syndrome	*CD40L* gene deletion
Hyper-IgE immunodeficiency syndrome	T-cell defects in production of IFN-γ and TNF-α
CVI disease	Helper T-cell defect in synthesis of IL-2, IL-4, and IFN-γ
HIV-related acquired immunodeficiency diseases	T-cell defects in production of immunostimulatory cytokines

Abbreviations: SCID = severe combined immunodeficiency disease; IL = interleukin; IFN = interferon; Ig = immunoglobulin; TNF = tumor necrosis factor; CVI = common variable immunodeficiency; HIV = human immunodeficiency virus.

- Severe combined immunodeficiency disease with eosinophilia (Omenn's syndrome) is associated with inadequate levels of IFN-γ and IL-2 but excessive production of IL-4, IL-5, and IL-10. Interferon-gamma treatment can normalize eosinophil counts and cytokine levels.[48]
- Hyperimmunoglobulin M immunodeficiency syndrome is associated with deletion of the *CD40L* gene. CD40L glycoproteins are ICAMs that promote contact between T cells and B cells. Their deficiency causes a failure of B-cell maturation and an inability to proceed with an IgM-IgG isotype switch.[49]
- Hyperimmunoglobulin E immunodeficiency (Job's) syndrome is associated with inadequate and/or defective T-cell production of IFN-γ and TNF-α, causing deficient cell-mediated immunity and unregulated IgE synthesis. Interferon-gamma replacement therapy has been effective in improving patients' immune status.[50]
- Common variable immunodeficiency (CVI) disease is associated with defective T-cell synthesis of IL-2, IL-4, and IFN-γ. Interleukin-2 replacement therapy can correct the hypogammaglobulinemia and restore immunocompetence.[51]
- Human immunodeficiency virus (HIV)–related acquired immunodeficiency diseases are associated with T-cell defects in the production of immunostimulatory cytokines.
- Chronic granulomatous disease (CGD) is a disease associated with defects in leukocyte phagocytosis. However, patients with CGD can improve with treatment with IFN-γ.[52] Examples of autoimmune diseases associated with cytokine excess and dysregulation (**Table 7-3**) include the following:
  - Rheumatoid arthritis (but not osteoarthritis) is associated with increased IL-1 and TNF-α levels in patient plasma and synovial fluid.[58,59]
  - Multiple sclerosis is associated with increased TNF-α levels in plasma and cerebrospinal fluid. Patients treated with anti-TNF-α show decreased demyelination and plaque formation.[60,61]
  - Patients with systemic autoimmune disease have increased levels of IL-1, IL-2, IL-6, IL-8, and TNF-α in plasma and eluates from the various immune-mediated tissue lesions.[62]
  - Type 1 diabetes is associated with IFN-γ–induced aberrant MHC class II expressions on islet cells. Such aberrant MHC expression by target cells has been implicated in the immunopathogenesis of type 1 diabetes.[63]
  - Autoimmune lymphocytic thyroiditis is associated with an increased number of Th[1]-cell infiltrates, as well as higher levels of IL-2 and TNF-α in the thyroid gland and other affected organs.[64]
  - Autoimmune "syndromes" may occur in immunodeficient patients who receive IFN-γ and IL-2 replacement therapy.[54]

Numerous studies have confirmed the pathogenic roles of IL-1 and TNF-α in autoimmune diseases by showing that these cytokines enhance and perpetuate the immune complex–mediated target tissue damage by stimulating local production of collagenase and protease. Clinical trials using commercially prepared IL-1ra, TGF-β, and monoclonal anti-TNF-α antibodies as immunosuppressive agents to rheumatoid arthritis, scleroderma, and inflammatory fibrotic diseases of lung and liver have been instituted.[65–67]

Laboratory Testing for Cytokines

Immunoassays, bioassays, and immunohistochemical methods are used to assess cytokine levels in various disease states and also to monitor effects of therapy (**Table 7-4**). The amount detected is reported in picograms or nanograms of cytokine protein per milliliter. Because clotting can induce blood leukocytes to release additional cytokines in vitro, plasma samples are preferred for assay use. The half-life of most cytokines in circulation is short (minutes). Healthy individuals usually have low to undetectable cytokine levels.[68–70] Increased levels of various cytokines are detected in the blood, body fluids, and tissue of patients with infections, neoplasms, and various types of immunologic diseases.

The commercial enzyme-linked immunosorbent assay (ELISA) and enzyme immunoassay kits currently available for measurement of cytokines use monoclonal or polyclonal anticytokine antibodies and enzyme-linked colorimetry as end point reactions. Most commercial reagents have the required specificity, but the test antibodies may bind to inactive cytokine fragments. Moreover, patient body fluids and tissue may contain immune and nonimmune binding proteins, rheumatoid factors, soluble

Table 7-3. Autoimmune Diseases Associated With Cytokine Dysregulation[54-63]

Disease	Dysregulation
Rheumatoid arthritis	Increased IL-1 and TNF-α levels in circulating and synovial fluid
Multiple sclerosis	Increased TNF-α levels in cerebrospinal fluid during active phase of disease
Systemic lupus erythematosus, Sjögren's syndrome, and systemic vasculitis	Increased levels of IL-1, IL-2, IL-6, IL-8, and TNF-α in the circulation
Autoimmune ulcerative colitis or Crohn's disease	Increased IL-1 and TNF-α levels in the circulation and bowel wall tissue
Type 1 diabetes and Graves' disease	Increased IFN-γ–induced aberrant MHC expression in target pancreatic islet and thyroid gland cells
Autoimmune syndromes in immunodeficient patients	Induced by IFN-γ or IL-2 cytokine replacement therapy, which exacerbates latent autoimmune diseases

Abbreviations: IL = interleukin; TNF = tumor necrosis factor; IFN = interferon; MHC = major histocompatibility complex.

Table 7-4. Laboratory Methods for Detection of Cytokines[68-80]

Method	Advantages	Disadvantages
Immunoassays (ELISA or EIA)	Commercial kits available for most cytokines (except IL-3, IL-5, IL-9, IL-11, IL-12) Technically simple Fast turnaround time (results within hours)	Specificity depends on monoclonal antibody used for testing Inactive cytokine fragments also measured Interference from plasma-binding proteins
Bioassays	Sensitive Only active forms of cytokine measured No interference by plasma proteins target cells	Tissue culture lines needed to provide target cells Confirmation by cytokine-specific neutralizing antibody needed for identification Not specific Labor intensive Slow turnaround time (at least a few days)
Hemolytic plaque assays*		
Peripheral blood mononuclear cell stimulation to assess cytokine profiles (see Table 7-6)*		
Tissue homogenate for ELISA or tissue sections for immunohistochemistry*		
RT-PCR or in situ hybridization to detect cytokine mRNA (cytokine gene expression)*		

Abbreviations: ELISA = enzyme-linked immunosorbent assay; EIA = enzyme immunoassay; IL = interleukin; RT-PCR = reverse-transcription polymerase chain reaction.

**Performed mostly by research laboratories.*

cytokine receptors, protease, and other biologic inhibitors, which can interfere with test results. Pretreatment of the test sample with polyethylene glycol can precipitate and remove some of these interfering and inhibitory substances.[71] Immunoassays have the advantage of technical simplicity and fast turnaround times.

Bioassays, on the other hand, are labor intensive and time consuming, although they may provide more clinically relevant information than immunoassays because they detect only the active forms of cytokines.[69,72] The target cells for each bioassay must be maintained in tissue culture, and identification of the tested cytokine requires additional confirmation by neutralizing cytokine-specific antibodies. Thus, the test turnaround time may be several days. Bioassays are currently used to measure IL-3, IL-5, IL-9, IL-11, and IL-12 because commercial immunoassay kits for these cytokines are not yet widely available.[1,68,69]

More recent methods of cytokine testing used by research centers include hemolytic plaque assays, ELISA using homogenized tissue in place of plasma, and immunostaining to detect cytokines in tissue lesions.[73,74] These methods cannot accurately differentiate intracellular cytokine storage from surface receptor binding.[69,74] The newest quantitation techniques for cytokines involve either measurement of mRNA (cytokine gene expression) in patient plasma by reverse-transcription polymerase chain reaction or in situ hybridization using isotope S–labeled cDNA probes on biopsy tissue cryostat sections.[75–77]

All cytokine assays should be calibrated against reference standards available from the World Health Organization through the Biological Response Modifier Program in Frederick, Maryland. Internal laboratory controls, calibrated against the reference standards, also should routinely be included in the cytokine assays to determine interassay variability. Each laboratory needs to establish its own normal ranges for the cytokines tested.[68,69]

Helper T-Cell Cytokines and Their Clinical Significance

Two helper T-cell cytokine production patterns (cytokine profiles) have been noted: Th^1 and Th^2. Testing involves in vitro stimulation of peripheral blood Th^1 and Th^2 cells with direct measurement of cytokine production by these activated helper cells.[78]

The Th^1 cytokines are IL-2, IFN-γ, and TNF-β. They participate mainly in "cellular immunity" activities, such as delayed hypersensitivity, defense against viral infections, and activation of macrophages and cytotoxic cells. The Th^2 cytokines are IL-4, IL-5, IL-6, IL-10, IL-13, and possibly IL-9; they participate mostly in "humoral immunity" activities such as allergic or atopic reactions, defense against parasites, induction of B-cell maturation to plasma cells, and IgE-IgA isotype switch.

Aberrant Th^1 and Th^2 cytokine profiles (excessive or defective production) have been noted in certain types of autoimmune and immunodeficiency diseases. Predominantly Th^1 cytokine activities are seen in organ-specific autoimmune diseases such as lymphocytic thyroiditis, type 1 diabetes, multiple sclerosis, and inflammatory bowel diseases. Systemic autoimmune diseases may show a predominance of either Th^1 or Th^2 cytokine activities, depending on the stage of the disease. Certain immunodeficiency diseases also are associated with defective Th^1 and/or Th^2 cytokine production.

At present, cytokine assays are mostly used for investigative studies to monitor patients receiving recombinant cytokines and anticytokine immunotherapy. Data from these studies will lead to the establishment of more disease-specific cytokine profiles for future reference and clinical use in patient management.[1,68] Due to the complexity and heterogeneity of cytokine effects and their pleotrophic properties, it is difficult to determine whether the abnormal levels of cytokines noted in various disease states reflect primary or secondary pathologic processes. The levels measured in vitro may not always reflect their in vivo activities. Thus, cytokine test results should be interpreted with caution, and isolated results should not be used as sole determinants in assessing a patient's clinical disease status.

Clinical Applications and Therapeutic Potentials of Cytokines

As researchers gain more knowledge and understanding of cytokine functions in health and disease states, it is found that cytokines can assume important roles in disease evaluation and monitoring, disease therapy, and disease prevention. For example, their functions in disease evaluation and monitoring include the following:

- Incipient septic shock can be forewarned by increasing levels of IL-1 and TNF-α in plasma.
- Intrauterine infection can be indicated by increased IL-6 in amniotic fluid.
- Psoriasis is associated with increased IL-8 levels in plasma.
- Cytokine profiles can be used for evaluation of immunocompetence in patients infected with HIV.
- Autoimmune diseases are associated with certain cytokine profiles (**Table 7-5**).

Table 7-5. Summary of Cytokine Profiles and Functional Overlap[2,4,81-83]

Almost all immunologically active cytokines perform multiple functions, inducing different effects on the same cell type or stimulating several cell types, often with diverse effects.
Cytokines made by one cell often have a number of coordinated functions that regulate a particular aspect of immune response.
The secretion of different sets of cytokines by different T-cell subsets is regulated at both the differentiation and activation stages by other cytokines.
Cytokine "networking" consists of positive and negative feedback cross-regulations. Such networking can induce various coordinated cascades of activities that have the advantage of immune response amplification. However, the consequence of such immune amplification can lead to exaggerated pathophysiologic events that cause extensive tissue damage and even death to the host.

- Certain immunodeficiency diseases are associated with defective production of IL-2, ICAMs, or IFN-γ (see Table 7-2).

Certain cytokines may be used in disease therapy as follows:

- Interferon-α to treat hepatitis B and C, human papillomatosis, HIV, and chronic fatigue syndrome
- Interferon-gamma to treat chronic granulomatous diseases
- Interleukin-2 and IL-4 to treat CVI disease
- Interferon-α and IL-2 to treat patients with acquired immunodeficiency syndrome and mycobacteria and toxoplasmosis[84]
- Granulocyte or macrophage colony-stimulating factor to correct neutropenias in HIV-infected, oncology, and transplant patients[85]
- Interleukin-2 to promote immune effector cell proliferation and activation for immunosuppressed patients with malignancy[53]

Cytokines also may be effective in disease prevention in several ways:

- Septic patients can benefit from prophylactic IL-1ra and anti–TNF-α treatment to avert complications of endotoxin shock.[86,87]
- Infants with intrauterine/neonatal infections may benefit from IFN-γ to increase their ability to defend against invading pathogens.
- Immunodeficient patients can benefit from the use of IL-2 as an immunoadjuvant to enhance their immune response to vaccines.[88]
- Patients with multiple sclerosis can be treated with IFN-β during the active phase of disease to decrease demyelination and plaque formation.
- Patients with rheumatoid arthritis may benefit from TGF-β and anti–TFN-α treatment to decrease the inflammatory and fibrotic destruction of joint tissue.[89]
- Patients with steroid-resistant Crohn's disease may benefit from anti–TNF-α therapy.[90,91]

Clinical trials of prophylactic/preventive IL-1ra therapy for crescentic glomerulonephritis, interstitial lung diseases, and graft-versus-host disease are ongoing. In addition to its use as an antitumor agent for metastatic melanoma and renal and breast carcinoma, IL-12 has been considered for antiviral therapy in certain chronic viral infections, such as HIV and hepatitis B and C.[4,6,11,25,39,81,92]

Summary

Cytokines are polypeptide products of activated immune cells, released during the effector phase of cellular stimulation. By acting as signaling molecules to promote intercellular communications, they contribute to immunoregulation and hematopoiesis. In vitro studies of isolated cells of the immune system have shown that cytokines affect cellular growth, maturation, differentiation, activation, and regulation. They are unique in that their functions overlap, they have synergistic and antagonistic effects, and they are capable of causing various types of both local and systemic pathologic events.

After their release from effector cells, cytokines can network among themselves and the immune system to initiate cascades of inflammatory, immunostimulatory, immunosuppressive, reparative, and destructive processes. This cytokine networking

Table 7-6. Cytokines and Cytokine Antagonists Studied in Ongoing Clinical Trials[1-4,10,14,81,89-92]

Cytokine/Antagonist	Use
Monoclonal anti–IL-1 antibodies	To treat sepsis and endotoxin shock
IL-10 and IFN-γ	To inhibit IL-1 activities by inducing IL-1ra synthesis
IL-1ra	To prevent crescentic glomerulonephritis and graft-versus-host disease
IL-1ra, TGF-β, and monoclonal anti–TNF-α antibodies	As immunosuppressive agents to rheumatoid arthritis, scleroderma, and various inflammatory fibrotic diseases
IL-2	To restore helper T-cell and B-cell functional defects in both congenital and acquired immunodeficiency diseases
IL-4	To treat Th[1]-related autoimmune diseases (can antagonize the inflammatory pathologic effects of Th[1] cytokines IL-1 and TNF-α)
IL-12	To treat certain chronic viral infections (eg, HIV, hepatitis B and C) and as an antitumor agent for metastatic melanoma and renal and breast carcinoma
Monoclonal anti–TNF-α antibodies	To treat steroid-resistant Crohn's disease
IFN-α and IFN-β	As antiviral, antiproliferative, and antiangiogenic agents; depending on dosage and administration schedule, can either enhance or suppress host immunity
IFN-γ	To increase host defense against invading pathogens and also to correct immunodeficiency in patients with chronic granulomatous disease

Abbreviations: IL = interleukin; IFN = interferon; ra = receptor antagonist; TGF = transforming growth factor; TNF = tumor necrosis factor; Th[1] = helper T.

contributes not only to natural immunity and tissue repair but also to pathologic autoimmunity (see Table 7-5). Several cytokines and their antagonists have been cloned and are currently being used in clinical trial studies as immunospecific therapeutic agents. Examples of these are listed in **Table 7-6**, and the preliminary phase I and II results are encouraging.

As cytokines assume greater clinical importance in disease evaluation, therapy, and prophylaxis, the laboratory will be required to offer accurate and expedient cytokine testing. Clinicians will use the test results as valuable guidelines for diagnosis and monitoring of patients' disease progress and the effects of various therapies.

References

1. Fox HS. Cytokines and adhesion molecules. In: Henry JB, ed. *Clinical Diagnosis and Management by Laboratory Methods*. 19th ed. Philadelphia, PA: WB Saunders Co; 1996:947–957.
2. Bellanti JA, Kaldlec JV, Escobar-Gutirrez A. Cytokines and the immune response. *Pediatr Clin North Am.* 1994;41:597–621.
3. Burke F, Stewart NM, Davies B, et al. Cytokine wall chart. *Immunol Today*. 1993;12:239.
4. Arend WP. Inhibiting the effects of cytokines in human diseases. *Adv Intern Med*. 1995;40:365–394.
5. Ward PA. Cytokines, inflammation, and autoimmune diseases. *Hosp Pract*. 1995;30:35–41.
6. Cronstein BN, Weissman G. The adhesion molecule in inflammation. *Arthritis Rheum*. 1993;36:147.
7. Brennan FM, Feldman M. Cytokines in autoimmunity. *Curr Opin Immunol*. 1992;4:754.
8. Voss SD, Hong R, Sondel PM. Severe combined immunodeficiency, interleukin (IL-2), and the IL-2 receptor: Experiments of nature continue to point the way. *Blood*. 1994;83:626–635.
9. Dinarello CA, Wolff SM. Mechanisms of disease: The role of IL1 in diseases. *N Engl J Med*. 1993;328:106–113.
10. Arend WP. IL-1 receptor antagonist. *Adv Immunol.* 1993;54:167–227.
11. Jenkins JK, Malyak M, Arend WP. The effects of IL-10 on IL-1ra and IL-1B production in human monocytes and neutrophils. *Lymphokine Cytokine Res*. 1994;13:47–54.
12. Lindermann A, Mertelsmann R. Interleukin-3: structure and function. *Cancer Invest*. 1993;11:609–623.
13. Lebman DA, Coffman RL. IL-4 causes isotype switching to IgE in T cell stimulated clonal B cell cultures. *J Exp Med*. 1988;168:853–857.

14. Rocken M, Racke M, Shevach EM. IL-4 induced immune deviation as antigen-specific therapy for inflammatory autoimmune disease. *Immunol Today*. 1996;17:225-230.

15. Sanderson CJ. Interleukin-5, eosinophils, and disease. *Blood*. 1992;79:3101-3109.

16. Mahanty S, Nutman TB. The biology of interleukin-5 and its receptor. *Cancer Invest*. 1993;11:624-634.

17. Akira S, Taga T, Kishimoto T. IL-6 in biology and medicine. *Adv Immunol*. 1993;5:1-78.

18. Kunisada T, Ogawa M, Hayashi S, et al. Interleukin-7 and B lymphopoiesis. *Chem Immunol*. 1992;51:205-235.

19. Picker LJ. Control of lymphocyte homing. *Curr Opin Immunol*. 1994;6:394-406.

20. Miller MD, Krangel MS. Biology and biochemistry of the chemokines: A family of chemotactic and inflammatory cytokines. *CRC Crit Rev Immunol*. 1992;12:17-46.

21. Yang YC. Human interleukin-9: A new cytokine in hematopoiesis. *Leuk Lymphoma*. 1992;8:441-447.

22. Moore KW, O'Garra A, de Waal Malefyt R, et al. Interleukin-10. *Annu Rev Immunol*. 1993;11:165-190.

23. Mosmann TR. Properties and functions of interleukin-10. *Adv Immunol*. 1994;56:1-26.

24. Neben S, Turner K. The biology of interleukin-11. *Stem Cells*. 1993;2:156-162.

25. Lamont AG, Adorini L. IL-12: A key cytokine in immune regulation. *Immunol Today*. 1996;17:214-217.

26. Manetti R, Parronchi P, Giudizi MG, et al. Natural killer cell stimulatory factor IL-12 induces TH1-specific immune response and inhibits the development of IL-4 producing TH2 cells. *J Exp Med*. 1993;177:199-204.

27. Ruddle NH. Tumor necrosis factor (TNF-alpha) and lymphotoxin (TNF-beta). *Curr Opin Immunol*. 1992;4:327-332.

28. Jacob CO. Tumor necrosis factor-alpha (TNF-alpha) in autoimmunity: Pretty girl or old witch. *Immunol Today*. 1992;13:122-125.

29. Wilson AG, di Giovine FS, Duff GW. Genetics of tumor necrosis factor-alpha in autoimmune, infectious, and neoplastic diseases. *J Inflamm*. 1995;45:1-12.

30. Wahl SM. TGF-beta inflammation: A cause and a cure. *J Clin Immunol*. 1992;12:61-74.

31. Border WA, Rusolatti E. TGF-beta in disease: The dark side of tissue repair. *J Clin Invest*. 1992;90:1-7.

32. Dubios CM, Ruscetti FW, Palaszynski EW, et al. Transforming growth factor (TGF)-beta is a potent inhibitor of IL-1 receptor expression: Proposed mechanism of inhibition of IL-1 action. *J Exp Med*. 1990;172:737-744.

33. Schattner, A. Review: Interferons and autoimmunity. *Am J Med Sci*. 1988;31:532-544.

34. Sarvetnick N, Shiruru J, Liggitt D, et al. Loss of pancreatic islet cell tolerance induced by beta-cell expression of interferon (IFN)-gamma. *Nature*. 1990;346:844–847.

35. Billiau A. Interferon-gamma: Biology and role in pathogenesis. *Adv Immunol*. 1996;62:61–129.

36. Bevilacqua MP. Endothelial-leukocyte adhesion molecules. *Annu Rev Immunol*. 1993;11:767–804.

37. Zimmerman GA, Prescott SM, McIntyre TM. Endothelial cell interaction with granulocytes: Tethering and signaling molecules. *Immunol Today*. 1992;13:9–11.

38. Anderson DC, Springer TA. Leukocyte adhesion deficiency: An inherited defect in the Mac-1, LFA-1, and glycoproteins (integrin). *Annu Rev Med*. 1987;38:175–194.

39. Fernandez-Botran R, Chilton PM, Ma YH. Soluble cytokine receptors: Their role in immunoregulation, diseases, and therapy. *Adv Immunol*. 1996;63:269–335.

40. Arend PW, Dayer JP. Cytokines and cytokine inhibitor or antagonists. *Arthritis Rheum*. 1990:33:305–315.

41. Jacobs CA, Beckman MP, Mohler K, et al. Pharmacokinetic parameters and blood distribution of soluble cytokine receptors. *Int Rev Exp Pathol*. 1993;34:123–135.

42. Jenkins JK, Arend WP. IL-1ra production in human monocytes is induced by IL-1a, IL-3, IL-4, and GM-CSF. *Cytokine*. 1993;5:407–415.

43. Svenson M, Hansen MB, Kayser L, et al. Effects of human anti-IL-1a autoantibodies on receptor binding and biological activities of IL-1. *Cytokines*. 1992;4:125–133.

44. Bendtzen K, Hansen MB, Ross C, et al. Cytokines and autoantibodies to cytokines. *Stem Cells*. 1995;13:206–222.

45. Takemura H, Suzuki H, Yoshizaki K, et al. Anti-IL-6 autoantibodies in rheumatic diseases. *Arthritis Rheum*. 1992;35:940–943.

46. Hession C, Decker JM, Sherblom AP, et al. Uromodulin (Tamm-Horsfall glycoprotein): A renal ligand for lymphokines. *Science*. 1987;237:1479–1484.

47. LaMarre J, Wollenberg GK, Gonias SL, et al. Biology of diseases: Cytokine binding and clearance properties of proteinase-activated alpha$_2$-macroglobulin. *Lab Invest*. 1991;65:3–14.

48. Schandene L, Ferster A, Mascart-Lemone F, et al. T helper type 2-like cells and therapeutic effects of IFN-gamma in SCID with hypereosinophilia (Omenn's syndrome). *Eur J Immunol*. 1993;23:56–60.

49. Fuleihan R, Ramesh N, Loh R, et al. Defective expression of the CD40 ligand in X-linked immunoglobulin deficiency with normal or elevated IgM. *Proc Natl Acad Sci U S A*. 1993;90:2170–2172.

50. Del Prete GF, Tiri A, Maggi E, et al. Defective in vitro production of g-IFN and TNF-α by circulating T cells from patients with hyper-IgE syndrome. *J Clin Invest*. 1989;84:1830–1835.

51. Cunningham-Rundles C, Mayer L, Sapira E, et al. Restoration of immunoglobulin secretion in vitro in CVI by in vivo treatment with polyethylene glycol-conjugated human recombinant IL2. *Clin Immunol Immunopathol*. 1992;64:46–56.

52. Bolinger AM, Taeubel MA. Recombinant interferon gamma for treatment of chronic granulomatous disease and other disorders. *Clin Pharm*. 1992;11:834–850.

53. Berstein ZP, Porter MM, Gould M, et al. Prolonged administration of low-dose IL-2 in HIV-associated malignancy results in selective expansion of innate immune effectors without significant clinical toxicity. *Blood*. 1995;86:3287–3294.

54. Schattner A. Lymphokines in autoimmunity. *Clin Immunol Immunopathol*. 1994;70:177–189.

55. Cope AP, Aderka D, Doherty M, et al. Increased levels of TNF receptors in the sera and synovial fluid of patients with rheumatic diseases. *Arthritis Rheum*. 1992;35:1160–1169.

56. Finkelman FD. Relationships among antigen presentation, cytokines, immune deviation, and autoimmune diseases. *J Exp Med*. 1995;182:279–282.

57. Del Prete GF, Tiri A, De Carli M, et al. High potential to TNF-α production of thyroid infiltrating lymphocytes in Hashimoto's thyroiditis: a peculiar feature of destructive thyroid autoimmunity. *Autoimmunity*. 1989;4:267–272.

58. Martinez C, Leonardo E, Cuende E. The role of cytokines in the pathogenesis of autoimmunity. In: Dayer JM, Spinas GA, eds. *Cytokine Congress Reports*. Basel, Switzerland: RECOM Publishers; 1994:3–5.

59. Eastgate JA, Symons JA, Wood NC, et al. Correlation of plasma interleukin 1 levels with disease activity in rheumatoid arthritis. *Lancet*. 1988;2:706–709.

60. Selmaj K, Raine CS, Cannella B, et al. Identification of lymphotoxin and TNF-α in multiple sclerosis lesions. *J Clin Invest*. 1991;87:949–954.

61. Chofflon M, Juillard C, Juillard P, et al. TNF production as possible predictor of relapse in patients with multiple sclerosis. *Eur Cytokine Netw*. 1992;3:523–531.

62. Al-Janadi M, Al-Balla S, Al-Dalaan A, et al. Cytokine profile in SLE, RA, and other rheumatic diseases. *J Clin Immunol*. 1993;13:58–67.

63. Gianani R. Sarvetnick N. Viruses, cytokines, antigens, and autoimmunity. *Proc Natl Acad Sci U S A*. 1996;93:2257–2259.

64. Romagnami S. Lymphokines production by human T cells in disease states. *Annu Rev Immunol*. 1994;12:227–257.

65. Tracey KJ, Cerami A. Tumor necrosis factor: A pleotrophic cytokine and therapeutic target. *Annu Rev Med*. 1994;45:491–503.

66. Roberts AB, Sporn MD. Physiological actions and clinical applications of transforming growth factor-beta (TGF-beta). *Growth Factors*. 1993;8:1–9.

67. Castilla A, Prieto J, Fausto N. TGF-Beta and alpha in chronic liver diseases. *N Engl J Med*. 1991; 324:933–940.

68. Whiteside TL. Cytokines and cytokine measurements in a clinical laboratory. *Clin Diagn Lab Immunol*. 1995;1:257–260.

69. Whiteside TL. Cytokines measurement and interpretation of cytokine assays in human disease. *J Clin Immunol*. 1994;14:327–339.

70. Grassi J, Roberge CJ, Frobert Y, et al. Determination of IL-1a, IL-1b, and IL-2 in biological media using specific enzyme immunometric assays. *Immunol Rev*. 1991;119:125–143.

71. Hopkins SJ, Humphreys M. Bioassay of IL-1 in serum and plasma following removal of inhibitory activity with polyethylene glycol. *J Immunol Methods*. 1990;133:127–131.

72. Hopkins SJ, Humphreys M, Jayson MV. Cytokines in synovial fluid, I: The presence of biologically active and immunoreactive IL-1. *Clin Exp Immunol*. 1988;72:422–426.

73. Lewis CE, McCracken D, Ling R, et al. Cytokine release by single immunophenotyped human cells: Use of the reverse plaque assay. *Immunol Rev*. 1991;119:23–39.

74. Vitolo D, Kanbour A , Dahl C, et al. Expression of mRNA for cytokines in tumor infiltrating mononuclear cells in ovarian adenocarcinoma and invasive breast carcinoma. *Int J Cancer*. 1992;51:573–580.

75. O'Gara A, Vieira P. Polymerase chain reaction for detection of cytokine gene expression. *Curr Opin Immunol*. 1992;4:211–215.

76. Bromley L, McCarthy S, Stickland JE, et al. Non-isotopic in situ detection of mRNA for interleukin-4 in archival human tissue. *J Immunol Methods*. 1994;167:47–54.

77. Vitolo D, Kanbour A, Johnson JT, et al. In situ hybridization for cytokine gene transcript in the solid tumor microenvironment. *Eur J Cancer*. 1993;3:371–377.

78. Friberg D, Bryant J, Shannon W, et al. In vitro cytokine production by normal human peripheral blood mononuclear cells as a measure of immunocompetence or the state of activation. *Clin Diagn Lab Immunol*. 1994;1:261–268.

79. Rossio JL, Rager HC, Goundry CS, et al. Cytokine testing in clinical trial monitoring. In: *Manual of Clinical Laboratory Immunology*. 4th ed. Washington, DC: American Society for Microbiology; 1992:924–927.

80. Paxton H, Cunningham-Rundles S, O'Gorman MRG. Laboratory evaluation of the cellular immune system. In: Henry JB, ed. *Clinical Diagnosis and Management by Laboratory Methods*. 19th ed. Philadelphia, PA: WB Saunders Co; 1996:877–912.

81. Cavallo G, Pozzilli P, Thorpe R. Cytokines and autoimmunity. *Exp Immunol*. 1994;96:1–7.

82. Durum SK, Muegge K. Cytokines linking the immune and inflammatory system: IL-1, TNF, IL-6, IFN-alpha/beta, and TGB-B. In: Rich RR, ed. *Clinical Immunology Principles and Practice*. Boston, MA: Mosby; 1996:350–362.
83. Mosmann T. Cytokines and immune regulation. In: Rich RR, ed. *Clinical Immunology Principles and Practice*. Boston, MA: Mosby; 1996:217–230.
84. Miles SA, Golde DW, Mitsuyasu RT. The use of hematopoietic hormones in HIV infections and AIDS related malignancies. *Hematol Oncol Clin North Am*. 1991;5:267–280.
85. Baldwin, GC, Gasson JC, Quan SG, et al. GM-CSF enhances neutrophil function in acquired immunodeficiency syndrome patients. *Proc Natl Acad Sci U S A*. 1988;85:2763–2766.
86. Fisher CJ Jr, Opal SM, Dhainault JF. Influence of an anti-TNF-α monoclonal antibody on cytokine levels in patients with sepsis. *Crit Care Med*. 1993;21:318.
87. Ohlsson K, Bjoerd P, Bergenfeldt M, et al. IL1 receptor antagonist reduces mortality from endotoxin shock. *Nature*.1990;348:550–552.
88. Meuer SC, Dumman H, Meyer zum Buschenfelde KH, et al. Low dose IL-2 induces systemic immune response against HBsAg in immunodeficient non-responders to hepatitis B vaccine. *Lancet*. 1989;1:15.
89. Elliot MJ, Maini RN, Feldmann M, et al. Treatment of RA with chimeric monoclonal antibodies to TNF-α. *Arthritis Rheum*. 1993;36:1681–1690.
90. Derkx B, Taiminian J, Radema S, et al. Tumor necrosis factor(TNF) antibody treatment in Crohn's disease. *Lancet*. 1993;342:173–174.
91. Van Dullemen HM, Hommes DW, Meenan J, et al. Complete remission of steroid refractory Crohn's diseases after administration of monoclonal anti-TFN antibody cA2. *Gastroenterology*. 1994;106:A1054.
92. Lan HY, Nikolic-Paterson DJ, Zarama M, et al. Suppression of experimental crescentic glomerulonephritis by the IL-1 receptor antigen. *Kidney Int*. 1993;43:479–485.

CHAPTER 8

General Considerations in the Diagnosis and Evaluation of Autoimmune Diseases

Robert M. Nakamura, MD, and David F. Keren, MD

General Approach to Diagnosis and Evaluation of Suspected Autoimmune Diseases

As discussed throughout this book, many autoantibody tests, such as that for antinuclear antibodies (ANAs), yield a significant number of positive results among asymptomatic controls. Therefore, careful selection of patients to be tested, as well as judicious selection of the tests themselves, are needed in the diagnostic process.[1] The first step is a careful and detailed history and physical examination.

History and Physical Examination

The clinician should search for evidence of an immunodeficiency disease and any possible immune dysfunction. He or she should then inquire about family history of diseases of immune pathogenesis, such as thyroiditis, systemic lupus erythematosus (SLE), myasthenia gravis, and so on. The clinician also should look for the coexistence of other diseases, such as tumors, because there is an increased incidence of autoimmune diseases in patients with neoplasms. A thorough physical examination—for enlarged thyroid glands, enlarged lymph nodes, arthritis, skin lesions, and so on—is critical.

Laboratory Findings That May Indicate Possible Autoimmune Disease

Results from several common laboratory tests, such as abnormal serum proteins by chemical or electrophoretic analysis, may suggest that further investigation for autoimmune disease is needed. These findings include

- Anemia with increased reticulocytosis may suggest autoimmune hemolytic anemia.
- Proteinuria and casts may indicate glomerulonephritis with immune pathogenesis.
- Hypogammaglobulinemia may indicate an immunodeficiency disorder.
- Elevated gamma globulin may indicate a wide variety of diseases, such as autoimmune liver disease or chronic systemic rheumatic disease.
- An abnormal liver profile with elevated gamma globulin may indicate chronic viral hepatitis and/or autoimmune liver disease.
- Hypertriglyceridemia may indicate an endocrine disease, such as Hashimoto's thyroiditis.
- Hyperglycemia is a classic feature of diabetes.

Immunologic Markers of Autoimmune Disease

Mackay and Burnet[2] have defined certain immunologic markers, which are often seen in autoimmune diseases. These markers include

- High level of serum gamma globulin
- Demonstration of autoantibodies in serum
- Demonstration of immune deposits in tissues
- Accumulation of lymphoid cells in the tissues involved in the autoimmune process
- Response to corticosteroid and immunosuppressive drugs
- Association with other autoimmune diseases, which may coexist in the patient or occur within his or her family
- Biologic false-positive serologic test for syphilis[3] (may be associated with SLE)

Classification of Autoimmune Diseases

There are numerous ways to classify the autoimmune diseases, as discussed in Chapter 1. However, the most useful and practical categories are the following[4]: endocrine organ–specific autoimmune diseases, systemic autoimmune diseases, organ system diseases, and other autoimmune diseases (**Table 8-1**).

Clinical Spectrum and Overlap of Autoimmune Diseases

Roitt[15] separated the autoimmune diseases into 2 broad categories: the organ-specific (thyrogastric) group and the lupus group. In the former, the common target organs include the thyroid, adrenals, stomach, and pancreas. This organ-specific group includes the following diseases[15,16]:

- Autoimmune thyroiditis (Hashimoto's disease, primary myxedema)
- Pernicious anemia with atrophic gastritis
- Primary Addison's disease
- Hypoparathyroidism
- Vitiligo

Table 8-1. Classification of Autoimmune Diseases

Disease	Antigen and Antibodies Involved
Endocrine Organ–Specific Autoimmune Diseases	
Autoimmune thyroiditis; primary myxedema; thyrotoxicosis	Thyroglobulin Cytoplasmic microsome thyroperoxidase enzyme
Graves' disease (diffuse toxic goiter)	TSI or anti-TSH antibody[5,6]
Addison's disease	Adrenal cell cytoplasm
Parathyroidism	Parathyroid cytoplasmic antigen
Insulin-resistant diabetes associated with acanthosis nigricans	Anti-insulin receptor
Insulin-resistant diabetes associated with ataxia-telangiectasia	Anti-insulin receptor
Allergic asthma; functional autonomic abnormalities	Antibodies to β_2-adrenergic receptors[7]
Type 1 diabetes	Antibodies to islet cells (cytoplasmic) Antibodies to GAD and IA-2
Premature ovarian failure	Interstitial cells and corpus luteum cells
Systemic Autoimmune Diseases	
Lupus erythematosus	Nuclear antigens (DNA, histone, Sm, RNP, SS-A, SS-B, nucleolar, etc)
Mixed connective tissue disease	RNP
Drug-induced lupus	Histone
Sjögren's syndrome	Nuclear antigens (nucleolar, SS-A, SS-B)
Scleroderma/CREST syndrome	Nuclear antigen (nucleolar DNA, RNP, Scl-70) centromere
Dermatomyositis/polymyositis	Nuclear antigens (DNA, PM-1), Jo-1
Rheumatoid arthritis	Altered γ-globulin; RA-associated nuclear antigen RA-33
Organ System Diseases	
Liver	
Autoimmune chronic active hepatitis	Smooth muscle (contractile proteins)
Primary biliary cirrhosis	Mitochondrial
Muscle	
Myasthenia gravis	Anti-AchR[8,9]
Blood	
Autoimmune hemolytic anemia	Red blood cell
Gastrointestinal	
Atrophic gastritis	Gastric cell microsomes
Pernicious anemia	Intrinsic factor Salivary duct cells Gastric parietal cells microsomes
Ulcerative colitis	Colon; lipopolysaccharide, atypical p-ANCA
Crohn's disease	Reticulin; epithelial antibodies, antisaccharomyces antibody
Celiac disease	Reticulin; gluten and/or gliadin; endomysium of smooth muscle
Nervous system	
Demyelinating diseases (eg, multiple sclerosis), amyotrophic lateral sclerosis, sensor motor neuropathy	Myelin; basic protein; myelin-associated glycoprotein, GM_1, GM_2, GD_1b ganglioside, SGPG[10]
Paraneoplastic syndromes	Purkinje's cell (Yo), ANNA-1 (Hu), ANNA-2 (Ri)[11-13]
Lambert-Eaton paraneoplastic syndrome (encephalomyeloneuropathy)	Calcium channel P/Q and N types[12,14]

(continued on next page)

Table 8-1. Classification of Autoimmune Diseases (continued)

Disease	Antigen and Antibodies Involved
Kidney	
Goodpasture's syndrome	Glomerular and lung basement membrane
Immune complex glomerulonephritis (many different types, including poststreptococcal, cryoglobulin, DNA–anti-DNA in SLE, etc)	Bacterial and viral antigens, cryoglobulins, DNA in SLE
Skin	
Pemphigus vulgaris	Prickle cell desmosomes
Bullous pemphigoid	Epithelial basement membrane
Cicatricial pemphigoid	Epithelial basement membrane
Dermatitis herpetiformis	Reticulin Endomysium of smooth muscle
Other Autoimmune Diseases	
Wegener's granulomatosis	Serine (proteinase-3)
Spontaneous male infertility	Sperm

Abbreviations: TSI = thyroid-stimulating immunoglobulin; TSH = thyroid-stimulating hormone; GAD = glutamic acid decarboxylase; IA-2 = islet cell antigen-2; RNP = ribonucleoprotein; RA = rheumatoid arthritis; AchR = acetylcholine receptor; SGPG = sulfate-3-glucuronylparagloboside; SLE = systemic lupus erythematosus.

- Primary ovarian failure
- Myasthenia gravis (found also in lupus group)

There is a definite interrelationship between the various endocrine organs and pernicious anemia with atrophic gastritis.[17,18] Patients with autoimmune thyroiditis have a 10% incidence of pernicious anemia, compared with 0.2% in the general population. The incidence of antiparietal cell antibodies in patients with autoimmune thyroiditis is 30%, and 50% of patients with pernicious anemia have thyroid antibodies.[17,18] The antibody reactivity in this group is organ specific. The lesions are localized to the specific organ, as in Hashimoto's thyroiditis.[3]

The lupus group is exemplified by the systemic rheumatic diseases that characteristically involve the skin, kidney, joints, and muscle. This group includes the following diseases[1,15]:

- Rheumatoid arthritis
- Dermatomyositis/polymyositis
- Sjögren's syndrome
- Scleroderma
- Chronic active hepatitis
- Myasthenia gravis

This second group of diseases induces autoantibodies directed against nuclear and cytoplasmic antigens that are neither organ nor species specific.

Of the many autoimmune diseases, there are remarkable overlaps at each end of the spectrum. For example, thyroid autoantibodies occur with high frequency in patients with pernicious anemia who have stomach autoimmunity. These patients have a higher incidence of thyroid autoimmunity than the normal population.[15,17,18] The cluster of rheumatologic diseases at the other end of the spectrum also shows significant overlap. Features of rheumatoid arthritis may be associated with the clinical picture of SLE.[19] In these diseases, immune complexes are deposited systemically in the kidneys, joints, and skin.

Special Laboratory Tests for Evaluating Autoimmune Diseases

The patient history and results of routine clinical laboratory tests help the pathologist select further tests. Test selection is critical in determining the positive predictive value of autoantibody tests.

A direct approach is tissue biopsy of the affected organ in a specific autoimmune disorder for histologic and immunohistochemical examination. This is most often used in autoimmune diseases that involve the kidney or skin. One can evaluate the tissue injury and determine the immunopathologic mechanism, for example, by immunofluorescent localization of immunoglobulin and complement components in the basement membrane of the skin, glomerular basement membrane, or blood vessels.

The most commonly ordered clinical laboratory tests for autoimmune diseases (**Table 8-2**) involve the detection of circulating antibodies. Cellular immune tests are rarely helpful. Immunofluorescence (IFM), enzyme-labeled antibody, and radioimmunoassay methods use primary antigen-antibody binding reactions and, because of high sensitivity, are preferred for the detection of circulating and tissue-bound antibodies and antigens. These test methods measure primary direct antibody-antigen binding and may be 1,000 times more sensitive than immunodiffusion and counterimmunoelectrophoresis (CIE) tests that require precipitin reactions between antibodies and tissue/cell extracts. Immunoblot assays can further identify polyspecific autoantibodies directed against multiple soluble and insoluble autoantigens. Immunodiffusion and immunoprecipitation, CIE, and immunoblot methods may be used to confirm positive IFM-ANA screens and to define the characteristics of targeted antigens.[21,22] The tests that involve secondary antigen-antibody preparations, such as complement fixation, agglutination, and precipitation in agar gel, are not as sensitive as IFM, enzyme immunoassays, or radioimmunoassay, but technically may be more suitable for the identification of certain autoantibodies.

In experimental settings, other methods have rarely proved useful in the epidemiologic studies of patients with suspected autoimmune disorders.[4] Cell-mediated immunity studies are too nonspecific to be helpful in individual cases. Other substances of diagnostic importance for which tests are commonly performed include rheumatoid factor, level of complement, and cryoglobulins.

Interpretation of Serum Autoantibody Levels in Autoimmune Diseases

Test results must be interpreted with reference to the patient's medical history and clinical disease states and with a clear understanding of the technical limitations of the test systems employed.

In general, the level of autoantibody is high in patients with autoimmune disorders and low in apparently healthy patients. A very high titer of autoantibody is significant, although a low or absent titer of autoantibody does not rule out the possibility of an autoimmune disorder. For example, at the height of severe thyroiditis, the gland may act as an immunoadsorbent and remove circulating antibody. In addition, thyroglobulin may be released into the circulation during the acute stage and neutralize circulating autoantibody. Therefore, the level or titer of a given antibody must be interpreted in relation to the stage or treatment of a particular disease.[4] In contrast, serum antibody levels in pemphigus correlate with the severity and course of the disease.[23]

The incidence of certain autoantibodies increases with age. In patients older than 60 years, 50% demonstrated low titers of 1 or more autoantibodies. Antinuclear, antiparietal cell, and antithyroid antibodies are age and sex dependent, with an increasing incidence in women and older people.[24–26] On the other hand, the incidence of smooth-muscle antibody and

Table 8-2. Method for Detection of Autoantibodies

Methods	Antigen Source	Use
Immunofluorescence	Tissue sections; cell lines	Sensitive assay for screening
Enzyme immunoassay	Pooled natural and/or recombinant nuclear antigens	Sensitive assay for screening*
Double immunodiffusion	Tissue and cell extracts	Requires precipitin reaction; high specificity but low sensitivity
Counterimmunoelectrophoresis	Tissue and cell extracts	Increased sensitivity and speed compared with immunodiffusion
Particle agglutination	Native or recombinant antigens	More sensitive than immunodiffusion
Immunoblotting	Cell extracts	Very sensitive, allowing detection of antibodies to soluble and insoluble antigens

**Confirmation of enzyme immunoassays by other tests such as immunofluorescence or Western blot are sometimes recommended.*[20]

rheumatoid factor does not correlate with age or sex and was similar in men and women. A study in Australia[26] tested a normal population for the presence of 13 autoimmune antibodies. Of 2,830 individuals tested, 22% displayed 1 or more autoantibodies. Several of these antibodies appeared to be persistent, lasting 6 years or longer. The parietal cell antibody persisted in 75.3% of the individuals. Antinuclear, thyroid microsomal, and smooth-muscle antibodies also were persistent.

Natural Autoantibodies in Nonautoimmune Conditions

Autoantibodies can be detected in nonautoimmune conditions such as infection, neoplasm, or physiologic stress. Furthermore, non–antigen-driven, spontaneously occurring, natural autoantibodies (NAAs) may be found in 20% to 50% of asymptomatic healthy individuals of all age groups, including neonates.[27,28] They are produced by CD5+ B cells from adult bone marrow precursor cells, fetal liver tissue, and cord blood. Most NAAs are low-avidity immunoglobulin (Ig) Ms, and their antigenic repertoire is similar to that seen in autoantibodies of various autoimmune diseases.[27,28] The targeted autoantigens include intracellular and membrane constituents such as DNA, Sm/ribonucleoprotein, actin, keratin, mitochondria, phospholipids, myelin basic protein, and acetylcholine receptors, as well as serum proteins such as IgG, lymphokines, and polypeptides of endocrine glands. Natural autoantibodies also show extensive cross-reactivity (polyreactivity) with environmental microbial antigens and chemical haptens; such polyreactivity is thought to reflect their "physiologic" immunoregulatory roles in the clearance of pathogens and catabolic wastes for maintaining homeostasis by forming immune complexes for efficient waste elimination.[28,29] Women have higher incidences of NAAs than do men.

Autoimmune Diseases in the Elderly Population

The majority of studies show that the prevalence of various autoantibodies increases in the elderly. However, there is no definite evidence of a parallel increase in autoimmune disease.[30,31] The majority of autoimmune diseases are characterized by onset in youth or early middle age. Onset of only a few autoimmune diseases occurs after the age of 50 years.

Late-Onset Systemic Lupus Erythematosus Versus Drug-Induced Lupus

Between 3% and 20% of patients with SLE may experience late onset of the disease.[20,32,33] Most authors define late onset as a diagnosis made at 50 years or older. Prognostically, late-onset SLE has a milder disease course than early-onset SLE.

In drug-induced lupus, patients experience the onset of symptoms at a mean age of 60 years and are diagnosed at a mean age of 62 years.[33] In spontaneous idiopathic SLE, the mean age of both onset and diagnosis is in the third decade of life.

These differences reflect the age range when the drugs known to initiate an autoimmune response are administered. Many patients receiving such drugs may develop positive ANAs; however, a smaller percentage develop drug-induced lupus. Ninety percent of patients taking procainamide for 2 years test positive for drug-induced lupus by IFM-ANA, but only 15% to 20% may develop symptoms of the disease.[34] Similarly, of patients receiving hydralazine for 3 years, 44% have positive results from an IFM-ANA test,[35] but only 5% to 10% develop signs of drug-induced lupus.[36]

Autoimmunity in the elderly may be manifested by the development of autoantibodies, which, in a vast majority of patients, have no pathophysiologic significance. Therefore, it is critical not to equate the detection of autoantibodies in the elderly with autoimmune diseases.[30,31]

Characteristics of Laboratory Testing

Value of Laboratory Tests

The value of a laboratory test depends on its ability to answer a specific clinical question important for patient management.[37] The clinical value of a new test should be determined not only by how well it performs but by how well it outperforms currently available tests and whether this performance can be justified economically. The cost-effectiveness of a new laboratory test in clinical practice should be determined.[38,39]

The predictive value of a test result is not a real measure of its clinical value, especially when it is used in the later stages of a diagnostic workup.[40] The clinical value can be determined by the amount of useful information that is provided by the test result.

Reasons for Requesting Laboratory Tests

Laboratory tests are used for many purposes, mainly disease detection, diagnosis, and monitoring.[38,41] Some of these reasons include

- Diagnosis
- Assessment of prognosis and severity of disease
- Monitoring of the disease course or the patient's response to therapy
- Screening of various populations (eg, high risk)
- Establishment of baseline values for assessment of future change
- Risk assessment
- Clinical research studies

Sensitivity, Specificity, and Predictive Values of Laboratory Tests

Several characteristics are used to describe laboratory tests. It is critical for the clinician to have some information on the sensitivity and specificity of the particular laboratory test.[42–46] Sensitivity can be defined as "positivity in disease," or the probability of a positive test given the presence of the disease. Specificity is often referred to as a "negative in health," or the probability of a negative test given the absence of the disease in question. Positive predictive value is the likelihood that the patient has the disease if the test is positive. Negative predictive value is the likelihood that the patient does not have the disease if the test result is negative.

Some important issues should be emphasized[43]:

- Positive and negative results must be well defined so they can be compared.
- The disease in question must be defined clearly and have relevance to decisions made in practice.
- The calculation of specificity should be done until the reference group
  - has been selected to exclude the disease in question, such as SLE, or
  - to obtain a "healthy" group, defined by the absence of any major illness.
- If the test is used to screen a population for a specific disease, the prevalence of the disease must be considered.
- If the test is used to distinguish options on the differential diagnosis of 2 diseases, the relative prevalence of these 2 conditions is more important than the prevalence of either condition in the population as a whole.

Diagnostic Testing Versus Evaluative Testing

Ward[47, 48] has emphasized that clinical laboratory tests may be categorized as diagnostic tests and evaluative tests.

Diagnostic Tests

The usefulness of a new test is determined by how the test categorizes diseased persons as diseased and unaffected persons as unaffected based on comparison with a gold standard indicator of disease. For a diagnostic test to be useful, it must be able to demonstrate high sensitivity and specificity on the differences between individual patients. Good diagnostic tests give reproducible results over time. A good example of a diagnostic test is the test for antibody to acetylcholine receptor in myasthenia gravis. The current radiolabeled test is sensitive, and a positive test result confirms the diagnosis.[8, 9]

Certain diagnostic tests may be useful as evaluative tests. Serum autoantibody levels often do not correlate and reflect the severity and course of the specific disease.[4]

Evaluative Tests

These tests are used to measure and assess changes in disease activity over time and are used to determine indexes of change.[49] Evaluative tests are used to compare the current status of a patient with his or her status at a previous point in time to determine whether there is improvement or a change for the worse. The value and accuracy of an evaluative test is determined by how it monitors changes in disease activity. Test results should be compared with changes in an accepted gold standard measurement of disease activity.

An example of a useful evaluative test would be to determine the serum level of the acute phase inflammatory C-reactive protein in rheumatic fever or rheumatoid arthritis. The C-reactive protein levels parallel the inflammatory activity during the course of the disease.[50]

Assessing New Evaluative Laboratory Tests

Before a new laboratory test is recommended for incorporation in clinical practice, the following points should be considered[47]:

- The test should be standardized so that its findings in clinical research studies can be reproduced and applied in a nonresearch setting.
- Test results should be made available in a timely manner for good patient care and clinical decision making.
- The new test should be more valid or more sensitive to change than evaluative tests already in use.
- The new test should be compared with existing tests by randomized trials to determine cost-effectiveness.[51]

Cutoff Values and Multiplicity of Laboratory Tests

Each clinical laboratory must define and establish cutoff values between normal and abnormal results. The assignment of the cutoff values determine the proportion of false-positive and false-negative results.[52] For example, does the "normal reference range" include 95%, 97.5%, or 99% of the "normal" population? Are age-related reference ranges assigned for certain autoantibodies?

For many clinical laboratory tests, the cutoff is made to include only 95% of the normal population, allowing a 5% false-positive rate. Thus, if someone without the specific disease has 1 test performed, there is a 5% chance the result will be abnormal. When multiple tests are performed, with a cutoff to include 95% of the normal population, the likelihood of obtaining a false-positive result rises dramatically with the number of tests performed. The likelihood of one abnormal result with 5 tests is 22%.[46,53] Therefore, abnormal results must be interpreted with caution if multiple tests have been performed.

In establishing normal reference ranges for autoantibody tests, one should consider cutoff values to include 97.5% or 99% of the normal population. Also, the test should include some form of quantitation.

Summary

Clinical evaluation and measures are preeminent in the diagnosis and management of autoimmune diseases, giving the laboratory an important role in the evaluation. Laboratory tests are useful in helping to establish diagnosis, monitor disease course, predict disease outcome, assess the need for and response to therapy, and gain insight into disease etiology or pathogenesis.[46,54]

The clinical laboratory should clearly state the immunologic test procedure performed, along with the definition of reference range to include the cutoff value and what percentage of the normal population is included in the reference range.

The clinical interpretation of a specific laboratory test can be influenced by many factors, including the sensitivity and specificity of the test, the clinical setting in which the test was requested, the reason the test was requested, and the number of tests performed.[46]

The clinician should order the test on the basis of what question he or she wants answered, as well as what he or she will do or recommend when the results are normal or definitely abnormal. The test request is unnecessary for patient care if the physician will not change either the clinical care or recommendation based on whether the results are normal or definitely abnormal.

References

1. Nakamura RM. General approach to diagnosis of autoimmune disorders. In: Nakamura RM, ed. *Immunopathology: Clinical Laboratory Concepts and Methods*. Boston, MA: Little Brown & Co; 1974:235–243.
2. Mackay IR, Burnet FM. *Autoimmune Diseases, Pathogenesis, Chemistry, and Therapy*. Springfield, IL: Charles C. Thomas; 1963:16–17.
3. Doniach D, Delhanty J, Lindquist HL, et al. Mitochondrial and other tissue autoantibodies in patients with biologic false positive reactions for syphilis. *Clin Exp Immunol*. 1970;6:871–884.
4. Nakamura RM, Binder WL. Current concepts and diagnostic evaluation of autoimmune disease. *Arch Pathol Lab Med*. 1988;112:869–877.
5. Vitti P, Chiovato L, Fiore E, et al. Use of cells expressing the human thyrotropin (TSH) receptor for the measurement of thyroid stimulating and TSH-blocking antibodies. *Acta Med Austriaca*. 1996;23:52–56.

6. Kim WB, Cho BY, Park HY, et al. Epitope for thyroid stimulating antibodies in Graves' sera: A possible link of heterogeneity to differences in response to anti-thyroid drug treatment. *J Clin Endocrinol Metab.* 1996;81:1758–1767.

7. Turki J, Liggett SB. Receptor specific functional properties of β_2-adrenergic receptor autoantibodies in asthma. *Am J Respir Cell Mol Biol.* 1995;12:531–539.

8. Wu JT, Astill M, Lloyd C, et al. Rhabdomyosarcoma cell line can be used for the isolation of soluble acetylcholine receptor and for assaying blocking and modulating autoantibodies. *J Clin Lab Anal.* 1993;7:11–18.

9. Kennel PR, Vilquin JT, Braun S, et al. Myasthenia gravis: Comparative autoantibody assays using human muscle, TE671, and glucocorticoid treated TE671 cells as sources of antigen. *Clin Immunol Immunopathol.* 1995;74:293–296.

10. Zeballos RS, McPherson RA. Update of autoantibodies in neurologic disease. *Clin Lab Med.* 1992;12:61–83.

11. Lennon VA. Views and reviews: Paraneoplastic autoantibodies: The case for a descriptive generic nomenclature. *Neurology.* 1994;44:2236–2240.

12. Lennon VA. Calcium channel and related paraneoplastic autoantibodies. In: Peter JB, Shoenfeld Y, eds. *Textbook of Autoantibodies.* Amsterdam, the Netherlands: Elsevier Science; 1996:139–147.

13. Dalmau J, Posner JB. Neurologic paraneoplastic antibodies (anti-yo; anti-Hu; anti-Ri): The case for a nomenclature based on antibody and antigen specificity. *Neurology.* 1994;44:2241–2246.

14. Lennon VA, Kryzer TJ, Griesmann GE, et al. Calcium-channel antibodies in Lambert-Eaton myasthenic syndrome and other paraneoplastic syndromes. *N Engl J Med.* 1995;332:1467–1474.

15. Roitt I. Autoimmunity and autoimmune disease. In: Roitt I, Brostoff D, Male D, eds. *Immunology.* St. Louis, MO: Mosby; 1993:1–12.

16. Ollier W, Symmons DPM. Introduction. In: Read AP, Brown TB, eds. *Autoimmunity.* Oxford, UK: BIOS Scientific Publishers; 1992:1–15.

17. Irvine WJ, Davies SH, Delamore IW, et al. Immunological relationship between pernicious anemia and thyroid disease. *Br Med J.* 1962;2:454–456.

18. Irvine WJ, Davies SH, Teitelbaum S, et al. The clinical and pathological significance of gastric parietal cell antibody. *Ann N Y Acad Sci.* 1965;124:657–691.

19. Lorber M, Gershwin E, Shoenfeld Y. The coexistence of systemic lupus erythematosus with other autoimmune disorders: The kaleidoscope of autoimmunity. *Semin Arthritis Rheum.* 1994;24:105–113.

20. Jaskowski TD, Schroder C, Martins TB, et al. Screening for antinuclear antibodies by enzyme immunoassay. *Am J Clin Pathol.* 1996;105:468–473.

21. Nakamura RM, Bylund DJ, Tan EM. Current status of available standards for quality improvement of assays for detection of autoantibodies to nuclear and intracellular antigens. *J Clin Lab Anal.* 1994;8:360–368.

22. Charles PJ, van Venrooij WJ, Maini RN. The consensus workshops for the detection of autoantibodies to intracellular antigens in rheumatic disease, 1989–1992. *Clin Exp Rheumatol.* 1992;10:507–511.

23. Beutner EH, Chorzelski TP, Kumar V. *Immunopathology of Skin.* 3rd ed. New York, NY: Churchill-Livingstone; 1987.

24. Whittingham S. Serological methods in autoimmune diseases in man. In: Kwapinski JBG, ed. *Research in Immunochemistry and Immunobiology.* Vol. 1. Baltimore, MD: University Park Press; 1972:121–176.

25. Hooper B, Whittingham S, Mathews JD, et al. Autoimmunity in a rural community. *Clin Exp Immunol.* 1972;12:79–87.

26. Hawkins BR, O'Connor KJ, Dawkins RL, et al. Autoantibodies in an Australian population, 1: Prevalence and persistence. *J Clin Lab Immunol.* 1979;2:211–215.

27. Youinou P, Buskila D, MacKenzie E, et al. CD5+ B cells and disease. In: Shoenfeld Y, Isenberg DA, eds. *Natural Autoantibodies: Their Physiological Role and Regulatory Significance.* Boca Raton, FL: CRC Press; 1993:142–158.

28. Abu-Shakra M, Shoenfeld Y. What are natural autoantibodies? In: Shoenfeld Y, Isenberg DA, eds. *Natural Autoantibodies: Their Physiological Role and Regulatory Significance.* Boca Raton, FL: CRC Press; 1993:15–33.

29. Louzir H, Ternynck T, Gorgi Y, et al. Enzyme immunoassay analysis of antibody specificities present in the circulating immune complexes of selected pathological sera. *J Immunol Methods.* 1988;114:145–153.

30. Weksler ME. The nature and significance of age-associated autoimmunity. In: Bona CA, Siminovitch KA, Zanetti M, et al, eds. *The Molecular Pathology of Autoimmune Diseases.* Chur, Switzerland: Harwood Academic Publishers; 1993:765–775.

31. Richmond GW, Yu BH. Autoantibodies, autoimmune diseases, and vasculitis in the aged. *Immunol Allergy Clin North Am.* 1993;13:647–672.

32. Hochberg MC, Boyd RB, Arnett FC, et al. Systemic lupus erythematosus: A review of clinical laboratory features and immunogenetic markers in 150 patients with emphasis on demographic subsets. *Medicine.* 1985;64:285–295.

33. Pistiner M, Wallace DJ, Nessim S, et al. Lupus erythematosus in the 1980's: A survey of 570 patients. *Semin Arthritis Rheum.* 1991;21:55–64.

34. Woosley RC, Drayer DE, Raidenberg MM, et al. Effect of acetylator phenotype on the rate at which procainamide induces antinuclear antibodies and the lupus syndrome. *N Engl J Med.* 1978;298:1157–1159.

35. Hughes GR, Rynes RI, Gharavi PFJ, et al. The heterogeneity of serological findings and predisposing host factors in drug induced lupus erythematosus. *Arthritis Rheum.* 1981;24:1070–1073.

36. Litwin A, Adams LE, Zimmer H, et al. Prospective study of immunologic effects of hydralazine in hypertensive patients. *Clin Pharmacol Ther*. 1981;29:447–456.

37. Robertson EA, Zweig MH, Van Steirteghem AC. Evaluating the clinical efficiency of laboratory test. *Am J Clin Pathol*. 1983;79:78–86.

38. Pannal P, Marshall W, Jabor A, et al. A strategy to promote the rational use of laboratory tests. International Federation of Clinical Chemistry. *Clin Chim Acta*. 1996;244:121–127.

39. Johnson HA. Diagnostic information as a commodity. *Clin Chem*. 1995;41:781–784.

40. Johnson HA. Predictive value and informational value of a diagnostic test. *Ann Clin Lab Sci*. 1993;23:159–164.

41. Nakamura RM, Bylund DJ. Factors influencing changes in the clinical immunology laboratory. *Clin Chem*. 1994;40:2193–2204.

42. Ealen RS, Gambino SR. *Beyond Normality: The Predictive Value and Efficiency of Medical Diagnosis*. New York, NY: Wiley; 1975.

43. Dawkins RL. Sensitivity and specificity of autoantibody testing. In: Rose NR, Mackay IR, eds. *The Autoimmune Diseases*. San Diego, CA: Academic Press; 1985:669–706.

44. Vecchio TJ. Predictive value of a single diagnostic test in unselected populations. *N Engl J Med*. 1966;274: 1171–1173.

45. Ransohoff DF, Feinstein AR. Problems of spectrum and bias in evaluating the efficacy of diagnostic tests. *N Engl J Med*. 1978;299:926–930.

46. Sibley J. Laboratory tests. *Rheum Dis Clin North Am*. 1995;21:407–428.

47. Ward MM. Evaluative laboratory testing—assessing tests that assess disease activity. *Arthritis Rheum*. 1995;38:1555–1563.

48. Ward MM. Clinical measurer in rheumatoid arthritis: Which are most useful in assessing patients? *J Rheumatol*. 1993;21:17–21.

49. Kirshner B, Guyatt G. A methodological framework for assessing health indices. *J Chronic Dis*. 1985;38:27–36.

50. Otterness IG. The value of C-reactive protein measurement in rheumatoid arthritis. *Semin Arthritis Rheum*. 1994;24:91–104.

51. Guyatt GH, Tugwell PX, Feeny DH, et al. A framework for clinical evaluation of diagnostic technologies. *Can Med Assoc* J. 1986;134:587–594.

52. Einstein AJ, Bodian CA. The relationship among performance measures in the selection of diagnostic tests. *Arch Pathol Lab Med*. 1997;121:110–117.

53. Cupples LA, Heeren T, Schatzkin A, et al. Multiple testing of hypothesis in comparing two groups. *Ann Intern Med*. 1984;100:122–219.

54. Sox HC. The evaluation of diagnostic tests: Principles, problems, and new developments. *Ann Rev Med*. 1996;47:463–471.

SECTION II

Systemic Autoimmune Diseases

9

CHAPTER

Clinical and Laboratory Evaluation of Systemic Lupus Erythematosus and Lupus-Related Disorders

Robert M. Nakamura, MD, and Eng M. Tan, MD

Introduction and Classification of Systemic Rheumatic Diseases

Systemic lupus erythematosus (SLE) is regarded as the prototype systemic rheumatic autoimmune disease with hyperactive and multiple abnormalities of the immune system.[1] The rheumatic diseases are characterized by the presence of 1 or more autoantibodies that may be directed against components of the surface, cytoplasm, or nucleus of the cell. The last group, autoantibodies to nuclear antigens (ANAs), is a hallmark of the systemic rheumatic diseases.[1–9]

Classification of the various rheumatic diseases has been difficult because of a lack of a firm etiologic basis for most of the diseases. A comprehensive classification was developed by Decker and the glossary subcommittee of the American College of Rheumatology.[10] The classification of systemic rheumatic diseases and related disorders used in this chapter is shown in **Table 9-1**.

Much progress was made during the last decade in the elucidation of the immune mechanisms involved in SLE and other rheumatic diseases. Many of the rheumatic diseases have a distinctive profile of autoantibodies with diagnostic specificities. Recently, the biochemical and biologic functions of many of the autoantigens have been defined and clarified. Many of the autoantigens are involved in important cellular functions, such as deoxyribonucleic acid (DNA) replication, the splicing of the precursors to messenger ribonucleic acid (RNA), and RNA processing.[4,11]

Systemic Lupus Erythematosus and Related Lupus-like Disorders

Systemic lupus erythematosus is a chronic disease that can affect any or every organ system of the body with different manifestations and presentations. It primarily affects younger women, with a median age onset in the third decade of life; the incidence ratio of SLE in women and men is 9:1.[12] Estimates of the overall prevalence of SLE in the general population range from 14.6 to 50.8 cases per 100,000 people; however, the disease prevalence varies according to sex and race.[13] There appears to be a higher incidence in black Americans and Hispanics.[7] Over 80% of cases occur during patients' childbearing years.[6,7] The annual incidence of SLE is estimated to be between 1.8 and 4.6 cases per 100,000 people.[12]

Systemic lupus erythematosus is characterized by the following significant features[1–6]:

- Tissue injury is mediated by DNA–anti-DNA immune complexes and other antigen-antibody complexes. The role of cell-mediated mechanisms is unclear but might be important in aggravating or perpetuating inflammation initiated by immune complexes.
- The disease presentation can be heterogeneous and characterized by frequent exacerbations and remissions.
- The disease demonstrates a hyperactive immune system with multiple abnormalities.
- Patients demonstrate a heterogeneous and polyclonal antibody response.
- Typically, an average of 3 different circulating antibodies are present simultaneously. The prevalence of antibodies varies widely, and more than 25 different types of autoantibodies have been identified in SLE.[4,5,6,14]

Etiologic Factors in Systemic Lupus Erythematosus

The exact etiology of this disease is still unclear. The causation is probably multifactorial and includes all factors contributing to the pathogenesis of the SLE.[1,15–17] There are 3 categories of factors: (1) host factors, which include sex, race, genetic, and immunologic abnormalities; (2) environmental factors, which include infection, ultraviolet irradiation, drugs, and chemicals; and (3) other factors, such as geography and diet.

Host Factors

Sex

The strongest risk factor for the development of SLE is female gender.[15,16] Hochberg and Kaslow[18] studied 74 women with SLE. These patients had a mean age of 30 years; 70% were white, 61% were married, and 78% were high school graduates. An equal number of neighborhood-matched control patients were studied. Researchers found that a history of pregnancy ending in miscarriage was associated with SLE.[16,18]

Race and Genetic Factors

Higher prevalence and morbidity of SLE have been seen in blacks, Asians, and Native Americans, relative to whites.[6,19] Genetic factors influence susceptibility to SLE and available data implicate multiple independent segregating genes.[20,21] Systemic lupus erythematosus tends

Table 9-1. Systemic Rheumatic Diseases and Related Disorders

Systemic lupus erythematosus
Discoid lupus erythematosus
Lupus-like syndrome
Drug-induced lupus erythematosus
Sjögren's syndrome
Scleroderma/CREST syndrome (calcinosis cutis, Raynaud's phenomenon, esophageal dysfunction, sclerodactyly, and telangiectasia)
Rheumatoid arthritis
Dermatomyositis and polymyositis
Mixed connective tissue diseases
Overlap syndromes
Connective tissue disease syndromes that have been poorly defined as to clinical category

to aggregate in families. About 10% to 12% of SLE patients have first-degree relatives with the disease, and up to 3% of all first-degree relatives of SLE patients develop the disease.[20] Studies have demonstrated a greater concordance rate of SLE among monozygotic and dizygotic twins.[22] The concordance for SLE was present in 11 (58%) of 19 monozygotic twins.

Systemic lupus erythematosus has been associated with HLA phenotypes. Excessive HLA-DR2, HLA-DR3, and HLA-DQwl are found in whites with SLE, compared with a similar control population. HLA-DR3–positive SLE patients produce high levels of tumor necrosis factor (TNF) and have a lower frequency of nephritis. HLA-DR2–positive patients produce little TNF and have a higher incidence of nephritis.[23]

Systemic lupus erythematosus can be viewed as a composite disease of multiple overlapping, autoimmune responses associated with a variety of different HLA-DQ polymorphisms.[20]

Immunologic Abnormalities

Immunologic abnormalities associated with SLE involve almost all components of the cellular, humoral, and antigen-presenting cell systems. In general, it can be stated that[1–6,14,24,25]

- Humoral immunity is enhanced.
- T-cell functions are suppressed.
- The regulatory and effector molecules produced and interaction between cells are extremely complex.
- The end result of immunologic abnormalities is polyclonal activation of B cells with production of a wide spectrum of antibodies.

Bach and Viard[24] have proposed that SLE can evolve in 3 steps: (1) polyclonal B-cell activation and proliferation by unknown etiologic factors (virus, chemicals, etc); (2) primary activation of natural antibody-producing clones, leading to the appearance of large amounts of natural autoantibodies in serum; and (3) secondary immunization against molecules synthesized in large amounts during lymphocytic proliferation released by dying cells. These molecules include nucleic acids, histones, and RNA splicing molecules, which are subsequently presented in an immunogenic form to T cells.

Environmental Factors

Infection

The presence of antinuclear antibodies was determined in female laboratory workers with varying degrees of exposure to blood from patients with SLE. The presence of anti-DNA antibodies was higher in laboratory workers than in an unexposed nonlaboratory group of women ($P < .001$).[26] These results help support a hypothesis that a transmissible agent that can cause autoantibody formation may exist in the blood of patients with SLE.

Systemic lupus erythematosus may have a viral etiology.[17,27] Despite increasing evidence that viruses (especially retroviruses) may be involved as etiologic factors in autoimmune diseases, clear-cut evidence for the definite role of these agents is missing.[28]

Ultraviolet Radiations

Ultraviolet radiation influences and exacerbates the clinical and immunopathologic expression of SLE lesions in the skin.[29] Autoimmunity involving photodenatured DNA has been shown experimentally.[9,30] Various studies suggest that ultraviolet radiation may contribute to the depressed T-cell function and enhanced B-cell activity observed in SLE.[31]

Chemicals

Certain chemicals have been implicated in SLE.[16] The syndrome of drug-induced lupus erythematosus (DLE) with hydralazine, procainamide, and isoniazid has been studied for clues to the pathogenesis of SLE. There have been varying reports that show the acetylation mechanism as a risk factor for this disease.

Alfalfa sprouts containing amino-acid L-canavanine, which demonstrate immunomodulatory properties in vitro, have been reported to induce an SLE-like syndrome in female monkeys.[32]

Other Factors

Geography

Systemic lupus erythematosus is considered rare in black Africans in contrast to the higher incidence of SLE among US blacks.[33] It has been postulated that malaria and other endemic infectious diseases may confer some protection against developing SLE.

Differential Diagnosis of Systemic Lupus Erythematosus

Systemic lupus erythematosus is a chronic multisystem disease and can be heterogeneous in its initial presentation. Several questions that should be answered are[34]

- What is SLE?
- What is a lupus-like disorder?
- What is not SLE?

What Is Systemic Lupus Erythematosus?

In 1971, the American College of Rheumatology (ACR), previously the American Rheumatism Association (ARA), published preliminary criteria for the classification of SLE.[35] Patients were then considered to have SLE if 4 of the criteria were met sequentially or simultaneously during any interval of observation.

In 1982, a subcommittee for SLE Criteria of ARA published revised criteria, which incorporated new immunologic knowledge and improved the disease classification of SLE.[36] The 1982 revised criteria included the 11 categories listed in Table 9-1. These criteria added (1) abnormal titer of antinuclear antibody by immunofluorescence or an equivalent assay and (2) antibody to native DNA and/or Sm antigen. In contrast to the 1971 listings, the 1982 criteria did not include Raynaud's phenomenon or alopecia because of their low sensitivity and specificity.

When the 1982 criteria for classification were compared with those from 1971, there was definite improvement in sensitivity and specificity. The 1982 criteria showed a 96.7% sensitivity and 96% specificity when evaluated with known SLE and control patients.[36] The 1982 ARA criteria considered patients to have SLE if 4 of the criteria were met sequentially or simultaneously during any period of observation. The criteria listed in **Table 9-2** may all be present at the same time or appear over a period of months to years.

What Is a Lupus-like Disorder?

Many diseases and syndromes may share certain clinical features with SLE but have differing etiologies and pathogenesis. Panush et al[34] have listed many such diseases, including vasculitis, cryoglobulinemia, polychondritis, lymphoproliferative diseases, rheumatic fever, glomerulonephritis, syphilis, lupoid hepatitis, DLE, and occult malignancy that are not SLE.

There is a very broad category of patients who demonstrate fewer than 4 of the 1982 ARA classification criteria for SLE[34,37–39] but are still considered to have lupus-like illnesses. These patients are classified as having one of the following conditions:

- Undifferentiated rheumatic disease
- Nonrheumatic disease
- Overlap syndrome
- Incomplete, latent, or incipient lupus

Undifferentiated Connective Tissue Disease

These patients have clinical, laboratory, and serologic features suggestive of more than a single rheumatic disease and do not fit the traditional classification criteria. Some patients may be diagnosed with mixed connective tissue disease (MCTD). The typical patient with MCTD demonstrates characteristically clinical features, together with high titers of antibody to nuclear ribonucleoprotein (nRNP).[40,41]

Overlap Syndrome

Patients with overlapping features of SLE and other rheumatic diseases such as rheumatoid arthritis have been observed.[39,42] It is uncertain whether overlap

Table 9-2. 1982 Revised American Rheumatism Association Criteria for Classification of Systemic Lupus Erythematosus*

Criterion	Definition
1. Malar rash	Fixed erythema, flat or raised, over the malar eminences, tending to spare the nasolabial folds
2. Discoid rash	Erythematous raised patches with adherent keratotic scaling and follicular plugging (atrophic scarring may occur in older lesions)
3. Photosensitivity	Skin rash as a result of unusual reaction to sunlight, by patient history or physician observation
4. Oral ulcers	Oral or nasopharyngeal ulceration, usually painless, observed by a physician
5. Arthritis	Nonerosive arthritis involving two or more peripheral joints, characterized by tenderness, swelling, or effusion
6. Serositis	a. Pleuritis-convincing history of pleuritic pain or rub heard by a physician, or evidence of pleural effusion or b. Pericarditis—documented by ECG or rub, or evidence of pericardial effusion
7. Renal disorder	a. Persistent proteinuria >0.5 g/day or >3+ if quantitation not performed or b. Cellular casts—may be red cell, hemoglobin, granular, tubular, or mixed
8. Neurologic disorder	a. Seizures—in the absence of offending drugs or known metabolic derangements (eg, uremia, ketoacidosis, or electrolyte imbalance) or b. Psychosis—in the absence of offending drugs or known metabolic derangements (eg, uremia, ketoacidosis, or electrolyte imbalance)
9. Hematologic disorder	a. Hemolytic anemia—with reticulocytosis or b. Leukopenia—<4,000/mm total on two or more occasions or c. Lymphopenia—<1,500/mm on two or more occasions or d. Thrombocytopenia—<100,000/mm in the absence of offending drugs
10. Immunologic disorder	a. Positive LE cell preparation or b. Anti-DNA—antibody to native DNA in abnormal titer or c. Anti-Sm—presence of antibody to Sm nuclear antigen or d. False-positive serologic test for syphilis known to be positive for at least 6 months and confirmed by *Treponema pallidum* immobilization or fluorescent treponemal antibody absorption test
11. Antinuclear antibody	An abnormal titer of antinuclear antibody by immunofluorescence or an equivalent assay at any point in time and in the absence of drugs known to be associated with drug-induced lupus syndrome

Abbreviations: ECG = electrocardiogram; LE = lupus erythematosus.

**The proposed classification is based on 11 criteria. For the purpose of identifying patients in clinical studies, a person is said to have systemic lupus erythematosus if 4 or more of the 11 criteria are present, serially or simultaneously, during any interval of observation.*

syndromes may represent the coexistence of 2 or more different diseases or whether the syndrome is a distinct entity. Studies by Lazaro et al[39] showed that the finding of high titers of antibody to nRNP did not allow identification of a particular subgroup.

Incipient or Latent Lupus

Another group of patients does not satisfy the 1971 or 1982 classification criteria for the diagnosis of SLE but has features suggestive of the disease.[43–45] Ganczarczyk et al[44] labeled this condition "incipient or latent lupus." Affected patients differ from those with classical SLE because they do not have renal and central nervous system (CNS) disease, decreased incidence of anti-DNA antibodies, fever, or positive Coombs' test. Latent or incipient lupus patients may represent a mild end of the spectrum of SLE or an evolutionary phase of the disease. To elucidate the significance of a specific case of latent or incipient lupus would require a long-term follow-up of the family and clinical course.

Incomplete Lupus

Patients with incomplete lupus erythematosus (ILE) syndrome are defined as meeting fewer than 4 of the ARA criteria. These patients, when compared with patients with SLE, are similar with respect to age, sex, and race. Other characteristics of ILE, compared with SLE, include the folowing[43–45]:

- Cutaneous manifestations are frequent among patients with ILE.
- Arthritis is common in both SLE and ILE patients.
- Patients with SLE have more visceral organ involvement than do patients with ILE.
- None of the ILE patients has immunologic abnormalities under the 1982 criteria other than a positive result for ANAs.
- The majority of patients with ILE continue to have symptoms of rheumatic disease and do not develop features of other rheumatic diseases.
- Most patients considered to have ILE do not develop classical SLE.

During 57 months of observation, 38 patients with ILE showed cutaneous and articular features and a positive ANA finding, and rarely had systemic diseases.[43,44] The ILE was not regarded as a subset of SLE and could have been labeled undifferentiated connective tissue disease.[45] However, it should not be confused with MCTD.[41]

Schur[46] recommended, similarly to the ARA criteria for the diagnosis of rheumatoid arthritis, that patients be diagnosed as having classic SLE (many criteria), definite SLE (4 or more criteria), probable SLE (3 criteria), or possible SLE (2 criteria). Patients meeting 2 or 3 criteria may be said to have incomplete, incipient, or latent, as well as possible and probable, lupus.[45] If these patients are monitored, a few may develop definite SLE.

The criteria should be used as guidelines to aid the clinician in making a diagnosis of SLE. The diagnosis of SLE should not be made without the presence of *both* clinical and laboratory findings of the disease.

Subsets of Lupus Erythematosus

Skin involvement is a common manifestation of SLE and occurs in approximately 85% of the patients.[41,47] Several of the subsets of lupus involve skin lesions.

Lupus Panniculitis/Lupus Erythematosus Profundus

This is a subset of SLE; approximately 2% of patients with SLE develop septal or lobular panniculitis with cellular infiltrates and vasculitis similar to Weber-Christian disease.[48,49] Immunofluorescent studies have demonstrated immune complexes in the walls of small and medium-sized vessels in patients with lupus panniculitis.

Subacute Cutaneous Lupus Erythematosus

Many patients with subacute cutaneous lupus erythematosus (SCLE) fulfill the classification criteria for SLE and have antibodies to Sjögren's syndrome B/La (SS-B/La), Sjögren's syndrome A/Ro (SS-A/Ro), and the HLA-DR3 phenotype.[47] Another similar group of lupus-like patients with discoid lesions associated with various complement deficiencies have been described.[50] Many of these patients do not satisfy the classification criteria for SLE and have low titers of antibodies to double-stranded DNA (dsDNA) and anti–SS-A/Ro antibodies with infrequent kidney involvement. An additional group of patients had some features of SLE, but differed from typical cases of SLE in terms of the clinical course and prognosis.

Chronic Discoid Lupus

A benign form of lupus may present as "discoid" (coin or disc shaped) cutaneous lesions without symptoms of systemic disease. This disorder is called chronic discoid lupus erythematosus (CDLE).[50] The clinical and laboratory characteristics of chronic discoid lupus have not been clearly delineated since adoption of the revised 1982 ACR Criteria for the Classification of SLE.

However, SLE can exist as a potentially fatal multisystemic disease with or without discoid lupus lesions. Thus, discoid skin lesions can occur in both benign cutaneous and systemic lupus erythematosus.[47,50,51] The skin lesions of chronic discoid lupus are[50]

- Persistent localized erythema
- Adherent scales
- Follicular plugging
- Telangiectasias
- Atrophy

Subacute cutaneous lupus erythematosus consists of papulosquamous or nonscarring lesions. Additional variants of chronic discoid lupus, such as lupus panniculitis and urticarial lupus, have also been described.[48,50]

Wallace et al[50] have defined CDLE as one of the variants of SLE in which the ACR criteria for SLE are not met.

Chronic discoid lupus erythematosus is a cutaneous autoimmune disorder that lacks any unifying diagnostic serologic abnormality. It is a mild form of lupus erythematosus that uncommonly disseminates to SLE.

There is considerable overlap between discoid lupus and SLE. Up to 15% of patients with SLE have cutaneous discoid lesions. About 6% to 12% of patients with SLE have discoid lupus for a varying number of years before the onset of systemic disease.[50] Antinuclear antibodies are commonly found, with estimates of prevalence in discoid lupus of 6% to 50% The ratio of women to men with discoid lupus (2:1) is much less biased toward women than is the systemic form.

Occult Systemic Lupus Erythematosus

Compared with younger patients, elderly patients with SLE have shown a female preponderance, more insidious onset, less frequent occurrence of classic SLE manifestations, and a more benign course. Occult lupus was reported in elderly men who presented with weight loss, fever, and polyarthritis; the diagnosis of SLE was delayed due to the pursuit of extensive diagnostic studies.[52] Most of the male patients responded favorably to corticosteroids.

Autoantibody Profile in Systemic Lupus Erythematosus

Characteristic of SLE is the presence of a broad spectrum of autoantibodies, including antibody to native DNA, Sm antigen, uridine-rich ribonucleoprotein (U_1RNP), SS-A/Ro. SS-B/La, and several other nonhistone protein or nonhistone protein–RNA complexes.[1–6] Polyclonality of antibodies is seen in SLE and scleroderma and to a lesser extent in the other systemic rheumatic diseases. Anti-DNA and anti-Sm are generally specific for SLE. Systemic lupus erythematosus is characterized by a heterogeneous and polyclonal antibody response, and in the typical patient with SLE, an average of 3 different circulating antibodies are present simultaneously.[53-55]

The prevalence of autoantibodies varies widely. Antibodies to native DNA and histones are detectable in up to 40% and 70% of patients, respectively, and antibodies to proliferating-cell nuclear antigen (PCNA) and cyclin or ALu RNA protein are detectable in 3% or less (**Table 9-3**).[1–6,14]

Antibodies to Double-stranded DNA and Single-stranded DNA

There are 2 general types of anti-DNA antibodies, 1 directed to dsDNA and the other directed to single-stranded DNA (ssDNA). The antibodies to dsDNA target base pair DNA; the epitope is often to the deoxyribose phosphate backbone or to some part of the helical conformation. Thus, the antibodies to dsDNA or native DNA also react to the deoxyribose phosphate backbone or to some aspect of the helical conformation on ssDNA. The epitope for specific ssDNA antibodies recognizes the exposed free purine and pyrimidine bases.

Patients with SLE have both dsDNA and ssDNA antibodies. However, those with autoimmune diseases other than SLE may have low levels of specific ssDNA antibodies and no definite antibodies reactive to dsDNA.

Anti-dsDNA antibodies are specific for SLE and are observed in SLE patients with active disease at a frequency of 75% to 90%.[56,57] There were many earlier reports of antibodies to dsDNA in diseases other than SLE. However, current thinking is that the reactive antibodies to DNA in the other diseases were actually anti-ssDNA antibodies. The dsDNA antibody tests often used dsDNA preparations contaminated with denatured or ssDNA.[57]

Antibody to DNA plays a definite role in the pathogenesis of SLE. In studies of affected patients, antibody to DNA is followed by the appearance of circulating DNA antigen, a sequence that results in the formation of immune complexes. Such DNA–anti-DNA–immune

Table 9-3. Antigens and Autoantibodies in Systemic Lupus Erythematosus*

Antigen	Molecular Structure	Autoantibody Frequency (%)
Native DNA	Double-strand DNA	40
Denatured DNA	Single-strand DNA	70
Histones	H1, H2A, H2B, H3, H4	70
Sm	Proteins, 29 (B^1), 28 (B), 16 (D), and 13 (E) kd, complexed with U1, U2 and U4-U6 snRNAs	30
Nuclear RNP (U^1 RNP)	Proteins, 70, 33 (A), and 22 (C) kd, complexed with U^1 snRNA; splicesome component	32
SS-A/Ro	Proteins, 60 and 52 kd, complexed with Y1-Y5 RNAs	35
SS-B/La	Phosphoproteins, 48 kd, complexed with Y1 nascent RNA Pol III transcripts	15
Ku	Proteins, 86 and 66 kd, DNA-binding proteins	10
Ki	Nuclear protein, 32 kd	31
PCNA/cyclin	Protein, 36 kd; auxiliary protein of DNA polymerase	3
Ribosomal RNP	Phosphoproteins, 38, 16, and 15 kd associated with ribosomes	10
Hsp 90	Heat-shock protein, 90 kd	50
ALu RNA protein	Protein, 68 kd, 11 complexed with ALu RNA	Rare
S10	Ribosomal small subunit protein, 20 kd	11
Cardiolipin	Anionic phospholipids	20-40

*There are many more autoantibodies. Over 50 have been reported to be present in SLE sera.

complexes are deposited in the kidney glomeruli and initiate kidney damage.[58,59]

Earlier methods for detection of DNA antibodies were precipitation, complement fixation, and passive hemagglutination,[57] which had lower sensitivity. Current methods are radioimmunoassay (RIA), indirect immunofluorescence microscopy (IFM) on *Crithidia luciliae*, and enzyme-linked immunosorbent assay (ELISA).[1–6] These DNA antibody assay methods can detect anti-DNA in 75% to 90% of patients with active, untreated SLE. Some of the available DNA antibody tests measure antibodies to both dsDNA and ssDNA because the preparations of dsDNA may be contaminated with ssDNA and vice versa.[57] However, the ssDNA can be removed from preparations of dsDNA by digestion with S_1 endonuclease, an enzyme with specificity for ssDNA.

One study showed that the indirect immunofluorescent assay with *C luciliae* was the most specific, whereas the radioimmunoassay for DNA was the most sensitive.[57] The ELISA was compared with radioactive Farr assay, and results showed a correlation between the 2 assay systems ($R^2 = 0.73$).[60]

Lafer et al[61] reported that in some patients with SLE, monoclonal antibodies derived from mice infected with SLE showed cross-reactivity between dsDNA and cardiolipin. However, the majority of patients demonstrated no cross-reactivity between anti-dsDNA and anticardiolipin antibodies.

Antibodies to Sm and Nuclear Ribonucleoprotein

Precipitating antibodies to Sm antigen have been considered highly specific markers for SLE.[14] Antibodies to both Sm and nRNP are found in patients with SLE. The Sm and nRNP antigens are clearly associated; the nRNP cannot be separated biochemically from the Sm antigen.[62,63] Lerner and Steitz[64] used the tools of molecular biology to show that Sm and nRNP antigens were subcellular particles composed of small nuclear RNAs (nRNAs) complexed with proteins. The particle bound by anti-nRNP is composed of an RNA component designated U_1 (uridine-rich), complexed to at least 7 proteins varying in molecular mass from 12 to 68 kd[4] and recently found in 20% to 40% of affected patients.[65,66]

The antigens of Sm consist of at least 4 proteins conventionally called B^1/B (28/29 kd), D (16 kd), and E (13 kd).[4] Purified anti-B^1/B antibodies cross-react with the D protein and vice versa, but no cross-reaction is observed in smaller percentages of SLE sera. Thus, at least 2 epitopes on the B^1/B protein are recognized by anti-Sm sera.[67] The antigens that react with anti-Sm and antinuclear RNA are therefore in assemblies of interactive proteins and RNAs engaged in precursor messenger RNP splicing.[4]

No characteristic clinical features are apparent in SLE patients with anti-Sm antibodies.[68,69] Patients who have antibodies to only nRNP have a low frequency of antibodies to DNA and a low frequency of clinically apparent renal disease.[65,66]

Patients with mixed connective tissue disease have heterogeneous clinical features, and the only uniform finding is the presence of antibodies to U_1RNP.[41,65,66] Antibodies to U_1RNP occur in a number of SLE patients who do not exhibit overlapping features with other systemic rheumatic diseases.

Antiribonucleoproteins (anti-nRNPs), referred to as anti-U_1RNP antibodies, are associated with mixed connective tissue disease and can occur in SLE in lower titers in 30% to 40% of patients with SLE.[66,68]

Anti-Sm and anti-nRNP antibodies may be detected by immunodiffusion, passive hemagglutination, or counterimmunoelectrophoresis. However, these methods do not accurately distinguish between antibodies against different small nRNA-associated polypeptides. The reactivities with individual RNAs and polypeptides can be best demonstrated by RNA immunoprecipitation and immunoblotting techniques, respectively. Immunoblotting has been found to be more sensitive than conventional methods for the detection of anti-Sm and anti-nRNP.

Currently, the most widely used laboratory tests for the detection of anti-Sm and anti-nRNP antibodies are immunodiffusion and ELISA. These tests can differentiate between Sm and nRNP antibodies but cannot define the specific antibody epitopes present in patient sera. The antibody specificity and epitopes are best determined by Western and Northern blotting methods.[70]

Antibodies to SS-A/Ro and SS-B/La

Patients with SLE can have antibodies to SS-A/Ro alone, or they may have both anti–SS-A/Ro and anti–SS-B/La. Having anti–SS-A/Ro alone is strongly associated with HLA-DR2 and is seen in younger patients with SLE (<22 years of age at onset). The presence of both anti–SS-A/Ro and anti–SS-B/La is associated with HLA-DR3 and is seen in older patients with SLE (>50 years of age at onset).[13,71] A study of 55 patients with SLE showed that those with anti–SS-A/Ro alone had far more serious renal disease.[13] They also had a higher incidence of concomitant anti-DNA antibodies than patients with both the anti–SS-A/Ro and anti–SS-B/La antibodies.[72]

Anti–SS-A/Ro autoantibodies have been closely associated with the appearance of nephritis, vasculitis, lymphadenopathy, and leukopenia in SLE patients.

Anti–SS-B/La antibodies, like anti–SS-A/Ro antibodies, are noteworthy for their strong association with Sjögren's syndrome, occurring in about 66% of patients with this disorder. The SS-B/La antigen is a cellular protein bound to a small RNA species and forming a small RNP that may function in processing RNA polymerase III transcripts.[72]

Clinical Subsets of Systemic Lupus Erythematosus Associated With SS-A/Ro Antibodies

Elevated levels of SS-A/Ro antibodies are related to several clinical autoimmune disorders, including[73,74]

- Neonatal lupus erythematosus syndrome
- Primary Sjögren's syndrome vasculitis
- Homozygous C2 and C4 deficiency with SLE-like disease
- Subacute cutaneous lupus erythematosus
- Patients with SLE who are ANA-negative
- Systemic lupus erythematosus with interstitial pneumonitis

Precipitating antibodies to SS-A/Ro are seen in 65% to 95% of patients with anti–SS-A/Ro associated subsets, and more than 90% of the patients have elevated anti–SS-A/Ro levels when ELISA methods are used.[14]

Neonatal Lupus Erythematosus

Neonatal lupus erythematosus (NLE) is a rare syndrome that occurs in a minority of infants delivered only by mothers who have anti–SS-A/Ro and/or anti–SS-B/La. The disease consists of transient rash in the newborn period, complete heart block, or both.[9,75–77]

About 33% of patients with SLE have antibodies to SS-A/Ro, SS-B/La, or both. However, it is not possible to predict which child of a mother with anti–SS-A/Ro or anti–SS-B/La will develop the skin abnormalities of NLE. The congenital heart block is caused by certain specific autoantibodies. Heart block occurs exclusively in a small number of infants whose mothers have antibodies to both SS-A/Ro (52 kd) and SS-B/La (48 kd) antigens. Infants of mothers without anti–SS-B/La or in whom the anti–SS-A/Ro is directed only at the 60-kd antigen and not at the 52-kd antigen are at low risk for NLE.[9,75–77] The occurrence and severity of NLE are unrelated to maternal disease activity or severity.

Vasculitis Associated With Sjögren's Syndrome

In a large group of patients with Sjögren's syndrome, 24 (86%) of 28 patients with vasculitis had anti–SS-A/Ro precipitins, whereas in 47 patients with no vasculitis, only 4 (8.5%) had anti–SS-A/Ro precipitins.[71]

Homozygous C2 and C4 Deficiency in Systemic Lupus Erythematosus

The anti–SS-A/Ro precipitating antibodies have been closely associated with homozygous C2 and C4 deficiency–associated SLE, which demonstrates SCLE and mild systemic disease associated with the presence of anti–SS-A/Ro antibodies.[6,78]

Subacute Cutaneous Lupus Erythematosus

The subset of SLE has been described by Sontheimer et al[47,51] and has the following features: widespread, nonscarring photosensitive form of histologically specific lupus erythematosus lesions of the skin; a high frequency of HLA-DR3; mild systemic clinical disease with minimal renal and nervous system involvement; and antibodies to SS-A/Ro and/or SS-B/La in 62% of patients.

The clinical features and serology of the many ANA-negative patients with SLE are very similar to those with SCLE.[50] The latter often demonstrate negative IF-ANA tests on mouse or rat tissue substrate, but are positive for ANA on HEp-2 human epithelial tissue culture lines.[4,79,80]

Antiphospholipid Antibodies in Systemic Lupus Erythematosus

Systemic lupus erythematosus is characterized by the presence of circulating antibodies to phospholipids, clinical features of arterial and venous thrombosis, and thrombocytopenia. The antiphospholipid antibodies are found frequently in patients with SLE and also in other disorders such as cancer, DLE, and infectious disorders.[81–88]

Antiphospholipid antibodies are found in up to 60% of patients with SLE. There is considerable recent evidence that antiphospholipid antibodies are heterogeneous and polyspecific.[80]

Cardiolipin (anionic phospholipid) has been used widely for the detection of antiphospholipid antibodies. The majority of anticardiolipin antibodies cross-react with other anionic phospholipids, but some also may react with zwitterionic phospholipids. Antibodies to anionic phospholipids may be IgG or IgM, whereas antibodies to zwitterionic phospholipids are more frequently IgM.[84,86]

Antibodies to phospholipids are identified in patients with SLE in 3 ways[87,89,90]:

- Serologic false-positive test for syphilis by a positive Venereal Disease Reference Laboratory test, a flocculation assay using carbon particles coated with cholesterol, lecithin (phosphatidylcholine), and cardiolipin
- The lupus anticoagulant assay, a prolongation of the kaolin partial thromboplastin time that is not corrected by normal plasma
- Cardiolipin immunoassay using cardiolipin or other negatively charged phospholipids as antigens

Patients with SLE usually react with a negatively charged phosphate group present in cardiolipin, phosphatidic acid phosphatidylserine, and phosphatidylinositol.

Several experimental attempts have been made to induce antiphospholipid antibody or lupus anticoagulant to develop an animal model of the disease[61,91,92]:

- When lipid A is combined with phospholipid and injected into rodents, highly specific antiphospholipid antibody is produced.
- When human monoclonal anti-DNA or mouse anti-idiotypic antibody is injected into mice, SLE and anticardiolipin antibodies are manifested.
- Cardiolipin combined with β_2-glycoprotein I induces antiphospholipid antibody in mice. Either substance alone does not induce antibody production.
- Hexagonal H_{11}, but not lamellar phospholipid, induces antiphospholipid antibodies in animals.

Viard et al[93] found that 17 (36%) of 47 patients with SLE had specific anti-β_2 glycoprotein I antibodies, which were statistically associated with anticardiolipin antibodies, thrombosis, and lupus anticoagulant. In addition, anti–β_2-glycoprotein I antibodies are closely associated with lupus anticoagulant activity.

In 1988, Harris and associates[94] developed a solid radioimmunoassay for anticardiolipin antibody. In 1987 and 1990, Harris et al[95,96] convened international workshops to improve the precision and accuracy of antiphospholipid antibody immunoassays. Reference sera were prepared, and standard units, GPL (IgG phospholipid) and MPL (IgM phospholipid), were defined: One GPL or MPL unit is equivalent to 1 mg/mL of an affinity-purified standard IgG or IgM sample. However, Lopez et al[97] recently suggested that an IgA-specific assay for antiphospholipid antibody is important in assessing antiphospholipid syndrome in patients with SLE.

More recently, evidence has shown that the major cardiolipin antibodies in patients with antiphospholipid antibody syndrome are directed against β_2-glycoprotein I.[98–100] Tincani et al[101] have demonstrated that anti–β_2-glycoprotein I autoantibodies in human antiphospholipid syndrome sera are directed to epitopes on native β_2-glycoprotein I.

Commercial manufacturers are developing ELISAs to detect autoantibodies to β_2-glycoprotein I. Erickson et al[102] have made available a reference calibrator for IgG antibodies to β_2-glycoprotein I.

Antiapolipoprotein AI

Apolipoprotein AI (ApoAI) is the major lipid-binding protein of high-density lipoprotein (HDL). Recently, the discovery of autoantibody reactive with ApoAI in SLE has aroused great interest.[103,104] The ApoAI has been observed to be immunogenic, and the ApoAI antibodies may play a role in the decreased HDL levels and ApoAI-ApoB ratios previously reported in subgroups of SLE.[105] The anti-ApoAI may be involved in the pathogenesis of accelerated atherosclerosis and myocardial disease observed with increased frequency in SLE patients.[10]

Anti-Ku and Anti-Ki Antibodies

The Ku antigen system consists of a pair of proteins called p70 and p80.[106,107] These proteins have a high affinity for DNA and are known to bind DNA. With the use of both immunoprecipitation and immunoblot assays, the Ku autoantibody was found in 10% of sera from patients with SLE and was not detected in 100 scleroderma sera examined.[106]

Autoantibodies to Ku protein were originally described in sera from patients with a polymyositis-scleroderma overlap syndrome, and the frequency of antibody by immunodiffusion assay was 3%.[108] In subsequent studies with an enzyme immunoassay (EIA), Reeves[108] showed that 39% of patients with SLE, 55% of those with MCTD, and 40% of those with scleroderma had low levels of antibodies to Ku protein. Yaneva and Arnett[109] used immunoaffinity-purified Ku protein in an immunoblot assay for Ku antibody. They found a significantly increased frequency of anti-Ku antibodies in patients with SLE (19%) and scleroderma (14%).

Anti-Ku antibodies were found in 23% of patients with primary pulmonary hypertension.[110] The patients with this disease frequently have Raynaud's phenomenon, serum antinuclear antibodies, and/or pulmonary vascular lesions similar to those seen in certain connective tissue diseases, such as scleroderma.

Anti-Ki antibody was first reported by Tojo et al[111] in 1981 and was observed in approximately 10% of patients with SLE. A relationship was observed between anti-Ki and the clinical features of arthritis, pericarditis, and pulmonary hypertension in these patients.

The Ki antigen was purified from rabbit thymus and had a molecular weight of 32,000 kd. Sakamoto et al[112] developed an ELISA and observed anti-Ki antibody in 30 (21.4%) of 140 SLE patients, while 11 (7.9%) were positive for anti-Ki by double immunodiffusion tests. The researchers also analyzed the clinical and serologic data and concluded that there is a higher prevalence of CNS involvement in patients with SLE and anti-Ki antibody.

The Ku autoantigen is a heterodimer complex consisting of 70- and 80-kd proteins that interact covalently with the ends of native DNA.[113,114] Autoantibodies to Ku have a nucleolar staining pattern and only 10% to 39% of patients with SLE have this antibody.

Antibodies to Proliferating Cell Nuclear Antigen and Heat Shock Protein 90

Antibodies to PCNA are detected in 3% of patients with SLE, who show no distinctive clinical features associated with the presence of these antibodies.[115] The PCNA protein has been characterized as cell cycle–related. The PCNA antibodies have been useful probes in the study of events regulating DNA replication, cell proliferation, and blast transformation. In one study, there was evidence of a higher frequency of diffuse proliferative glomerulonephritis in anti-PCNA–positive patients.[116]

Autoantibody to a mammalian heat shock protein (Hsp-90) has been observed.[117,118] The Hsp-90 (90 kd) is a cytoplasmic and plasma membrane protein.[117] The autoantibody to Hsp-90 was observed in 50% of patients with SLE and 2 of 6 patients with polymyositis.

Antibodies to Ribosomal Ribonucleoprotein and Systemic Lupus Erythematosus with Central Nervous System Involvement

Autoantibodies to ribosomal proteins of the cytoplasm have been recognized in patients with SLE.[119,120] About 10% of SLE patients appear to have autoantibodies that stain the cytoplasm by indirect immunofluorescence. Frequently, the nucleoli also are stained. Three autoantigenic phosphoproteins (36, 16, and 15 kd) are present in ribosomal ribonucleoprotein (rRNP).[4] These 3 proteins are components of the large ribosomal subunit and are often referred to as ribosomal P proteins.

An association has been reported between psychotic syndromes in SLE and autoantibodies to RNP.[121] In a study of 32 SLE patients with autoantibodies to rRNP, 18 (56%) had psychotic syndromes. Many other factors are probably associated with this phenomenon.

Autoantibodies directed against a ribosomal small subunit protein of 20,000 kd were found in the sera of 5 (11%) of 44 SLE patients.[122] The ribosomal protein was identified as S10 on the basis of two-dimensional gel electrophoresis and immunoblotting. Anti-S10 antibodies were observed more frequently in SLE patients who also had anti-Sm and antiribosomal P protein antibodies. In sera from 31 patients with other autoimmune diseases, the immunoblotting assay detected the S10 autoantibody in only 1 patient who had primary Sjögren's syndrome.[121]

Schneebaum et al[123] have reported elevated levels of autoantibodies to the C-terminal region of ribosomal P proteins, which appears to be a specific marker for SLE. Overall, 27 (10%) of 269 patients with SLE demonstrated elevated levels of IgG or IgM antibodies, including 26 (14%) of 187 patients without and 24 (29%) of 82 patients with neuropsychiatric manifestations. The antiribosomal P antibodies are associated with both severe depression and psychosis in patients with SLE.[123–125]

There have been conflicting reports regarding the usefulness of antiribosomal P protein levels in the evaluation of neuropsychiatric systemic lupus erythematosus (NPSLE).[124,126] Teh and Isenberg[126] reviewed and reappraised these reports and discussed several possible reasons for the discrepancies. The studies mainly disagreed in regard to the usefulness of antiribosomal P protein antibody levels as a single measurement for determining whether the patient has lupus psychosis. A major factor in the disparate results reported may have been due to differences in the methods and criteria used to define NPSLE.[126]

One study has documented a rise and rapid fall in antiribosomal P protein levels just before the onset of recurrent psychosis such that the antibody levels were no longer normal by the time the patient presented for care.[127] Such a rapid decline in antiribosomal antibody level may account for some of the conflicting data already described.

Central Nervous System Systemic Lupus Erythematosus

Much of the pathogenesis of CNS disease in SLE is unknown. It may be a combination of microvascular injury and interference with normal cortical function as a result of antibodies reacting with membranes of neuronal cells.[125]

Neuropsychiatric manifestations may occur in as many as 70% of SLE patients.[128,129] Autoantibodies that react with neuronal cell membranes or cross-react with lymphocytes have been found in the cerebrospinal fluid of patients with SLE.[130]

Robbins et al[131] studied cytoskeletal protein from bovine neural extracts by Western blot methods. They demonstrated that 22 SLE patients with neuropsychiatric manifestations had an increased incidence of antineurofilament antibody when compared with 34 SLE patients without neuropsychiatric symptoms, 78 patients with other diseases, and 22 normal control patients. Fifty-eight percent (7/12) of patients with SLE and diffuse neuropsychiatric manifestations had antineurofilament antibody when compared with the healthy control group with an incidence of 18% (4/22).

Patients with SLE and negative antineurofilament antibody results had significantly elevated levels of anticardiolipin antibody. Antiphospholipid antibodies are associated with venous and arterial thrombosis in SLE patients. These antibodies also are associated with neurologic and ophthalmologic manifestations, regardless of whether the mechanism of neurologic involvement is thrombotic.[83–85,126]

The following points can be observed in SLE patients with neuropsychiatric disease[125,129]:

- Eighty percent of patients with active CNS SLE have abnormal electroencephalograms.
- Elevated levels of serum antiribosomal P antibody are seen in 40% to 90% of SLE patients with psychosis or major depression.
- Antiribosomal P protein antibodies are seen in patients with diffuse rather than focal CNS involvement.
- Serum levels of anti-DNA, complement, and immune complex do not correlate with the activity of CNS SLE. The antineuronal antibody assays are difficult to perform and are not available in most diagnostic clinical laboratories. In the complete evaluation of NPSLE, the antineuronal antibody is helpful but not necessary.
- Analysis of the cerebrospinal fluid in CNS SLE may show
    - — an elevated cell count and increased protein concentration in 33% of SLE patients.
    - — abnormal IgG, IgM, or IgA indices with a combination of oligoclonal bands in diffuse neuropsychiatric disease (this is not specific for CNS SLE).

Antibodies to Nuclear Lamina

The nuclear lamina is the proteinaceous meshwork lining the inner surface of the nuclear envelope of eukaryotic cells. In mammalian cells, the nuclear lamina is composed of 3 major polypeptides called lamins A, B, and C.[132,133] In addition, minor lamin polypeptides D and E have been identified.

Predominant lamin B antibody specificity in the sera from SLE patients was reported.[133] Antibodies to lamin B or lamins A and C have been noted in patients with chronic autoimmune diseases such as SLE, rheumatoid arthritis, and undifferentiated connective tissue disease.[134] Predominant anti–lamin A and anti–lamin C antibodies were observed in 12 (75%) of 16 patients with active autoimmune chronic active hepatitis.[135]

With the antilamina antibodies detected by immunoblot tests using purified rat liver lamina, peripheral staining patterns were identified by indirect immunofluorescence on HEp-2 cells using fluorescein isothiocyanate–conjugated goat antihuman IgG, IgM, and IgA. The patterns were similar to those from reference sera with anti-DNA antibodies.[132,136,137]

Chronic fatigue syndrome (CFS) is a clinically defined condition consisting of profound fatigue associated with a variety of nonspecific symptoms.[138–140] Investigations demonstrated that 31 (52%) of 60 patients with CFS had serum autoantibodies to nuclear envelope antigens. The autoantibodies were of the IgG isotype and reacted to B_1 nuclear lamin.[141] The B_1 nuclear lamin autoantibodies were detected by an immunoblot assay and confirmed with immunoprecipitation of radiolabeled in vitro translated product of complementary DNA encoding human lamin B_1.

Antilymphocyte Autoantibodies

Antilymphocyte autoantibodies are commonly observed in patients with SLE.[142,143] The question that remains is whether the antilymphocyte antibody contributes to the development of autoimmunity, or whether it is produced by the immune system to restore homeostasis as a result of aggressive autoimmune stimulation.[142]

The antilymphocyte autoantibodies in SLE vary in titer with disease activity, similar to dsDNA autoantibodies, and are associated with depletion of circulating T cells.[144] The presence of these antilymphocyte antibodies correlates closely with the spectrum of immune system functional abnormalities observed in patients with SLE.[143]

Autoantibodies to Chromatin (Nucleosomes)

Chromatin is the native histone-DNA complex associated with nonhistone proteins and RNA found in living cells (**Figure 9-1**). Nucleosome is the fundamental repeating unit of chromatin (**Figure 9-2**). Tan[145] emphasized that it could be a major autoantigen in SLE. Circulating nucleosome oligomers have been demonstrated in the plasma of patients with SLE.[146]

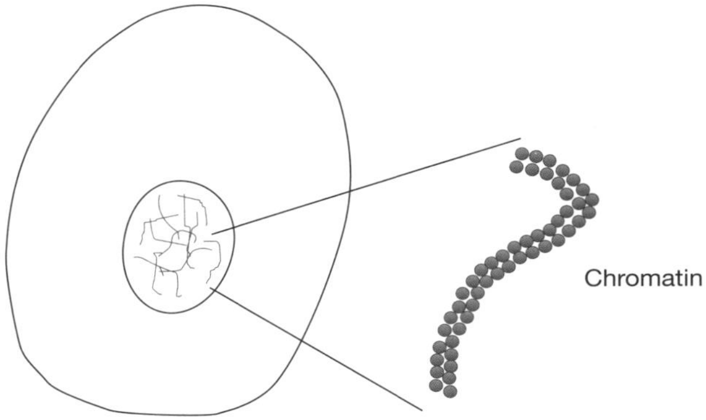

Figure 9-1. Cell showing nucleus with segments of nuclear chromatin, which is the native histone-DNA complex associated with non-histone proteins and RNA.

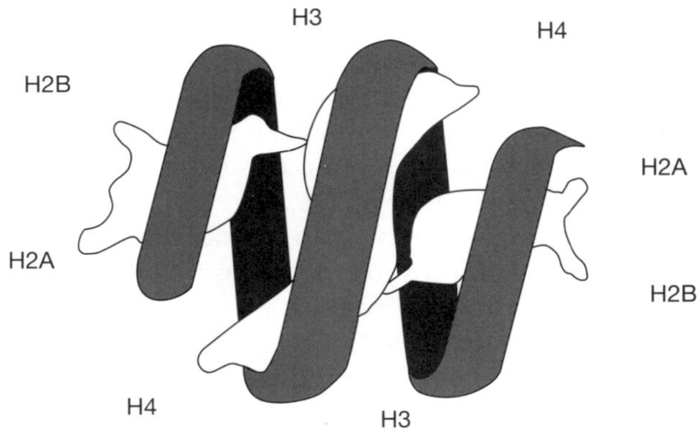

Figure 9-2. Nucleosome is the fundamental repeating unit of the chromatin. Diagram shows the structural association with histones 2A, 2B, H3, and H4.

An ELISA has been developed for the detection of antibodies to chromatin.[147,148] The chromatin-reactive antibodies recognize epitopes that are unique to the native histone-DNA complex, and other antibodies recognize individual histones or native dsDNA.[148,149]

Chabre et al[148] demonstrated with an ELISA method that SLE patients have nucleosome-restricted antibodies. These antibodies react with the whole nucleosome or chromatin particle but not with its individual components, such as dsDNA and histones. Sixteen of 40 sera samples from patients with SLE displayed anti-dsDNA and/or antihistone activity, which was always associated with antinucleosome activity. However, 3 samples showed antinucleosome activity that was not associated with concomitant anti-dsDNA or antihistone activity.

The presence of antibodies to chromatin in SLE patients has been well documented. The incidence of antichromatin autoantibodies in SLE has been reported to be 50% to 97%.[148–152] In cases of active SLE, between 85%[142] and 100%[148] of patients test positive. In SLE, the majority of the chromatin-reactive antibodies recognize epitopes that require the native histone-DNA complex, and the antibodies to individual histones or native dsDNA constitute only a small portion of the antichromatin reactivity.[148,149]

Historically, the LE cell test was one of the first useful for diagnosis.[153–155] The LE cell phenomenon is the result of the reaction between patient serum autoantibodies and nuclei released from dead cells, with subsequent phagocytosis by living polymorphonuclear cells. Several early studies indicated that antibodies to chromatin and not anti-dsDNA were responsible for this phenomenon.[155–157]

Strong reactivity on the antichromatin ELISA and the LE cell test are found in the same groups of patients with SLE and DLE. The LE cell test is difficult to perform and not highly reproducible. The ELISA for antichromatin has shown good diagnostic sensitivity, given that 78% of patients with SLE are antibody positive.[151] The ELISA for antichromatin is more sensitive than the LE cell test. Patients with SLE and DLE may show evidence of autoantibodies to chromatin, which is discussed in the next section.[158]

Drug-Induced Lupus Erythematosus and Antihistone Antibodies

Drug-induced lupus erythematosus is a syndrome resembling mild SLE, a similarity that can complicate treatment. The most common drugs involved are hydralazine and procainamide. Drugs less frequently associated with DLE are chlorpromazine, isoniazid, methyldopa, penicillamine, quinidine, and sulfonamides.[159]

The presence of histone antibodies is characteristic of DLE. Histones are basic proteins containing high molar ratios of positively charged amino acids, lysine, and arginine. They are found in eukaryotic cells associated with DNA in chromatin. The subunit of this histone-DNA complex is called a nucleosome (Figure 9-2), which has 2 molecules of each of the "core" histones (H2A, H2B, H3, and H4) and 1 molecule of H1, along with DNA of about 200 base pairs in length.[160,161]

The dominant antihistone antigenic determinants in SLE are the C-terminal of H1 and the trypsin-sensitive N-terminal of H2B.[162] However, autoantibodies also may be found to trypsin-sensitive N and C terminals of H4[162] and to the complex of (H2A-H2B)-DNA.[163,164]

Two patterns of autoantibody reactivity were observed in drug-induced antihistone autoantibodies[158]:

1. All 21 patients (100%) with procainamide-induced lupus and 7 (58%) of 12 patients with quinidine-induced lupus had IgG autoantibodies reactive with the (H2A-H2B)-DNA complex and with chromatin.

2. Eighteen (95%) of 19 chlorpromazine-treated patients and 14 (82%) of 17 patients with hydralazine-induced lupus had IgM antibodies, which were more reactive to DNA-free histone and corresponding histone-DNA complexes, and almost no binding to H1-stripped chromatin.

In studies of DLE, the liver enzyme acetyltransferase was found to acetylate drugs such as hydralazine and procainamide and to play a role in detoxification and excretion of those drugs. Patients with low levels of acetyltransferase activity were more prone to develop ANAs and clinical symptoms than patients with phenotypically high levels of acetyltransferase activity. Patients with high levels of enzyme who were rapid acetylators were not immune to the development of ANAs. These patients, however, took a longer and larger cumulative dose of hydralazine before developing disease. These findings concerning acetyltransferase phenotypes have been confirmed in patients treated with procainamide.[165]

Procainamide is the most common drug involved in drug-induced autoimmunity, although hydralazine, quinidine, and other drugs also have been implicated. In DLE, antibodies to ssDNA and histones are present. In SLE, on the other hand, antibodies to native dsDNA, Sm, and U_1RNP antigens are often present, in addition to the antibodies to histones. Procainamide is used to treat patients with cardiac arrhythmias, and most patients eventually develop antihistone antibodies. However, only 10% to 20% of procainamide-treated patients develop symptomatic autoimmune disease.[4,166] In asymptomatic patients, the antihistone antibody is predominantly IgM and displays broad reactivity with all of the individual histones.

Patients with symptomatic disease develop a unique type of IgG antihistone antibody, which, rather than reacting with individual histones, shows specific reactivity with the histone H2A-H2B dimer complex.[161] Thus, the IgG anti-(H2A-H2B) is a useful diagnostic marker, with high sensitivity and specificity for symptomatic diseases, in contrast to the benign form of procainamide-induced autoimmunity with IgM antibodies to the individual histone.

In hydralazine-induced lupus erythematosus, the complex of H2A-H2B is an important target antigen, but the H3-H4 complex appears to be more reactive.[161,163] In both types of DLE (hydralazine and procainamide), IgM antibodies are present in higher concentrations than are IgG antibodies.

In one study, 50% of all patients treated with procainamide developed ANAs after 1 year of treatment.[3] The slow acetylators developed ANAs more rapidly than the rapid acetylators.[165] All patients on prolonged procainamide treatment developed a positive ANA response irrespective of acetylator phenotype.

Assays for Antihistone Antibodies

One of the first assays was a microcomplement fixation test developed by Stollar.[167] This assay was not very sensitive and was difficult to perform accurately to detect antihistone antibodies.[168] Subsequently, Tan et al[169] and Fritzler and Tan[170] developed an immunofluorescent procedure with the use of mouse kidney substrate. This assay is very specific for antihistone antibodies but cannot be used with sera that contain high levels of anti-DNA antibodies, which display background binding to acid-extracted nuclei. Sera containing predominant antihistone activity to H3 and H4 showed negligible reactivity in the immunofluorescence assay.[171] The immunofluorescence assay was largely selective for antibodies to H2A, H2B, and/or H2A-H2B complex if epitopes on the histones were not blocked by DNA.[168,171]

More recently, ELISAs and immunoblots of histones have been used. Subnucleosome structures have been employed in an ELISA format to measure autoantibodies to specific structures of histones and in chromatin.[147]

Clinical Evaluation of Suspected Cases of Systemic Lupus Erythematosus

The prevalence of SLE has been estimated to be 50.8 cases per 100,000 people.[172] The prevalence of SLE in white women younger than 15 years is 0 per 100,000. The incidence of SLE in 10- to 20-year-old women is 4.4 per 100,000 in whites, 31 per 100,000 in Asians, 19.8 per 100,000 in blacks, and 13 per 100,000 in Hispanics.[173,174]

The diagnostic workup includes the following steps:

1. Completion of a patient history and physical examination
2. Correlation of the clinical and physical examination findings with the ARA criteria for definite SLE[36]
3. Laboratory evaluation
   - Complete blood cell count, erythrocyte sedimentation rate, urinalysis
   - Appropriate panel of chemistry tests, depending on history and physical examination
   - Tests for autoantibodies to nuclear and cytoplasmic antigens

Most physicians rely on the 1982 ARA criteria for the classification of SLE. It should be emphasized that these criteria were developed for the classification of SLE patients when such patients were compared with those having other systemic rheumatic diseases. When the criteria are used to test against other diseases, the sensitivity and specificity for SLE have been 96%.[46]

As discussed earlier, Schur[46] suggested classifying SLE patients as classic, definite, probable, and possible. If patients with possible SLE are monitored long term, few develop SLE. Other cases of possible SLE may evolve into another illness or symptoms may disappear.[175]

Certain diseases, such as idiopathic thrombocytopenic purpura, isolated hemolytic anemia, and isolated proteinuria may have a positive result with an IFM-ANA test without other evidence of SLE.[12,174] Some patients with these diagnoses may develop SLE when monitored over a period of time. Thus, such patients should be monitored and periodically reevaluated to establish the correct diagnosis.

Laboratory Evaluation of Systemic Lupus Erythematosus and Related Disorders

The laboratory assessment of a patient suspected of having SLE or another systemic rheumatic disorder begins with a sensitive screening test for nuclear and cytoplasmic antibodies. Currently, the most widely used test is the IFM-ANA test with HEp-2 cells as the substrate. Different autoantibodies produce characteristic morphologic patterns of fluorescent staining. These patterns indicate the presence of specific ANAs, which should be identified by specific secondary tests.[176]

Most laboratories have noted that if the IFM-ANA test results are negative or the end point titer is less than 160, the follow-up secondary tests yield positive results in less than 5% of patients.[177] Further testing for disease-specific autoantibodies is indicated if the ANA titer is 160 or greater. An exception to this would be if a strong cytoplasmic staining of HEp-2 cells is noted at lower titers, in which case specific tests for certain cytoplasmic autoantibodies, such as Jo-1 and RNP, should be considered.

Immunofluorescence-based ANA determinations using tissue culture cells as the antigen-containing substrate for universal detection of antitissue autoantibodies will remain the staple method for some time to come. Many improvements or modifications of this technique have been introduced in the past few years. They include advances in instrumentation and immunologic reagents and manufacturers' use of tissue culture cells in the log phase of growth and/or in mitosis to detect antibodies to proliferation-associated antigens such as PCNA and cell cycle–related antigens. The cumulative effect of such technologic modifications has resulted in imperceptible and hitherto undocumented changes in the sensitivity and specificity of IFM-ANA.

To address these issues, the ANA Standardization Committee of the International Union of Immunological Societies conducted an international multicenter study in which coded samples of "normal" sera and sera from several disease categories were analyzed at 1:40, 1:80, 1:160, and 1:320 dilutions.[178] The results are presented in **Table 9-4**. It can be seen that at 1:40 dilution only 68.3% of normal sera were negative by IFM-ANA; it was only at 1:160 dilution that 95% of normal sera were negative. Clear distinctions could be made between sera from patients with SLE, scleroderma, and Sjögren's syndrome on the one hand and normal sera on the other at any of the 4 dilutions studied. The suggestion was made that IFM-ANA readings should be made at both 1:40 and 1:60 dilutions, because although statistically significant differences could not be made between normal sera and sera from patients with rheumatoid arthritis and soft-tissue rheumatism,

Table 9-4. Operating Characteristics of Immunofluorescence Microscopy-Antinuclear Antibody Tests[178]

Disease	Cutoff Dilution	Sensitivity* (%)	Specificity† (%)
SLE	1:40	97.4	68.3
	1:80	97.4	87.6
	1:160	94.7	95.0
	1:320	86.8	96.7
Scleroderma	1:40	100.0	68.3
	1:80	94.6	86.7
	1:160	86.5	95.0
	1:320	83.8	96.7
Sjögren's syndrome	1:40	84.2	68.3
	1:80	76.3	86.7
	1:160	73.7	95.0
	1:320	71.1	96.7
Rheumatoid arthritis	1:40	48.6	68.3
	1:80	37.8	86.7
	1:160	13.5	95.0
	1:320	2.70	96.7
STR	1:40	38.5	68.3
	1:80	23.1	86.7
	1:160	7.70	95.0
	1:320	3.80	96.7

Abbreviations: SLE = systemic lupus erythematosus; STR = soft-tissue rheumatism.
**Sensitivity is the percentage of patients with the disease for whom the assay was positive at the indicated cutoff.*
†Specificity is the percentage of normal patients for whom the assay was negative at the indicated cutoff.

there was still a trend toward higher percentages of positive tests in the latter. No differences in positive and negative results were observed in normal sera from patients aged 20 to 60 years.

If the IFM-ANA test is negative, the patient has a less than 0.14% probability of having SLE. Thus, the IFM-ANA test is useful to rule out the diagnosis of SLE.[1,46,179] A negative IFM-ANA test does not, however, rule out the possibility of all systemic rheumatic diseases. Polymyositis/dermatomyositis, rheumatoid arthritis, and scleroderma may have negative IFM-ANA results and still show evidence of specific antibodies by other methods.[1,2,5]

A positive IFM-ANA test has a predictive value of 20% to 35% for SLE.[46] The IFM-ANA test is positive in up to 74% of patients with Sjögren's syndrome, 40% to 87% of patients with scleroderma (especially those with a speckled pattern of ANAs), 16% of patients with juvenile rheumatoid arthritis, and 25% to 50% of patients with rheumatoid arthritis (especially those with a diffuse pattern of ANAs).[178–181] Antinuclear antibodies tend to be present in higher titers in patients with SLE than in patients with other disorders.

Normal Versus Abnormal Level of Autoantibodies to Nuclear Antigens

The incidence of positive IFM-ANA results in people older than 40 years gradually increases with age in the normal population, and low positive titers by IFM-ANA in patients younger than 40 years (especially women) can be significant.[176,182,183] However, the data from the multicenter study described earlier[178] do not agree with the first section of these reports.

The ANAs in the normal population aged 65 years or older was 11.4% versus 3.6% in the younger population.[184] A total of 419 people (270 men and 144 women) were studied. The ANA positivity was observed in these individuals in titers of 1:40 or higher with the IFM-ANA test, using the HEp-2 cell as substrate. In the multicenter study,[178] the normal population older than 65 years was not included.

In another study[185] of 485 healthy volunteers, ranging in age from 18 to 70 years, 62 (13%) of 485 tested positive by IFM-ANA with HEp-2 cells at a dilution of 1:40. However, 42 (68%) of those 62 healthy blood donors had a titer of 1:80 or lower.

Fritzler et al[186] reported on a study of 2500 female blood donors between the ages of 20 and 50 years. When sera were tested by IFM on HEp-2 cells, 15.9% and 1.1% had ANA titers greater than 1:20 and 1:80, respectively.

The IFM test at 1:160 dilution of serum may be positive in as many as 5% of so-called normal individuals with no signs and symptoms of a rheumatologic disease.[178,187] Although a positive IFM result suggests the possibility of a rheumatologic disease, the test is not diagnostic and therefore should prompt initiation of tests to determine the specificity of ANAs when they are at titers of 1:160 or greater and other clinical evaluations or laboratory tests.[187]

In a follow-up study of the IFM-ANA after 4 years, most initial ANA-positive individuals remained positive without significant variation in their titer levels.[184] Hawkins et al[183] demonstrated that the 1,237 (43.6%) ANA-positive results persisted during a 6-year period in an Australian population of 2,838 adults older than 18 years.

In the interpretation of the IFM-ANA test, the clinician must know what substrate was used in the assay procedure: rodent epithelial tissues (liver or kidney) or human tissue culture cell lines, which have a higher "background" with normal sera. Today, most tests are performed with HEp-2 tissue culture cell lines (the substrate of choice).[176,188] With mouse (rodent tissue) substrate, 5% to 10% of the normal population has a positive result at a screening dilution of 1:20, and 1% tests positive at 1:320.[188]

Enzyme Immunoassay Tests for Antinuclear Antibodies

Enzyme immunoassay kits using natural and recombinant antigens to screen simultaneously for a panel of autoantibodies to nuclear antigens are available from several commercial sources.[189,190] These tests claim to detect autoantibodies responsible for homogeneous, speckled, peripheral, centromeric, and nucleolar immunofluorescent patterns, as well as to detect specific autoantibodies to SS-A, SS-B, Sm, RNP, Scl-70/DNA-topoisomerase I, histone, and dsDNA. These EIA kits are promoted as alternative methods for both the screening and detection of "total" antinuclear antibodies, to be used as a replacement for the IFM-ANA test.

Although such EIA-ANA tests are less labor-intensive and can be used to screen and detect a panel of common specific autoantibodies usually observed in the systemic rheumatic diseases, they are not 100% sensitive when compared with IFM-ANA. They also may fail to detect certain ANAs with atypical and classic immunofluorescent patterns. A comprehensive comparative analysis of commercial EIA-ANA kits done in 1995 recommended that the titers and patterns of EIA-positive sera be confirmed with IFM-ANA on HEp-2 cells.[190]

Thus, reporting of negative EIA-ANA results should state that autoantibodies to specific antigens in the test (eg, SS-A, SS-B, Sm, RNP, Scl-70/DNA-topoisomerase I, histone, dsDNA) were not detected. This clarification helps alert clinicians that a negative EIA-ANA result is not the equivalent of "negative for all nuclear antibodies."

Secondary Tests for Autoantibodies in Systemic Lupus Erythematosus

It is extremely important to confirm and further identify the immunologic/antigenic specificity of a positive ANA result. The tests for specific autoantibodies include ELISA, RIA, agglutination, immunoblot, and immunodiffusion.[192]

Further recommended secondary tests for the detection of autoantibodies in SLE are[1,2,5,6,53,54]

- dsDNA
- nRNP
- Sm
- SS-A/Ro
- SS-B/La

Antibodies to both dsDNA and Sm are highly diagnostic of SLE, although they are found in only about 75% and 25% of patients, respectively.[1,46,57] Antibodies to ssDNA and nucleoprotein are frequently found in patients with SLE and rheumatoid arthritis; antibodies to nRNP are frequently found in patients with SLE and scleroderma. Antibodies to SS-A/Ro and SS-B/La are frequently found in patients with SLE or Sjögren's syndrome.[1–6]

Spontaneous Systemic Lupus Erythematosus Versus Drug-Induced Lupus

The important features of spontaneous SLE are[1]

- If the IFM-ANA is negative, the patient has a minimal possibility of having SLE.

- In SLE patients, the IFM-ANA test is seen in usually higher titers than in patients with other disorders.
- The presence of both autoantibodies to dsDNA and Sm antigen are highly diagnostic of SLE.
- In SLE, the patient often has a multitude of autoantibodies to nuclear and cytoplasmic antigens. The antibody response is heterogeneous and polyclonal, and there is usually an average of 3 different circulating antibodies present simultaneously.[1]

The differential diagnosis between DLE and spontaneous SLE is based on the clinical symptoms and immune profile. The noteworthy features are[159–168]

- Both conditions are associated with the presence of ANA. However, antibodies to dsDNA and Sm are very rare in DLE.
- Antibodies to histones are frequent in DLE but are also seen in approximately 60% to 75% of patients with spontaneous SLE.
- In DLE, the presence of histone antibodies and antibodies to ssDNA may be present. However, in SLE, antibodies to dsDNA, Sm, and U[1]RNP antigens are often present in addition to the histone antibodies.
- In procainamide-induced lupus, the antihistone antibodies are mainly directed to the H2A-H2B complex. In hydralazine-induced lupus, the histone antibodies are directed to the H1 and H3-H4 complex.

Antinuclear Antibody–Negative Systemic Lupus Erythematosus

The standardization of IFM-ANA tests has been extremely difficult, and several recommendations have been made to improve their reproducibility, reliability, and consistency.[176,178,191–194] In the past, there have been reports that the prevalence of ANA-negative SLE may be 5% or more of the total population of patients with SLE.[74,79,80] Today, most investigators feel that ANA-negative SLE patients may occasionally be seen, but with better diagnostic tests the number of patients who have untreated SLE and are negative by IFM-ANA are rare and constitute a small percentage. The IFM-ANA test may be negative in some cases of SLE when patients have antibodies restricted to cytoplasmic constituents.[192]

It has been brought to the attention of clinical laboratories that quality assurance programs designed to detect SS-A/Ro antibodies with IFM-ANA tests are needed.[195] The inability to detect SS-A/Ro antibodies may account for a significant percentage of so-called ANA-negative SLE patients.[195,196]

Autoantibody to SS-A/Ro is frequently present in SCLE. Many affected patients have been falsely labeled as having ANA-negative SLE. These misdiagnosed patients demonstrate a positive IFM-ANA result on substrate of HEp-2 or other cells containing enriched SS-A/Ro antigen.[195]

Another study showed that certain patients with SLE and prominent cutaneous disease who test negative by IFM-ANA possess only anti-ssDNA antibodies.[197] These anti-ssDNA antibodies are directed toward the presence of a pyrimidine base buried in native DNA. These antigenic determinants are not detected in routine IFM-ANA tests because ssDNA determinants are not normally expressed in intact cell nuclei of the tissue substrate.

Maddison et al[74] reported on 66 patients in whom clinical features of SLE developed and who had repeated negative IFM-ANA test results in their sera over an extended period of time. Only 24 (36%) of the 66 patients described fulfilled 4 or more of the 1971 ARA criteria for SLE. The researchers found that 41 (62%) of the 66 patients had precipitating antibodies to SS-A/Ro, and 18 (72%) of the remaining 25 patients had antibody to ssDNA. Further studies of sera from patients with SLE who have demonstrated negative IFM-ANA results with mouse liver substrates showed that 66% of patients tested positive for nuclear staining by a more sensitive human KB epithelial tissue culture substrate.

It should be noted that ANA negativity does not preclude the diagnosis of SLE. Systemic lupus erythematosus represents a wide spectrum of clinical and immunologic features. It is possible that among most large series of SLE patients, some could be persistently ANA negative.[80]

Status of the Lupus Erythematosus Cell Test

The LE cell test was first described by Hargraves et al[153] in 1948, and the test was based on an in vitro immune reaction between the patient's autoantibodies to nuclear antigens and damaged nuclei in the test medium. The test was not very sensitive and was subject to numerous variables.

Today, most clinical laboratories have discontinued use of the LE cell test in favor of more definitive and specific immunologic tests for specific nuclear and cytoplasmic autoantibodies.[198]

In theory, a positive IFM-ANA test should include all patients who also may have a positive LE cell result. However, there have been several documented cases of patients with a positive LE cell result and a negative ANA reported from reliable clinical laboratories. Wallace and Metzger[199] reported positive LE cell tests and negative ANA tests in brothers with SLE and reviewed the literature. They proposed the following 3 indications for ordering an LE cell test:

- To confirm suspected SLE in a patient who fulfills 3 other ACR criteria for SLE
- In an ANA-negative patient who has symptoms or signs highly suspicious of SLE
- To examine serous fluids

The authors felt that these 3 indications would make the LE cell test useful for diagnosis under limited circumstances. It has been observed that an SLE patient can develop specific antibodies to nucleosomes.[148,149]

Other Laboratory Tests for the Evaluation of Systemic Lupus Erythematosus

Skin Lesions

Three tests are usually performed for patients presenting with skin lesions: a routine histologic examination, an autoantibody test for nuclear and cytoplasmic antigens, and an immunofluorescent lupus band test.

Burnham et al,[200] Cormane,[201] and Tan and Kunkel[202] first described the deposition of immunoglobulin at the basement membrane zone (BMZ) of involved skin of lupus erythematosus patients. Similar findings were found along the BMZ of uninvolved skin of SLE patients.[203] Since then, direct immunofluorescence of normal skin of SLE patients has become known as the lupus band test. This test is used to differentiate SLE from benign cutaneous lupus because deposition of immunoglobulin and complement in uninvolved skin is not observed in benign cutaneous lupus.[71,201–203]

In a study of patients with chronic discoid lupus erythematosus (CDLE) and SCLE, direct immunofluorescent studies showed the following[204]:

- Eight of 11 CDLE patients and all of the SCLE patients had staining with IgG and/or IgM in lesional biopsies.
- In CDLE, the pattern of staining of Ig was always particulate at the dermoepidermal junction (DEJ).
- In SCLE, the IgG pattern of staining at the DEJ was particulate epidermal staining. Immunoglobulin M staining also was observed at the DEJ.
- Deposition of IgG and C3 in uninvolved skin was noted only in patients with SLE.
- Patients with SCLE usually had IgM staining at the DEJ in nonlesional unexposed skin.
- Antibodies to SS-A/Ro are present in most patients with SCLE. Direct immunofluorescence studies of skin on these patients demonstrated discrete speckled IgG deposits in the basal cell cytoplasm, which is associated with the presence of anti–SS-A/Ro autoantibodies in serum.[205]

Helm and Peters[206] showed that the membrane attack complex (MAC) C5b-9 of complement is localized in the BMZ of cutaneous lesions of patients with SLE. Direct immunofluorescence for MAC deposition in lesional skin is sensitive, is a specific marker for cutaneous LE, and may be a useful adjunct to the lupus band test. Membrane attack complex was detected in lesions of patients with CDLE and SLE.

Serologic Markers of Disease Activity

Serologic markers for disease activity in SLE vary in their degree of usefulness.[207–209] For example, changes in serum levels (measured monthly) of anti-dsDNA predicts disease activity, but measurement of U_{Sm}-RNP, anti–SS-A/Ro, and histone antibody levels is of limited value in monitoring disease activity.

Autoantibodies to C1q in SLE patients may contribute to the progression of renal disease with proliferative glomerulonephritis.[210–213] The mechanism by which autoantibodies to C1q contribute to nephritis is uncertain. However, one possibility is that these autoantibodies amplify the inflammatory response by binding to C1q, which has bound to immune complexes in the glomeruli.[211]

Levels of complement factors, such as C3, C4, and CH50, are helpful for monitoring disease activity. However, the cost-effectiveness and clinical usefulness of monitoring complement levels in patients with SLE is controversial.[214]

There are more than 40 different non–antigen-specific methods to detect immune complexes, and immune complexes can be found in a wide variety of diseases. In SLE, no particular clinical manifestations correlate with the presence of non–antigen-specific immune complexes as detected by the solid phase C1q binding assay. The question of whether immune complex assays can help predict future SLE disease activity has resulted in conflicting answers.[214]

Esdaile et al[208] have claimed that fluctuations in laboratory test values are poor predictors of disease exacerbations in SLE, but also that the tests are important in diagnosis and their role in long-term prognosis and prediction of disease response to therapy needs further studies.

Tests for Evaluation of Kidney Disease Associated With Systemic Lupus Erythematosus

Patients with active SLE often have active and progressive glomerulonephritis mediated by immune complex injury that is primarily mediated by DNA and DNA-immune complexes.[7,8,214] The following points should be noted[207,209,215,216]:

- Serologic abnormalities in SLE may develop many months before evidence of renal involvement and should alert the clinician to the need for testing urinary sediments and protein excretion in urine to detect renal injury.
- Persistent depression of C3, C4, or CH50 are often associated with progression of kidney diseases.
- In SLE patients with follow-up renal biopsies in excess of 7 years, the best predictors of long-term outcome were
  - — the ultrastructural variables of mesangial, subendothelial, and subepithelial deposits.
  - — an observed decrease in the amount of mesangial or subendothelial deposits, which was best at predicting a lower risk of renal impairment, renal insufficiency, and mortality.
- Patients with diffuse proliferative nephritis have higher anti-DNA antibody levels than do patients with focal proliferative and membranous nephritis.
- C3 and DNA binding (anti-DNA antibody) levels correlate with the severity of clinical lupus nephritis.
- Complement levels of C4 do not correlate with the severity of lesions seen by kidney biopsies.
- The elevated levels of complement split products and products of alternative and terminal pathway activation more accurately reflect disease activity of SLE than do conventional measurements of complement.

The traditional measurements of complement C3, C4, and CH50 levels correlate with disease activity in SLE. However, an elevated level of C4d has the most sensitivity with regard to subsequent flare in SLE, and an elevated Bb (the proteolytic active cleavage fragment of factor B) level has the highest specificity and the greatest predictive value.[207] Assay of Bb levels is performed with a specific monoclonal antibody and represents activation of factor B of the alternative complement pathway.

Evaluation of Suspected Cases of Neuropsychiatric Systemic Lupus Erythematosus

The effective diagnostic evaluation steps for NPSLE are[124,217]

1. Patient history and physical examination
2. Complete blood cell count, appropriate chemistry analyses, urinalysis
3. Cultures of bodily fluids to exclude secondary causes of CNS dysfunction (eg, infection), when appropriate
4. Serologies, such as complement levels and dsDNA antibodies, which may help in assessing SLE activity but are of little benefit in the evaluation of NPSLE
5. For patients with progressive cognitive impairment or acute diffuse CNS symptoms,
   - — an electroencephalogram
   - — cerebrospinal fluid analysis with IgG index and oligoclonal band study
   - — magnetic resonance imaging (MRI) studies of the brain
6. Serum antiribosomal P protein antibody assay for patients with psychosis or major depression
7. Antiphospholipid antibodies for patients with dementia or seizures
8. Antiphospholipid antibodies and MRI studies for SLE patients with focal NPSLE manifestations
9. An echocardiogram for patients with embolic strokes

Patients with a combination of diffuse manifestations may require extensive diagnostic testing. It is unlikely that one clinical sign or diagnostic test will be abnormal in all patients with NPSLE.[217]

Summary

Systemic lupus erythematosus is a non–organ-specific autoimmune disease with immune dysregulation characterized by polyclonal activation of B cells and production of a large spectrum of autoantibodies with a marked preference for nuclear and intracellular antigens. The etiology of SLE is still unknown, but it is considered multifactorial. Several endocrine-metabolic, environmental, and genetic factors play a role in the triggering and perpetuation of SLE.

Systemic lupus erythematosus is the prototypic systemic rheumatic disease involving multiple organs. It affects people of all ages and both sexes, but is most prevalent in women during childbearing years.

In the diagnosis of SLE, most physicians rely on the 1982 ARA Criteria for the Classification of SLE.[36] The diagnosis of SLE is usually made if 4 or more of the criteria are met either serially or simultaneously during any interval of observation. When these criteria are tested against other diseases, the sensitivity and specificity for the diagnosis of SLE have been approximately 96%.

Lupus-like diseases that meet fewer than 4 of the criteria have variously been labeled probable, possible, latent, incipient, or incomplete lupus. A few affected patients may develop definite SLE (with 4 or more criteria) if monitored long term. However, many patients may develop other diseases with better prognoses.

The IFM-ANA test is the best screening test for SLE. If the results are negative, the patient has a minimal probability of having SLE. In SLE patients, ANAs are usually seen in higher titers than in patients with other disorders. Antibodies to dsDNA and Sm antigen are highly diagnostic of SLE. In SLE, patients often have a multitude of various autoantibodies to nuclear and intracellular antigens.

In CDLE, antibodies to histone and ssDNA may be present. However, in SLE, antibodies to dsDNA, Sm, and U_1RNP antigens are often present, in addition to antibodies to histones. It is important to identify clinical subsets of SLE to understand the prognosis and clinical course of the disease. Subsets of SLE may demonstrate manifestations related to the presence of specific autoantibodies. The differential diagnosis of SLE, lupus-like diseases, and clinical subsets of SLE have been described along with the correlation with specific autoantibodies to certain intracellular antigens.

References

1. Nakamura RM, Bylund DJ. Contemporary concepts for the clinical and laboratory evaluation of systemic lupus erythematosus and "lupus-like" syndromes. *J Clin Lab Anal*. 1994;8:347–359.
2. Nakamura RM, Tan EM. Update on auto-antibodies to intracellular antigens in systemic rheumatic diseases. *Clin Lab Med*. 1992;12:1–23.
3. Tan EM. Autoantibodies to nuclear antigens (ANA): Their immunobiology and medicine. *Adv Immunol*. 1982;33:167–240.
4. Tan EM. Antinuclear antibodies: Diagnostic markers for autoimmune diseases and probes for cell biology. *Adv Immunol*. 1989;44:93–151.
5. Nakamura RM, Tan EM. Recent advances in laboratory tests and the significance of autoantibodies to nuclear antigens in systemic rheumatic diseases. *Clin Lab Med*. 1986;6:41–53.
6. Lahita RG, ed. *Systemic Lupus Erythematosus*. 2nd ed. New York, NY: Churchill Livingstone; 1992.
7. Mills JA. Systemic lupus erythematosus. *N Engl J Med*. 1994;330:1871–1879.
8. Boumpas DT, Austin HA III, Fessler BJ, et al. Systemic lupus erythematosus: Emerging concepts, Part 1: Renal, neuropsychiatric, cardiovascular, pulmonary, and hematologic disease. *Ann Intern Med*. 1995;122:940–950. Review.
9. Boumpas DT, Fessler BJ, Austin HA III, et al. Systemic lupus erythematosus: Emerging concepts, Part 2: Dermatologic and joint disease, the antiphospholipid antibody syndrome, pregnancy and hormonal therapy, morbidity and mortality, and pathogenesis. *Ann Intern Med*. 1995;123:42–53. Review.
10. Decker JL. Glossary subcommittee of ARA committee on rheumatologic practice. *Arthritis Rheum*. 1986;26: 1029.
11. von Muhlen CA, Tan EM. Autoantibodies in diagnosis of systemic rheumatic diseases. *Semin Arthritis Rheum*. 1995;24:323–358.
12. Emlen W. Systemic lupus erythematosus and mixed connective tissue disease. *Immunol Allergy Clin North Am*. 1993;13:291–311.
13. Hochberg MC, Boyd RE, Ahearn JM, et al. Systemic lupus erythematosus: A review of clinical-laboratory features and immunogenetic markers in 150 patients with emphasis on demographic subsets. *Medicine*. 1985;64:285–295.

14. Reichlin M. Systemic lupus erythematosus. In: Bijazzi PE, Reichlin M, eds. *Systemic Autoimmunity*. New York, NY: Marcel Dekker; 1991:163–199.

15. Jacob L, Viard JP, Louvard D, et al. Recent advances in pathogenesis of systemic lupus erythematosus. *Adv Nephrol*. 1990;19:237–256.

16. Hochberg MC. Systemic lupus erythematosus. *Rheum Dis Clin North Am*. 1990;16:617–639.

17. Phillips PE. The potential role of microbial agents in the pathogenesis of systemic lupus erythematosus. *J Rheumatol*. 1981;8:344–347.

18. Hochberg MC, Kaslow RA. Risk factors for the development of systemic lupus erythematosus. *Clin Res*. 1983;31:732A.

19. Esdaile JM. Prognosis in systemic lupus erythematosus. *Springer Semin Immunopathol*. 1994;16:337–355.

20. Arnett FC. Genetic aspects of human lupus. *Clin Immunol Immunopathol*. 1992;63:4–6.

21. Kono DH, Theofilopoulous AN. Genetic contributions to SLE. *J Autoimmun*. 1996;9:437–452.

22. Block SR, Winfield JB, Lockshin MC, et al. Studies of twins with systemic lupus erythematosus: A review of the literature and presentation of 12 additional sets. *Am J Med*. 1975;59:533–552.

23. Schur PH. Third international conference on systemic lupus erythematosus. *Arthritis Rheum*. 1992;35:1238–1240.

24. Bach JF, Viard JP. Hypothesis: Systemic lupus erythematosus as a disease secondary to polyclonal lymphocyte activation. *Clin Exp Rheumatol*. 1990;8(suppl 5):57–64.

25. Dayal AK, Kammer GM. The T cell enigma in lupus. *Arthritis Rheum*. 1996;39:23–33.

26. Zambinski MA, Messner RP, Mandel JS. Anti-dsDNA antibodies in laboratory workers handling blood from patients with systemic lupus erythematosus. *J Rheumatol*. 1992;19:1380–1384.

27. Pincus T. Studies regarding a possible function for viruses in the pathogenesis of systemic lupus erythematosus. *Arthritis Rheum*. 1982;25:847–856.

28. Kalden JR, Gay S. Retroviruses and autoimmune rheumatic diseases. *Clin Exp Immunol*. 1994;98:1–5.

29. Norris DA. Pathomechanisms of photosensitive lupus erythematosus. *J Invest Dermatol*. 1993;100(suppl):58S–68S.

30. Tan EM, Stoughton RB. Ultraviolet light alteration of cellular DNA in vivo. *Proc Natl Acad Sci U S A*. 1969;62:708–714.

31. Crow MK, Christian CL. Etiologic hypothesis for systemic lupus erythematosus. In: Lahita RG, ed. *Systemic Lupus Erythematosus*. 2nd ed. New York, NY: Churchill Livingstone; 1992:51–64.

32. Malinow MR, Bardana DJ Jr, Pirofsky B, et al. Systemic lupus erythematosus-like syndrome in monkeys fed alfalfa sprouts: role of a nonprotein amino acid. *Science*. 1982;216:415–417.

33. Greenwood BM. Autoimmune disease and parasitic infections in Nigerians. *Lancet*. 1968;2:380–382.

34. Panush RS, Greer JM, Morshedian KK. What is lupus? What is not lupus? *Rheum Dis Clin North Am*. 1993;19:223–234.

35. Cohen AS, Reynolds WE, Franklin EC, et al. Preliminary criteria for the classification of systemic lupus erythematosus. *Bull Rheum Dis*. 1971;21:643–648.

36. Tan EM, Cohen AS, Fries JF, et al. The 1982 revised criteria for the classification of systemic lupus erythematosus. *Arthritis Rheum*. 1982;25:1271–1277.

37. Lockshin MD. What is SLE? *J Rheumatol*. 1989;16:419–420.

38. Lom-Orta H, Alarcon-Segovia D, Diaz-Jouanen E. Systemic lupus erythematosus: Differences between patients who do and who do not fulfill classification criteria at the time of diagnosis. *J Rheumatol*. 1980;7:831–837.

39. Lazaro MA, Maldonado-Cocco JA, Catoggio LJ, et al. Clinical and serological characteristics of patients with overlap syndrome: Is mixed connective tissue disease a distinct clinical entity? *Medicine*. 1989;68:58–65.

40. Nimelstein SH, Brody S, McShane D, et al. Mixed connective tissue disease: A subsequent evaluation of the original 25 patients. *Medicine*. 1980;59:239–248.

41. Sharp GC, Irvin WS, Tan EM, et al. Mixed connective tissue disease: An apparently distinct rheumatic disease syndrome associated with a specific antibody to extractable nuclear antigen (ENA). *Am J Med*. 1972;52:148–159.

42. Panush RS, Edwards NG, Longley S, et al. "Rhupus" syndrome. *Arch Intern Med*. 1988;148:1633–1636.

43. Asherson RA, Cervera R, Lahita RG. Latent, incomplete or lupus at all? *J Rheumatol*. 1991;18:1783–1786.

44. Ganczarczyk L, Urowitz MB, Gladman DD. "Latent lupus." *J Rheumatol*. 1989;16:475–478.

45. Greer JM, Panush RS. Incomplete lupus erythematosus. *Arch Intern Med*. 1989;149:2473–2476.

46. Schur PH. Clinical features of SLE. In: Kelly WN, Harris ED, Ruddy S, et al, eds. *Textbook of Rheumatology*. 4th ed. Philadelphia, PA: WB Saunders Co; 1993;2:1017–1042.

47. Sontheimer RD, Gilliam JN. Systemic lupus erythematosus and the skin. In: Lahita RG, ed. *Systemic Lupus Erythematosus*. 2nd ed. New York, NY: Churchill Livingstone; 1992:657–681.

48. Tuffanelli DL. Lupus erythematosus panniculitis (profundus): Clinical and immunologic studies. *Arch Dermatol*. 1971;103:231–242.

49. Diaz-Jouanen E, Del Iorazius RJ, Alarcon-Segovia D, et al. Systemic lupus erythematosus presenting as panniculitis (lupus profundus). *Ann Intern Med*. 1975;82:376–379.

50. Wallace DJ, Pistiner M, Nessim S, et al. Cutaneous lupus erythematosus without systemic lupus erythematosus: clinical and laboratory features. *Semin Arthritis Rheum*. 1992;21:221–226.

51. Sontheimer RD, Maddison PJ, Reichlin M, et al. Serologic and HLA associations in subacute cutaneous lupus erythematosus. *Ann Intern Med*. 1982;97:664–671.

52. Baer AN, Pincus T. Occult systemic lupus erythematosus in elderly men. *JAMA*. 1983;249:3350–3352.

53. Notman DD, Kurata N, Tan EM. Profiles of antinuclear antibodies in systemic rheumatic diseases. *Ann Intern Med*. 1975;83:464–469.

54. Tan EM, Chan EKL, Sullivan KF, et al. Antinuclear antibodies (ANAs): Diagnostically specific immune markers and clues toward the understanding of systemic autoimmunity. *Clin Immunol Immunopathol*. 1988;47:121–141.

55. Mongey AB, Hess EV. Antinuclear antibodies and disease specificity. *Adv Intern Med*. 1991;36:151–169.

56. Tomer Y, Buskila D, Shoenfeld Y. Pathogenic significance and diagnostic value of lupus autoantibodies. *Int Arch Allergy Immunol*. 1993;100:293–306.

57. Buskila D, Shoenfeld Y. Anti-DNA antibodies. In: Lahita RG, ed. *Systemic Lupus Erythematosus*. 2nd ed. New York, NY: Churchill Livingstone; 1992:205–236.

58. Wallace DJ, Hahn BH, Klippel J. Lupus nephritis. In: Wallace DJ, Hahn BH, eds. *Dubois Lupus Erythematosus*. Philadelphia, PA: Lea & Febiger; 1993:542–549.

59. Okamura M, Kanayama Y, Amastu K, et al. Significance of enzyme linked immunosorbent assay (ELISA) for antibodies to double stranded and single stranded DNA in patients with lupus nephritis: Correlation with severity of renal histology. *Ann Rheum Dis*. 1993;52:14–20.

60. Firer MA, Shoenfeld Y, Isenberg DA, et al. I. The use of ELISA for the measurement of autoantibodies to nuclear antigens: Comparison with other methodologies. *Isr J Med Sci*. 1988;24:747–750.

61. Lafer EM, Rauch J, Andrzejewski JR, et al. Polyspecific monoclonal lupus autoantibodies reactive with both polynucleotides and phospholipids. *J Exp Med*. 1981;153:897–909.

62. Northway JD, Tan EM. Differentiation of antinuclear antibodies giving speckled staining patterns in immunofluorescence. *Clin Immunol Immunopathol*. 1972;1:140–154.

63. Mattioli M, Reichlin M. Physical association of two nuclear antigens and mutual occurrence of their antibodies. The relationship of the Sm and RNA protein (Mo) systems in SLE sera. *J Immunol*. 1973;110:1318–1324.

64. Lerner MR, Steitz JA. Antibodies to small nuclear RNAs complexed with proteins are produced by patients with systemic lupus erythematosus. *Proc Natl Acad Sci U S A*. 1979;76:5495–5499.

65. Kasukawa R. Preliminary diagnostic criteria for classification of mixed connective tissue disease. In: Kasukawa R, Sharp GC, eds. *Mixed Connective Tissue Disease and Anti-nuclear Antibodies*. Amsterdam, the Netherlands: Excerpta Medica; 1987:41–47.

66. ter Borg EJ, Groen H, Horst G, et al. Clinical association of antiribonucleoprotein antibodies in patients with systemic lupus erythematosus. *Semin Arthritis Rheum*. 1990;20:164–173.

67. Habets WJ, Berden JHM, Hoch SO, et al. Further characterization and subcellular localization of Sm and U1 ribonucleoprotein antigens. *Eur J Immunol*. 1985;15:992–997.

68. Munves EF, Schur PH. Antibodies to Sm and RNA. *Arthritis Rheum*. 1983;26:848–853.

69. Barada FA, Andrews BS, Davis JS, et al. Antibodies to Sm in patients with systemic lupus erythematosus. Correlation of Sm antibody titers with disease activity and other laboratory parameters. *Arthritis Rheum*. 1981;24:1236–1244.

70. Takeda Y, Wang GS, Wang RJ, et al. Enzyme-linked immunosorbent assay using isolated (U) small nuclear ribonucleoprotein polypeptides as antigens to investigate the clinical significance of autoantibodies to these polypeptides. *Clin Immunol Immunopathol*. 1989;50:213–230.

71. Weiss RA, Mogavero HS, Synkowski DR, et al. Diagnostic tests and clinical subsets in systemic lupus erythematosus: Update 1983. *Ann Allergy*. 1983;51:135–146.

72. Chan EK, Tan EM. Epitopic targets for autoantibodies in systemic lupus erythematosus and Sjögren's syndrome. *Curr Opin Rheumatol*. 1989;1:376–381.

73. McCauliffe DP, Lux FA, Lieu TS, et al. Ro/SS-A and the pathogenic significance of its antibodies. In: Talal N, ed. *Sjögren's Syndrome: A Model for Understanding Autoimmunity*. 2nd International Symposium. San Diego, CA: Academic Press; 1989:67–73.

74. Maddison P, Reichlin M, Provost T. Association of autoantibodies to certain cytoplasmic antigens with systemic lupus erythematosus. *Arthritis Rheum*. 1977;20:126. Abstract.

75. Watson RM, Lane AT, Barnett NK, et al. Neonatal lupus erythematosus: A clinical, serological and immunogenetic study with review of the literature. *Medicine*. 1984;63:362–370.

76. Behan WMH, Behan PO, Reid JM, et al. Family studies in congenital heart block associated with Ro antibody. *Br Heart J*. 1989;62:320–324.

77. Derksen RHWN, Meilof JF. Anti-Ro/SS-A and anti-La/SS-B autoantibody levels in relation to systemic lupus erythematosus disease activity and congenital heart block. *Arthritis Rheum*. 1992;35:176–189.

78. Provost TT, Arnett FC, Reichlin M. Homozygous C2 deficiency, lupus erythematosus and anti-Ro (SSA) antibodies. *Arthritis Rheum*. 1983;26:1279–1282.

79. Bohan A. Seronegative systemic lupus erythematosus. *J Rheumatol*. 1979;6:534–540.

80. Urowitz MB, Gladman DD. Antinuclear antibody negative systemic lupus erythematosus. In: Lahita RG, ed. *Systemic Lupus Erythematosus*. 2nd ed. New York, NY: Churchill Livingstone; 1992:561–567.

81. Alarcon-Segovia D, Sanchez-Guerrero J. Primary antiphospholipid syndrome. *J Rheumatol*. 1989;16: 482–488.

82. Asherson RA, Baguley E, Pal C, et al. Antiphospholipid syndrome: Five year follow-up. *Ann Rheum Dis*. 1991;50:805–810.

83. Lockshin MD. Antiphospholipid antibody syndrome. *JAMA*. 1992;268:1451–1453.

84. McNeil HP, Chesterman CN, Krilis SA. Immunology and clinical importance of antiphospholipid antibodies. *Adv Immunol*. 1991;49:193–280.

85. Sammaritano LR, Gharavi AE, Lockshin MD. Antiphospholipid antibody syndrome: Immunologic and clinical aspects. *Semin Arthritis Rheum*. 1990;20:81–96.

86. Piette JC, Wechsler B, Francis C, et al. Systemic lupus erythematosus and the antiphospholipid syndrome: Reflections about the relevance of ARA criteria. *J Rheumatol*. 1992;19:1835–1837.

87. Roubey RAS. Immunology of the antiphospholipid antibody syndrome. *Arthritis Rheum*. 1996;39:1444–1454. Review.

88. Emlen W. Antiphospholipid antibodies: New complexities and new assays. *Arthritis Rheum*. 1996;39:1441–1443. Editorial.

89. Alarcon-Segovia D, Perez-Vasquez ME, Villa AR, et al. Preliminary classification criteria for the antiphospholipid syndrome within systemic lupus erythematosus. *Semin Arthritis Rheum*. 1992;21:275–286.

90. Creagh MD, Greaves M. Lupus anticoagulant. *Blood Rev*. 1991;5:162–167.

91. Harris EN. Immunology of phospholipid antibodies. In: Lahita RG, ed. *Systemic Lupus Erythematosus*. 2nd ed. New York, NY: Churchill Livingstone; 1992:305–325.

92. Schwartz RS, Stollar DB. Origins of anti-DNA autoantibodies. *J Clin Invest*. 1985;75:321–327.

93. Viard JP, Amoura Z, Bach JF. Association of anti-β_2 glycoprotein I antibodies with lupus-type circulating anticoagulant and thrombosis in systemic lupus erythematosus. *Am J Med*. 1992;93:181–186.

94. Harris EN, Phil M, Asherson RA, et al. Antiphospholipid antibodies—autoantibodies with a difference. *Ann Rev Med*. 1988;39:261–271.

95. Harris EN, Gharavi AE, Patel SP, et al. Evaluation of the anticardiolipin test: Report of an international workshop held 4 April, 1986. *Clin Exp Immunol*. 1987;68:215–222.

96. Harris EN. The second international anticardiolipin standardization workshop/the Kingston antiphospholipid antibody study (KAPS) group. *Am J Clin Pathol*. 1990;94:476–484.

97. Lopez LR, Santos ME, Espinoza LR, et al. Clinical significance of immunoglobulin A versus immunoglobulins E and M anticardiolipin antibodies in patients with systemic lupus erythematosus—correlation with thrombosis, thrombocytopenia, and recurrent abortion. *Am J Clin Pathol*. 1992;98:449–454.

98. Matsuura E, Igarashi Y, Yasuda T, et al. Anticardiolipin antibodies recognize β_2-glycoprotein I structure altered by interacting with an oxygen modified solid phase surface. *J Exp Med*. 1994;179:457–462.

99. Roubey RAS, Eisenberg RA, Harper MF, et al. "Anticardiolipin" autoantibodies recognize β_2-glycoprotein I in the absence of phospholipid: Importance of antigen density and bivalent binding. *J Immunol*. 1995;154:954–960.

100. Roubey RAS, Pratt CW, Buyon JP, et al. Lupus anticoagulant activity of autoimmune antiphospholipid antibodies is dependent upon β_2-glycoprotein I. *J Clin Invest*. 1992;90:1100–1104.

101. Tincani A, Spatola L, Prati E, et al. The anti-β_2-glycoprotein I activity in human anti-phospholipid syndrome sera is due to monoreactive low-affinity autoantibodies directed to epitopes located on native β_2-glycoprotein I and preserved during species' evolution. *J Immunol*. 1996;157:5732–5738.

102. Erickson EN, Najmev SS, Keil LB, et al. Reference calibrators for IgG antibodies to β_2-glycoprotein I: Preparation, properties, and availability to investigators. *Clin Chem*. 1996;42:1116–1117.

103. Rivkin E, Lahita RG. Isolation of a cDNA clone with homology to apolipoprotein AI using sera from an SLE patient. *Arthritis Rheum*. 1991;34(suppl):S162.

104. Lahita RG, Rivkin E, Wallace DJ, et al. Low HDL-cholesterol and apolipoprotein AI levels in patients with SLE and IgG cardiolipin antibodies: A possible etiologic factor in atherosclerosis. *Arthritis Rheum*. 1991;34(suppl):S42.

105. Merrill JT, Rivkin E, Shen C, et al. Selection of a gene for apolipoprotein AI using autoantibodies from a patient with systemic lupus erythematosus. *Arthritis Rheum*. 1995;38:1655–1659.

106. Francoeur AM, Peebles CL, Gomper PT, et al. Identification of Ki(Ku, p70/p80) autoantigens and analysis of anti-Ki autoantibody reactivity. *J Immunol*. 1986;136:1648–1653.

107. Mimori T, Akizuku M, Yamagata H, et al. Characterization of a high molecular weight acidic nuclear protein recognized by autoantibodies in sera from patients with polymyositis-scleroderma overlap. *J Clin Invest*. 1981;68:611–620.

108. Reeves WH. Use of monoclonal antobodies for the characterization of novel DNA-binding proteins recognized by human autoimmune sera. *J Exp Med*. 1985;161:18–39.

109. Yaneva M, Arnett FC. Antibodies against Ku protein in sera from patients with autoimmune diseases. *Clin Exp Immunol*. 1989:76:366–372.

110. Isern RA, Yaneva M, Weiner E, et al. Autoantibodies in patients with primary pulmonary hypertension: Association with anti-Ku. *Am J Med*. 1992;93:307–312.

111. Tojo T, Kaburaki J, Hayakawa M, et al. Precipitating antibody to a soluble nuclear antigen "Ki" with specificity for systemic lupus erythematosus. *Ryumachi*. 1981;21(suppl):129–134.

112. Sakamoto M, Takasaki Y, Yamanaka K, et al. Purification and characterization of Ki antigen and detection of anti-Ki antibody by enzyme-linked immunosorbent assay in patients with systemic lupus erythematosus. *Arthritis Rheum*. 1989;32:1554–1562.

113. Mimori T, Hardin JA, Steitz JA. Characterization of the DNA-binding protein Ku recognized by autoantibodies from patients with rheumatic disorders. *J Biol Chem*. 1986;261;2274–2278.

114. Nikaido T, Shimada K, Shibata M, et al. Cloning and nucleotide sequence of cDNA for Ki antigen, a highly conserved nuclear protein detected with sera from SLE patients. *Clin Exp Immuno*l. 1990;79:209–214.

115. Miyachi K, Fritzler MJ, Tan EM. Autoantibody to a nuclear antigen in proliferating cells. *J Immunol*. 1978;121:2228–2274.

116. Fritzler MJ, McCarty GA, Ryan JP, et al. Clinical features of patients with antibodies directed against proliferating cell nuclear antigen (PCNA). *Arch Rheum*. 1983;26:140–145.

117. Koyasu S, Nishida E, Kadowski T, et al. Two mammalian heat-shock proteins, Hsp 90 and Hsp 100 re actin-binding proteins. *Proc Natl Acad Sci U S A*. 1986;83:8054–8058.

118. Minota S, Koyasu S, Yahara I, et al. Autoantibodies to the heat-shock protein hsp90 in systemic lupus erythematosus. *J Clin Invest*. 1988;81;106–109.

119. Gordon J, Towbin H, Rosenthal M. Antibodies directed against ribosomal protein determinants in the sera of patients with connective tissue disease. *J Rheumatol*. 1982;9:247–252.

120. Miyachi K, Tan EM. Antibodies reacting with ribosomal ribonucleoproteins in connective tissue disease. *Arthritis Rheum*. 1979;22:87–93.

121. Bonfa E, Golombek SJ, Kaufman LD, et al. Association between lupus psychosis and anti-ribosomal P protein antibodies. *N Engl J Med*. 1987;317:265–271.

122. Bonfa E, Parnassa AP, Rhodes DD, et al. Antiribosomal S10 antibodies in humans and MRL/1 pr mice with systemic lupus erythematosus. *Arthritis Rheum*. 1989;32:1252–1261.

123. Schneebaum A, Singleton JC, West SG, et al. Association of psychiatric manifestations with antibodies to ribosomal P proteins in systemic lupus erythematosus. *Am J Med*. 1991;90:54–62.

124. Teh LS, Bedwell AE, Isenberg DA, et al. Antibodies to protein P in systemic lupus erythematosus. *Ann Rheum Dis*. 1992;51:489–494.

125. West SG, Emlen W, Wener MH, et al. Neuropsychiatric lupus erythematosus: A 10 year prospective study on the value of diagnostic tests. *Am J Med*. 1995;99:153–163.

126. Teh LS, Isenberg DA. Antiribosomal P protein antibodies in systemic lupus erythematosus. A reappraisal. *Arthritis Rheum*. 1994;37:307–315.

127. Spezialetti R, Bluestein HG, Peter JB, et al. Neuropsychiatric disease in Sjögren's syndrome: Anti-ribosomal P and anti-neuronal antibodies. *Am J Med*. 1993;95:153–160.

128. Bluestein HG, Woods VL Jr. Antineuronal antibodies in systemic lupus erythematosus. *Arthritis Rheum*. 1982;25:773–778.

129. Bluestein HG. The central nervous system in systemic lupus erythematosus. In: Lahita RG, ed. *Systemic Lupus Erythematosus*. 2nd ed. New York, NY: Churchill Livingstone; 1992:639–655.

130. How A, Dent PB, Liao SK, et al. Antineuronal antibodies in neuropsychiatric systemic lupus erythematosus. *Arthritis Rheum*. 1985;28:789–795.

131. Robbins ML, Kornguth SE, Bell CL, et al. Antineurofilament antibody evaluation in neuropsychiatric systemic lupus erythematosus. *Arthritis Rheum*. 1988;31:623–631.

132. Senecal JL, Raymond Y. Autoantibodies to major and minor nuclear lamins are not restricted to autoimmune diseases. *Clin Immunol Immunopathol*. 1992;63:115–125.

133. Lassoued K, Guilly MN, Danon F, et al. Antinuclear autoantibodies specific for lamins. *Ann Intern Med*. 1988;108:829–833.

134. Lassoued S, Oksman F, Fournie B, et al. Autoantibodies to lamins in rheumatoid arthritis. *Arthritis Rheum*. 1990;33:877–879.

135. Wesierska-Gadek J, Penner E, Hitchman E, et al. Antibodies to nuclear lamins in autoimmune liver disease. *Clin Immunol Immunopathol*. 1988;49:107–115.

136. Senecal JL. Are there subsets of autoantibodies to nuclear lamins? *Arch Rheum*. 1992;35:1407–1408.

137. Senecal JL, Raymond Y. Autoantibodies to DNA, lamins, and pore complex proteins produce distinct peripheral fluorescent antinuclear antibody patterns on the HEp-2 substrate. *Arthritis Rheum*. 1991;34:249–251. Letter.

138. Holmes GP, Kaplan JE, Gantz NM, et al. Chronic fatigue syndrome: A working case definition. *Ann Intern Med*. 1988;108:387–389.

139. Schulvederberg A, Straus SE, Peterson P, et al. Chronic fatigue research. *Ann Intern Med*. 1992;117:325–331.

140. McKenzie R, Straus SE. Chronic fatigue syndrome. *Adv Intern Med*. 1995;40:119–153.

141. Konstantinov K, von Mikecz A, Buchwald D, et al. Autoantibodies to nuclear envelope antigens in chronic fatigue syndrome. *J Clin Invest.* 1996;98:1888–1896.

142. Winfield JB, Mimura T. Pathogenetic significance of anti-lymphocyte autoantibodies in systemic lupus erythematosus. *Clin Immunol Immunopathol.* 1992;63:13–16.

143. Winfield JB, Mimura T. Antilymphocyte autoantibodies. In: Lahita RG, ed. *Systemic Lupus Erythematosus.* 2nd ed. New York, NY: Churchill Livingstone; 1992:293–304.

144. Tsokos GC. Lymphocyte abnormalities in human lupus. *Clin Immunol Immunopathol.* 1992;63:7–9.

145. Tan EM. Autoantibodies in pathology and cell biology. *Cell.* 1991;67:841–842.

146. Rumore PM, Steinman CR. Endogenous circulating DNA in systemic lupus erythematosus: Occurrences as multimeric complexes bound to histones. *J Clin Invest.* 1990;86:471–477.

147. Burlingame RW, Rubin RL. Subnucleosome structures as substrates in enzyme-linked immunosorbent assays. *J Immunol Methods.* 1990;134:187–199.

148. Chabre H, Amoura Z, Piette J-C, et al. Presence of nucleosome-restricted antibodies in patients with systemic lupus erythematosus. *Arthritis Rheum.* 1995;38:1485–1491.

149. Burlingame RW, Boey ML, Starkebaum G, et al. The central role of chromatin in autoimmune responses to histones and DNA in systemic lupus erythematosus. *J Clin Invest.* 1994;94:184–192.

150. Robitaille P, Tan EM. Relationship between deoxyribonucleoprotein and deoxyribonucleic acid antibodies in systemic lupus erythematosus. *J Clin Invest.* 1973;52:316–323.

151. Halbert SP, Karsh J, Anken M. Studies on autoantibodies to deoxyribonucleic acid and deoxyribonucleoprotein with enzyme-immunoassay (ELISA). *J Lab Clin Med.* 1981;97:97–111.

152. Karsh J, Halbert SP, Anken M, et al. Anti-DNA, anti-deoxyribonucleoprotein and rheumatoid factor measured by ELISA in patients with systemic lupus erythematosus, Sjögren's syndrome and rheumatoid arthritis. *Int Arch Allergy Appl Immunol.* 1982;68:60–69.

153. Hargraves MM, Richmond H, Morton R. Presentation of two bone marrow elements: The "tart" cell and the "LE" cell. *Proc of the Staff Meetings of the Mayo Clinic.* 1948;23:25–28.

154. Haserick JR, Bortz DW. A new diagnostic test for acute disseminated lupus erythematosus. *Cleve Clin Q.* 1949;16:158–164.

155. Holman H, Deicher HR. The reaction of the lupus erythematosus (LE) cell factor with deoxyribonucleoprotein of the cell nucleus. *J Clin Invest.* 1959;38:2059–2072.

156. Lachmann PJ. An attempt to characterize the lupus erythematosus cell antigen. *Immunology.* 1961;4:153–163.

157. Rekvig OP, Hannestad K. Lupus erythematosus (LE) factors recognize both nucleosomes and viable human leukocytes. *Scand J Immunol.* 1981;13:597–604.

158. Burlingame RW, Rubin RL. Drug induced antihistone autoantibody display two patterns of reactivity with substructure of chromatin. *J Clin Invest.* 1991;88:680–690.

159. Price EJ, Venables PJ. Drug-induced lupus. *Drug Saf.* 1995;12:283–290.

160. Klug A, Finch JT, Richmond TJ. Crystallographic structure of the octamer histone core of the nucleosome. *Science.* 1985;229:1109–1110.

161. Rubin RL, McNally EM, Nusinow SR, et al. IgG antibodies to the histone complex H2A-H2B characterize procainamide-induced lupus. *Clin Immunol Immunopathol.* 1985;36:49–59.

162. Thomas JO, Wilson CM, Hardin JA. The major core histone antigenic determinants in systemic lupus erythematosus are in the trypsin-sensitive regions. *FEBS Lett.* 1984;169:90–96.

163. Rubin RL, Waga S. Antihistone antibodies in systemic lupus erythematosus. *J Rheumatol.* 1987;14(suppl 13):118–126.

164. Rubin RL, Bell SA, Burlingame RW. Autoantibodies associated with lupus induced by diverse drugs target a similar epitope in the (H2A-H2B)-DNA complex. *J Clin Invest.* 1992;90:165–173.

165. Woosley RL, Drager DE, Reidenber MM, et al. Effect of acetylator phenotype on the rate at which procainamide induces antinuclear antibodies and the lupus syndrome. *N Engl J Med.* 1987;298:1157–1159.

166. Rubin RL. Autoimmune reactions induced by procainamide and hydralazine. In: Kammuller M, Bloksma M, Siemen W, eds. *Autoimmunity and Toxicology: Immune Disregulation Induced by Drugs and Chemicals.* Amsterdam, the Netherlands: Elsevier Science; 1988:119–150.

167. Stollar BD. Reactions of systemic lupus erythematosus sera with histone fractions and histone-DNA complexes. *Arthritis Rheum.* 1971;14:485–492.

168. Rubin RL. Antihistone antibodies. In: Lahita RG, ed. *Systemic Lupus Erythematosus.* 2nd ed. New York, NY: Churchill Livingstone; 1992:247–271.

169. Tan EM, Robinson J, Robitaille P. Studies on antibodies to histones by immunofluorescence. *Scand J Immunol.* 1976;5:811–818.

170. Fritzler MJ, Tan EM. Antibodies to histones in drug induced and idiopathic lupus erythematosus. *J Clin Invest.* 1978;62:560–567.

171. Rubin RL, Joslin FJ, Tan EM. A solid phase radioimmunoassay for antihistone antibodies in human sera: Comparison with an immunofluorescent assay. *Scand J Immunol.* 1982;15:63–70.

172. Moore P, Lisak RP. Systemic lupus erythematosus: Immunopathogenesis of neurological dysfunction. *Springer Semin Immunopathol.* 1995;17:43–60.

173. Lehman TJA, McCurdy DK, Bernstein BH, et al. Systemic lupus erythematosus in the first decade of life. *Pediatrics.* 1989;83:235–239.

174. Lehman TJA. A practical guide to systemic lupus erythematosus. *Pediatr Clin North Am.* 1995;42:1223–1238.

175. Greer JM, Panush RS. Incomplete lupus erythematosus. *Arch Intern Med.* 1989;149:2473–2476.

176. Nakamura RM, Ivor L, Hannon WH, et al. Quality assurance for the indirect immunofluorescence test for autoantibodies to nuclear antigens (IF-ANA): approved guideline. *NCCLS Document 1/LA-2-A.* 1996;16:1–15.

177. Homburger HA. Cascade testing for autoantibodies in connective tissue diseases. *Mayo Clin Proc.* 1995;70:183–184.

178. Tan EM, Feltkamp TEW, Smolen JS, et al. Range of antinuclear antibodies in "healthy" individuals. *Arthritis Rheum.* 1997;40:1601–1611.

179. Griner PF, Mayewski RJ, Mushlin AI, et al. Selection and interpretation of diagnostic tests and procedures. *Ann Intern Med.* 1981;94:553–600.

180. Liang MH, Meenan RF, Cathcart ES, et al. A screening strategy for population studies in systemic lupus erythematosus: Series design. *Arthritis Rheum.* 1980;23: 152–157.

181. Shiel WC Jr, Jason M. The diagnostic associations of patients with antinuclear antibodies referred to a community rheumatologist. *J Rheumatol.* 1989;16:782–785.

182. Hooper B, Whittingham S, Mathews JD, et al. Autoimmunity in a rural community. *Clin Exp Immunol.* 1972;12:79–87.

183. Hawkins BR, O'Connor KJ, Dawkins RL, et al. Autoantibodies in an Australian population, 1: Prevalence and persistence. *J Clin Lab Immunol.* 1979;2:211–215.

184. Xavier RM, Yamauchi Y, Nakamura M, et al. Antinuclear antibodies in healthy aging people: A prospective study. *Mech Ageing Dev.* 1995;78:145–154.

185. De Vlam K, De Keyser F, Verbruggen G, et al. Detection and identification of antinuclear autoantibodies in the serum of normal blood donors. *Clin Exp Rheumatol.* 1993;11:393–397.

186. Fritzler MJ, Pauls JD, Kinsella TD, et al. Antinuclear, anticytoplasmic and anti-Sjögren's syndrome antigen A (SS-A/Ro) antibodies in female blood donors. *Clin Immunol Immunopathol.* 1985;36:120–128.

187. Pisetsky DS. Antinuclear antibodies. *Immunol Allergy Clin North Am.* 1994;14:371–385.

188. Reichlin M. ANA's and antibodies to DNA: Their use in clinical diagnosis. *Bull Rheum Dis.* 1993;42:3–5.

189. Moncé NM, Bogusky RT, Cappel NN. An enzyme immunoassay screening test for the detection of total antinuclear antibodies. *J Clin Lab Anal.* 1991;5:439–442.

190. Jaskowski TD, Schroder C, Martins TB, et al. Screening for antinuclear antibodies by enzyme immunoassay. *Am J Clin Pathol.* 1996;105:468–473.

191. Nakamura RM, Bylund DJ, Tan EM. Current status of available standards for quality improvement of assays for detection of autoantibodies to nuclear and intracellular antigens. *J Clin Lab Anal.* 1994;8:360–368.

192. Fritzler MJ. Immunofluorescent antinuclear antibody test. In: Rose NR, Conway de Marco E, Fahey JC, et al, eds. *Manual of Clinical Immunology.* 4th ed. Washington, DC: American Society of Microbiology; 1992:724–729.

193. Nakamura RM, Peebles CL, Rubin RL, et al. Autoantibodies to nuclear antigens. In: *Advances in Laboratory Tests and Significance in Systemic Rheumatic Diseases.* 2nd ed. Chicago, IL: ASCP Press; 1985:43-65.

194. Nakamura RM, Rippey JH. Quality assurance and proficiency testing for autoantibodies to nuclear antigen. *Arch Pathol Lab Med.* 1985;109:109–114.

195. Bylund DJ, Nakamura RM. Importance of detection of SS-A/Ro autoantibody in screening immunofluorescence tests for autoantibodies to nuclear antigens. *J Clin Lab Anal.* 1991;5:212–218.

196. Harmon C, Deng JS, Peebles CL, et al. The importance of tissue substrate in the SS-A/Ro antigen-antibody system. *Arthritis Rheum.* 1984;27:166–173.

197. Deng JS, Sontheimer RD, Gilliam JN. Relationships between antinuclear and anti-Ro/SS-A antibodies in subacute cutaneous lupus erythematosus. *J Am Acad Dermatol.* 1984;11:494–499.

198. Conn RB. Practice parameter—the lupus erythematosus cell test. *Am J Clin Pathol.* 1994;101:65–66.

199. Wallace DJ, Metzger AL. Positive LE preps and negative ANA in brothers with SLE: Is there still a role for the LE cell prep? A literature review. *J Rheumatol.* 1992;19:497.

200. Burnham TK, Neblett TR, Fine G, et al. The application of the fluorescent antibody technique to the investigation of lupus erythematosus and various dermatoses. *J Invest Dermatol.* 1963;41:451–456.

201. Cormane RH. "Bound" globulin in the skin of patients with chronic discoid lupus erythematosus and systemic lupus erythematosus. *Lancet.* 1964;1:534–537.

202. Tan EM, Kunkel HG. An immunofluorescent study of the skin lesions in systemic lupus erythematosus. *Arthritis Rheum.* 1966;9:37–46.

203. Provost TT, Andres G, Maddison PJ, et al. Lupus band test in untreated SLE patients: Correlation of immunoglobulin deposition in the skin of the extensor forearm with clinical renal disease and serological abnormalities. *J Invest Dermatol.* 1980;74:407–412.

204. David-Bajar KM, Bennion SD, De Spain JD, et al. Clinical, histologic, and immunofluorescent distinctions between subacute cutaneous lupus erythematosus and discoid lupus erythematosus. *J Invest Dermatol.* 1992;99:251–257.

205. Valeski JE, Kumar V, Forman AB, et al. A characteristic cutaneous direct immunofluorescent pattern associated with Ro (SS-A) antibodies in subacute cutaneous lupus erythematosus. *J Am Acad Dermatol.* 1992;27:194–198.

206. Helm KF, Peters MS. Deposition of membrane attack complex in cutaneous lesions of lupus erythematosus. *J Am Acad Dermatol.* 1993;28:687–691.

207. Buyon JP, Tamerius J, Belmont HM, et al. Assessment of disease activity and impending flare in patients with systemic lupus erythematosus—comparison of the use of complement split products and conventional measurements of complements. *Arthritis Rheum.* 1992;35:1028–1037.

208. Esdaile JM, Abrahamowicz M, Joseph L, et al. Laboratory tests as predictors of disease exacerbations in systemic lupus erythematosus. *Arthritis Rheum.* 1996;39:370–378.

209. Porcel JM, Ordi J, Castro-Salomo A, et al. The value of complement activation products in the assessment of systemic lupus erythematosus flares. *Clin Immunol Immunopathol.* 1995;74:283–288.

210. Lefkowith JB, Gilkeson GS. Nephritogenic autoantibodies in lupus. *Arthritis Rheum.* 1996;39:894–903.

211. Uwatoko S, Mannik M. Low-molecular weight C1q-binding immunoglobulin G in patients with systemic lupus erythematosus consists of autoantibodies to the collagen-like region of C1q. *J Clin Invest.* 1988;82:816–824.

212. Siegert C, Daha M, Westedt M, et al. IgG autoantibodies against C1q are correlated with nephritis, hypocomplementemia, and dsDNA antibodies in systemic lupus erythematosus. *J Rheumatol.* 1991;18:230–234.

213. Siegert CEH, Daha MR, Tseng CMES, et al. Predictive value of IgG autoantibodies against C1q for nephritis in systemic lupus erythematosus. *Ann Rheum Dis.* 1993;52:851–856.

214. Ruddy S, Moxley G. Clinical utility of assays for immune complexes and complement. *Immunol Allergy Clin North Am.* 1994;14:387–400.

215. Houssiau FA, D'Cruz D, Veanna J, et al. Lupus nephritis: The significance of serological tests at the time of biopsy. *Clin Exp Immunol.* 1991;9:345–349.

216. Esdaile JM, Lawrence J, MacKenzie T, et al. The pathogenesis and prognosis of lupus nephritis: Information from repeat biopsy. *Semin Arthritis Rheum.* 1993;23:135–148.

217. West SG. Neuropsychiatric lupus. *Rheum Dis Clin North Am.* 1994;20:129–158.

CHAPTER 10

Clinical and Laboratory Evaluation of Rheumatoid Arthritis

Robert I. Fox, MD, PhD

In recent years, there has been increased recognition of the poor long-term functional outcome and increased mortality among a subset of rheumatoid arthritis (RA) patients. However, other RA patients have limited disease that may spontaneously remit in the absence of aggressive therapy. The key challenge for the diagnostic laboratory is to identify patients destined for a poor outcome in order to allow early initiation of aggressive therapy. Commonly used clinical laboratory studies for diagnosis include rheumatoid factor (RF), erythrocyte sedimentation rate (ESR), C-reactive protein (CRP), and radiographs of the involved joints. However, these tests do not adequately predict long-term clinical outcome, response to a particular therapy, or likelihood of toxicity to particular medications. Recent studies of RA patients have examined additional autoantibodies (especially antifilaggrin antibodies responsible for antiperinuclear factors), genetic polymorphisms (including HLA-DR4 and genes related to monocyte activation), agalactosyl immunoglobulin (Ig) G isoforms, cytokines and their receptors, other acute phase reactants (APRs), and collagen breakdown products for their potential to predict outcome in RA patients. None of the markers (taken alone) has proven to have adequate specificity and sensitivity, but a combination of these markers may define clinical subsets of RA patients with regard to response to therapy and long-term prognosis. Furthermore, a careful definition of RA patient subsets by their laboratory markers and their response to therapy will provide insight into the pathogenetic mechanisms of RA.

Clinical Features of Rheumatoid Arthritis

"If you don't have any new therapeutic bullets, you should learn to aim your existing bullets more carefully." Dr Oliver Wendell Holmes, Jr, in his address to Harvard Medical School, Class of 1880.

Articular and Extra-articular Manifestations

Rheumatoid arthritis is a systemic autoimmune disorder of unknown etiology. Its major distinctive feature is a chronic symmetric swelling of the peripheral joints. The main diagnostic dilemma is that the group of patients currently termed RA is heterogeneous in its long-term outcome. About 50% of RA patients have an acute onset of joint symptoms characterized by pain and swelling, while another group of RA patients have less dramatic onset of joint symptoms that initially may be intermittent and can be controlled by over-the-counter pain relievers. Almost 25% of patients in each group may undergo spontaneous remission, but more than 50% of each group develop a progressive, erosive joint disease.[1,2] Once an RA patient has established "erosive" disease, none of the current therapies is curative, and most patients slowly progress through a series of different medications toward further joint destruction. Each medication appears to temporarily slow the disease but ultimately is discarded after 2 to 3 years due to lack of continuing efficacy or toxicity.

Outcome measures have traditionally been based on radiographically evident changes in the joints, but recent evidence indicates the importance of functional status as an outcome measure. This variable correlates best with loss of employment, the need for medical/ancillary services, and other overall costs to the patient and health care system. Furthermore, an increased level of functional disability in RA patients correlates with increased mortality rates when compared with age- and sex-matched controls.[3]

Among many scientists involved in basic research, pharmaceutical companies designing drugs, and even primary care physicians, there are several significant misconceptions about RA, including the following[4–6]:

- Patients with RA are a relatively homogeneous group who share a particular genotype (HLA-DR4) and respond to the new miracle drug (ie, methotrexate).
- Existing laboratory studies (RF, ESR, CRP) adequately identify RA patients and allow all therapy to be rationally selected and monitored.

As basic science, pharmaceutical drug developers, and clinical laboratory specialists move farther from practicing rheumatologists (and RA patients) into their own "private domains of research," these fallacies become more prevalent. A critical fact is that RA patients are heterogeneous in their genetics, methods of clinical presentations, and response to therapy.[3,7]

Therefore, no single animal model can be expected to fulfill the pathogenetic key steps for all patients, nor can any single drug be expected to

Table 10-1. American Rheumatism Association 1987 Revised Criteria for the Classification of Rheumatoid Arthritis

Criterion	Definition
1. Morning stiffness	Morning stiffness in and around the joints, lasting at least 1 hour before maximal improvement.
2. Arthritis of 3 or more joint areas	At least 3 joint areas simultaneously have had soft tissue swelling or fluid (not bony overgrowth alone) observed by a physician. The 14 possible areas are right or left , PIP, MCP, wrist, elbow, knee, ankle, and MTP joints.
3. Arthritis of hand joints	At least 1 area swollen (as defined above) in a wrist, MCP, or PIP joint.
4. Symmetric arthritis	Simultaneous involvement of the same joint areas (as defined in 2) on both sides of the body (bilateral involvement of PIPs, MCPs, or MTPs is acceptable without absolute symmetry).
5. Rheumatoid nodules	Subcutaneous nodules, over bony prominences or extensor surfaces, or in juxta-articular regions, observed by a physician.
6. Serum rheumatoid factor	Demonstration of abnormal amounts of serum rheumatoid factor by any method for which the result has been positive in <5% of normal control subjects.
7. Radiographic changes	Radiographic changes typical of rheumatoid arthritis on posteroanterior hand and wrist radiographs, which must include erosions or unequivocal bony decalcification localized in or most noticeable adjacent to the involved joints (osteoarthritis changes alone do not qualify).

Abbreviations: PIP = proximal interphalangeal; MCP = metacarpophalangeal; MTP = metatarsophalangeal.

**For classification purposes, a patient is said to have rheumatoid arthritis if he or she has satisfied at least 4 of these 7 criteria. Criteria 1 through 4 must have been present for at least 6 weeks. Patients with 2 clinical diagnoses are not excluded. Designation as classic, definite, or probable rheumatoid arthritis is not to be made based on these criteria.*

help all patients. Although methotrexate has greatly improved the lives of many RA patients, it (at best) slows the rate of progression, and attempts to discontinue the drug lead to a predictable recurrence of disease. In fact, fewer than 50% of RA patients on methotrexate show a response in at least 50% of involved joints at 2-year follow-up and are simply continued on this drug for lack of other options. Thus, RA, the most common and debilitating of diseases treated by rheumatologists, remains poorly treated (ie, only controlled and not cured), and current laboratory measurements have not altered the blind "empiric" approach of trying a medicine for a few months, and, if it does not work, trying another.

Estimates of RA prevalence depend on the criteria used to define the illness. This is a difficult problem, because there is no established etiologic agent or unique clinical or laboratory feature that can be used to define the disease, particularly in its early stages. Diagnosis is usually based on the presence of clinical signs (joint pain and swelling) and laboratory abnormalities (RF, ESR, and CRP). The most widely used criteria are the American College of Rheumatology (ACR) 1987 Revised Criteria (**Table 10-1**). The subdivision of RA into early, moderate, and severe stages on the basis of radiographic changes is presented in **Table 10-2**. Unfortunately, clinical assessments are subject to measurement variation and there is significant controversy about the criteria for early changes of RA on joint radiographs (as will be discussed below). Estimates of prevalence based on current ACR criteria indicate that between 1% and 2% of the adult population in every part of the world is affected with definite or classic RA. The prevalence is higher in women than in men for each age group; although the ratios vary in different studies, the general estimates are about 2.5:1 (women-men). The conditions most commonly confused with RA are systemic lupus erythematosus (SLE), psoriatic arthritis, and rheumatoid factor–negative spondyloarthropathies.

In addition to articular manifestations of arthritis, the RA patient may have other organs affected by the autoimmune process. Associated nonarticular manifestations may include subcutaneous nodules, vasculitis, pericarditis, pulmonary nodules or

Table 10-2. Criteria for Determining the Progression and Remission of Rheumatoid Arthritis and Functional Capacity of Patients With the Disease Classification of Progression of Rheumatoid Arthritis[8]

Stage	Criteria
I. Early	1. No destructive changes on radiographic examination.* 2. Radiographic evidence of osteoporosis may be present.
II. Moderate	1. Radiographic evidence of osteoporosis, with or without slight subchondral bone destruction; slight cartilage destruction may be present.* 2. No joint deformities, although limitation of joint mobility may be present.* 3. Adjacent muscle atrophy. 4. Extra-articular soft tissue lesions, such as nodules and tenosynovitis, may be present.
III. Severe	1. Radiographic evidence of cartilage and bone destruction, in addition to osteoporosis.* 2. Joint deformity, such as subluxation, ulnar deviation, or hyperextension, without fibrosis or bony ankylosis.* 3. Extensive muscle atrophy. 4. Extra-articular soft tissue lesions, such as nodules and tenosynovitis, may be present.
IV. Terminal	1. Fibrous or bony ankylosis.* 2. Criteria of stage III.

**These criteria must be present to permit classification of a patient in any particular stage or grade.*

interstitial fibrosis, mononeuritis, episcleritis, or (less commonly) scleritis. Sjögren's syndrome (keratoconjunctivitis sicca) and Felty's syndrome (leukopenia and often splenomegaly) are also found in association with RA.[9]

Current Controversy Over Early Versus Late Therapy

The poor long-term prognosis for many RA patients has led to a popular view that there may be a "window" of therapeutic opportunity for treatment of RA within the first 2 to 3 years following disease onset. Therefore, there is a recent trend toward aggressive therapy for all RA patients early in the course of their disease. The obvious risk to such an approach is that some patients can be expected to go into remission without aggressive therapy.[10] For example, over 10% of RA patients in a community-based study had a spontaneous remission during the first year of disease in the absence of specific antirheumatic treatment.[11] Furthermore, some rheumatologists do not believe that early institution of aggressive therapy changes the long-term outcome in RA patients.[1,7] This debate about the benefit or nonbenefit of aggressive therapy in early RA probably reflects clinicians' inability to identify subsets of RA patients who will undergo spontaneous remission or respond to a particular drug. Therefore, the key question for the clinical laboratory is how to identify which patient group will have a particular outcome and thus allow a more rational use of early aggressive therapy.

A final problem in studying the long-term outcome of RA is the substantial delay in diagnosis and beginning of therapy in some patients. In one study at a health maintenance organization,[12] a median lag time of 36 weeks occurred before diagnosis of RA was made by a primary care physician and several more months before referral to a specialist for treatment. This demonstrates that primary care providers should be educated about the need for early diagnosis of RA. At present, an increasing proportion of the population enters health maintenance organizations and referral to specialists and laboratory testing is discouraged for fiscal reasons.[13] Thus, an important window of therapeutic opportunity for some RA patients may be lost. Even if a new "perfect" laboratory test to predict poor outcome in an RA patient were developed, a key task would be the education of primary care physicians and the medical health insurance community that such testing is cost-efficient in the long run.

Patients with limited education or financial resources may be less compliant, unable to afford medications, and unable to participate in required clinical follow-up. Thus, an improved medical education structure will be required to implement the advantages of improved laboratory testing. Furthermore, these social and educational factors must be considered when evaluating the value of a laboratory test to predict long-term outcome. For example, a perfect laboratory test cannot accurately predict outcome if the patient cannot afford the necessary medications. Thus, long-term follow-up of studies must include the socioeconomic status of the patient as well as other measures of RA activity.

Laboratory Features Currently Used in Evaluating Rheumatoid Arthritis

Serologic Markers

Rheumatoid Factors and Other Autoantibodies

Rheumatoid factors are immunoglobulins that react with the Fc portion of IgG molecules. In vivo, RF binds to immune complexes (IgG molecules bound to antigens), activates complement, and facilitates removal of immune complexes by the reticuloendothelial system.[14] The most common laboratory test for RF is latex fixation in which different dilutions of patient sera are tested for their ability to agglutinate (cross-link) latex spheres coated with denatured IgG. Due to their large size (ie, pentameric molecules), IgM RFs most efficiently cross-link the IgG-coated latex beads. Immunoglobulin A RF (ie, IgA anti-IgG Fc) is best detected by enzyme-linked immunosorbent assay and has been proposed to correlate better with long-term outcome in RA than does IgM RF.[15,16] Immunoglobulin G RF (an IgG anti-IgG Fc antibody) is difficult to measure due to self-aggregation, because the IgG reacts with the Fc receptor of other IgG molecules. It is sometimes termed "cryptic RF," and results of studies that measure IgG RF have been difficult to reproduce.

In clinical practice, RF is associated with many diseases other than RA, including subacute bacterial endocarditis, hepatitis B and C, and other autoimmune diseases (**Table 10-3**). Also, the signs and symptoms of RA may precede the development of RF by up to 6 months in some patients. Nevertheless, RF remains one of the key methods used to subdivide arthritis patients into RF-positive (seropositive) and RF-negative (seronegative) subclasses. The absence of RF in an RA patient triggers a search for other causes of arthritis, such as spondyloarthropathies (psoriatic, Reiter's syndrome, ankylosing spondylitis), SLE, or other causes, such as infections or metabolic etiologies. However, RF is frequently absent in childhood onset RA, a condition termed *juvenile RA*. It has been proposed that some adult RF-negative RA patients experience adult onset of juvenile RA.[17]

Table 10-3. Selected Diseases Associated With Elevated Serum Rheumatoid Factor

Chronic bacterial infections
Subacute bacterial endocarditis
Leprosy
Tuberculosis
Syphilis
Lyme disease
Viruses
Hepatitis B and C
Parvovirus
Cytomegalovirus
Infectious mononucleosis (Epstein-Barr virus)
Hematologic diseases
Waldenström's macroglobulinemia
Myeloma
Lymphoma
Mixed cryoglobulinemia (type II)
Hypergammaglobulinemic purpura
Chronic inflammatory diseases of uncertain etiology
Sarcoidosis
Pulmonary interstitial disease
Autoimmune liver disease

Antinuclear antibodies (ANAs) have traditionally been associated with SLE, but also are present in almost 50% of RA patients. The pattern of ANAs on human epithelial tissue (HEp-2 cells) is often finely speckled and may have titers greater than 1:640. The nuclear antigens associated with RA in HEp-2 cells have not been well defined by either Western blot or gene cloning, in contrast to the careful characterization of multiple autoantigens associated with SLE, Sjögren's syndrome, and polymyositis. When ANA testing is performed using WIL-2 cells (or other lymphoblastoma cells transformed by Epstein-Barr virus), reactivity of the RA cell with the EBNA-1 antigen has been noted consistently; this antigen was initially termed *RA nuclear antigen* but was later shown to be identical to EBNA-1. Further characterization of the nuclear antigens recognized in RA patients may provide an important prognostic marker.

Antineutrophil cytoplasmic antibodies (ANCAs) are useful markers in patients with vasculitis, such as Wegener's granulomatosis and other autoimmune disorders. They are subdivided into c-ANCA (most closely associated with Wegener's granulomatosis) and p-ANCA (which is found in other diseases, including polyarteritis nodosa). Antineutrophil cytoplasmic antibodies have been found in the synovial fluid of adult RA[18] and juvenile RA[19] patients. For example, ANCAs were detected in the synovial fluid of 39.3% of patients with RA and 5.9% of those with osteoarthritis.[19] However, in RA patients, synovial ANCA was not associated with extra-articular manifestations or vasculitis.[20] Nor were ANCAs detected at a significant level in the sera of RA patients.

Immunoglobulin G antiperinuclear factor (APF) has been proposed as a marker to provide prognostic information in RA patients in addition to RF and ESR.[21,22] The APF seropositivity in RA patients is neither altered by the use of corticosteroids nor influenced by patient age or gender, the duration of illness, or the number of joints affected. Antiperinuclear factor is an IgG antibody generally detected by immunofluorescence assay using buccal mucosa epithelial cells. Attempts to purify the APF antigen from these cells have been unsuccessful due to the proposed lability of the antigen.[22] Furthermore, APF assays by immunofluorescence have been technically difficult to replicate, and few laboratories currently perform the test. The recent identification of the APF antigen as a 200-kd molecule identical to filaggrin[21] may allow development of more reproducible assays. It appears that a particular epitope on filaggrin is responsible for the APF reactivity.

Antibodies against cytokeratins (AKAs) are measured in immunofluorescence assays using the stratum corneum of various cornified epithelia. These assays also are difficult to perform due to technical artifacts and thus not widely employed. However, the recent demonstration that the AKA also detects filaggrin may lead to more reliable assays using purified antigen.[21] A different epitope on filaggrin is detected by AKA than by APF. Using multivariate analysis, both AKA and APF had statistically significant value in addition to latex RF for predicting active RA at 24 months.

Aberrant glycosylation of serum proteins has been reported in RA and patients with other chronic diseases.[23] In particular, agalactosyl IgG [Gal(o)] is an immunoglobulin lacking terminal galactose on the oligosaccharides situated in the Fc region. There is a decrease in the galactosylation of specific proteins, including autoantibodies (such as IgM and IgA RF), and of irrelevant IgG (such as antitetanus toxoid), as well as other serum proteins.[23] The glycosylation defect is not specific for RA; it is found in other chronic diseases such as tuberculosis.[21] In 2 recent studies,[24,25] the level of agalactosyl IgG [Gal(o)] was found to correlate with disease activity in RA patients and predict radiologic progression at 3 years. The aberrant glycosylation may play a role in the pathogenesis of RA by affecting the function of IgM RF.[26,27] In normal IgM molecules, the 2 highly conserved oligosaccharides of the Fc region are found buried between the CH2 domains, where they may restrain the Fc region from binding complement C1q or binding to monocyte Fc receptors.[26] Thus, the more mobile Fc region of agalactosyl RF may more easily participate in the activation of complement, bind to monocyte Fc receptors, or be recognized by lectin-like proteins present on the surface of vascular cells.[28] From the clinical laboratory point of view, the production of Gal(o) antibodies may reflect a part of the pathogenetic process in RA that is not well measured by cytokines or APRs.

Acute Phase Reactants

Acute phase reactants can be produced by many cell types, but their principal site of production is the liver. In response to any systemic inflammatory process, cytokines are released into the circulation and travel to the liver, where they stimulate production of APRs such as fibrinogen, CRP, and serum amyloid A (SAA). Thus, elevation of these APRs implies a systemic inflammatory process that provides valuable clues to the activity of RA. However, some patients with active RA do not exhibit elevation of all APRs or may show elevation of only particular APRs. This is a key limitation to using the reactants in monitoring therapy in RA. This complex response of APR production in patients is shown in **Figure 10-1**. Cytokines may exert either a proinflammatory or anti-inflammatory pattern of APR. The net balance of these activities is measured in clinical assays of APRs.

The ESR is considered a measure of acute disease activity in RA. An elevated ESR can result from many processes but predominantly reflects increased fibrinogen production in the liver by interleukin-6 (IL-6) and leukemia inhibitory factor (see Figure 10-1). In comparison, IL-1 and tumor necrosis factor (TNF) tend to inhibit fibrinogen production. Decreases in ESR may occur in RA patients after the start of either corticosteroid or other antirheumatic medications.[29] However, elevation of ESR at the time of acute arthritis onset does not adequately predict the development of erosive disease at follow-up 2 years later.

In comparison, elevated CRP at the onset of disease correlates with progressive erosion in the RA

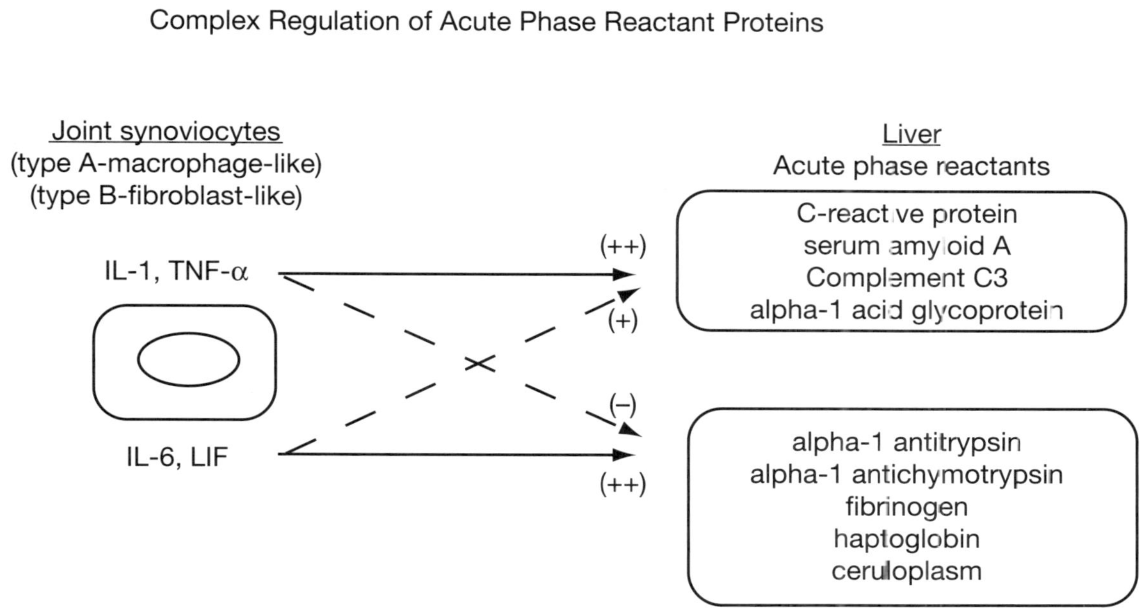

Figure 10-1. Regulation of acute phase reactants by cytokines. Cytokines are produced at the inflammatory site, travel through the blood stream, and induce synthesis of acute phase reactants in other tissues, particularly the liver.

patient.[29] The different prognostic values of these 2 APRs may be related to the preferential induction of CRP by particular cytokines, because CRP is more closely related to IL-1 and TNF-α (see Figure 10-1). Serum amyloid A has predictive values similar to those of CRP.[29] Although elevated CRP and SAA at disease onset are relatively specific predictors of poor outcome, they are not sufficiently sensitive. For example, some RA patients with low or normal CRP at disease onset still develop a slowly progressive erosive disease. This is particularly true of RA patients with a gradual onset of polyarthritis. Despite the limitation of ESR and CRP to detect active disease in all RA patients, these mea-surements remain a mainstay of clinical management. An important future goal for the clinical laboratory is the development of prognostic markers for those RA patients in whom ESR, CRP, and SAA are not elevated.

Complement components are synthesized in the liver by APRs as well as by other cell types.[30] However, complement may be "consumed" by immune activation so the net level of complement components reflects the balance of production and consumption. Measurements of complement activation (eg, C3a, C4a, C4d, C5a) have shown active consumption in synovial fluid and in the plasma of RA patients with extra-articular manifestations, such as vasculitis.[31,32] Therefore, measurement of complement activation has been proposed as a sensitive method to monitor disease activity.

Although these tests have worked admirably in the research laboratory, they have not gained widespread acceptance in general rheumatologic practice. Part of the problem is that complement may be artifactually activated during either collection or processing, leading to false-positive results. New methods of sample collection, including inhibitors that prevent artifactual activation of complement (after sample collection), may overcome these problems.[33]

Cytokines, Soluble Cytokine Receptors, Chemokines, Monoinflammatory Proteins, and RANTES

Proinflammatory cytokines, such as IL-1,[34] TNF-α, and IL-6,[35] are present at higher levels in synovial fluid and blood of RA patients than of normal controls. These elevated levels correlate with clinical measurements of the number of inflamed joints.[29] Although IL-1 and IL-6 seem to correlate more closely to original pathogenetic processes of RA than do ESR or CRP, the direct measurement of these cytokines has not provided more therapeutic information than the measurement of their derivative acute phase proteins.[29] The poor correlation of proinflammatory cytokines (IL-1, IL-6, TNF-α) in serum with long-term prognosis also may reflect their complicated interactions on different organs of the body. For example, IL-1 and TNF-α may act on the hypothalamus to induce prostaglandin E_2 synthesis and upregulation of adrenocorticotropic hormone, leading to increased levels of the anti-inflammatory glucocorticoids. Furthermore, the cost of these cytokine measurements and their reliability and reproducibility in the routine clinical laboratory has not been established, limiting their use to the research laboratory and perhaps specific clinical trials.

A family of cytokines known as chemokines, which chemoattract various leukocytes, have been identified in the synovial fluid and sera of RA patients.[36] The chemokines are a family of low-molecular-weight (8- to 10-kd) proteins with specificity for various types of inflammatory cells. Chemokine peptides contain 4 cysteine groups linked either directly (C-C) or with intervening amino acids (C-X-C). The C-C chemokines primarily attract monocytes and include monocyte-chemotactic and activating factor, monocyte inflammatory proteins (MIP-α1, MIP-α2, MIP-β), interferon gamma inducible protein 10 (IP-10), and RANTES (regulated on activation, normal T expressed) (**Table 10-4**). The C-X-C chemokines include IL-8, growth-regulated gene product, and platelet factor 4. Some, but not all, of these chemokines have been detected in synovial fluid at levels much higher than those in osteoarthritis joint fluids.[37–39] In comparison, RANTES and IP-10 are not significantly elevated in either joint fluid or serum. T-cell–derived cytokines, such as IL-2, interferon gamma, or IL-4, are not detected at elevated levels in joint or sera of RA patients in any consistent pattern.[40] The pattern of cytokines found in synovial fluid suggests a monocytic (synoviocyte type A) and/or fibroblastic (synoviocyte type B) origin.

In the liver, serum α_1-antitrypsin is an acute phase glycoprotein containing 3 carbohydrate side chains, linked by *N*-glycoside to the asparagine molecules (Asn46, Asn83, and Asn247) of the single polypeptide unit. "Microheterogeneity" in the glycosylation of α_1-antitrypsin has been observed in various inflammatory states, including RA. In a recent study of RA patients,[41] high concentrations of α_1-antitrypsin with altered glycosylation were found. Future studies of RA patients will be required to determine whether measurements of these α_1-antitrypsin variants provide information superior to the IgG Gal(o) levels described earlier.

Hyaluronic Acid and Collagen Breakdown Products

A crucial part of the joint destruction in RA is the erosion of articular cartilage and the associated release of mucopolysaccharides. Therefore, markers of connective tissue destruction in the joint could be useful in monitoring RA patients. For example, soluble fragments of hyaluronic acid (HA) can be elevated 10 to 20 times in the sera of RA patients. The elevated serum levels are presumed to derive from leakage into the blood from the inflamed tissues, resulting in draining lymph and a possible defect in the receptor-mediated

Table 10-4. Comparison of Chemokine Levels in Synovial Fluid of Patients With Either Rheumatoid Arthritis or Osteoarthritis

Chemokine	Rheumatoid Osteoarthritis	Responsive Arthritis	Cell Type
IL-8	+	++++	PMN, T cells
GRO	+++	(–)	PMN
ENA-78	+	+++	PMN
MCAF		+++	Monocytes, T cells
MIP-1a	+	++++	Monocytes, T cells
RANTES		+	Monocytes, T cells
IP-10		+	Monocytes, T cells

Abbreviations: IL-8 = interleukin-8; GRO = growth-regulated gene product (detected as mRNA); ENA-78 = epithelial neutrophil-activating peptide-78; MCAF = monocyte-chemotactic and activating factor; MIP-1a = macrophage inhibitory protein-1a; RANTES = regulated on activation-normal T-cell expressed and presumably secreted; IP-10 = interferon-inducible protein-10.

clearance by liver endothelial cells in RA patients.[42] Serum HA levels correlated closely with clinical disease activity in patients with RA in one study.[42] However, in another study,[43] the diagnostic value of HA was questioned because the level was found to vary markedly during the day, corresponding to physical activity. Increased HA levels also are seen in other inflammatory diseases, particularly those involving the liver, and in patients with infections. Thus, further studies on HA levels will be required to determine whether HA is a useful marker in RA patients.

In one study,[44] an increased concentration of circulating cartilage oligomeric protein (COMP) was found in patients with rapid joint destruction, and COMP levels were correlated with APRs such as CRP. In comparison, elevated levels of chondroitin sulfate (a marker of cartilage aggregan synthesis) were found in patients with a slow rate of joint destruction and may provide a marker for this subset of RA. The urinary excretion of collagen cross-links, pyridinoline, and deoxypyridinoline can be measured using high-performance liquid chromatography and are elevated in patients with RA.[45] These markers also indicate increased "turnover" and may be an important future method for monitoring disease. However, the value of these measurements in monitoring RA therapy or prognosis remains to be demonstrated.

Genetic Markers

There has been a great deal of interest in the diagnostic use of alleles for major histocompatibility complex (MHC) antigens on chromosome 6, in particular, the increased frequency of the class II MHC allele *DR4* (particularly alleles *DRB1*0401* or *DRB1*0404*) in white patients with RA. In nonwhite populations, an increase in *DR1* (particularly allele *DRB1*1001*) is noted. These different *DR* alleles share a stretch of similar amino acids from positions 70 to 74 in the third hypervariable region. This "shared epitope" also appears to be responsible for the previously defined serologic specificities called Dw4, Dw14, and Dw15 associated with RA. Approximately 70% of white patients with RA in the United States and Western Europe possess *HLA-DR4*, compared with 25% of healthy white individuals. However, 42% of the healthy white population has one or more of the alleles "predisposing to susceptibility." Thus, oligotyping for these *DR* alleles would not be a very specific test in clinical practice for the prediction of RA in the general population.[46]

Recent retrospective studies have suggested that *HLA-DR4* may serve as a severity factor in RA. These studies have examined the presence of a single copy of *DR4* (heterozygote), 2 copies of *D4* (homozygote) and "mixed *DR4*/shared epitope" (one copy of *DR4* and a shared epitope allele on the other chromosome). A single copy of *DR4* or a single shared epitope does not confer more prognostic information than does clinical examination and CRP at the time of diagnosis.[47] Homozygous *DR4* is associated with extra-articular manifestations, including Felty's syndrome.[48] Studies involving RA patients with one copy of *DR4* and one "shared epitope allele" have given different results at different centers.[6,49]

At present, the role of *HLA-DR* typing in RA is limited to research applications, such as studies of new therapeutic agents, to determine whether particular alleles allow for selection of therapy. One preliminary report has indicated that *DR4* patients may be relatively resistant (or have only transient response) to therapy with methotrexate alone but have improved response to combined therapy (O'Dell, personal communication). If these preliminary observations are confirmed, *HLA-DR4* typing will become an important part of routine clinical management.

Among non-HLA genes, genetic predisposition to RA has been associated with a particular allele of the gene-encoding macrophage factor NRAMP1[50]; this gene regulates the priming and activation of macrophages for enhanced TNF-α and IL-1β production. The same study identified 4 other genetic loci associated with a subset of RA, including genes located at 2q34 (*TNP1*) and 2q35 (*IL8R*, *VIL1*, *DES*). A separate study[51] noted a high frequency of a particular polymorphism of the 70-kd heat shock protein 70-1 promoter in RA patients. Further studies will be required to determine whether these new polymorphic markers provide prognostic information.

Radiographic Studies

The radiograph of the hand or foot is generally considered the gold standard for diagnosis and progression in RA. Therefore, it is surprising to internists that the evaluation and scoring of radiographs for early RA remains a subject of controversy among bone radiologists.[4,52] The significance of this debate is indicated in a large retrospective study of RA,[53] where 26% of affected patients had radiographic changes of the joint consistent with early RA, but did not progress substantially during a 5-year follow-up period in the absence of aggressive therapy. Most of the debate centers on the criteria for early joint changes specific for RA.[52,54] In later stages of the disease, there is good agreement on the scoring of erosive lesions using the methods of Pincus, et al,[54] or Sharp.[55]

Other methods used to assess RA joint damage include ultrasonography, bone densitometry, and magnetic resonance imaging (MRI). However, the reproducibility of joint ultrasonography may be limited by artifacts (especially during early or mild disease stages) and MRI remains too costly for routine use. Scintigraphy with technetium 99 and bone densitometry of peripheral joints show promise in identifying a subgroup of early RA patients with higher risk for progressive joint erosion and have comparable cost to multiple joint radiographs.[56]

Hand bone mineral density (BMD) measurement by dual-energy x-ray absorptiometry has potential as a marker of progression in early RA. Hand BMD correlates with measures of disease activity and the loss of functional capacity and precedes a loss of bone density in the lumbar spine.[57] Loss of bone density in the hand has been found to occur early in the disease and may progress in the absence of other laboratory markers of systemic disease. Hand BMD has the potential to be an outcome measure in early disease. Other promising tests are cytokines, genetic typing, improved bone imaging methods, and measurement of collagen breakdown products. It is likely that a combination of these tests will provide greater sensitivity and specificity than any single test.

In a practical sense, the best way to quickly evaluate the best laboratory measures will be to access the stored serum banks of commercial pharmaceutical companies that have collected "storage samples" during their clinical drug trials. In these drug studies, patient compliance with medication, as well as careful collection of associated clinical and radiologic data, are available, making further correlation of clinical response to a particular therapy possible. Therefore, the most practical hope for classifying subsets of RA is the establishment of a liaison among pharmaceutical companies (to share existing samples or to prospectively collect suitable samples), academic research institutions studying RA, and biotechnology companies with the expertise to develop or run unique assays. The success of workshops sponsored by the National Institutes of Health in coordination with other laboratory and clinical studies serves as a model for workshops to predict prognostic markers in RA.

Current Questions Regarding the Use of the Clinical Laboratory and Future Directions

Myriad studies have been published about the correlation of specific laboratory variables and clinical outcomes over a short time (2 to 3 years) in RA patients. However, these studies have generally used a panel of patients evaluated at tertiary referral centers. In comparison, the community physician generally sees a different population of new onset arthritis patients. To gain acceptance by clinicians and insurance providers, laboratory tests for the general practitioner must have the simplicity and low cost of an RF. New tests to help predict outcomes might be found by examining the specific isotype of RF (eg, IgA-RF) or by improving detection methods for antibodies against filaggrin (eg, to replace APF or AKA assays using immunofluorescence).

Acknowledgments

This study was made possible by grants from the National Institutes of Health M01 RR00833 and RO133983 and was partially supported by the Scripps-Stedham, Kovler, Ramsdell, and Hennings Charitable Foundations.

After this chapter was submitted, several recent papers have addressed additional diagnostic tests to help predict prognosis in rheumatoid arthritis. These papers are reviewed in the July 2002 issue of Laboratory Medicine *(33:7).*

References

1. Kushner I, Dawson NV. Aggressive therapy does not substantially alter the long-term course of rheumatoid arthritis: So what else is new? *Rheum Dis Clin North Am*. 1993;19:163–172.
2. Harris E. Rheumatoid arthritis: Pathophysiology and implications for therapy. *N Engl J Med*. 1990;322:1277–1289.
3. Pincus T. The underestimated long-term medical and economic consequences of rheumatoid arthritis. *Drugs*. 1995;50:1–14.
4. van Riel PL, van Gestel AM, van de Putte LB. Development and validation of response criteria in rheumatoid arthritis: Steps towards an international consensus on prognostic markers. *Br J Rheumatol*. 1996;35(suppl 2):4–7.
5. O'Dell J, Haire CK, Moore G. Treatment of rheumatoid arthritis with methotrexate alone, sulfasalazine, and hydroxychloroquine or a combination. *N Engl J Med*. 1996;334:1287–1291.

6. Emery P, Salmon M, Gooi J. Should patients with recent onset of rheumatoid arthritis be offered genetic screening? *Ann Rheum Dis*. 1996;55:934–935. Letter.

7. Iannuzzi L, Dawson N, Zein N, et al. Does drug therapy slow radiographic progression in RA? *N Engl J Med*. 1983;309:1023–1028.

8. Steinbrocker O, Traeger CH, Batterman RC. Therapeutic criteria in rheumatoid arthritis. *JAMA*. 1949;140:659–662.

9. Harris E. Rheumatoid arthritis: Clinical features. In: Kelly W, Harris E, Ruddy S, et al, eds. *Textbook of Rheumatology*. Philadelphia, PA: WB Saunders; 1995:874–901.

10. Wilske K, Healey L. The need for aggressive therapy in RA. *Med Clin North Am*. 1993;19:153–163.

11. Van Heidge D, van Leewen M, Rijswijkm V. Biannual radiographic assessments of hands and feet in a three-year prospective follow-up of patients with early RA. *Arthritis Rheum*. 1992;35:26–34.

12. Chan K, Felson D, Yood R, et al. The lag time between onset of symptoms and diagnosis of RA. *Arthritis Rheum*. 1994;37:814–820.

13. Weinblatt M. Rheumatoid arthritis: Treat now, not later. *Ann Intern Med*. 1996;124:773–774.

14. Carson DA, Chen PP, Fox RI, et al. Rheumatoid factors and the immune networks. *Annu Rev Immunol*. 1987;5:109–126.

15. Jonsson T, Arinbjarnarson S, Thorsteinsson J, et al. Raised IgA rheumatoid factor (RF) but not IgM RF or IgG RF is associated with extra-articular manifestations in rheumatoid arthritis. *Scand J Rheumatol*. 1995;24:372–375.

16. Elkon K, Gharavi E, Patel E. IgA and IgM rheumatoid factors in serum, saliva and other secretions: Relationship to rheumatoid arthritis. *Clin Exp Immunol*.1983;52:75–84.

17. Fong S, Chen PP, Fox RI, et al. The diversity and idiotypic pattern of human rheumatoid factors in disease. *Concepts Immunopathol*. 1988;5:168–191.

18. Afeltra A, Sebastiani GD, Galeazzi M, et al. Antineutrophil cytoplasmic antibodies in synovial fluid and in serum of patients with rheumatoid arthritis and other types of synovitis. *J Rheumatol*. 1996;23:10–15.

19. Speckmaier M, Rother E, Terreri T, et al. Prevalence of anti-neutrophil cytoplasmic antibodies (ANCA) in juvenile chronic arthritis. *Clin Exp Rheumatol*. 1996;14:211–216.

20. Rother E, Schochat T, Peter HH. Antineutrophil cytoplasmic antibodies (ANCA) in rheumatoid arthritis: A prospective study. *Rheumatol Int*. 1996;15: 231–237.

21. Sebbag M, Simon M, Vincent C, et al. The antiperinuclear factor and the so-called antikeratin antibodies are the same rheumatoid arthritis-specific autoantibodies. *J Clin Invest*. 1995;95:2672–2679.

22. Manera C, Franceschini F, Cretti L, et al. Clinical heterogeneity of rheumatoid arthritis and the antiperinuclear factor. *J Rheumatol*. 1994;21:2021–2025.

23. Pilkington C, Yeung E, Isenberg D, et al. Agalactosyl IgG and antibody specificity in rheumatoid arthritis, tuberculosis, systemic lupus erythematosus and myasthenia gravis. *Autoimmunity*. 1995;22:107–111.

24. Lacki JK, Porawska W, Mackiewicz U, et al. Changes in agalactosyl IgG levels correlate with radiological progression in early rheumatoid arthritis. *Ann Med*. 1996;28:265–269.

25. Bodman-Smith K, Sumar N, Sinclari H, et al. Agalactosyl IgG [Gal(o)]—An analysis of its clinical utility in the long-term follow-up of patients with rheumatoid arthritis. *Br J Rheumatol*. 1996;35:1063–1066.

26. Dwek RA, Lellouch AC, Wormald MR. Glycobiology: The function of sugar in the IgG molecule. *J Anat*. 1995;187:279–292.

27. Ezekowitz RA. Agalactosyl IgG and mannose-binding proteins: Biochemical nicety or pathophysiological paradigm? *Nat Med*. 1995;1:207–208. Comment.

28. Malhotra R, Wormald MR, Rudd PM, et al. Glycosylation changes of IgG associated with rheumatoid arthritis can activate complement via the mannose-binding protein. *Nat Med*. 1995;1:237–243. Published erratum appears in *Nat Med*. 1995;1:599.

29. Badolato R, Oppenheim J. Role of cytokines, acute phase proteins and chemokines in the progression of rheumatoid arthritis. *Semin Arthritis Rheum*. 1996;26:526–538.

30. Barland P, Lipstein E. Selection and use of laboratory tests in the rheumatic diseases. *Am J Med*. 1996;100:16S–23S.

31. Osterland CK. Laboratory diagnosis and monitoring in chronic systemic autoimmune diseases. *Clin Chem*. 1994;40:2146–2153.

32. Sato Y, Watanabe H, Kogure A, et al. Complement-activating properties of IgM rheumatoid factors reacting with IgG subclasses. *Clin Rheumatol*. 1995;14:425–428.

33. Hugli TE. Protease inhibitors: Novel therapeutic application and development. *Trends Biotechnol*. 1996;14:409–412.

34. Eastgate J, Symons J. Wood N. Correlation of plasma interleukin-1 levels with disease activity in RA. *Lancet*. 1988;2:706–709.

35. Houssiau F, Devogelaer J, Van Damme J. Interleukin–6 in synovial fluid and serum of patients with rheumatoid arthritis and other inflammatory arthritis. *Arthritis Rheum*. 1988;31:784–788.

36. Robinson E, Keystone E, Schall T, et al. Chemokine expression in rheumatoid arthritis (RA): Evidence of RANTES and macrophage inflammatory protein (MIP)-1 beta production by synovial T cells. *Clin Exp Immunol*. 1995;101:398–407.

37. Koch A, Kunkel S, Burrows J. Synovial tissue macrophages as a source of chemotactic cytokine IL-8. *J Immunol*. 1991;147:2187–2195.

38. Koch A, Kunkel S, Harlow L. Enhanced production of monocyte chemoattractant protein-1 in rheumatoid arthritis. *J Clin Invest*. 1992;90:772–779.

39. Koch A, Kunkel K, Harlow L. Macrophage inflammatory protein-1 alpha. A novel chemotactic cytokine for macrophages in rheumatoid arthritis. *J Clin Invest*. 1994;93:921–928.

40. Berhelot J, Bataille R, Maugar Y, et al. Rheumatoid arthritis as a bone marrow disorder. *Semin Arthritis Rheum*. 1996;26:505–514.

41. Hrycaj P, Nayyar S, Stanworth DR, et al. Micro-heterogeneity of alpha-1-antitrypsin in relation to the concentration of its complex with immunoglobulin A in the sera of patients with rheumatoid arthritis. *Clin Exp Rheumatol*. 1996;14:119–123.

42. Emlen W, Niebur J, Flanders G, et al. Measurement of serum hyaluronic acid in patients with rheumatoid arthritis: Correlation with disease activity. *J Rheumatol*. 1996;23:974–978.

43. Laurent TC, Laurent UB, Fraser JR. Serum hyaluronan as a disease marker. *Ann Med*. 1996;28:241–253.

44. Mansson B, Carey D, Alini M. Cartilage and bone metabolism in RA: Differences between rapid and slow progression of disease identified by serum markers of cartilage metabolism. *J Clin Invest*. 1995;95:1071–1077.

45. Graverand MP, Tron AM, Ichou M, et al. Assessment of urinary hydroxypyridinium cross-links measurement in osteoarthritis. *Br J Rheumatol*. 1996;35:1091–1095.

46. Arnett F. Histocompatibility typing in the rheumatic diseases: Diagnostic and prognostic implications. *Med Clin North Am*. 1994;20:371–387.

47. Hall FC, Weeks DE, Camilleri JP, et al. Influence of the HLA-DRB1 locus on susceptibility and severity in rheumatoid arthritis. *Q J Med*. 1996;89:821–829.

48. Weyland C, Hicok K, Conn D. The influence of HLA-DRB1 genes on disease severity in rheumatoid arthritis. *Ann Intern Med*. 1992;117:801–806.

49. Gough A, Faint J, Salmon M, et al. Genetic typing of patients with inflammatory arthritis at presentation can be used to predict outcome. *Arthritis Rheum*. 1994;37:1166–1170.

50. Shaw MA, Clayton D, Atkinson SE, et al. Linkage of rheumatoid arthritis to the candidate gene NRAMP1 on 2q35. *J Med Genet*. 1996;33:672–677.

51. Quadri SA, Taneja V, Mehra NK, et al. HSP70-1 promoter region alleles and susceptibility to rheumatoid arthritis. *Clin Exp Rheumatol*. 1996;14:183–185.

52. Wassenberg S, Rau R. Problems in evaluating radiographic findings in rheumatoid arthritis using different methods of radiographic scoring: Examples of difficult cases and a study design to develop an improved scoring method. *J Rheumatol*. 1995;22:1990–1997.

53. Fex E, Jonsson K, Johnson U, et al. Development of radiographic damage during the first 5–6 years of rheumatoid arthritis. A prospective follow-up study of a Swedish cohort. *Br J Rheumatol*. 1996;35:1106–1115.

54. Pincus T, Callahan LF, Fuchs HA, et al. Quantitative analysis of hand radiographs in rheumatoid arthritis: Time course of radiographic changes, relation to joint examination measures, and comparison of different scoring methods. *J Rheumatol*. 1995;22:1983–1989.

55. Sharp JT. Scoring radiographic abnormalities in rheumatoid arthritis. *Radiol Clin North Am*. 1996;34:233–241.

56. Bohndorf K, Schalm J. Diagnostic radiography in rheumatoid arthritis: Benefits and limitations. *Baillieres Clin Rheumatol*. 1996;10:399–407.

57. van Rield P, Van Heidge D, van Putte L. Radiographic progression in RA: Results of three comparative trials. *J Rheumatol*. 1995;22:1797–1799.

58. Devlin J, Lilley J, Gough A, et al. Clinical associations of dual-energy X-ray absorptiometry measurements of hand bone mass in rheumatoid arthritis. *Br J Rheumatol*. 1996;35:1256–1262.

CHAPTER 11

Advances in the Diagnosis and Laboratory Evaluation of Systemic Rheumatic Diseases Other Than Rheumatoid Arthritis

Henry A. Homburger, MD

The systemic rheumatic diseases (SRDs), also called connective tissue diseases, include systemic lupus erythematosus (SLE), rheumatoid arthritis, Sjögren's syndrome, systemic sclerosis (scleroderma), CREST (calcinosis, Raynaud's phenomenon, esophageal dysfunction, sclerodactyly, telangiectasia) syndrome, mixed connective tissue disease (MCTD), and polymyositis. This group of diseases is also referred to collectively as non–organ-specific autoimmune diseases, a name that reflects the fact that each disease may involve several different organ systems simultaneously. The pathogenesis of SRDs is presumed to be autoimmune, although the precise immunologic mechanisms are not known.

Collectively, these diseases are important because many patients present with signs and symptoms compatible with one or more of them. For this reason, clinicians are often called on to rule out the diagnosis of an SRD, and the clinical laboratory plays an important role in the diagnostic evaluation of affected patients.

This chapter discusses the role of the clinical laboratory in performing tests for autoantibodies as markers of SRDs. Separate sections are devoted to laboratory tests for autoantibodies that are useful in the clinical evaluation of SRDs, the analytic methods used to perform these tests, and a suggested approach to the use of sequential tests for autoantibodies to evaluate patients for the presence of SRDs.

Overview of Laboratory Tests for Autoantibodies in Systemic Rheumatic Diseases: Antinuclear Antibodies and Antibodies to Extractable Nuclear Antigens

The most commonly performed screening test for SRDs is the test for antinuclear antibodies (ANAs). Antinuclear antibodies are particularly common in the following diseases: SLE, discoid lupus erythematosus, drug-induced lupus erythematosus, MCTD, Sjögren's syndrome, scleroderma/CREST syndrome, rheumatoid arthritis, and polymyositis/dermatomyositis. Antinuclear antibodies also occur in many organ-specific autoimmune diseases, such as autoimmune thyroiditis and autoimmune chronic active liver disease. All these diseases are characterized by the presence of autoantibodies that react with one or more antigens found in the nucleus or cytoplasm of mammalian cells.[1,2] Testing for ANAs, therefore, is commonly performed early in the diagnostic evaluation of patients suspected of having an SRD.

The most commonly used analytic method to test for ANAs is indirect immunofluorescence performed on substrate slides made from mounted tissue sections, such as mouse liver, or tissue culture cells, such as human epithelioid cells (HEp-2 or KB cells).[2] Many different specificities of ANA are identified by immunofluorescence as distinct morphologic patterns of staining; some patterns of immunofluorescence suggest the presence of specific antibodies that are strongly associated with particular diseases.

The following patterns are commonly reported in positive ANAs for patients with SRDs: homogeneous (diffuse) staining of the nucleus; speckled staining of the nucleus; nucleolar staining; and centromeric (discrete speckled) staining of the nucleus. Antibodies to double-stranded DNA (dsDNA, or native DNA), histones, and deoxyribonucleoprotein characteristically demonstrate homogeneous nuclear staining.[3] The homogeneous pattern on the HEp-2 cell substrate demonstrates uniform staining of the nuclei. Nucleoli appear as negatively stained areas. Mitotic cells and their chromosomes stain as irregularly shaped masses. The rim (peripheral) pattern is often seen with significant levels of anti-dsDNA antibodies. The nuclei stain predominantly at their periphery. The speckled pattern is the most commonly observed ANA pattern. Speckled patterns of fine, discrete, or clumpy consistency have been described. A uniform (true speckled) pattern is seen with anticentromere antibodies in cells not in division. A clumpy speckled pattern is seen with antibodies to the extractable nuclear antigens uridine-rich ribonucleoprotein (U_1RNP), Sm (Smith), and Sjögren's syndrome-B/La (SS-B/La). Sera that contain anti–SS-A/Ro produce a pattern of discrete nuclear speckles on a wide variety of human cell substrates.[4] The centromere pattern consists of discrete and uniform speckles scattered throughout the nucleus. Mitotic cells are positive, demonstrating a clustering of the centromeres in the chromosomes in different arrangements according to the mitotic stage. The centromere pattern is associated with the CREST syndrome, a milder variant of scleroderma. The nucleolar pattern is characterized by homogeneous or speckled staining of the nucleolus. This pattern is often associated with dull, homogeneous fluorescence in the rest of the nucleus, and the chromosomes in mitotic cells are unstained. The nucleolar pattern suggests autoantibodies to 4-6S RNA. Nucleolar autoantibodies occur primarily in the sera of patients with scleroderma, SLE, Sjögren's syndrome, or Raynaud's phenomenon.[5]

In addition to these commonly observed patterns, a number of other fluorescent staining patterns have been described on ANA test substrates, including the proliferating-cell nuclear antigen (PCNA) pattern, the nuclear membrane pattern, and several cytoplasmic staining patterns. The PCNA pattern consists of fine-to-coarse nuclear speckling in 30% to 60% of the cells in interphase, with negative staining of the chromosome region of mitotic cells. This pattern is very specific for patients with SLE and has been reported in SLE patients with diffuse glomerulonephritis.[6] The antinuclear membrane pattern appears as a rim around the nucleus; it resembles a peripheral pattern, but is distinguished by the fact that the metaphase chromosome stage is negative. This autoantibody has recently been recognized in patients with autoimmune liver disease.

Results of the ANA test are reported as negative or positive. If positive, the result includes the end point titer and a description of the immunofluorescence pattern observed morphologically. Examples of the most common morphologic patterns of ANA already described are shown in **Figure 11-1**. As noted previously, the pattern of ANA often suggests the presence of a specific antibody that can be identified by follow-up testing.

Several notes of caution are indicated to avoid inappropriate use of the ANA test. This test should be requested only if there is clinical suspicion of an SRD, because positive results occur in some healthy individuals. This is particularly true in adults older than 40 years.[7] Weakly positive results (titers of 80 or less) are usually not strongly predictive of an SRD. In addition, different substrates frequently yield different end point titers and may produce different patterns with the same ANA-positive serum.[8]

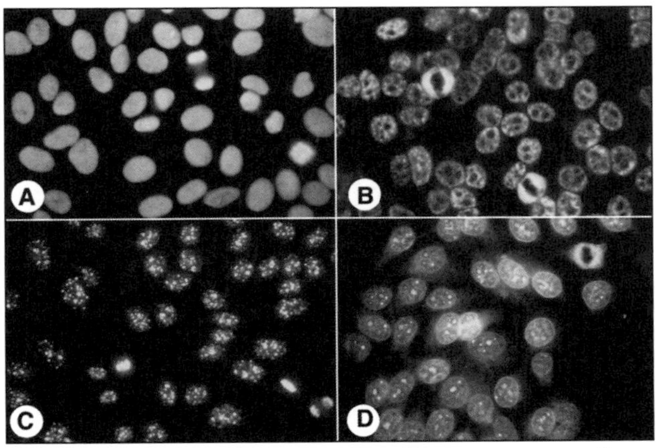

Figure 11-1. Common morphologic patterns of antinuclear antibodies in HEp-2 substrates. A, homogeneous; B, speckled; C, centromere; D, nucleolar and nuclear membrane.

Table 11-1. Autoantibodies Associated With Systemic Rheumatic Diseases

Antibody Detected	Disease Association
dsDNA	Systemic lupus erythematosus
Sm	Systemic lupus erythematosus
Centromere	CREST variant of scleroderma
RNA polymerases I-III	Scleroderma
Topoisomerase I	Scleroderma
Histidyl-tRNA synthetase (Jo-1)	Polymyositis
Signal recognition particles	Polymyositis
U_1RNP	Mixed connective tissue disease
SS-A/Ro, SS-B/La	Sjögren's syndrome; lupus erythematosus

Abbreviations: CREST = calcinosis, Raynaud's phenomenon, esophageal dysfunction, sclerodactyly, telangiectasia; dsDNA = double-stranded DNA; U_1RNP = uridine-rich ribonucleoprotein.

To ensure the reliability of ANA testing, it is recommended that each laboratory test and establish the frequencies of positive ANA results in healthy individuals younger and older than 40 years. In addition, laboratories are encouraged to test reference sera that contain ANAs reactive with dsDNA, SS-A/Ro, SS-B/La, U_1RNP, and Sm, as well as nucleolar antigens, periodically as a quality control activity. These reference sera are available from the Arthritis Foundation/CDC Reference Laboratory, Immunology Branch 1-1202, A25, Centers for Disease Control and Prevention, Atlanta, Georgia.

Disease-Specific Autoantibodies

A number of specific autoantibodies are strongly associated with particular SRDs (**Table 11-1**). The presence in serum of immunoglobulin (Ig) G autoantibodies to dsDNA is characteristic of SLE.[1] These antibodies, which characteristically produce a homogeneous or peripheral pattern of fluorescence on substrates used in the ANA test, are rarely found in patients with other SRDs. Nevertheless, care must be exercised to perform testing by a method specific for antibodies for dsDNA. Antibodies to single-stranded

Table 11-2. Antigenic Proteins of the Extractable Nuclear Antigens

Antigen	Protein	Sources*
U_1RNP	68 kd†	Calf thymus
Sm	Several (B, B1, D, E, F, G) ranging in molecular size from 11 to 26 kd	Bovine thymus or spleen
SS-A/Ro	52 kd†, 60 kd†	
SS-B/La	47 kd†	
Topoisomerase I (Scl-70)	75 kd†	

Abbreviations: U_1RNP = uridine-rich ribonucleoprotein; SS = Sjögren's syndrome.

**All extractable nuclear antigens cannot be prepared from a single tissue source. Topoisomerase I is found in thymus but not spleen. SS-A/Ro is found in spleen but not thymus.*

†These proteins are available as recombinant molecules.

DNA (ssDNA) are common in both healthy individuals and patients with a variety of diseases and may cause false-positive results in poorly controlled immunoassays (enzyme or immunoradiometric).[9] Similarly, low titers of IgM antibodies to dsDNA are found in patients who do not have SLE, and these antibodies may cause false-positive results when tests are performed by immunofluorescence on the substrate *Crithidia lucillae*. This method is based on the binding of anti-dsDNA antibodies to circular dsDNA in the kinetoplast of *C lucillae*, which are then detected by use of a fluorochrome-conjugated antihuman immunoglobulin antibody.

Testing for autoantibodies to extractable nuclear antigens (ENAs) is useful to categorize several SRDs. These antigens, which can be eluted from substrate cells by washing with saline, are structurally unique ribonucleoprotein autoantigens. The ENAs include several different antigens, of which 4 are particularly important clinically: U_1RNP, Sm, SS-A/Ro, and SS-B/La. These antigens are composed of one or more proteins associated with small nuclear (or small cytoplasmic) RNA species (snRNP). The RNA species range in size from 80 to approximately 350 nucleotides and are ubiquitous components of eukaryotic cells.[10] Some autoantibodies to ENAs react with molecules of the uridine-rich U family of snRNPs, notably the U_1RNP and Sm molecules. Anti-ENA autoantibodies recognize the proteins associated with snRNP particles, and reactivity persists after chemical separation of the protein and RNA components of the snRNP particle.[11,12] **Table 11-2** includes a list of ENA protein antigens, their molecular sizes, and tissue sources.

Anti-ENA autoantibodies characteristically produce a coarse, speckled pattern of immunofluorescence in the ANA test.[1] These autoantibodies are present in relatively high concentrations in serum and can be detected by double immunodiffusion (**Figure 11-2**) or immunoassay. Immunodiffusion methods are entirely dependent on the availability of monospecific antisera to define ENA-specific precipitins. More recently,

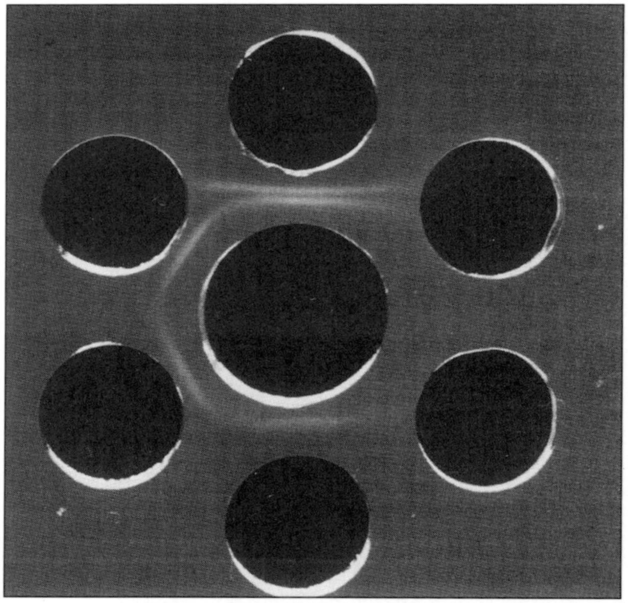

Figure 11-2. Double immunodiffusion for autoantibodies to extractable nuclear antigens U_1RNP and Sm. The center well was loaded with U_1RNP/Sm antigen. The outside wells were loaded with control sera or patient sera as follows (counterclockwise from top well): anti-U_1RNP and anti-Sm control, patient 1 in duplicate, anti-U_1RNP control, patient 2 in duplicate. Precipitin formed with serum from patient 1 shows a line of identity (fusion of precipitins) with anti-U_1RNP control sera.

immunoassay methods have been developed to measure anti-ENA autoantibodies. These methods use purified or recombinant ENA proteins adsorbed to the wells of microtiter plates to capture specific antibodies in patient sera. The enzyme immunoassay method is more sensitive than double immunodiffusion, but may generate false-positive results in some sera with above-normal concentrations of immunoglobulins due to increased nonspecific binding to the microtiter wells. Immunoassays based on recombinant U_1RNP, Sm, SS-A/Ro, and SS-B/La protein antigens are commercially available.

Autoantibodies to U_1RNP and Sm occur in patients with SLE; and anti-Sm antibodies are considered a marker for this disease.[1] Although anti-Sm antibodies occur in a minority (5% to 30%) of patients with SLE, the specificity of anti-Sm antibodies for this disease is extremely high when tests are performed by double immunodiffusion. Similarly, unequivocal positive anti-Sm results obtained by immunoassays are found only in patients with SLE. Care must be taken in interpreting the results of anti-Sm tests performed by immunoassays, however, because weakly positive results (absorbencies slightly above the cutoff for positive results) may occur in patients who do not have SLE.[13]

Anti-U_1RNP autoantibodies occur in patients with several of the SRDs; detection of anti-U_1RNP antibodies is useful in establishing the diagnosis of MCTD, SLE, and Sjögren's syndrome.[1] The presence of anti-U_1RNP, often in high concentration in the absence of anti-dsDNA and other anti-ENA autoantibodies, strongly suggests the diagnosis of MCTD.[14] Mixed connective tissue disease has clinical features similar to SLE, scleroderma, and polymyositis. Arthritis and arthralgias, Raynaud's phenomenon, esophageal dysfunction, and myositis are common in MCTD, but renal involvement is infrequent. The finding of anti-U_1RNP is important in establishing the diagnosis of MCTD and in ruling out other SRDs. A positive test for anti-U_1RNP autoantibodies in the context of positive tests for other autoantibodies, such as anti-dsDNA and anti–SS-A/Ro antibodies or anti–Scl-70 antibodies, is inconsistent with MCTD, and other diagnoses must be considered.

Anti–SS-A/Ro is an important marker autoantibody found in patients with SLE or Sjögren's syndrome.[15–17] Its importance is its strong association with childhood and neonatal SLE and with congenital heart block in neonates born to mothers with SLE. In patients with Sjögren's syndrome, anti–SS-A/Ro is associated with features of extraglandular inflammation, including vasculitis, purpura, cytopenias, and adenopathy.[18] Testing for anti–SS-A/Ro is performed by double immunodiffusion or enzyme immunoassay. The 2 methods are comparable, although enzyme immunoassay has greater analytic sensitivity. As with other tests for autoantibodies performed by this method, care must be taken to avoid false-positive results associated with increased nonspecific binding to antigen-coated immunosorbents. Anti–SS-B/La also is found in the sera of patients with SLE or Sjögren's syndrome, although somewhat less frequently than anti–SS-A/Ro. This autoantibody is a helpful marker for SRDs, and the finding of anti–SS-B/La or anti–SS-A/Ro in a patient with some clinical findings compatible with SLE or Sjögren's syndrome, such as Raynaud's phenomenon, may antedate full clinical expression of these diseases.[19]

A number of other autoantibodies are useful as disease-specific markers for the SRDs scleroderma and polymyositis/dermatomyositis. The ANA test performed on the HEp-2 substrate is positive in nearly all patients with scleroderma; predominant patterns are speckled, the fine speckled or anticentromere pattern, and the nucleolar pattern.[1] Autoantibodies to the saline ENA type I topoisomerase, a 70-kd protein also called Scl 70, are specific for scleroderma.[20] The DNA topoisomerase group comprises a ubiquitous class of enzymes that change the binding of closed-circular DNA molecules by catalyzing transient breaks in the phosphatide backbones of DNA. Topoisomerase I antigen is extractable from chicken erythrocytes, calf thymus, and rat liver and has been produced by recombinant DNA technology. Autoantibodies to topoisomerase I in serum are detectable in 20% to 60% of patients with scleroderma, depending on the technique. Lower frequencies are obtained with the double immunodiffusion method performed using crude antigen extracts, and somewhat higher frequencies are obtained with immunometric methods, such as enzyme immunoassay. Anti–topoisomerase I autoantibodies are usually found in patients with extensive cutaneous involvement and interstitial pulmonary fibrosis.[20]

Anticentromere autoantibodies are a marker for a less aggressive form of scleroderma called the CREST variant. The CREST variant is characterized by reduced incidences of diffuse cutaneous and renal involvement and increased incidences of calcinosis and telangiectasia.[21] Anticentromere autoantibodies produce a characteristic fine speckled pattern on

HEp-2 substrate cells in the ANA test (see Figure 11-1C). Many patients with scleroderma also have autoantibodies that react with nucleoli in the ANA test. These autoantibodies react with 4 to 6S RNA and also are found in some patients with SLE, Sjögren's syndrome, or Raynaud's phenomenon. More rarely, in patients with scleroderma, nucleolar staining may indicate autoantibodies to RNA polymerase I, II, and III. These patients are reported to have an increased likelihood of diffuse cutaneous and cardiac involvement.[22]

Detection of disease-specific autoantibodies is useful in the diagnosis and classification of inflammatory myopathies, including polymyositis and dermatomyositis. Autoantibodies to nuclear or cytoplasmic antigens occur in 80% to 90% of such patients; more than 50% have a positive ANA, and approximately 30% have a myositis-specific autoantibody.[23,24] Diffuse homogeneous staining of the cytoplasm of HEp-2 cells in the ANA test suggests the presence of a myositis-specific autoantibody, such as antisynthetase or antibodies to signal recognition particles (SRPs).[25] Antisynthetase antibodies react with aminoacyl–transfer RNA synthetase enzymes. These enzymes catalyze the attachment of amino acids to specific tRNA molecules and include histidyl-, threonyl-, alanyl-, isoleucyl-, and glycyl-tRNA synthetase. The most frequent marker autoantibody in patients with polymyositis is anti–histidyl-tRNA synthetase (also called anti–Jo-1). This autoantibody is detected by double immunodiffusion or enzyme immunoassay and occurs in a subgroup (approximately 20%) of patients with polymyositis who have an increased incidence of interstitial pulmonary fibrosis and symmetrical polyarthritis.[24] Anti-SRP autoantibodies react with proteins of the signal recognition complex, a cytoplasmic complex that mediates translocation of polypeptides across the endoplasmic reticulum, and occur in a small subset of myositis patients with acute onset disease often complicated by cardiac involvement.[25]

Analytic Methods of Testing for Autoantibodies: Double Immunodiffusion, Indirect Immunofluorescence, and Immunometric Assays

A universal feature of immunoassay methods for detecting autoantibodies is the use of antigens as reagents in the analytic systems. The nature of the reagent antigen defines the specificity of the antibodies that are detected and measured.[26,27] Reagent antigens may be crude preparations that contain the antigens of clinical interest or highly purified or recombinant molecules. The clinical applications of tests for autoantibodies often are directly related to the nature of the reagent antigens. Tests that employ crude or complex antigen preparations, such as whole cells or tissue substrates, are useful primarily as screening tests, whereas tests that employ highly purified or recombinant antigens, such as tests for antibodies to the ENAs, may detect antibodies that are disease-specific markers.[1]

The nature of the reagent antigen also influences the precision and accuracy of tests used to quantitate the level or concentration of specific autoantibodies. Quantitation performed using crude antigen as a reagent tends to be semiquantitative and imprecise with the result expressed as a titer, or the reciprocal of the dilution of the test specimen used in the assay. Highly purified antigens may be used to prepare a pure preparation of specific antibodies by affinity chromatography, which enables calibration of the test system either in mass units (eg, mg of antibody protein/mL) or in arbitrary quantitative units.[28]

Double Immunodiffusion

A modification of the classic immunoprecipitation technique that has already been mentioned, double immunodiffusion, is most commonly used to detect autoantibodies.[29] In this method, an aqueous solution of reagent antigen is placed in the center well of an agar slide, and positive control sera and specimens to be tested for the presence of specific antibodies are pipetted into surrounding wells. After incubating for 24 to 48 hours to permit diffusion of the antigen and antibodies throughout the gel, precipitin lines form, which are detected visually. Specific antibodies in the test specimens are identified by lines of identity formed with control sera known to contain antibodies of the same specificity. An example of a double immunodiffusion gel for autoantibodies to the extractable nuclear antigens U_1RNP and Sm is shown in Figure 11-2.

The double immunodiffusion method is simple to perform and requires no special equipment; however, the technique is qualitative and is insensitive to concentrations of antibodies less than 0.1 to 1.0 mg/mL. The relative lack of sensitivity of this method limits its application in the clinical laboratory to situations in which patient sera contain relatively high concentrations of specific autoantibodies.[30] Results of double immunodiffusion tests also are subject to errors in interpretation. False-negative results may occur if the concentration of antigen is not carefully adjusted to produce a zone of equivalence with the concentration of antibodies usually encountered in patient specimens. In addition, multiple precipitin lines of unknown specificity may be seen with clinical specimens, and these precipitins may obscure identification of specific antibodies of clinical interest.

Indirect Immunofluorescence

Indirect immunofluorescence is the technique most commonly used in clinical laboratories to screen for specific antibodies that react with cellular antigens. It is more sensitive than double immunodiffusion and faster to perform. The increased sensitivity of indirect immunofluorescence enables detection of human autoantibodies at concentrations of less than 0.1 mg/mL.[31,32] The technique is semiquantitative, with results expressed in titers, and is readily adaptable to detection and measurement of many clinically important specific antibodies.[1]

Indirect immunofluorescence tests are performed by incubating diluted patient sera with thin sections of animal or human tissues or cultured cells that have been fixed chemically to allow penetration of specific antibodies. After incubation with patient sera, unbound antibodies and serum proteins are washed off the slide and a second-stage antibody (eg, fluorochrome-conjugated antihuman immunoglobulin) is pipetted onto the substrate tissue. This reagent antibody binds to any specific antibodies that have been captured by antigens in the substrate. Bound antihuman immunoglobulin antibody is visualized by using a fluorescent microscope. Incident light at a wavelength optimal to excite the fluorochrome is directed at the substrate slide, and light emitted by the fluorochrome is isolated by appropriate filters and transmitted to the microscope objective, where it can be visualized by a technologist. The presence of specific antibodies is indicated by fluorescence of the tissue or cells on the substrate slide. The sequential steps of an indirect immunofluorescence test for specific antibodies are shown in **Figure 11-3**.

Accurate performance of indirect immunofluorescence for autoantibodies requires careful attention to quality control of the test specimen, substrate slides, and fluorochrome-conjugated antihuman immunoglobulin antiserum.[33] Sera from fasting patients are optimal for testing; hyperlipidemic or hemolyzed sera may produce increased background

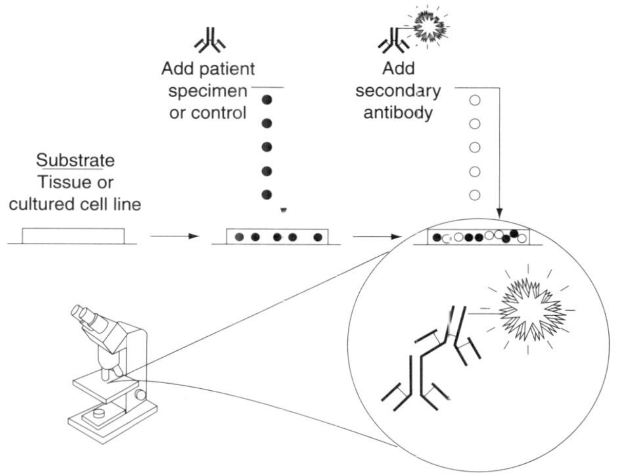

Figure 11-3. Steps in the indirect immunofluorescence technique.

fluorescence. In addition, each batch of tests on patient sera must include known negative and positive control sera. Long-term quality control requires comparison testing of successive lots of substrate slides with known negative and positive control sera to ensure that there is minimal nonspecific binding of human immunoglobulins in the negative sera and comparable binding of specific antibodies as defined by similar end point titers (plus or minus one dilution) for the positive control sera. Successive lots of antihuman immunoglobulin antisera also are compared to ensure reproducibility of the analytic system. These reagents are characterized in terms of their antibody-to-total protein content, fluorochrome-protein ratio (typically in the range of 3:1) and the dilution of reagent antiserum that yields maximum specific-nonspecific fluorescence as demonstrated using well-characterized positive and negative control sera.[34,35] In most indirect immunofluorescence assays, it also is desirable to test a weakly reactive (positive) control serum periodically to ensure that there has been no loss of analytic sensitivity due to storage of the substrate slides or fluorochrome-conjugated antiserum.

Immunoassays

Immunoassay methods are widely used and versatile for detecting and measuring autoantibodies. These methods, also called sandwich immunoassays, make use of a solid phase conjugate of reagent antigen (the immunosorbent) to capture specific antibodies from patient specimens. Specific antibodies bound to the immunosorbent in the first stage of the assay are detected in the second stage by incubation with a polyclonal or monoclonal antihuman immunoglobulin antibody that has been labeled with an enzyme, radionuclide, or luminescent molecule.[36] In the final stage, the amount of labeled second-stage antibody that has bound to the immunosorbent is determined by measuring a colored or fluorescent product generated by the enzyme label or by counting radioactivity. The enzyme immunoassay, a popular version of the basic immunoassay technique for measurement of specific antibodies, is shown in **Figure 11-4**.

Antigen immunosorbents can be prepared from crude antigen mixtures for use in screening tests like the antinuclear antibody test or from highly purified antigens for use in the measurement of marker autoantibodies. Immunoassays are very sensitive compared with the precipitin technique. Analytic sensitivity is in the range of 1 to 10 ng of antibody protein/mL. The increased sensitivity is largely a result of amplification of the signal produced by the binding of labeled, second-stage anti-immunoglobulin antibody. As noted earlier, the second-stage antibody typically is labeled with an enzyme or radionuclide. Commonly used enzyme labels, such as alkaline phosphatase, generate many moles of measurable product for each mole of second-stage antibody bound to the immunosorbent, and radionuclides emit measurable radiation that can be counted to a predetermined end point of total counts. The analytic sensitivity of immunoassays is primarily limited by the ratio of specific-to-nonspecific binding of immuno-globulin in the first stage of the assay.[36,37] Immunosorbents with low levels of nonspecific binding afford maximum sensitivity.

The most common immunoassay for specific antibodies is the enzyme immunoassay. In this technique, an antigen is adsorbed noncovalently to the wells of a microtiter plate. Enzyme immunoassay may be used to detect specific antibodies qualitatively or to make semiquantitative measurements of specific autoantibodies by use of a standard curve calibrated in units. For qualitative applications, the absorbance in wells incubated with diluted patient serum is compared with a negative (nonimmune) control serum pool. Positive results are indicated by absorbencies significantly greater than that of the negative control pool, typically at least twice the negative control (background) level. For more quantitative applications, the absorbance in wells that contain diluted patient serum is compared with a standard curve. In either application, positive and negative control sera must be run with each plate to ensure that all steps in the procedure have been performed properly.

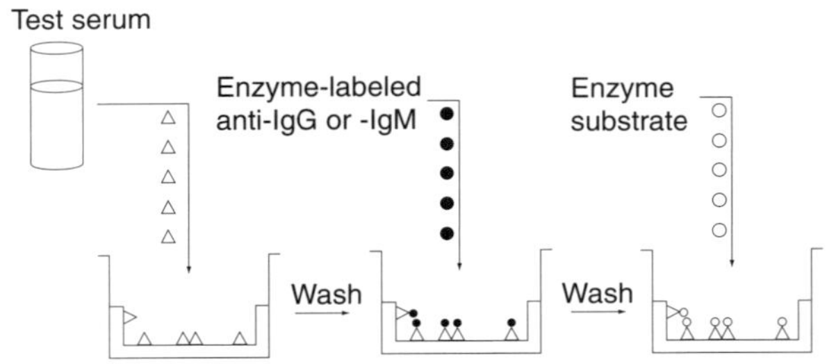

Figure 11-4. Steps in the enzyme immunoassay technique.

The accuracy and precision of semiquantitative tests performed by enzyme immunoassay also have limitations. The methods are inherently variable, and successive tests on the same serum often yield results that vary by as much as 15% to 20%.[36,37] In addition, the standard curve of absorbance versus antibody level is usually nonlinear. Consequently, even though results are often reported on a continuous scale in units, it is best to regard them as semiquantitative. Results are often interpreted as falling within ranges (eg, negative, borderline, weakly positive, and strongly positive) with each category defined by a range of values expressed in units.

A Laboratory Approach to Diagnosis of Systemic Rheumatic Diseases: Consideration of Cascade Testing

Patients with SRDs often present with constitutional signs and symptoms or with inflammatory signs involving virtually any organ system. Because of the diversity of clinical signs that accompany the onset of these diseases, clinicians often attempt to exclude an SRD early in the diagnostic process. In this context, appropriate laboratory testing can have an important role in establishing an accurate diagnosis, whereas inappropriate testing can lead to an overlooked or mistaken diagnosis. The cascade described here is a diagnostic algorithm based on the use of laboratory tests for autoantibodies, which attempts to optimize the detection of disease in previously undiagnosed patients by using the fewest number of tests.

The laboratory assessment of a patient suspected of having an SRD begins with testing for antinuclear antibodies.[38] As already noted, these autoantibodies are regarded as diagnostic markers of SRDs, although the frequency and diagnostic specificity of positive ANA results vary considerably among patients with different diseases.[39] In addition, weakly positive ANA results occur in many healthy people older than 40 years and in patients with nonrheumatic diseases. Consequently, effective use of the ANA test in this diagnostic algorithm is based on established empiric relationships between various test results and their associated predictive values for establishing or excluding the diagnosis of an SRD.

The initial test for ANA is usually performed by indirect immunofluorescence with the use of substrate slides prepared from HEp-2 cells. Different autoantibodies produce characteristic morphologic patterns of fluorescent staining. The patterns suggest the presence of particular ANA specificities, which can be distinguished by appropriate second-order tests for autoantibodies (**Table 11-3**). The approximate concentrations of autoantibodies are determined by the end point titers. Thus, 2 pieces of information derived from the ANA test result—the morphologic pattern and the end point titer—are useful in determining the need for additional tests for disease-specific autoantibodies. In this regard, available data suggest that testing for specific autoantibodies is not useful if the ANA test result is negative or the end point titer is less than 160[40]; such follow-up testing yields positive results in fewer than 5% of cases. With the exception of sera that produce strong cytoplasmic staining of HEp-2 cells, this algorithm calls for no further testing of sera with negative or weakly positive ANA results.

Further testing for disease-specific autoantibodies is indicated if the ANA titer is 160 or more. The choice of appropriate second-order tests for specific autoantibodies is determined by the morphologic patterns of positive ANA results (see Table 11-3). Two frequently observed patterns of positive ANA test results are the so-called homogeneous and peripheral patterns. As noted earlier, these patterns are associated with autoantibodies to dsDNA and nuclear histone proteins. Anti-dsDNA autoantibodies of the IgG class are characteristically found in patients with idiopathic lupus erythematosus and drug-induced lupus erythematosus. Thus, the algorithm includes testing for IgG anti-dsDNA autoantibodies on all sera that produce homogeneous or peripheral staining of HEp-2 cells if the end point ANA titer is 160 or more. It is not necessary to routinely test for antihistone autoantibodies as part of the algorithm, because drug-induced autoantibodies can be suspected clinically from the medical history, and determination of antihistone autoantibodies adds little to the assessment of patients suspected of having idiopathic lupus erythematosus.

The most common pattern of positive ANA results is the coarsely speckled pattern. It often indicates the presence of autoantibodies to one or more ENAs.[41,42] Autoantibodies to ENAs are present in relatively high concentrations in serum, especially in patients with high-titered ANAs of the coarsely speckled pattern. Autoantibodies to U_1RNP and Sm occur in patients with lupus erythematosus, and seropositivity for anti-Sm is considered diagnostic for the disease. Anti-U_1RNP autoantibodies are present with several SRDs, and detection of such autoantibodies helps to distinguish among MCTD, SLE, and Sjögren's syndrome. The presence of anti-U_1RNP in high concentration in the absence of other autoantibodies strongly suggests the diagnosis of MCTD, which clinically may resemble SLE, scleroderma, and polymyositis. The finding of anti-U_1RNP alone is important information for establishing the diagnosis of MCTD and for excluding other SRDs. The finding of anti-U_1RNP autoantibodies coexisting with other autoantibodies is inconsistent with MCTD, and other diagnoses must be considered.

Table 11-3. Morphologic Patterns of Antinuclear Antibodies by Immunofluorescence Testing and Recommended Second-Order Tests for Specific Autoantibodies

Pattern	Second-Order Tests
Homogeneous, peripheral, or speckled	Anti-dsDNA Anti-ENA (U_1RNP, Sm, SS-A/Ro, SS-B/La, and anti-Scl 70)
Nucleolar	Anti–Scl 70 (type I topoisomerase)
Centromere	None
Cytoplasmic	Anti–Jo-1 (histidyl-tRNA synthetase)

Abbreviations: dsDNA = double-stranded DNA; ENA = extractable nuclear antigens; U_1RNP = uridine-rich ribonucleoprotein; tRNA = transfer RNA.

Anti–SS-A/Ro is an important marker autoantibody for SLE or Sjögren's syndrome. Although anti–SS-B/La is not diagnostic for any single SRD, the finding of anti–SS-B/La with or without anti–SS-A/Ro in a patient with clinical findings suggestive of SLE or Sjögren's syndrome helps to establish these diagnoses.

Two additional autoantibodies, anti–Scl 70 and anti–Jo-1, are identifiable in ANA-positive sera and serve as disease-specific markers for scleroderma and polymyositis/dermatomyositis, respectively[24,43] The ANA test performed by indirect immunofluorescence on HEp-2 substrate cells shows positive results in almost all patients with scleroderma; predominant patterns are speckled (coarsely or anticentromere) and nucleolar. Autoantibodies to the ENA Scl 70 (type I topoisomerase) are specific for scleroderma and show a speckled nuclear staining pattern in HEp-2 cells. Another type of speckled ANA pattern, the anticentromere, also is found in the sera of patients with scleroderma. Typically, anticentromere autoantibodies are a marker for a less aggressive type of scleroderma—the CREST variant. This type is characterized by decreased occurrences of diffuse cutaneous and renal involvement and increased occurrences of calcinosis and telangiectasia. No further testing is indicated in patients with a positive ANA and a centromere pattern.

As previously noted, the disease-specific autoantibody anti–Jo-1 (anti–histidyl-tRNA synthetase) is a useful marker of polymyositis. Autoantibodies to nuclear or cytoplasmic antigens are present in 80% to 90% of patients with polymyositis, and more than 50% of patients with myositis have a positive ANA test result. Approximately 30% of such patients have a myositis-specific autoantibody, most commonly anti–Jo-1. Diffuse staining of the cytoplasm of HEp-2 cells in the ANA test suggests the presence of anti–Jo-1, which is associated with an increased incidence of pulmonary fibrosis in patients with polymyositis. Thus, in this algorithm, testing for anti–Jo-1 autoantibodies is performed automatically on sera that produce characteristic cytoplasmic staining of HEp-2 cells.

Although algorithm testing for autoantibodies is useful in the initial laboratory assessment of patients suspected of having an SRD, such diseases are diagnosed primarily on clinical criteria. In some patients with clinically unambiguous features of an SRD and a positive ANA result, a specific marker autoantibody is undetectable. Conversely, patients with nonrheumatic diseases may be seropositive for ANAs, but such patients rarely have positive results for marker autoantibodies on second-order tests. Therefore, the finding of a positive ANA result with negative results for marker autoantibodies is inconclusive, and an SRD must be diagnosed on the basis of other criteria.

Algorithm testing is not recommended in patients with an established diagnosis of an SRD. Although testing for certain autoantibodies, including ANAs and anti-dsDNA, is occasionally useful for monitoring the clinical course of such patients, these tests should be performed individually rather than in sequence. The decision to repeat tests for autoantibodies depends on the clinical course of the disease. A stable clinical course usually obviates the need for retesting, whereas clinical exacerbation or new manifestations of disease may prompt the search for additional autoantibodies.

As stated previously, the ANA test serves as a screen to detect many different specific antibodies. Clinical laboratories often report only the dominant pattern observed by indirect immunofluorescence at the end point dilution and may not report other patterns observed at lesser dilutions. For this reason, and because patients may develop additional autoantibodies during the course of disease, it may be useful to repeat the ANA test periodically to ensure that all important disease-specific autoantibodies are detected. Several of the autoantibodies found by the ANA test and by follow-up testing are useful in identifying subsets of patients with SRDs that are heterogeneous in their clinical course. In this sense, individual disease-specific autoantibodies also are useful as prognostic indicators.

In patients with SLE, it is common to repeat the test for anti-dsDNA antibodies at periodic intervals or when there is an apparent exacerbation of disease. Anti-dsDNA antibodies participate in the formation of immune complexes that promote vasculitis and glomerular injury in SLE, and increased concentrations of anti-dsDNA antibodies in serum often precede clinical exacerbations. Immunoassays for anti-dsDNA antibodies are capable of detecting changes in the serum concentrations of these autoantibodies that accompany disease exacerbations; however, the assays are semiquantitative and results on control sera may vary by as much as 20% or more from day to day. Small changes in the concentrations of antibodies (ie, changes of less than 20% of the test result in U/mL) are often the result of analytic variability and do not indicate real changes. In patients with other SRDs, it is rarely necessary to repeat tests for marker autoantibodies unless there is a marked change in the clinical course of disease or the ANA test reveals an additional pattern not detected previously.

References

1. Tan EM. Antinuclear antibodies: Diagnostic markers for autoimmune diseases and probes for cell biology. *Adv Immunol*. 1989;44:93–151.

2. Tan EM. Autoantibodies to nuclear antigens (ANA): Their immunobiology and medicine. *Adv Immunol*. 1982;33:167–240.

3. Tan EM. Relationship of nuclear staining patterns with precipitating antibodies in systemic lupus erythematosus. *J Lab Clin Med*. 1967;70:800–812.

4. Harmon C, Deng JS, Peebles CL, et al. The importance of tissue substrate in the SS-A/Ro antigen-antibody system. *Arthritis Rheum*. 1984;27:166–173.

5. Bernstein RM, Steigerwald JC, Tan EM. Association of antinuclear and antinucleolar antibodies in progressive systemic sclerosis. *Clin Exp Immunol*. 1982;48:43–51.

6. Miyachi K, Fritzler MJ, Tan EM. Autoantibody to a nuclear antigen in proliferating cells. *J Immunol*. 1978;121:2228–2234.

7. Anhalt JP, Kenny GE, Rytel NW. Detection of microbial antigens by counter-immunoelectrophoresis. In: Gavan TL, ed. *Cumulative Techniques and Procedures in Clinical Microbiology, No.8*. Washington, DC: American Society for Microbiology; 1978:3–8.

8. Cleymaet JE, Nakamura RM. Indirect immunofluorescent antinuclear antibody tests: Comparison of sensitivity and specificity of different substrates. *Am J Clin Pathol*. 1972;58:388–393.

9. Brinkman K, Termaat R, Van den Brink H, et al. The specificity of the anti-dsDNA ELISA: A closer look. *J Immunol Methods*. 1991;139:91–100.

10. Pettersson I, Hinterberger M, Mimori T, et al. The structure of mammalian small nuclear ribonucleoproteins. *J Biol Chem*. 1984;259:5907–5914.

11. Conner GE, Nelson D, Wisniewolski R, et al. Protein antigens of the RNA-protein complexes detected by anti-Sm and anti-RNP antibodies found in serum of patients with systemic lupus erythematosus and related disorders. *J Exp Med*. 1982;156:1475–1485.

12. Wooley JC, Zukerberg LR, Chung SY. Polypeptide components of human small nuclear ribonucleoproteins. *Proc Natl Acad Sci U S A*. 1983;80:5208–5212.

13. Froelich CJ, Wallman J, Skosey JL, et al. Clinical value of an integrated ELISA system for the detection of 6 autoantibodies (ssDNA, dsDNA, SM, RNP/Sm, SSA, and SSB). *J Rheumatol*. 1990;17:192–200.

14. Sharp GC, Irvin WS, Tan EM, et al. Mixed connective tissue disease: an apparently distinct rheumatic disease syndrome associated with a specific antibody to an extractable nuclear antigen (ENA). *Am J Med*. 1972;52:148–159.

15. Clark G, Reichlin M. Tomasi T. Characterization of a soluble cytoplasmic antigen reactive with sera from patients with systemic lupus erythematosus. *J Immunol*. 1969;102:117–122.

16. Mattioli M, Reichlin M. Heterogeneity of RNA protein antigens reactive with sera of patients with systemic lupus erythematosus. *Arthritis Rheum*. 1974;17:421–429.

17. Alspaugh M, Tan EM. Antibodies to cellular antigens in Sjögren's syndrome. *J Clin Invest*. 1975;55:1067–1073.

18. Alexander EL, Arnett FC, Provost TT, et al. Sjögren's syndrome: Association of anti-Ro (SS-A) antibodies with vasculitis, hematologic abnormalities, and serologic hyperactivity. *Ann Intern Med*. 1983;98:155–159.

19. Reichlin M, Friday K, Harley JB. Complete congenital heart block followed by anti-Ro/SSA in adult life: Studies of an informative family. *Am J Med*. 1988;84:339–344.

20. Shero JH, Bordwell B, Rothfield NF, et al. High titers of autoantibodies of topoisomerase I (Scl-70) in sera from scleroderma patients. *Science*. 1986;231:737–740.

21. Earnshaw WC, Machlin PS, Bordwell BJ, et al. Analysis of anticentromere autoantibodies using cloned autoantigen CENP-B. *Proc Natl Acad Sci U S A*. 1987;84:4979–4983.

22. Kuwana M, Kaburaki J, Mimori T, et al. Autoantibody reactive with three classes of RNA polymerases in sera from patients with systemic sclerosis. *J Clin Invest*. 1993;91:1399–1404.

23. Plotz PH, Dalakas M, Leff RL, et al. Current concepts in the idiopathic inflammatory myopathies: Polymyositis, dermatomyositis, and related disorders. *Ann Intern Med*. 1989;111:143–157.

24. Arnett FC, Hirsch TJ, Bias WB, et al. The Jo-1 antibody system in myositis: Relationships to clinical features and HLA. *J Rheumatol*. 1981;8:925–930.

25. Targoff IN, Johnson AE, Miller FW. Antibody to signal recognition particle in polymyositis. *Arthritis Rheum*. 1990;33:1361–1370.

26. Benjamin DC, Berzofsky JA, East IJ, et al. The antigenic structure of proteins: A reprisal. *Annu Rev Immunol*. 1984;2:67–101.

27. Sela M. Antigenicity: Some molecular aspects. *Science*. 1969;166:1365–1374.

28. Tijssen P. *Practice and Theory of Enzyme Immunoassays*. Amsterdam, the Netherlands: Elsevier Science Pub. Co.; 1985.

29. Ouchterlony O, Nilsson LA. Immunodiffusion and immunoelectrophoresis. In: Wier DM, ed. *Handbook of Experimental Immunology*. Oxford, England: Blackwell; 1986:1.

30. Wilson MR, Sanders RD. Immunodiffusion assays for antibodies to small nuclear ribonucleoproteins and other cellular antigens. In: Rose NR, deMacario EC, Fahey JC, et al, eds. *Manual of Clinical Laboratory Immunology.* 4th ed. Washington DC: American Society for Microbiology; 1992:741–746.

31. Nakamura RM, Tan EM. Recent advances in laboratory tests and the significance of autoantibodies to nuclear antigens in systemic-rheumatic diseases. *Clin Lab Med.* 1986;6:41–53.

32. Molden DP, Nakamura RM, Tan EM. Standardization of the immunofluorescence test for autoantibody to nuclear antigens (ANA): Use of sera of defined antibody specificity. *Am J Clin Pathol.* 1984;82:57–66.

33. Nakamura RM, Rippey JH. Quality assurance and proficiency testing for autoantibodies to nuclear antigen. *Arch Pathol Lab Med.* 1984;109:109.

34. Tan EM, Fritzler MJ, McDougal JS, et al. Reference sera for antinuclear antibodies: Antibodies to native DNA, Sm, nuclear RNP, and SS-B/La. *Arthritis Rheum.* 1982;25:1003–1005.

35. McDougal JS, Kennedy S, McDuffie FC. Standards and quality assurance for immunologic tests. In: Rippey JH, Nakamura RM, eds. *Diagnosis Immunology: Technology Assessment and Quality Assurance.* Skokie, IL: College of American Pathologists; 1983:147–155.

36. Carter JH. Enzyme immunoassays: Practical aspects of their methodology. *J Clin Immunoassay.* 1984;7:64–72.

37. Gosling JP. A decade of development of immunoassay methodology. *Clin Chem.* 1990;36:1408–1427.

38. Tan EM. Antinuclear antibodies: Diagnostic markers for autoimmune diseases and probes for cell biology. *Adv Immunol.* 1989;44:93–151.

39. Condemi JJ. The autoimmune diseases. *JAMA.* 1992;268:2882–2892.

40. Jacob GL, Homburger HA. Autoantibodies to extractable nuclear antigens: Frequency of occurrence in ANA-positive and ANA-negative sera. Presented at the 6th Annual AMLI Meeting; July 28–August 1, 1993; San Diego, CA. [Abstract]

41. Conner GE, Nelson D, Wisniewolski R, et al. Protein antigens of the RNA-protein complexes detected by anti-Sm and anti-RNP antibodies found in serum of patients with systemic lupus erythematosus and related disorders. *J Exp Med.* 1982;156:1475–1485.

42. Alexander EL, Arnett FC, Provost TT, et al. Sjögren's syndrome: Association of anti-Ro (SS-A) antibodies with vasculitis, hematologic abnormalities, and serologic hyperreactivity. *Ann Intern Med.* 1983;98:155–159.

43. Shero JH, Bordwell B, Rothfield NF, et al. High titers of autoantibodies to topoisomerase I (Scl-70) in sera from scleroderma patients. *Science.* 1986;231:737–740.

CHAPTER 12

Laboratory Testing in Women With Silicone Breast Implants

David F. Keren, MD, and Henry N. Claman, MD

In the past few years, the use of an important medical product, polydimethylsiloxane (silicone), was curtailed owing to concerns about its safety, and many patients with silicone prostheses, predominantly women with silicone breast implants, are worried about their personal safety. This chapter reviews the use of silicone and the controversy over its safety and provides recommendations for laboratory testing in affected patients.

Use of Silicone

Silicone has been used for medical applications since 1962, first as tubing for shunts in hydrocephalic patients and in myringotomy, and more recently as devices for joint, penile, testicular, and breast prostheses.[1] Its use was "grandfathered in," because regulations for premarket approval of such medical devices were not established until well over a decade after its introduction. Everyone is exposed to silicone in a variety of substances, including cosmetics, hand lotions, hair sprays, caulking materials, processed foods, antacids, needle coatings, syringe lubricants, and many medical devices.[2] Patients with type 1 diabetes may inject up to 50 g of silicone along with their insulin over their lifetimes.[3]

There is no one standard form of breast implant; therefore, the type of implant being reported about in any particular paper is often unclear. Early on (in the 1950s and 1960s), primarily in Japan, substances such as paraffin and liquid silicone were injected directly into breast tissue. Later, silicone hardened by fumed silica was used to encase the silicone gel. The resulting implants could consist of as much as 35% silica in the implant envelope.[4] Before 1991, polyurethane was used to coat some implants to decrease the likelihood of capsular contraction. However, due to concern about the long-term effects of polyurethanes (which break down to release 2,4-toluene diamine—a carcinogen in experimental animals), it has not been used in this capacity since then.[2] Currently, 3 main types of implants are used: silicone gel-filled, saline-filled, and double-lumen implants (which contain saline in one lumen and silicone in the other). All are lined with hardened silicone.

Although silicone is a very stable polymer, it is far from inert. The body develops an inflammatory reaction to it, as it does with almost any foreign solid substance. The degree of the inflammation varies from individual to individual and from one silicone preparation to another. The term *inflammation* is sometimes confused with the term *immunologic reaction*. When reading articles about this subject, it is necessary to determine whether the authors distinguish the nonspecific process of inflammation from the specific process of recognition inherent in immunologic reactions.

All implant capsules leak, and the phenomenon of progressive oozing of the silicone gel through the capsule has been well-documented in vitro and in vivo.[5–8] Yu et al[6] estimated that about 1 mg of silicone per day may be released into body fluid at 37°C. As silicone is released, it is taken up by macrophages and dispersed into progressively smaller droplets that, by virtue of increased surface area compared to larger droplets, are more readily hydrolyzed and oxidized into a variety of siloxane oligomers.[9] This hydrolysis continues in the tissue for years.[5] In addition to hydrolysis, oxidation of silicone results from removal of a methyl group from a silicone side chain.[5] This may cause formation of a silicone gel, which replaces the silicone liquid. The silicone content of the leakage may be demonstrated by nuclear magnetic resonance spectroscopy.[10]

Approximately 60% to 80% of breast implants have been used for augmentation; the remainder have been used for reconstruction after surgery (for breast cancer, congenital defects, or trauma).[2] There is no record of the precise number of women in the US who have silicone implants; some estimates suggest 1 to 2 million women, whereas others place the total slightly below 1 million. In 1995, Cook et al[11] published the results of a 1989 mail survey of 40,000 households chosen as being representative of the US population at that time. They found a breast implant prevalence of 8.08 per 1,000 women and found that the procedure was most common in white women of higher socioeconomic classes. They also noted that approximately 60% of the implants were placed for cosmetic reasons.

Federal Regulations and Silicone Implants

Because the use of silicone implants antedated the Medical Device Amendments written into law by Congress in 1976, they were exempt from the rigorous pre–market approval process that new devices must now undergo.[12] In July 1991, many anecdotal reports of breast implants being associated with connective tissue diseases, especially scleroderma, reached the attention of the lay press. Because there were no controlled or epidemiologic studies available, this information was given to the public in an uncritical manner. This resulted in a general panic that caused the Food and Drug Administration (FDA) to demand that companies manufacturing implants submit pre–market approval applications.[12] In the meantime, David Kessler (former FDA commissioner) proposed a moratorium on the use of silicone gel breast implants until they could be shown to be safe. This moratorium was widely misinterpreted to indicate that they were not safe, despite Kessler's care in noting that it is the responsibility of the manufacturer to prove the devices are safe, not the responsibility of the FDA to prove that they are not.

Capsule Formation

A capsule forms around all implants as a result of the foreign body inflammatory reaction to the continuous leakage of silicone gel through the silicone rubber envelope. Although the envelope around the implant seems to be relatively inert, it only appears so because it is in equilibrium with the silicone gel it contains. Some of the gel is absorbed into the envelope, causing swelling of the envelope and, possibly, breaks in the noncovalent bonds of the polymer.[13] As a result, some silicone gel leaks into the surrounding tissue, where it may be hydrolyzed. The silicone is also phagocytosed by macrophages, by which it may be further hydrolyzed and oxidized. The capsule that forms around implants consists largely of fibrous connective tissue, macrophages, a few lymphocytes, and plasma cells.[13] Approximately 25% of women develop a noticeable contracture as this fibrous capsule constricts with time. The amount of contracture can be estimated using the Baker scale.

The lymphocytes within the capsule are sparse and have proved difficult to isolate and characterize. Because of this, most researchers have looked at the peripheral blood as an easy-to-obtain sample of breast-implant patient lymphocytes. One immunologic study[14] used 9 monoclonal antibody markers and found a modest increase in the number of CD57+ cells in the peripheral blood. Furthermore, a greater frequency of in-vitro response (composed mainly of natural killer cells) to a silicone extract was found in patients with higher levels of contracture than in those with a lower level of contracture. However, the standard deviations in this study were very high (50% of the signal—ie, for the "severe" group, they counted 307 ± 150, or one standard deviation). Although this evaluation is of interest for epidemiologic and experimental studies, such large standard deviations preclude any practical use of this information in individual patients. Furthermore, it is of interest that no difference was found in the number of CD19, CD3, CD4, CD8, CD25, CD16, CD3+DR+, CD4+DR+, or CD8+DR+ cells in higher-contracture patients compared with minimal-contracture patients and controls. These data argue strongly against using flow cytometry studies on peripheral blood lymphocytes for routine assessment of these patients. Immunohistologic evaluation of the capsule has failed to disclose antibody deposition or complement activation in this tissue, arguing against the presence of a type I or type II immunopathologic event as its etiology.[15]

A minority (about 5%) of women are "significantly bothered" by the contracture.[12] In some cases, the capsule has epithelialized, and one case of squamous cell carcinoma has been identified in a capsule.[16] As already mentioned, prior to 1991, polyurethane coating was used in some implants to decrease the contracture effect. It is no longer used because experimental studies have shown that 2,4-toluene diamine (a breakdown product of polyurethane) can cause hepatocellular carcinoma in rats. Some researchers[13] noted that fewer plasma cells and lymphocytes were present in the fibrous connective tissue and inflammatory cells around implants coated with polyurethane, although this observation was not quantified. Other researchers[17] saw increased numbers of cells with expression of HLA-DR in lymphocytes associated with the capsule, compared with lymphocytes from peripheral blood. Although this implies immune activation, no controls with lymphocytes from other periprosthetic capsules were performed. Although of interest for experimental work, there is no indication for performing such studies on explanted material. Indeed, the authors reported great difficulty in collecting sufficient numbers of lymphocytes for their studies.

Implant Rupture With Leakage and Migration of Silicone

Methods have been devised to quantify the amount of "bleeding" of the silicone gel from both new and explanted implants.[5] The surface of silicone implants is permeable to small amounts of silicone. In addition, implants may rupture from trauma (automobile accidents) or spontaneously. When this occurs, the gel may spread outside the capsule. The likelihood of rupture increases the longer implants are in place[18]; that is, implants seem to age badly. Even if the implant has not ruptured, the silicone usually finds its way beyond the confines of the implant surface. Typically, foreign body granulomas surround most of these particles.[19] Some of them, however, make their way to distant sites, such as lymph nodes. Electron probe microanalysis has identified elemental silicon in the synovia, skin, and alveolar macrophages of some women with implants.[20]

Carcinogenicity

The largest age-matched controlled epidemiologic study on the effect of silicone implants on breast cancer was conducted at the University of California–Los Angeles Medical Center.[21] In 3,112 women with silicone implants who were followed for an average of 11 years, researchers found a slightly lower rate of breast cancer in women with implants compared with women without implants. A similar study by Petit et al[22] in France found no increased incidence of a second primary breast cancer or death in patients who received gel-filled silicone implants after mastectomy for a primary breast cancer, and Bryant and Brasher[23] found no increase or decrease of breast cancer among breast implant patients. There have been anecdotal reports of carcinoma and lymphoproliferative disease in implant patients, but these reports should be viewed in the context of the overall occurrence of neoplasms in the general population.[24] As far as the polyurethane issue is concerned, the FDA has estimated that the lifetime risk of developing hepatocellular carcinoma for a woman with a polyurethane-coated implant is less than 1 in 1 million and therefore has not recommended the removal of existing implants.

Experimental studies have shed little light on the risk of developing other types of cancers in humans exposed to silicone breast implants. Rodents are known to develop a variety of neoplasms under a variety of circumstances. Approximately 25% of rats exposed to silicone rubber develop malignant fibrous histiocytomas.[25] Genetically susceptible mice may also develop plasma cell tumors after being injected with silicone; however, existing data are too weak to document a significant threat to women with implants.[26,27] Larger epidemiologic studies must be performed before a link with human myeloma can be seriously considered.

Information Available to Physicians and the Public

Although this issue has created a public furor and resulted in several large legal settlements for the plaintiffs, there is little objective evidence that silicone breast implants lead to an increased incidence of any definable autoimmune disease. The studies available in this area can be divided into 3 categories:

- Anecdotal reports of a few patients who developed some form of autoimmune disease (A large portion of the published material falls into this category.)
- A few carefully conducted, large, controlled studies
- A few studies involving immunopathogenetic mechanisms associated with silicone implants and disease

The quality of methods used in these animal studies, case reports, and immunologic studies has been characterized as generally inferior.[28]

Another source of information comes from a few commercial laboratories that provide physician practices with one-sided, inflammatory literature coercing the physicians into ordering expensive, unproven, almost certainly useless, and potentially alarming tests on asymptomatic patients with silicone implants.

Autoimmune Disease and Silicone Breast Implants

Definable Connective Tissue Diseases

Autoimmune complaints can be divided into definable connective tissue diseases, such as scleroderma, rheumatoid arthritis, and systemic lupus erythematosus (SLE), and vague complaints that may be consistent with fibromyalgia or other nonspecific conditions.

One startling feature of some early, uncontrolled, anecdotal reports was the seemingly high rate of scleroderma (a relatively uncommon connective tissue disease). Spiera and Kerr[29] reported 11 cases of individuals who received silicone implants and who also developed scleroderma. Interestingly, 2 of the patients had had chin implants rather than breast implants. Furthermore, one had a medical history of Raynaud's phenomenon that predated the insertion of the implant. Of 5 patients who had the implants removed, 2 improved clinically, but 3 died of complications of scleroderma. The authors did not report precisely how the patients were selected for the study, but they compared them with the number of nonimplant patients with scleroderma seen in their clinic (both authors are from rheumatology departments and would be expected to have patients with diseases such as scleroderma). They saw 11 patients with silicone implants with scleroderma in this period, the first 5 of whom presented to them "randomly," for an incidence of 4% among this nonrandom population. The other 6 patients were influenced by the authors' publicized interest in rheumatic disease among silicone implant patients.

Large, controlled epidemiologic studies in the years following these early papers have not found a significant association between the presence of silicone breast implants and the development of scleroderma. Looking at the number of patients with scleroderma who had implants, Hochberg et al[30] found that 1% of the 210 scleroderma patients they followed for a mean of 11 years had implants. Sanchez-Guerrero et al[2] noted that when the Hochberg et al data are combined with a larger series of 741 women they followed with scleroderma, the percentage of female scleroderma patients who had breast implants (0.66%) was similar to the percentage of women in the general population estimated to have silicone breast implants.[31] Englert et al[32] found no association between this disease and silicone gel implants. They noted an adjusted odds ratio of 1.00, with a 95% confidence interval of 0.16 to 6.16. Although Spiera et al[33] complained that the epidemiologic studies had not followed patients for a long enough period of time, they noted that "there is as yet inadequate epidemiologic data to definitively establish causality." To date, no large, controlled epidemiologic studies have determined any clear-cut relationship between other defined connective tissue diseases and silicone breast implants. They found no association between the development of SLE and silicone breast implants. A recent meta-analysis of nine cohort studies, nine case-control studies, and two cross-sectional studies concluded that there was no evidence of an association between the implants and any of the individual connective tissue diseases, or even of other autoimmune or rheumatic conditions.[34]

Sanchez-Guerrero et al[2] summarized anecdotal reports of 292 patients through June 1993 who developed rheumatic symptoms after receiving silicone gel–filled breast implants (**Table 12-1**). The summary clearly documents that scleroderma was the most commonly reported of the defined autoimmune diseases. In the general population, rheumatoid arthritis and SLE are much more common than scleroderma. If

Table 12-1. Reported Cases of Connective Tissue Disease 1964–1993[2]

Condition	Diagnosis (Number of Patients)
Definite autoimmune disease	Scleroderma (38)
	Rheumatoid arthritis (5)
	SLE (5)
	MCTD (2)
	PM/DM (3)
	Raynaud's phenomenon (2)
	Phospholipid syndrome (1)
Possible autoimmune disease	Sjögren's syndrome (4)
	Rheumatoid arthritis (4)
	SLE (3)
	DM (2)
	Still's disease (1)
	Osteoarthritis (1)
Other diagnosis	Connective tissue–like disease* (56)
	Human adjuvant disease (1)
	Rheumatic symptoms (164)

Abbreviations: SLE = systemic lupus erythematosus; MCTD = mixed connective tissue disease; PM = polymyositis; DM = dermatomyositis.
**Connective tissue–like disease includes patients not meeting enough classification criteria for a specific connective tissue disease.*

the anecdotal reports represented the general population of patients with silicone implants, the results may suggest that a subset of women who receive these implants may have an unusual reaction (possibly related to genetic factors that are somehow accelerated by the implants) that results in the development of a rare clinical condition. This impression, however, has not been confirmed by larger, controlled epidemiologic studies (as will be discussed below). The largest number of the reported Sanchez-Guerrero cases did not fit into any specific category due to the vagueness of the complaints. Therefore, 221 patients were classified as "other diagnosis." Of course, some of these patients would have developed symptoms without implants, and some of them (including one of the more famous legal cases—*Hopkins v Dow Corning* [1991]) had had their symptoms for years before the implants were inserted.[1] Nonetheless, the unusual distribution of connective tissue disease suggests that more than chance is involved.

One early large cohort study[35] followed for 11 years 378 patients who had silicone breast prostheses implanted. Only 125 patients stayed with the study until its end, but none developed a defined connective tissue disease during the period of observation. Unfortunately, these data are weakened by the large number of patients who were not followed.

A large, carefully controlled epidemiologic study by Gabriel et al[36] followed 749 women with breast implants for a mean of 7.8 years and compared them with 1,498 community controls. The researchers found connective tissue disease in 5 case subjects and in 10 control subjects. Twenty-five of the case subjects had signs of arthritis, compared with 39 of the control subjects. The researchers concluded that there was no association between breast implants and defined connective tissue diseases. The study also looked at symptoms of less definable disease and again found no direct association with silicone breast implants. However, the authors noted that even larger and longer studies are needed to rule out a more subtle effect.

Another large study[37] used a questionnaire method to follow up on 287 women with silicone breast implants; 235 of the case subjects and 210 control subjects returned the questionnaires. Although there were more rheumatic complaints after silicone implantation than in controls, there was no evidence for an increased prevalence of definable rheumatic diseases. Another questionnaire-based study was reported by Englert and Brooks,[38] who interviewed patients with scleroderma and control subjects to determine the exposure to silicone. They found that there were comparable rates of silicone implants in the 2 populations, but failed to demonstrate an association between silicone breast implants and scleroderma.

In 1995, Sanchez-Guerrero et al[39] published a comprehensive cohort study that provided highly reliable data refuting the claimed association between silicone breast implants and either defined connective tissue diseases or an increased incidence of signs and symptoms of such diseases. The authors used data from the Nurses' Health cohort study begun in 1976. Every 2 years since the study's inception, questionnaires were sent to a selected cohort of nurses. Out of 109,750 women participating, 89,376 returned their survey in 1992. The information was gathered at the time of massive media attention in 1991 that made it difficult to obtain objective information. Among the women, 1,183 had had silicone breast implants for an average of 9.9 ± 6.4 (standard deviation) years of follow-up. Only 3 had a definable connective tissue disease (rheumatoid arthritis in all 3). Therefore, the early anecdotal reports about a link between silicone breast implants and scleroderma are clearly refuted by this and other data discussed earlier.

A slightly larger retrospective cohort study published by Hennekens et al[40] included data recorded after the media attention became pronounced in 1991 and 1992. Nonetheless, the study agreed with the other large epidemiologic studies in excluding an increased risk of women with silicone implants developing connective tissue disease. However, possibly because they used data gathered after the media attention and after letters suggesting that large financial settlements were possible if patients had complaints of connective tissue diseases, the authors were unable to exclude small increased risks of connective tissue disease among these patients.

An extensive review article from the FDA[41] concluded that the studies of defined connective tissue diseases, including scleroderma, suggest that there is no substantially increased risk for women with silicone breast implants to develop these disorders. The article noted, however, that there is insufficient information in the available literature to conclusively evaluate the possibility of a link between breast implants and the vague connective tissue disease–like syndromes. With the current emotional environment, it may be impossible to craft a study that will deal conclusively with this issue.

Poorly Defined Connective Tissue Conditions

Some authors have used terms such as "human adjuvant disease" to describe women who describe nonspecific complaints. Unfortunately, human adjuvant disease is not clearly defined. The symptoms patients describe are difficult to diagnose because they are so common among the general population. Cohen and Rohrich[42] note that approximately 40 million people in the United States have some type of musculoskeletal disease. Although osteoarthritis is the most prevalent, vague complaints of fibromyalgias occur with great frequency. Autoimmune diseases are more common in women than in men and usually occur in the second through fifth decades. Some researchers[43] who have reported studies on these symptoms complain about the lack of inclusion of women with vague, nonspecific symptoms in the larger epidemiologic studies. Yet studies such as that by Liang et al[44] have recorded atypical connective tissue diseases by reporting the prevalence of 41 signs and symptoms, including vague complaints that are difficult to quantify. As mentioned previously, these large, controlled studies have failed to record a significant relationship even between these vague symptoms and silicone breast implants that have been in place for an average of almost 10 years.[39]

Human adjuvant disease is not a new notion. It was first reported by Miyoshi et al[45] in 1964. The 2 women they reported developed arthritis-like symptoms after their breasts were directly injected with paraffin. The most deleterious rheumatic effects have been reported on women who have had direct injections with paraffin and/or silicone gels of unknown purity. The term "adjuvant disease" was used because these symptoms were similar to those of an experimental condition induced in rats by subcutaneously injecting them with complete Freund's adjuvant (CFA).[46] This adjuvant is used to augment the immune response in experimental animals (never humans) to antigens that are emulsified in CFA prior to injection. About 25% of rats injected with CFA develop adjuvant disease. No association with adjuvant as such is seen in humans, however, making the term "human adjuvant disease" misleading. The manifestations described by authors who use this term include vague rheumatic symptoms, fever, malaise, and weight loss. Because of the imprecision of the diagnosis, a panel of rheumatologists, epidemiologists, and plastic surgeons has recommended that the term not be used.[46]

Potential Hazard to Infants

Levine and Ilowite[47] reported that 6 children who had been breast-fed by mothers who had silicone implants exhibited abnormal esophageal motility. The researchers did not find this in 2 other breast-fed infants, nor in 3 control babies who were bottle-fed. There was, however, no significant difference in the incidence of autoantibodies between breast-fed and bottle-fed infants. Both groups of babies had some nonspecific rheumatologic symptoms. Subsequent letters to the editor[48,49] noted that Levine and Ilowite should have excluded mothers with scleroderma from their study, and that one of the children had been misclassified (when seen by another practitioner, the child was determined to have a neurologic disorder rather than true muscle dysfunction). The original authors[50,51] agreed that they had misclassified one infant, disagreed with the need to exclude mothers with scleroderma, and confirmed a relationship between at least one author and an anti-implant organization called Children Afflicted by Toxic Substances (CATS).

Levine et al[52] also recorded a modest increase in urinary nitric oxide metabolites and neopterin in approximately 33% of the children who were breast-fed by mothers with implants and noted a relationship among the presence of these substances, macrophage activation, and decreased esophageal motility. Two other breast-fed infants of mothers with silicone breast implants were reported to have myalgias and arthralgias.[53] Both of these children had antinuclear antibody (ANA) activity, and one child had antibodies against denatured type II collagen in high titer. This child's mother also had ANA activity and rheumatic complaints. Although some European physicians have cautioned against breast-feeding by mothers with silicone breast implants, the evidence that it may harm their infants is meager; Flick[54] and Williams[55] caution that insufficient evidence exists for such a recommendation. It is noteworthy that many nipples for baby bottles are made from silicone.

Laboratory Findings Related to Autoimmunity

As with nonimplant patients, when patients with silicone implants present with symptoms of a definable connective tissue disease, they are likely to demonstrate a specific autoantibody. Press et al[56]

Table 12-2. Breast Implant Patients With Defined Autoimmune Disorders[55]

Patient	Diagnosis	Age at Implant	Year to Symptoms	ANA Titer	RF Titer
A	d-Scl	46	7	640	640
B	l-Scl	39	20	640	640
C	CREST	20	14	640	—
D	Raynaud's	34	11	320	—
E	l-Scl	30	2	640	—
F	l-Scl	32	12	320	—
G	Scl/SLE/MCTD	37	5	640	320
H	SLE	26	14	320	—
I	SLE/RA/MCTD	32	6	640	1,280
J	RA	35	8	80	640
K	Seronegative RA	28	9	—	—

Abbreviations: ANA = antinuclear antibody; RF = rheumatoid factor; d-Scl = diffuse scleroderma; l-Scl = limited scleroderma; CREST = calcinosis, Raynaud's phenomenon, esophageal dysfunction, sclerodactyly, telangiectasia; SLE = systemic lupus erythematosus; MCTD = mixed connective tissue disease; RA = rheumatoid arthritis.

reported on 11 patients who were referred to the division of rheumatology at Scripps clinic because of a combination of silicone implants and signs and symptoms of SLE, scleroderma, rheumatoid arthritis, or overlap syndrome. Ten of the 11 patients had high ANA titers, and the ANA specificities were similar to those found in the idiopathic forms of each particular autoimmune disease (**Table 12-2**). In contrast, 13 other women who had less clearly defined autoimmune phenomena had lower titers of ANA, and in many cases the specificities could not be identified.

In yet another small, anecdotal series, Silver et al[57] reported on 3 women who had implants and some "serologic" evidence of connective tissue disease. Patient 1 had negative results for ANA and rheumatoid factor; Patient 2 had an anti–double-stranded DNA (anti-dsDNA) titer of 1:80 before removal of the implant. After removal, the anti-dsDNA was undetectable. Patient 3 had an ANA result initially described as 1:20 and diffuse, but as 1:80 and speckled later in the same report. It is unknown whether Patient 3 was studied further after the implant was removed.

Bridges et al[58] reported on 156 women with silicone implants who had rheumatic complaints, comparing their serologic data with those of women with implants who had no rheumatic complaints and those of women without silicone implants who had fibromyalgia. Most of the women had normal serology, and there was no difference in the levels of immunoglobulins, ANAs, rheumatoid factor, and C-reactive protein between control subjects and women with either joint and muscle pain or joint swelling, regardless of whether they had silicone implants. The authors suggested that some women with implants may develop atypical immunologic reactions, but noted that their assertion could not be proven from their data. The lack of an association between autoantibodies and joint swelling or muscle pain argue against routine screening with these tests unless the patient has specific symptoms of a defined connective tissue disease.

Claman and Robertson[59] conducted a pair of cross-sectional analyses of women with implants and control subjects. The only autoantibody tested was ANA. All women were given a physical examination by the researchers. There were 19 healthy control subjects (group 0), 38 women with implants who appeared healthy (group I), 82 women with implants and various symptoms such as fatigue and musculoskeletal aches and pains (group II), and 11 women with implants who had developed classical autoimmunity subsequent to implantation (group III). More women than would be expected in group III had scleroderma. An ANA of 1+ at 1:256 (HEp-2 cells) was considered positive. Sixty-four percent of group III and 26% of group II were ANA-positive. These results were not surprising. However, 18% of the apparently healthy women in group I were ANA-positive, compared with 0% of those in control group 0 ($P < .05$). This result was not expected and was the first to suggest that implantation in apparently healthy women may be accompanied by some indication of

Table 12-3. Autoantibody Tests in Implant Patients With Clinical Systemic Lupus Erythematosus and All Implant Patients (Including Those With Vague Symptoms)[2]

Test	Positive Results	
	Implant and Clinical SLE	All Implant Patients
ANA	71%	23%
Anti-dsDNA	80%	3%
Anti-Sm	25%	1%

Abbreviations: ANA = antinuclear anitbody; dsDNA = double-stranded DNA.

autoimmunity (eg, a weakly positive ANA). Although there was undoubtedly ascertainment bias (because the sample was collected after news reports in the popular press became prevalent) in the acquisition of groups II and III, this was not the case in groups 0 and I.

The results were sufficiently disturbing to warrant a confirmatory study,[60] so additional women were recruited for groups 0 and I, and the ANA test was performed in a different laboratory in which a positive result was scored at a level of 1+ at 1:80. In the second study, there was a prevalence of positive ANA in 6% of the 18 women in group 0 and in 35% of the 37 women in group I. When the results were pooled, there was a prevalence of positive ANAs in 3% of healthy women without implants and 27% of 75 apparently healthy women with implants ($P = .002$).

It is unclear why asymptomatic women with implants have an increased prevalence of weakly positive ANA, because ANAs are not often drawn on healthy women who are then followed clinically with repeat evaluations. A possible analogy occurs in follow-up studies of apparently healthy people with chronic biologic false-positive tests (BFPs) for syphilis. If the chronic BFP subjects are women, there is a considerable risk for later development of SLE or questionable connective tissue disease; this is not true in men.[61] Whether the presence of a positive ANA in an apparently healthy woman with silicone breast implants is analogous to a chronic BFP for syphilis in an apparently healthy woman is still open to question. In the current managed care environment, it is hoped that women with implants will be followed adequately.

In a comprehensive summary of the scientific literature on the subject of laboratory tests from silicone breast implant patients, Sanchez-Guerrero et al[2] found that among patients with definite or possible autoimmune disease, 38% had rheumatoid factor activity, 62% were positive for ANA, and 30% had anti-dsDNA. If results are limited to those with definite connective tissue disease, the percentage of laboratory abnormalities is similar to those with connective tissue disease who do not have implants. The authors found that 71% of implant patients with clinical SLE had positive ANA (95% expected), 80% had anti-dsDNA (80% expected), and 25% had anti-Sm (25% expected) (**Table 12-3**). However, when all implant patients (including those in the "other diagnosis" category) were included, the percentage of positive ANA results dropped to 23% (typically, at least 10% of controls with no rheumatic complaints have a positive ANA), positive anti-dsDNA dropped to 3% (1% to 2% are positive in a normal population), and positive anti-Sm dropped to 1%. Also, 87.5% of implant patients with clinical rheumatoid arthritis had rheumatoid factor in their serum, whereas when patients with less specific symptoms were included, only 14% were positive. The patients with clinical mixed connective tissue disease had anti-ribonucleoprotrein (anti-RNP) (100%), whereas only 2% of the larger group had this antibody. Clearly, the small numbers allow few conclusions. It does seem clear, however, that the usefulness of autoantibody testing seems to be confined to patients with specific symptoms.

Some anecdotal reports[62–65] of other laboratory findings in patients with silicone implants include a patient with fatigue and increased immunoglobulin (Ig) A in the serum, a patient with Kikuchi's histiocytic necrotizing lymphadenitis and a ruptured implant, a patient with *Mycobacterium avium-intracellulare* mastitis, and 2 patients with possible silicone allergy. Some of the researchers used their situations to learn something about other diseases, such as the observation by Sever et al[63] about the ruptured-implant case that the transient abnormal immune reaction seen supports the relationship between Kikuchi's disease and T-cell immunity. However, the authors of this book do not advocate measuring immunoglobulin levels in asymptomatic women with silicone implants.

The most recent studies on clinical immunology tests in patients with silicone breast implants comes from Karlson et al[66] at Harvard Medical School. They studied serum from 200 women who had been exposed to silicone breast implants and who had not reported problems with defined autoimmune diseases. They compared them with 200 age-matched controls (women not exposed to implants) and found no difference in ANA, anti-dsDNA, anti-Sm/RNP, anti-SSA/Ro, anti-SSB/La, anti-Scl-70 (topoisomerase), rheumatoid factor, IgG, IgA, IgM, serum complement, C-reactive protein, anticardiolipin, antithyroglobulin, antithyroid microsomal (thyroid peroxidase), and antisilicone antibodies.[66] An increase was found in the frequency of anti-ssDNA in the women with silicone implants compared with the healthy controls (41% vs 29%, $P = 0.012$). The authors commented that the increase in anti-ssDNA has unknown clinical relevance.

Other Immunologic Studies in Humans

Results from cellular immune studies in implant patients have been heterogeneous. Ojo-Amaize et al[67,68] found elevated concentrations of both IL-1 beta and IL-1 receptor antagonist in plasma samples from women with silicone breast implants. These findings are consistent with the ongoing fibrosis and foreign-body response in the capsule surrounding virtually all implants. Although these assays are interesting in explaining some of the inflammatory effects, they are not necessary to follow up patients with implants. The lack of these mediators and receptor antagonists will not provide information to aid in patient care.

Some researchers[13] have suggested that adsorption of proteins on the surface of silicone may result in humoral immunologic reactivity to serum proteins. Bonfield and Anderson[69] recorded an increase in IL-1 beta secreted by monocytes cultured on silicone rubber if the surface was precoated with IgG or fibrinogen. The implication is that implant patients may have altered immunoreactivity because of the increased IL-1 beta. This speculation may deserve further experimental studies, but it is not required for routine evaluation of implant patients.

Reports lacking basic details such as how patient populations were selected for immunologic studies still abound, even though such information is important in understanding the significance of the data to the general population of women with silicone breast implants. One study[70] on monocyte infiltrates in salivary glands of women with silicone breast implants stated that ". . . more than half the women we saw with silicone breast implants had a Sjögren's-like syndrome." This would be stunning information if it represented all women with implants, but it obviously does not. The report said only "From the first 24 women that were seen. . . ." How were the patients chosen? Were these women referred by their primary care physicians because of rheumatic disease complaints, dry eyes, or dry mouth? The reader of the article is unable to tell. Therefore, it is necessary to be critical when reviewing the literature; to demand details about patient selection, controls, and methods; and to try to separate phenomenology from relevant science.

Immune Response to Silicone in Humans

Antisilicone and antisilicate antibodies have been described in women with silicone implants. However, this phenomenon was first reported in hydrocephalic children with silicone shunts.[71] Randall[72] used the antisilicone antibody assay on sera from 79 women with breast implants who had various problems, including local reactions and systemic symptoms. The binding assay involved a prolonged incubation with the putative antigen. This suggests that the antibodies were probably of low affinity. Randall found that about 50% of these women had antibody levels greater than 2 standard deviations above the mean of the control group without implants. However, other women were well within the normal range.

Recent studies have found that diabetics with daily exposure to low levels of silicone from needles and syringes have the same low level of antisilicone antibodies as a control population. Presumably, control subjects are exposed to silicone in the environment. Wolf et al[73] noted, however, that IgG antisilicone levels correlated directly with the amount of silicone exposure and suggested that the highest titers were present in patients with ruptured silicone breast implants, making this a possibly useful screening test for ruptured implants. There is no evidence, however, that the antisilicone antibody level correlates with the development of autoimmune phenomena.

A report by Shen et al[74] demonstrated the presence of IgG or IgM antisilicate antibodies in plasma from both symptomatic and asymptomatic women with silicone breast implants. Women described as symptomatic were more likely to have these antibodies (12 of the 40 women studied) than were asymptomatic women (8 of the 91 women studied). Surprisingly, reactivity was found in one woman who had SLE but no implant and in 1 of 50 healthy control women. Another interesting feature of this study is the depiction of assay results that showed the median and mode of the responses in 50 healthy women to be higher than the median and mode for asymptomatic women with implants. Further, a large number of the healthy women had results by enzyme immunoassay (EIA) that were quite close to the cutoff. Although the study of antisilicate antibodies may be useful for research, it is unlikely that this assay will be of clinical use for individual patients.

Cell-mediated immunity to silicone has been studied by several groups. Ojo-Amaize et al[68] compared the silicone-specific peripheral blood responses of women categorized into 4 groups: healthy women with no implants, healthy women with implants, those with nonspecific symptoms (chronic fatigue, musculoskeletal symptoms, and skin disorders), and those with explanted implants and clinical symptoms. In all groups, the majority of the patients were within the normal range. None of the patients had defined connective tissue diseases such as scleroderma or SLE. The explanted group included 4 patients with modestly increased stimulation indices. Six of the 21 patients with nonspecific symptoms did not overlap the control population. Although the authors asserted this was an "apparently specific screening blood test," it is doubtful that any information from it could be used in patient care in a way that would justify the expense. This publication has been criticized for many of its methods and conclusions.[75]

Smalley et al[76] reported increased in vitro proliferation of peripheral blood lymphocytes in women with silicone implants compared with controls when the lymphocytes were stimulated by silicon dioxide. Both symptomatic and asymptomatic women had significantly increased proliferation indices compared with controls. Unfortunately, this study's description of materials and methods is not explicit enough to allow replication of its experiments by an independent researcher. This study and those conducted in animals (described in the next section) are consistent with a cell-mediated immune recognition of silicon dioxide or silicone hapten groups (almost certainly attached to carrier proteins). Symptomatic women seemed to have a stronger stimulation response in the study by Smalley et al[76]; however, no statistically significant difference was noted between the 2 groups. A similar proliferative response by peripheral blood lymphocytes to silicone was reported by Ciapetti et al.[77] This area of research investigation may be useful; however, it is doubtful that an isolated stimulation index will be of use in managing a patient with silicone breast implants.

Animal Models and Theories

A wide variety of experimental animal models have been reported, but often only in abstract form. However, some offer straightforward findings related to inflammation found around the implants. For instance, injection of silicone into experimental animals consistently produces a chronic inflammatory (usually granulomatous) response. Silicone inclusions are typically present in giant cells and monocytes. Plasma cells, lymphocytes, and neutrophils also may be present in inflammatory lesions in laboratory animals, which is similar to the findings in capsules around human silicone breast implants.[78] Some animal models have been devised to test hypotheses about the relevance of silicone to autoimmune disease.

One important hypothesis is that silicone may act as an adjuvant (not to be confused with the term *human adjuvant disease*) that augments the humoral immune response against a variety of antigens. Studies in rats have shown that silicone gel can act as an immunologic adjuvant that augments the antibody response to coadministered antigens.[79] Such studies have demonstrated increased antibody responses to coadministered antigens such as bovine serum albumin, rat thyroglobulin, and bovine collagen II.[80,81] In fact, the adjuvant activity of silicone gel is at least equal to that of CFA. The molecular weight and specific gel preparations used in the studies have been found to be important in the humoral adjuvant effects obtained.[82]

Another frequently tested hypothesis is that silicone may act as a hapten to elicit a cellular or humoral immune response. A humoral response must occur to some extent, because many patients with silicone-based implants (as well as individuals with chronic Silastic tubing shunts) develop detectable antibodies to silicone. Whether or how this could cause damage to tissues is completely unknown. Repeated exposure to silicone gel has been shown to induce cutaneous delayed hypersensitivity in sheep.[83] This finding is consistent with the modest numbers of lymphocytes surrounding the capsule in women with silicone breast implants. However, no relationship has been shown between this cell-mediated immune event and autoimmune disease. McDonald et al[84] found that silicone gel injected into the peritonea of several strains of mice elicited peritoneal cells that could stimulate a modest T-cell proliferation by lymphocytes.

Other researchers have hypothesized that silicone may alter endogenous tissues, thereby inducing an immune response to the body's tissues.[85] There is evidence to support some of these ideas. For instance, workers in the sandblasting industry who are exposed to crystalline silicon dioxide have an increased incidence of scleroderma. There is no evidence, however, that silicone degrades to silicon dioxide in sufficient quantities in vivo to cause a similar problem.[86] Indeed, the epidemiologic evidence already cited largely refutes this possibility.

Because silicone gel may be a product of the oxidative degradation of silicone, such gel formation could be relevant to the issue of altered immune reactivity.[5] However, in studies using the DA rat (an animal highly susceptible to the development of arthritis), injection of silicone gel alone produced no cases of arthritis, although mineral oil alone did.[81]

The Positions of Professional Organizations

The American College of Rheumatology states: "there is no convincing evidence that these implants cause any generalized disease."[86] The American Medical Association and the FDA concluded that data are insufficient to prove an association between silicone gel implants and any immune disorder. Furthermore, the FDA advisory panel declined to recognize the term *human adjuvant disease* as a defined clinical entity.[87]

The College of American Pathologists adopted the following position concerning this area of testing in 1993[88]:

> *It is the position of the College of American Pathologists that laboratory tests measuring blood, urine or tissue silicon, silicone, toluene diamines, or related substances are not currently indicated or useful for purposes of medical care of individual breast implant recipients. Research interests may be served by investigation of the measurement of these materials in controlled studies. Serum autoantibody tests or panels are useful in the evaluation of individual patients suspected of having collagen vascular disease, whether or not they have received breast implants, but such tests provide no findings uniquely indicative or supportive of purported silicone induced autoimmune disease in implant recipients. Interpretation of such panels as "consistent with silicone reaction" for example, is not supported by the current medical literature.*
>
> *The sale or distribution in commerce of diagnostic tests or instruments intended for use in evaluating patients with silicone implants should depend on FDA evaluation and approval. To date, the FDA has not approved any such tests, instruments, or systems. If FDA were to give approval, the approval would likely be for investigational purposes only until sufficient data were available to justify approval for general use. Without approval by the FDA, the use of diagnostic tests, instruments, or test systems intended for the evaluation of patients with silicone implants would be excluded from coverage under the Medicare program and could subject the user to an increased risk of medical malpractice liability.*

Implant Removal

The FDA panel[87] noted that an asymptomatic woman who has no indication of a ruptured implant is at greater risk from the implant removal procedure than from any known pathologic danger. Nemecek and Young[12] noted that a small number of women with symptoms such as arthralgia or myalgia, unusual rheumatic symptoms, and chronic fatigue may benefit from implant removal, as may a woman with a definitive diagnosis of a rheumatologic condition such as scleroderma, SLE, or rheumatoid arthritis. It should be noted that although some women have been reported to benefit from implant removal under these circumstances,[89] other women have experienced no demonstrable benefit.[90] Furthermore, there are no data indicating that any laboratory test in an asymptomatic woman would be a useful guide to therapy or follow-up.

Slavin and Goldwyn[91] reported on 46 women who requested removal of their implants over a one-year time period. The reasons for the requests varied: 17 feared possible long-term consequences; 14 were concerned about esthetic problems related to encapsulation; 8 had systemic symptoms; 7 had ruptured implants (determined by mammography); and 4 were concerned about the interference of the implant with mammography or clinical examination for cancer. Of the 7 patients with severe systemic symptoms, only one became asymptomatic and none had changes in autoantibody levels after removal of the implant.

The question is more problematic in symptomatic women, some of whom have shown improvement after implant removal whereas others have not. Elberg et al[92] recommended that "in patients with severe connective tissue disease, removal of the implant must be seriously considered." They further recommend that patients with symptoms of connective disease should not receive implants. Houpt and Sontheimer[93] summarized reports of 27 patients with connective tissue disease and silicone implants; 15 experienced substantial-to-complete recovery after implant removal, 7 had partial improvement, and 5 had no benefit.

Laboratory Testing for Asymptomatic Women With Silicone Implants

All women with silicone implants who present with symptoms of connective tissue disease should undergo the same serologic tests performed for women without such implants. However, some laboratories and anecdotal reports advocate laboratory testing, often in monumental proportions, in all women with silicone implants, even in the absence of clinical symptoms. Sanchez-Guerrero et al[2] point out that this may not be a wise choice. First, because many tests such as the ANA (antinuclear antibody) may show positive results even among healthy individuals (depending on where the cutoff is set), psychological distress may result from positive results that have no clinical correlation with symptoms. Second, negative ANAs have been reported in women with symptoms of connective tissue disease. Thus, neither result is conclusive.

The cost of such testing is also a factor in the current era of managed care. This is not to say that large, carefully controlled studies of immune responses in these individuals should not be conducted. On the contrary, such studies, supported by research grants and performed by competent investigators using protocols approved by human use committees and investigational review boards, would be very valuable. Furthermore, the fact that some patients with clinical symptoms of connective tissue disease have had decreases in ANA titers after implant removal suggests a relationship that needs to be pursued by independent investigators. A recent report from Bridges et al[58] found that asymptomatic women with silicone implants did not demonstrate antibodies to known disease-related polypeptides when the Western blot assay was used.

One weakness in many studies on ANA activity is the lack of attention to details such as the control group. Depending on the cutoff titer used, ANA activity may be found in as many as 20% to 30% of healthy middle-aged women, and its presence is expected to be higher in patients with symptoms of connective tissue disease. Indeed, it would be surprising if a patient population selected by rheumatic complaints did not have a higher frequency of ANA reactivity than a general population of women. This is true regardless of the presence of silicone breast implants. Therefore, interesting studies such as those by Cuellar et al[94] that record ANA positivity in 30% of individuals using a mouse kidney substrate and 57.8% of individuals using an HEp-2 cell line are difficult to interpret without knowing precisely how the patients were selected. (Were they self-referred or referred by attorneys, generalists in the community, plastic surgeons, or rheumatologists?) It also must be known whether the referrals differed from those of 264 women with whom they were compared and who were also sent to the laboratory for ANA testing. The latter group had a surprisingly low positivity rate of only 7.6% (although the study does not specify by which assay—HEp-2 or mouse kidney). Interestingly, none of the 813 women with silicone breast implants were reported to have highly significant Sm reactivity. Six who were referred for rheumatic complaints had SSA reactivity, 6 had dsDNA activity, and only 1 had Scl-70 activity. The researchers' review of the literature notes several abstracts that report no ANA control at all. When reading this literature, it is best to pay close attention to the selection of the population studied and the controls used as well as the methods of the study.

The FDA has not cleared (by the 510k process) any of the tests that have been marketed to measure blood levels of silicone, toluene diamines, antibodies against silicone or silica, or autoantibodies to host proteins claimed to be modified by silicone.[95]

Some laboratories have reported a variety of strange requests. For instance, Nuttall et al[96] noted a dramatic increase in laboratories asked to perform urinary platinum determinations. The rationale is that platinum catalysts are used during preparation of the silicone polymer (described earlier). However, there are no data to support the usefulness of such a study. The authors noted that the half-life of platinum is less than 3 days and that any remaining amounts of platinum would bind to adipose tissue. When they compared the platinum levels in 150 implant patients with 25 control women and 21 control men, none of the implant patients had a level higher than the control reference population (<4 μg/L). Platinum assays should be used for their intended purpose—ie, monitoring patients on cisplatin therapy (where platinum in urine is often 100 to 1,000 μg/L).

Public Aspects of the Breast Implant Controversy

The possibility that silicone breast implantation might be related to an increased incidence of scleroderma is a scientific problem of considerable importance. If it were found to be true, it could lead to insights into the etiology and pathogenesis of idiopathic scleroderma, a frequently devastating disease about which little is known. The epidemiologic data appear to show that there is either a very small relationship or no relationship between implants and any clearly defined connective tissue disease. This should come as a relief and reassurance to the many women with implants.

Nevertheless, the circus-like, media-saturated atmosphere in which these epidemiologic studies were carried out has not made the research easier. Angell[97] reviewed this dilemma and concluded that no one involved had helped the situation. This included the media, the manufacturers, the medical profession, many litigating attorneys, and even some patients and advocate groups. After all, the question of whether silicone implants "cause" autoimmune disease is a medical rather than a legal question and should therefore be decided by carefully controlled scientific studies.

Summary

Although silicone clearly elicits a local, chronic inflammatory response, the data linking it to connective tissue disease are unproven and weak. Additional controlled studies performed over long periods are needed to study this issue. At the present time, the use of extensive laboratory testing on asymptomatic women who happen to have silicone breast implants is wasteful, potentially misleading, and useful only when performed as part of a controlled research protocol. Symptomatic patients should have tests directed to their specific symptoms.

References

1. Cook RR, Harrison MC, LeVier RR. The breast implant controversy. *Arthritis Rheum*. 1994;37:153–157.
2. Sanchez-Guerrero J, Schur PH, Sergent JS, et al. Silicone breast implants and rheumatic disease. Clinical, immunologic, and epidemiologic studies. *Arthritis Rheum*. 1994;37:158–168.
3. Fisher JC. The silicone controversy: When will science prevail? *N Engl J Med*. 1992;326:1696–1698.
4. Hirmand H, Latrenta GS, Hoffman LA. Autoimmune disease and silicone breast implants. *Oncology*. 1993;7:17–28.
5. Peters W, Smith D, Lugowski S. Silicon assays in women with and without silicone gel breast implants. *Ann Plast Surg*. 1999;43:324-330.
6. Yu LT, Latorre G, Marotta J, et al. In vitro measurement of silicone bleed from breast implants. *Plast Reconstr Surg*. 1996;97:756–764.
7. Brody G. Fact and fiction about breast implant 'bleed.' *Plast Reconstr Surg*. 1977;3:615–616. [Editorial]
8. Bergman R, van der Ende A. Exudation of silicone through the envelope of gel-filled prostheses: An in vitro study. *Br J Plast Surg*. 1979;32:31–34.
9. Garrido L, Bogdanova A, Cheng LL, et al. Detection of silicone migration and biodegradation with NMR. *Curr Top Microbiol Immunol*. 1996;210:49–58.
10. Garrido L, Young VL. Analysis of periprosthetic capsular tissue from women with silicone breast implants by magic-angle spinning NMR. *Magn Reson Med*. 1999;42:436-444.
11. Cook RR, Delongchamp RR, Woodbury M, et al. The prevalence of women with breast implants in the United States—1989. *J Clin Epidemiol*. 1995;48:519–525.
12. Nemecek JA, Young V. How safe are silicone breast implants? *South Med J*. 1993;86:932–944.
13. Kossovsky N, Freiman CJ. Silicone breast implant pathology. Clinical data and immunologic consequences. *Arch Pathol Lab Med*. 1994;118:686–693.
14. Granchi D, Cavedagna D, Ciapetti G, et al. Silicone breast implants: The role of immune system on capsular contracture formation. *J Biomed Mater Res*. 1995;29:197–202.

15. Sanger JR, Komorowshi RA, Larson DL, et al. Tissue humoral response to intact and ruptured silicone gel-filled prostheses. *Plast Reconstr Surg*. 1995; 95:1033–1038.

16. Kitchen SB, Paletta CE, Shehadi SI, et al. Epithelialization of the lining of a breast implant capsule. Possible origin of squamous cell carcinoma associated with a breast implant capsule. *Cancer*. 1994;73:1449–1452.

17. Katzin WE, Feng L, Abbuhl M, et al. Phenotype of lymphocytes associated with the inflammatory reaction to silicone gel breast implants. *Clin Diagn Lab Immunol*. 1996;3:156–161.

18. Phillips JW, de Camara KL, Lockwood MD, et al. Strength of silicone breast implants. *Plast Reconstr Surg*. 1996;97:1215–1225.

19. van Diest PJ, Beekman WH, Hage JJ. Pathology of silicone leakage from breast implants. *J Clin Pathol*. 1998;51:493–497.

20. Greene WB, Raso DS, Walsh LG, et al. Electron probe microanalysis of silicon and the role of the macrophage in proximal (capsule) and distant sites in augmentation mammaplasty patients. *Plast Reconstr Surg*. 1995;95:513–519.

21. Deapen MD, Pike MC, Casagrande P, et al. The relationship between breast cancer and augmentation mammaplasty: An epidemiologic study. *Plast Reconstr Surg*. 1986;77:361–367.

22. Petit J-Y, Monique GL, Mouriesse H, et al. Can breast reconstruction with gel-filled silicone implants increase the risk of death and second primary cancer in patients treated by mastectomy for breast cancer? *Plast Reconstr Surg*. 1994;94:115–119.

23. Bryant H, Brasher P. Breast implants and breast cancer—reanalysis of a linkage study. *N Engl J Med*. 1995;332:1535–1539.

24. Duvic M, Moore D, Menter A, et al. Cutaneous T-cell lymphoma in association with silicone breast implants. *J Am Acad Dermatol*. 1995;32:939–942.

25. Hatanaka S, Oneda S, Okazaki K, et al. Induction of malignant fibrous histiocytoma in female Fisher rats by implantation of cyanoacrylate, zirconia, polyvinyl chloride or silicone. *In Vivo*. 1993;7:111–115.

26. Potter M, Morrison S, Wiener F. Induction of plasmacytomas with silicone gel in genetically susceptible strains of mice. *J Natl Cancer Inst*. 1994;86:1058–1065.

27. Rabkin CS, Silverman S, Tricot G, et al. The National Cancer Institute silicone implant/multiple myeloma registry. *Curr Top Microbiol Immunol*. 1996;210:385–387.

28. Angell M. Shattuck Lecture—evaluating the health risks of breast implants: The interplay of medical science, the law and public opinion. *N Engl J Med*. 1996;334:1513–1516.

29. Spiera H, Kerr LD. Scleroderma following silicone implantation: A cumulative experience of 11 cases. *J Rheumatol*. 1993;20:958–961.

30. Hochberg MC, Miller R, Wigley FM. Frequency of augmentation mammaplasty in patients with systemic sclerosis: Data from the Johns Hopkins–University of Maryland Scleroderma Center. *J Clin Epidemiol*. 1995;48:565–569.

31. Wigley FM, Miller R. Augmentation mammaplasty in patients with systemic sclerosis. Data from the Baltimore Scleroderma Research Center and Pittsburgh Scleroderma Data Bank. *Arthritis Rheum*. 1992;35(suppl):S46. [Abstract]

32. Englert H, Morris D, March L. Scleroderma and silicone gel breast prostheses—the Sydney study revisited. *Aust N Z J Med*. 1996;26:349–355.

33. Spiera RF, Gibofsky A, Spiera H. Silicone gel filled breast implants and connective tissue disease: An overview. *J Rheumatol*. 1994;21:239–245.

34. Janowsky EC, Kupper LL, Hulka BS. Meta-analyses of the relation between silicone breast implants and the risk of connective-tissue diseases. *N Engl J Med* 2000;342:781–790.

35. Weisman MH, Vecchione TR, Albert D, et al. Connective tissue disease following breast augmentation: A preliminary test of the human adjuvant disease hypothesis. *Plast Reconstr Surg*. 1988;82:626–630.

36. Gabriel SE, O'Fallon WM, Kurland LT, et al. Risk of connective tissue diseases and other disorders after breast implantation. *N Engl J Med*. 1994;330:1697–1702.

37. Gilray EJ, Moens JHB, Riley AH, et al. Silicone breast prostheses and rheumatic symptoms: A retrospective follow up study. *Ann Rheum Dis*. 1994;53:194–196.

38. Englert JH, Brooks P. Scleroderma and augmentation mammaplasty—a causal relationship. *Aust N Z J Med*. 1994;24:74–80.

39. Sanchez-Guerrero J, Colditz G, Karlson EW, et al. Silicone breast implants and the risk of connective-tissue diseases and symptoms. *N Engl J Med*. 1995;332:1666–1670.

40. Hennekens CH, Lee I, Cook NR, et al. Self-reported breast implants and connective-tissue diseases in female health professionals. A retrospective cohort study. *JAMA*. 1996;275:616–621.

41. Silverman BG, Brown SL, Bright RA, et al. Reported complications of silicone gel breast implants: An epidemiologic review. *Ann Intern Med*. 1996;124:744–756.

42. Cohen SB, Rohrich RJ. Evaluation of the patient with silicone gel breast implants and rheumatic complaints. *Plast Reconstr Surg*. 1994;94:120–125.

43. Vasey FB, Aziz N. Breast implants and connective tissue diseases. *N Engl J Med*. 1995:333:1423. [Letter]

44. Liang MH, Karlson EW, Sanchez-Guerrero J. Breast implants and connective tissue diseases. *N Engl J Med*. 1995:333:1424. [Reply]

45. Miyoshi K, Miyamune T, Kobayashi Y, et al. Hypergammaglobulinaemia by prolonged adjuvanticity in man: Disorders developed after augmentation mammaplasty. *Jpn J Med*. 1964;2122:9–14.

46. Brody GS, Conway DO, Deapen DM, et al. Consensus statement on the relationship of breast implants to connective tissue disorders. *Plast Reconstr Surg*. 1992;90:1102–1105.

47. Levine JJ, Ilowite NT. Sclerodermalike esophageal disease in children breast-fed by mothers with silicone breast implants. *JAMA*. 1994;27:213–216.

48. Bartel DR. Sclerodermalike esophageal disease in children of mothers with silicone breast implants. *JAMA*. 1994;272:767. [Letter]

49. Epstein WA. Silicone breast implants and sclerodermalike esophageal disease in breast-fed infants. *JAMA*. 1996;275:184. [Letter]

50. Levine JJ, Ilowite NT. Sclerodermalike esophageal disease in children of mothers with silicone breast implants. *JAMA*. 1994;272:769–770. [Reply]

51. Levine JJ, Ilowite NT. Silicone breast implants and sclerodermalike esophageal disease in breast-fed infants. *JAMA*. 1996;275:184–185. [Letter]

52. Levine JJ, Ilowite NT, Pettei MJ, et al. Increased urinary NO3– and NO2– and neopterin excretion in children breast fed by mothers with silicone breast implants: Evidence for macrophage activation. *J Rheumatol*. 1996;23:1083–1087.

53. Teuber SS, Gershwin ME. Autoantibodies and clinical rheumatic complaints in two children of women with silicone gel breast implants. *Int Arch Allergy Immunol*. 1994;103:105–108.

54. Flick JA. Silicone implants and esophageal dysmotility. Are breast-fed infants at risk? *JAMA*. 1994;271: 240–241.

55. Williams AF. Silicone breast implants, breastfeeding and scleroderma. *Lancet*. 1994;343:1043–1044.

56. Press RI, Peebles CL, Kumagai Y, et al. Antinuclear autoantibodies in women with silicone breast implants. *Lancet*. 1992;340:1304–1307.

57. Silver RM, Sahn EE, Allen JA, et al. Demonstration of silicon in sites of connective-tissue disease in patients with silicone-gel breast implants. *Arch Dermatol*. 1993;129:63–68.

58. Bridges AJ, Conley C, Wang G, et al. A clinical and immunologic evaluation of women with silicone breast implants and symptoms of rheumatic disease. *Ann Intern Med*. 1993;116:929–936.

59. Claman HN, Robertson AD. Antinuclear antibodies and breast implants. *West J Med*. 1994;160:225–228.

60. Claman HN, Robertson AD. Antinuclear antibodies in apparently healthy women with breast implants. In: Potter M, Rose NR, eds. *Immunology of Silicones*. Berlin, Germany: Springer-Verlag; 1996:265–268.

61. Moore JE, Lutz WO. Natural history of systemic lupus erythematosus: An approach to its study through chronic biological false-positive reactors. *J Chronic Dis*. 1955;1:297.

62. Levenson T, Greenberger PA, Murphy R. Peripheral blood eosinophilia, hyperimmunoglobulinemia A and fatigue: Possible complications following rupture of silicone breast implants. *Ann Allergy Asthma Immunol*. 1996;77:119–122.

63. Sever CE, Leight CP, Appenzeller J, et al. Kikuchi's histiocytic necrotizing lymphadenitis associated with ruptured silicone breast implant. *Arch Pathol Lab Med*. 1996;120:380–385.

64. Lee D, Goldstein EJC, Zarem HA. Localized *Mycobacterium avium-intracellulare* mastitis in an immunocompetent woman with silicone breast implants. *Plast Reconstr Surg*. 1995;95:142–144.

65. Kirwan L. Two cases of apparent silicone allergy. *Plast Reconstr Surg*. 1995;96:236–237.

66. Karlson EW, Hankinson SE, Liang MH, et al. Association of silicone breast implants with immunologic abnormalities: a prospective study. *Am J Med*. 1999;106:11-19.

67. Ojo-Amaize EA, Lawless OJ, Peter JB. Elevated concentrations of interleukin-1 beta and interleukin-1 receptor antagonist in plasma of women with silicone breast implants. *Clin Diagn Lab Immunol*. 1996;3:257–259.

68. Ojo-Amaize EA, Conte V, Lin H, et al. Silicone-specific blood lymphocyte response in women with silicone breast implants. *Clin Diagn Lab Immunol*. 1994;1:689–695.

69. Bonfield TL, Anderson JM. Functional versus quantitative comparison of IL-1beta from monocytes/macrophages on biomedical polymers. *J Biomed Mater Res*. 1993;27:1195–1199.

70. Freundlich B, Sandorfi N, Altman C, et al. Monocyte/macrophage infiltrates in the salivary glands of women with silicone breast implants. *Curr Top Microbiol Immunol*. 1996;210:323–326.

71. Goldblum RM, Pelley RP, O'Donell AA, et al. Antibodies to silicone elastomers and reactions to ventriculoperitoneal shunts. *Lancet*. 1992;340:510–513.

72. Randall T. Antibodies to silicone detected inpatients with severe inflammatory reactions. *JAMA*. 1992;268:1821–1822.

73. Wolf LE, Lappe M, Peterson RD, et al. Human immune response to polydimethylsiloxane (silicone): Screening studies in a breast implant population. *FASEB J*. 1993;7:1265–1268.

74. Shen G, Ojo-Amaize EA, Agopian MS, et al. Silicate antibodies in women with silicone breast implants: Development of an assay for detection of humoral immunity. *Clin Diagn Lab Immunol*. 1996;3:162–166.

75. Cohen JJ. T cell response in women with silicone breast implants. *Clin Diagn Lab Immunol.* 1995;2:253–254. [Letter]

76. Smalley DL, Shanklin DH, Hall MF, et al. Immunologic stimulation of T lymphocytes by silica after use of silicone mammary implants. *FASEB J.* 1995;9:424–427.

77. Ciapetti G, Granchi D, Stea S, et al. Assessment of viability and proliferation of in vivo silicone-primed lymphocytes after in vitro re-exposure to silicone. *J Biomed Mater Res.* 1995;29:583–590.

78. Picha GJ, Goldstein JA. Analysis of the soft-tissue response to components used in the manufacture of breast implants: Rat animal model. *Plast Reconstr Surg.* 1991;87:490–500.

79. Naim J, Lanzafame RJ. The adjuvant effect of silicone-gel on antibody formation in rats. *Immunol Invest.* 1993;22:151–161.

80. Naim JO, van Oss CJ, Lanzafame RJ. The induction of auto-antibodies to thyroglobulin in rats with silicone as adjuvant. *Surg Forum.* 1993;64:676–678.

81. Naim JO, Ippolito KML, Lanzafame RJ, et al. Induction of type II collagen arthritis in the DA rat using silicone gel as adjuvant. *Curr Top Microbiol Immunol.* 1996;210:103–111.

82. Naim JO, Ippolito KML, Lanzafame RJ. The effect of molecular weight and gel preparation on humoral adjuvancy of silicone oils and silicone gels. *Immunol Invest.* 1995;24:537–547.

83. Narini PP, Semple JL, Hay JB. Repeated exposure to silicone gel can induce delayed hypersensitivity. *Plast Reconstr Surg.* 1995;96:371–380.

84. McDonald AH, Weir K, Sanger JR. Silicone-induced T cell proliferation in mice. *Curr Top Microbiol Immunol.* 1996;210:190–198.

85. Touchette N. Silicone implants and autoimmune disease: Studies fail to gel. *J NIH Res.* 1992;4:49–52.

86. Sergent JS. Silicone gel breast implants and rheumatic disease. *Hotline: Newsletter of the American College of Rheumatology*, February 27, 1992.

87. Council on Scientific Affairs, American Medical Association. Silicone gel breast implants. *JAMA.* 1993;270:2602–2606.

88. CAP position statement. College of American Pathologists, Chicago, IL, 1993.

89. Walsh FW, Solomon DA, Espinoza LR, et al. Human adjuvant disease: A new cause of chylous effusions. *Arch Intern Med.* 1989;149:1194–1196.

90. Varga J, Schumacher HR, Jimenez SA. Systemic sclerosis after augmentation mammaplasty with silicone implants. *Ann Intern Med.* 1989;111:377–383.

91. Slavin SA, Goldwyn RM. Silicone gel implant explantation: Reasons, results and admonitions. *Plast Reconstr Surg.* 1995;95:63–69.

92. Elberg JJ, Kjoller KH, Krag C. Silicone mammary implants and connective tissue disease. *Scand J Plast Reconstr Surg Hand.* 1993;27:243–248.

93. Houpt KR, Sontheimer RD. Autoimmune connective tissue disease and connective tissue disease-like illnesses after silicone gel augmentation mammaplasty. *J Am Acad Dermatol.* 1994;31:626–642.

94. Cuellar ML, Scopelitis E, Tenenbaum SA, et al. Serum antinuclear antibodies in women with silicone breast implants. *J Rheumatol.* 1995;22:236–240.

95. CDC Report. Diagnostic tests for silicone breast disease. *JAMA.* 1996;275:680. [Editorial]

96. Nuttall KL, Gordon WH, Ash KO. Breast implants and urinary platinum. *Clin Chem.* 1994;40:1787.

97. Angell M. *Science on Trial.* New York, NY: WW Norton; 1996.

CHAPTER 13

Guidelines for Selecting and Using Laboratory Tests for Autoantibodies to Nuclear, Nucleolar, and Other Related Cytoplasmic Antigens

Carlos Alberto von Mühlen, MD, PhD, and Robert M. Nakamura, MD

After the basic steps of history taking and routine physical examination, a correct diagnosis and clinical evaluation are achieved with further use of clinical laboratory and imaging tests. In such testing, autoantibody determination is essential when an autoimmune disease is suspected. In distinct entities, such as systemic vasculitis and diffuse connective tissue diseases, testing for autoantibodies helps in one of the following ways:

- Confirming the suspected disease using sets of diagnostic criteria in which autoantibodies are one of the items to be fulfilled.[1–4]
- Monitoring activity and severity of the disease.
- Monitoring therapy. For example, a high titer of anti–double-stranded DNA (anti-dsDNA) is characteristic of systemic lupus erythematosus (SLE). A fall in anti-dsDNA or antihistone serum concentration, along with increasing serum complement levels, may be associated with decreased serum immune complexes and no new kidney lesions.[5] In the absence of immune complexes and kidney glomerulonephritis a low titer of dsDNA antibodies indicates improvement in disease activity.
- Classifying a patient in a better or worse prognostic subgroup of a diffuse connective tissue disease. For example, Jo-1 autoantibodies are associated with a subgroup of polymyositis patients with increased frequency of lung fibrosis, poor response to corticosteroid treatment, and a bad prognosis.[6,7] However, polymyositis-scleroderma (PM-Scl) autoantibodies identify a white population carrying an overlap syndrome with clinical features of polymyositis and systemic sclerosis, with a survival rate approaching 100% in 10 years.[8–11]

The most commonly ordered clinical laboratory tests in autoimmune diseases involve the detection of serum-circulating autoantibodies. Cellular immune tests generally are impractical and only helpful in certain diseases that are mediated by cellular immune mechanisms. Good screening tests in diffuse connective tissue disease have high sensitivity, a characteristic found in both the rheumatoid factor test and the antinuclear antibody (ANA) test by immunofluorescence microscopy (IFM).[12] The selection of further tests heavily depends on clinical findings and on the screening for ANAs. Methods such as immunoblot, enzyme-linked immunosorbent assay (ELISA), counterimmune electrophoresis, double immunodiffusion, and immunoprecipitation should be used to confirm a positive ANA screen, showing the specific antigen-autoantibody system involved (**Table 13-1**).

Table 13-1. Methods for Autoantibody Detection in Autoimmune Systemic Rheumatic Diseases[13]

Disease	Antigen Involved	Methods for Detection of Autoantibodies
Systemic lupus erythematosus	Nuclear antigens (DNA, histone, Sm, RNP, SS-A/Ro, SS-B/La, PCNA, Ku), cytoplasmic ribosomal RNP	IFM on cells or tissue-section substrates, ELISA, immunoblot, agglutination, immunoprecipitation, immunodiffusion
Mixed connective tissue disease	U_1RNP	Immunoprecipitation, agglutination, ELISA, immunoblot, immunodiffusion
Drug-induced SLE	Histones, chromatin	IFM, ELISA, immunoblot
Sjögren's syndrome	Nuclear antigens (SS-A/Ro, SS-B/La)	IFM on cell substrates, ELISA, immunoblot, immunoprecipitation, immunodiffusion
Scleroderma/CREST syndrome	Nuclear/nucleolar antigens (Th/To, fibrillarin, nRNP, topoisomerase I, RNA polymerases); centromeres A, B, and C	IFM on cells or tissue-section substrate, immunoprecipitation, ELISA, immunoblot
Dermatomyositis/polymyositis	Nucleolar antigens (PM-Scl), cytoplasmic (Jo-1 and other tRNA synthetases)	IFM on cells or tissue-section substrate, immunoprecipitation, ELISA, immunoblot
Rheumatoid arthritis	Altered gamma globulin, RA-associated nuclear antigen, RA-33, APF	IFM, latex agglutination or laser nephelometry (rheumatoid factor), immunoprecipitation, immunoblot, ELISA
Systemic vasculitis	Neutrophil granular components (aANCA, cANCA, pANCA)	IFM, ELISA

Abbreviations: RNP = ribonucleoprotein; PCNA = proliferating-cell nuclear antigen; IFM = immunofluorescence microscopy; ELISA = enzyme-linked immunosorbent assay; U_1RNP = uridine-rich ribonucleoprotein; SLE = systemic lupus erythematosus; CREST = calcinosis, Raynaud's, esophageal dysmobility, sclerodactyly, telangiectasia; PM = polymyositis; Scl = scleroderma; RA = rheumatoid arthritis; ANCA = antineutrophil cytoplasmic antibody; APF = antiperinuclear factor.

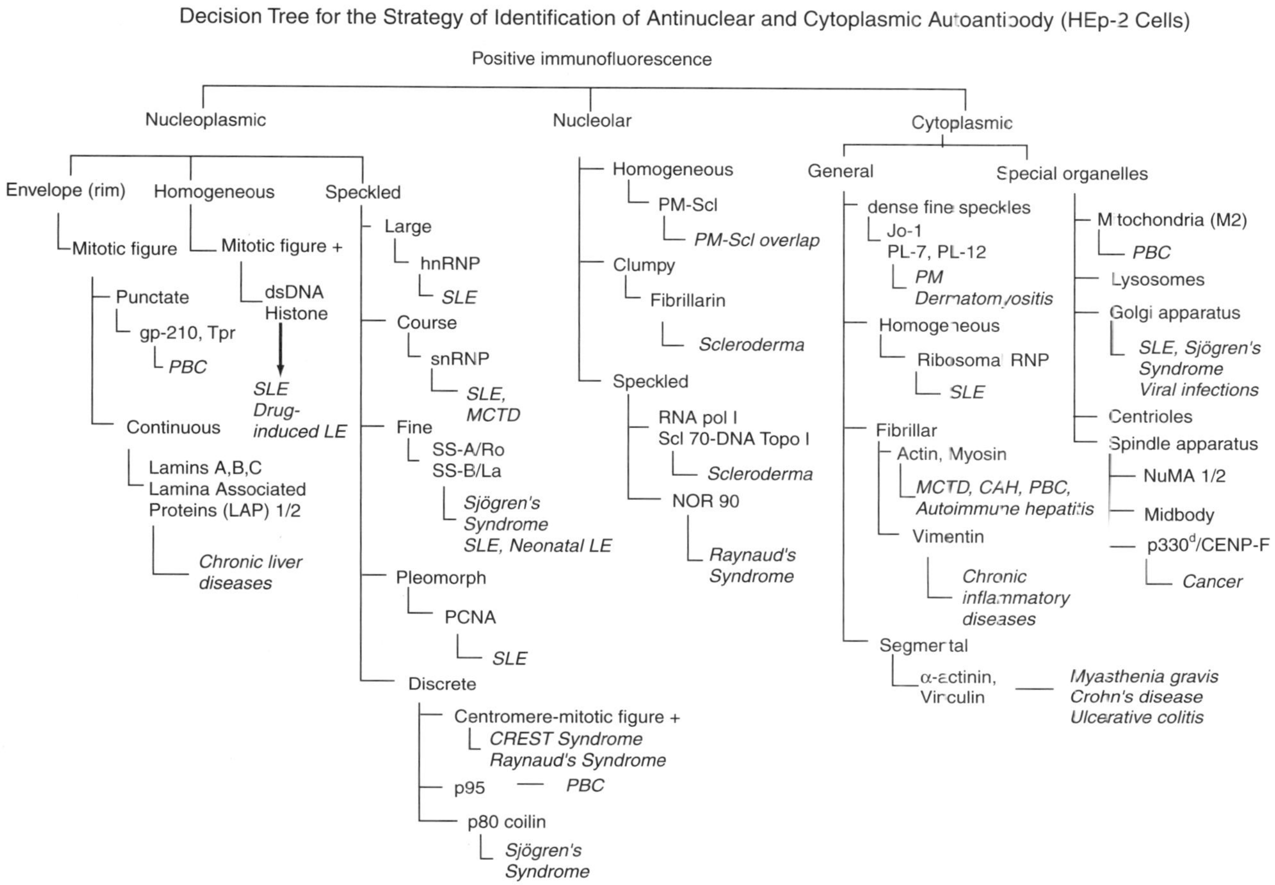

Figure 13-1. Decision tree. Abbreviations: SLE = systemic lupus erythematosus; SS = Sjögren's syndrome; MCTD = mixed connective tissue disease; NOR = nucleolar organizing region; NuMA = nuclear mitotic associated protein; PBC = primary biliary cirrhosis; CAH = chronic active hepatitis; CREST = calcinosis, Raynaud's phenomenon, esophageal dysfunction, sclerodactyly, and telangiectasia; hnRNP = heteronuclear ribonucleoprotein; PM = polymyositis; Scl = scleroderma; PCNA = proliferating-cell nuclear antigen. Reproduced with permission from: Krapf AR, von Mühlen CA, Krapf FE, Nakamura RM, Tan EM, eds. *Atlas of Immunofluorescent Autoantibodies*. Munich, Germany: Urban & Schwarzenberg; 1996.

Decision Tree for the Identification of Antinuclear and Cytoplasmic Antibodies in HEp-2 Cells

The indirect IFM assay is a comprehensive test for screening autoantibodies. A decision tree to correctly identify autoantibodies in the clinical laboratory has been published.[14] **Figure 13-1** shows that a positive immunofluorescence using HEp-2 cells as substrate may elicit 3 main patterns: nucleoplasmic, nucleolar, or cytoplasmic. Special organelles involved in cell division (eg, centrioles) or proteins that are integral components of the spindle apparatus, such as nuclear mitotic-associated protein (NuMA) or proteins of the midbody, also may be recognized.

This decision tree may be used as a general guide to correlate any immunofluorescence pattern to a known disease and to consider the possible antigen or antigens involved. Normally, the antigen gives name to its respective autoantibody (eg, Jo-1, Jo-1 autoantibody). In some instances, a synonym may be used (Scl-70, DNA-topoisomerase I autoantibody). The correct next steps in autoantibody identification using other tests depend entirely on the results of ANA screening by IFM,[15,16] as well as on the clinical presentation. In other words, staining patterns are indicative of antibody specificities, and further definitive tests should be performed to determine the specificity of the antibodies.[17]

Patterns Elicited by Immunofluorescence Microscopy in HEp-2 Cells

The HEp-2 human larynx epithelioma cancer cell line is used in most reference laboratories.[18,19] Six main patterns of fluorescence may be recognized[20–23]:

- Homogeneous nucleoplasmic with a homogeneous pattern of chromosomes in dividing cells (**Image 13-1**), suggesting the presence of histone or dsDNA autoantibodies.
- Peripheral nuclear, seen with autoantibodies to nuclear membrane proteins (eg, lamins)[23–29] or proteins of the pore complex (eg, gp210).[30,31]
- Speckled nuclear, with autoantibodies targeting nonhistone antigens. Several distinct speckled patterns may be observed: autoantibodies to Sm (**Image 13-2**) and uridine-rich ribonucleoprotein (U_1RNP) (**Image 13-3**) show coarse speckles; anti–Sjögren's syndrome-A/Ro (anti–SS-A/Ro) and anti–SS-B/La show fine speckles. The possibilities in this regard are manifold, including distinct speckles varying in number, seen with anti–p80-coilin, or anti-p95, an antigen commonly seen in primary biliary cirrhosis.[32]
- Homogeneous, granular, or clumpy nucleolar specificities mostly seen in patients with scleroderma or overlap syndromes with scleroderma features: anti–Scl-70 (**Image 13-4**), PM-Scl (**Image 13-5**), fibrillarin, NOR-90, and RNA polymerase I.[8,10,33–35]
- Centromeric, seen with antibodies in the CREST (calcinosis, Raynaud's phenomenon, esophageal dysfunction, sclerodactyly, and telangiectasia) syndrome (limited systemic sclerosis) and in primary biliary cirrhosis.[9,27,29,34,36–39]
- Different cytoplasmic staining patterns (**Images 13-6** to **13-8**).[21,22,40–44]

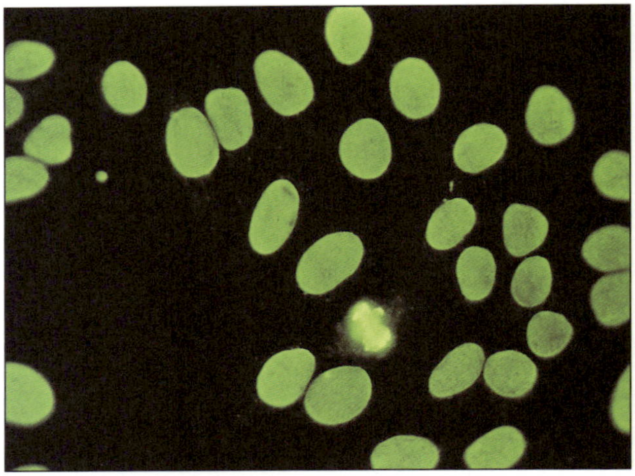

Image 13-1. Homogeneous nuclear pattern in HEp-2 cells caused by antihistone antibodies.

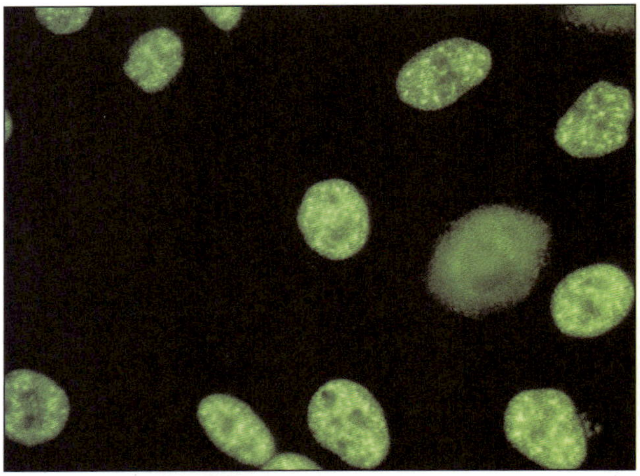

Image 13-2. Coarse granular nuclear pattern with Sm antibodies. Note the negative dividing cell.

Antinuclear Antibody Testing in Normal People and in Other Clinical Situations

It is important to note that normal individuals,[45–51] as well as patients with many nonrheumatic conditions,[14,52–55] such as chronic liver diseases, many neoplasms, or active infections, may exhibit similar autoantibodies. They are generally in lower titers than the specificities detected in patients with autoimmune diseases. Also, low titers of autoantibodies may frequently precede the onset of overt clinical disease in asymptomatic individuals by many years.[55] The diagnostic value of any autoantibody determination directly depends on the clinical presentation of the patient and should be considered only in the context of other clinical and physical findings.[14,15]

Specific Tests for Autoantibodies

Enzyme-linked immunosorbent assay, immunoblot, immunoprecipitation, and radioimmunoassay methods use primary antigen-antibody binding reactions and, because of their high sensitivity, are preferred for the detection of circulating and tissue-bound antibodies and antigens. Tests that involve secondary antigen-antibody preparations, such as

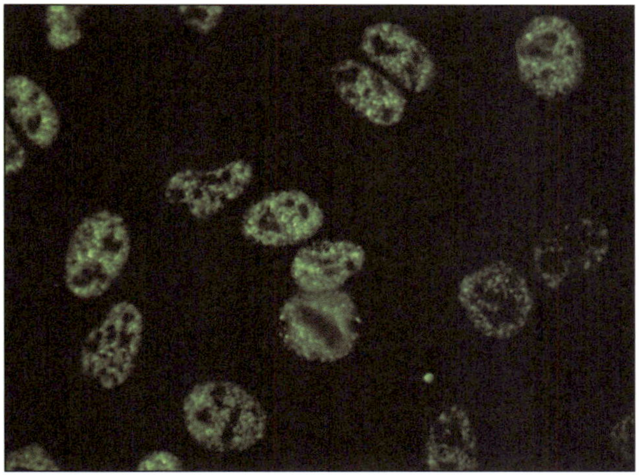

Image 13-3. Coarse granular nuclear pattern with U_1RNP antibodies.

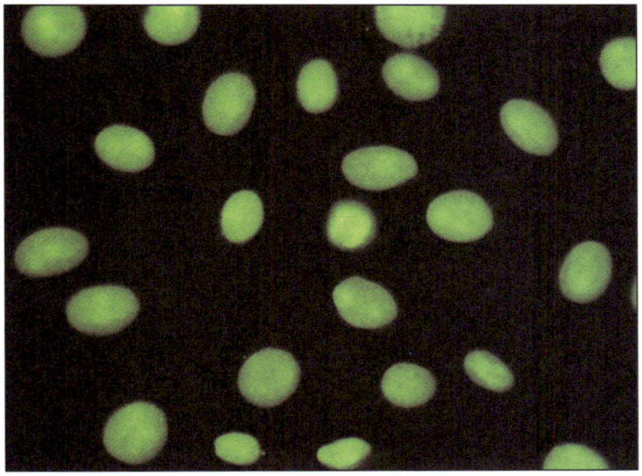

Image 13-4. Faint nucleolar staining and homogeneous nuclear pattern caused by anti–Scl-70 antibodies.

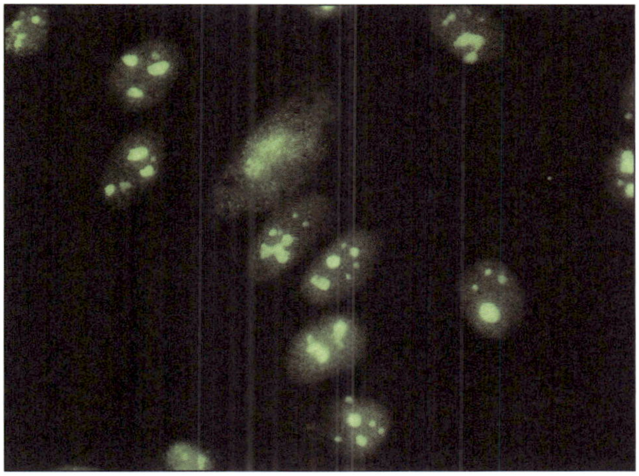

Image 13-5. Strong homogeneous nucleolar staining with PM-Scl antibodies.

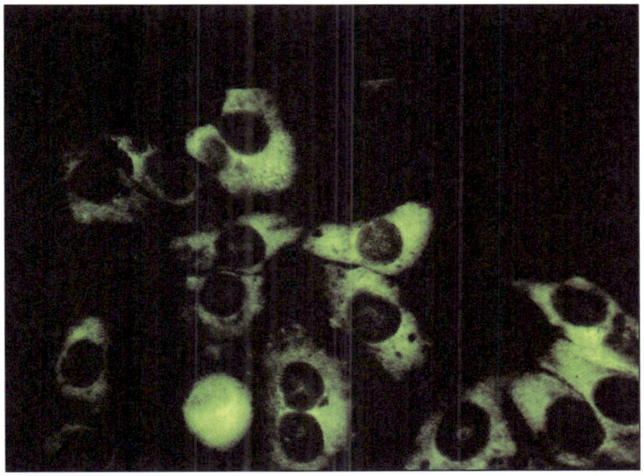

Image 13-6. Homogeneous cytoplasmic pattern with rRNP antibodies.

complement fixation, agglutination, and precipitation in agar gel, may not be as sensitive as immunofluorescence or radioimmunoassay in some circumstances, but may be more technically suitable for the specific identification of certain autoantibodies.[56]

New ELISA kits claiming to detect a variety of autoantibodies are being released for autoantibody screening. However, it is technically impossible at this time to have "total" fractions of ANAs in these preparations, so they are not 100% sensitive for the screening of ANAs when compared with fluorescence microscopy with HEp-2 cells. Furthermore, they cannot detect certain autoantibodies (eg, proliferating-cell nuclear antigen or NuMA) with either atypical or classical fluorescence patterns. After screening with such reagents, it is recommended that results be reported stating that autoantibodies to specific antigens contained in the test (eg, SS-A/Ro, Scl-70, U_1RNP) were not detected. Only then will the clinician be aware that a negative result by this technique does not imply "negative for all ANAs." One publication stressed the marginal agreement between ANA testing by immunofluorescence and by 6 different commercial ELISAs.[57]

Immunoblotting

The immunoblot assay allows specific characterization of many autoantibody systems. Proteins from cultured cells are separated by gel electrophoresis,[58,59] and then electrotransferred to nitrocellulose paper, a solid support for antigens. The paper is cut in strips,

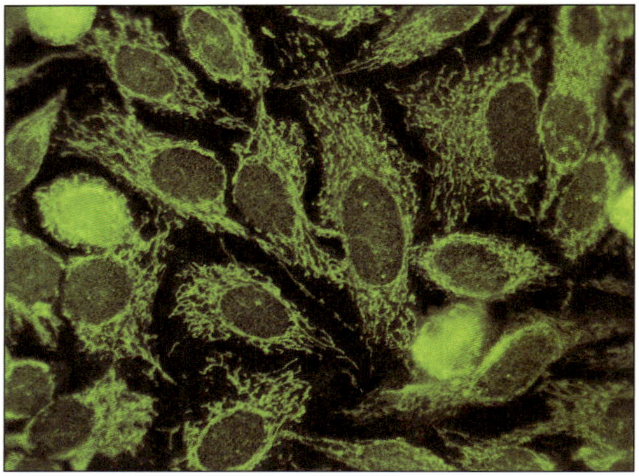

Image 13-7. A reticular cytoplasmic pattern indicating mitochondrial antibodies.

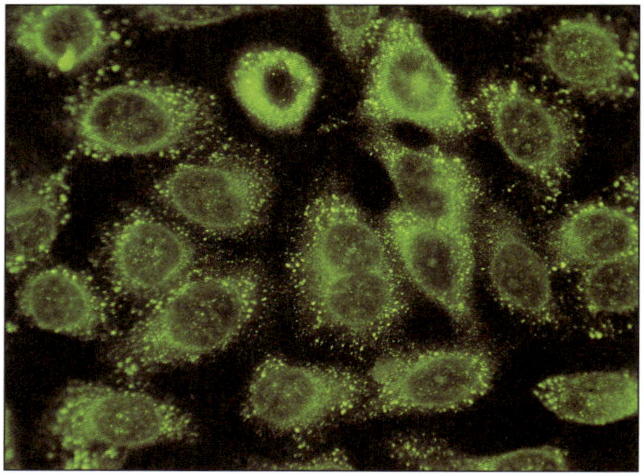

Image 13-8. Multiple cytoplasmic dots recognized by Jo-1 antibody-positive serum.

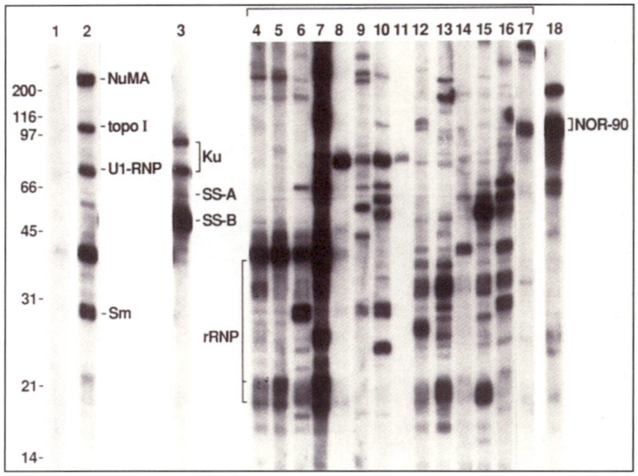

Image 13-9. Western blot showing heterogeneous reaction from juvenile SLE sera (lanes 4 to 18). Lane 1 = negative control; lanes 2 and 3 = autoantibody-positive controls identified by their cognate antigen names.

and each strip is incubated with a proband serum. Many methods may be used for detecting a positive reaction, including a radiolabeled probe, most commonly ^{125}iodine–protein A incubation[60] followed by autoradiography[61]; a colorimetric method with enzymes, such as alkaline phosphatase or horseradish peroxidase, acting on their chromo-genic substrates and giving visible colors; or chemiluminescence reaction.[62] Molecular markers and controls should be used in each assay procedure (**Image 13-9**).

Sjögren's Syndrome

Sjögren's syndrome is an autoimmune exocrinopathy, characterized by polyarthritis, purpura, and sicca symptoms—xerophthalmia and xerostomia.[63] More than 90% of affected patients exhibit autoantibodies targeting SS-A/Ro and/or SS-B/La, and high-titer immunoglobulin (Ig) M rheumatoid factor is commonly observed.[15,16,64,65] The most important tests to be applied in Sjögren's syndrome sera are indirect immunofluorescence in HEp-2 cells, immunoblot, double immunodiffusion, or ELISA.

The immune response to SS-B/La appears to be linked to the one directed to SS-A/Ro, so if anti–SS-B/La is positive, both autoantibodies appear together in patients with primary Sjögren's syndrome. Nevertheless, SS-A/Ro antibodies are commonly observed without anti–SS-B/La. Both systems of autoantibodies are clinically associated with an increased frequency of purpura, hypergammaglobulinemia, severe salivary gland dysfunction, parotid swelling, high titers of rheumatoid factor, lymphopenia, and leukopenia.[16,66]

No more than 4% of patients with primary Sjögren's syndrome have p80-coilin autoantibodies, a specificity infrequently seen in patients with SLE or primary biliary cirrhosis. Antibodies to p80-coilin have been described with a characteristic staining pattern of distinct nuclear speckles in HEp-2 cells. The 80-kd band is evident in many immunoblot preparations using whole cell lysates.[67,68]

The diagnosis of primary Sjögren's syndrome is best achieved with a constellation of tests. Classification criteria were defined in 1993 for patients who enter scientific research.[1] The oral component is best evaluated with salivary gland scintigraphy and biopsy of the accessory labial salivary glands.[69–71] Salivary gland scintigraphy is a quantitative method, comparing radioisotope scintillation over the parotid and submandibular glands with that over the thyroid gland after intravenous injection of technetium Tc 99m.[72,73] Lower concentration over the salivary glands is proportional to lymphocyte infiltration and inflammatory parenchyma destruction. Toward the end of the procedure a final challenge is normally executed: the patient swallows some citric juice to stimulate saliva flow into the oral cavity. Reduced scintillation within the mouth is observed in patients with Sjögren's syndrome. Biopsy of the parotid glands is almost never performed due to the risk of facial nerve sectioning. A reasonable alternative is to biopsy the sublingual or lower lip small accessory salivary glands under local anesthesia.[70,74]

The overall performance of this test is less than optimal. The authors have been using Saxon's test[75–77] for screening. In Saxon's test, the patient chews 4 preweighted sterilized gauzes for 2 minutes without swallowing any saliva; the final weight of the gauzes is then measured. A difference greater than 1.6 g from pretest values is considered normal saliva production for patients younger than 60 years. For older people, the cutoff is 0.7 g,[78] because there is a physiologic reduction in salivary gland function with advancing age.

The ocular component of Sjögren's syndrome may be readily evaluated by 3 standard procedures normally conducted by an ophthalmologist—Schirmer's test, tear breakup time, and the rose bengal dye test of the corneal surface.[79] Schirmer's test uses 2 strips of filter paper placed inside the lower eyelid of both eyes for 5 minutes. Wetting of more than 10 mm is considered normal, between 5 and 10 mm is borderline, and less than 5 mm is abnormal. An abnormal test suggests abnormal function of the lacrimal glands. The time necessary for the lacrimal film over the cornea to break up after blinking may be measured in seconds. A quick breakup time indicates loss of protein substances in the lacrimal fluid due to lacrimal gland dysfunction. Punctate pigmentation of the corneal surface may be observed with a slit lamp after application of a drop of rose bengal dye to each eye, when a loss of tears has led to corneal erosions.

Polymyositis and Dermatomyositis

Polymyositis is an autoimmune condition leading to inflammatory changes of the striated muscle cells, sometimes associated with skin erythema (dermatomyositis).[80–82] Negative results from indirect immunofluorescence with HEp-2 cells as substrate may occur in many sera from patients with inflammatory muscle disease. This screening test may not be useful for these patients, as it is for the diagnosis of other diffuse connective tissue diseases. Antibodies to tRNA synthetases have been described[6,7,83–88] and are considered a hallmark of polymyositis. Unfortunately, the demonstration of their presence may be achieved only by using more elaborate tests, such as immunoblot or immunoprecipitation. The tRNA synthetases are a group of cytoplasmic enzymes responsible for the complexing of each amino acid to its cognate tRNA: histidyl (Jo-1), threonyl (PL-7), alanyl (PL-12), isoleucyl (OJ), and glycyl (EJ). The prevalence of antisynthetase antibodies may be as high as 37% in patients with autoimmune muscle inflammatory disease.[83]

Many commercial vendors offer an ELISA for Jo-1 antibodies. Autoantibodies targeting Jo-1, previously known as PM-1, characterize a syndrome of polymyositis with lung fibrosis and poor response to corticosteroid treatment[7,89]; therefore, they are considered the most important synthetase autoantibodies to be detected in this particular disease (sensitivity = 20% to 40%, specificity > 95%). The Jo-1 autoantibody is clinically useful in the differential diagnosis and follow-up of patients with polymyositis, sometimes appearing even before the onset of interstitial lung disease.

Other autoantibodies described in polymyositis patients may also characterize distinct subgroups of the disease. Antibodies to signal recognition particle (SRP) are seen in adult black women with polymyositis who have severe myositis and/or a rapid onset of muscle symptoms; no cutaneous features; low frequency of either interstitial lung disease, arthritis, or Raynaud's phenomenon; and no clinical overlap with other diffuse connective tissue diseases.[83,90] KJ and other antisynthetase autoantibodies identify this same clinical group of patients.[88] Mi-2 antibodies are mainly found in adult (22%) and pediatric (14%) dermatomyositis patients, in patients with overlap syndromes with dermatomyositis, or in those who have malignancy with myositis. The Mi-2 specificity is considered the most significant marker autoantibody for dermatomyositis at this time.[7,91–93]

Classification criteria have been developed for polymyositis and dermatomyositis.[81] The diagnosis is achieved by using 3 different tests: neurophysiologic studies, serum enzymes, and muscle biopsy. The most characteristic patient has proximal weakness in the extremities, high serum levels of creatine phosphokinase and lactic dehydrogenase (sometimes aldolase is also elevated), and a distinct pattern of short positive waves in the neurophysiologic study. It is very important to keep in mind that many other diseases may cause similar clinical and laboratory presentation,[94] so a differential diagnosis that includes infections and metabolic and paraneoplastic disturbances is essential. A pathologic specimen should be obtained from an affected muscle, stained with hematoxylin and eosin, and sent for histochemical analyses. The histologic examination and analyses may help elicit metabolic conditions caused by defective transport mechanisms in the mitochondria,[95–97] a group of diseases with clinical findings similar to polymyositis.

Scleroderma

Scleroderma (systemic sclerosis) is a disease of unknown origin affecting the dermis with abnormal proliferation of collagen and affecting internal organs, such as the esophagus, lungs, and kidneys. Classification criteria for scleroderma were developed and tested many years ago.[2] Raynaud's phenomenon, although present in more than 90% of affected patients, may not be considered a criterion for diagnosis due to lack of specificity. Autoantibodies may be detected in more than 95% of patients with scleroderma.[10] The most useful tests for screening scleroderma sera are immunofluorescence with HEp-2 cells, immunoblot, double immunodiffusion, and ELISA. Immunoprecipitation is essential for the detection of autoantibodies targeting the RNA polymerases.

Testing for ANAs with HEp-2 cells is very important in patients with suspected scleroderma.[98] Most commonly observed are the centromeric and nucleolar patterns. Centromeres are positive in the majority (50% to 70%) of patients with the limited form of the disease, sometimes called CREST syndrome. Centromere antibodies characterize a group of patients with better prognosis and less systemic involvement.[10,15,99–101] Other clinical associations with centromere antibodies are with joint pain, Raynaud's phenomenon, telangiectasia, lung involvement, and a significantly young age at disease onset. Anticentromere antibodies may also be seen in primary biliary cirrhosis,[29,39,102] and in rare instances other patients may test positive with either indirect immunofluorescence or immunoblot. Positive results in low titers have been reported in patients with isolated pulmonary hypertension, SLE, primary Sjögren's syndrome, or undifferentiated connective tissue disease with Raynaud's phenomenon.[14,16] In female blood donors without apparent disease, the frequency was less than 0.1%.[47] In immunoblot assays of whole-cell extracts, 3 bands may be detected: 16 kd (CENP-A), 80 kd (CENP-B), and 120 kd (CENP-C). Centromere autoantibodies may be present in patients with Raynaud's phenomenon before full clinical development of the disease.

Autoantibodies recognizing nucleolar structures target many different autoantigens, from anti–Scl-70 (anti–topoisomerase I) to antifibrillarin, among many others.[103] Anti–topoisomerase I antibodies may be detected readily by immunoblot, with a characteristic band around 95 to 100 kd, or by ELISA. They characterize a subgroup of scleroderma patients with bad prognosis due to progressive systemic involvement.[34,36,104] These patients present with widespread skin involvement, so they are said to have the diffuse form of the disease. They tend to have more urgent and earlier organic manifestations, such as renal crisis, interstitial lung disease, and intestinal involvement. Anti–topoisomerase I autoantibodies may be present in patients with Raynaud's phenomenon before the full development of scleroderma, so the test may be very useful in early diagnosis.

It may be important to detect other autoantibody systems, in particular subsets of scleroderma. Antibodies to fibrillarin (U_3snRNP) are seen in no other diffuse connective tissue disease and are mostly observed in young men with scleroderma and a lower frequency of joint involvement.[10,33,34,105,106] The autoantibodies are frequent in black patients with diffuse cutaneous systemic sclerosis and a higher frequency of skeletal muscle and small bowel involvement. The characteristic pattern in HEp-2 cells is that of clumpy nucleolar staining. Autoantibodies to the RNA polymerases I and II (sensitivity = 24% and 5%, respectively; specificity = 100%) and III (sensitivity = 45% in diffuse scleroderma, 6% in limited scleroderma; specificity = 100%)[98,107] tend to occur together in the same patient and identify individuals with diffuse cutaneous disease. A high prevalence of internal organ involvement, mainly heart and kidney, with renal crisis, seems to be responsible for the poor survival rate in these patients. Other clinical characteristics in this subset of scleroderma are a predominance in men, older age at onset, less cutaneous vasculitis, and a lower frequency of lung fibrosis.

Because more than 90% of patients with scleroderma have esophageal motor disturbances and more than 50% have lung fibrosis, it is recommended that the diagnostic workup begin with lung radiographs or computerized tomography, as well as with a scintigraphic study of esophageal function.[108] The distal two thirds of the esophagus are dilated, with cardiac valve incompetence leading to reflux of stomach contents. Barium study of the esophageal transit is too insensitive, especially in the first years of the disease. Esophageal manometry may be an alternative, but costs and poor patient tolerance are major concerns.

A useful test for scleroderma is nailfold capillary microscopy, in which a distinct pattern may be observed.[99,109,110] Typical findings of the "SD pattern" (standing for scleroderma, or scleroderma-dermatomyositis) are vast disorganization of the capillary architecture, megacapillaries, deletion areas, and multiple hemorrhages. This test is positive even in the early stages of the disease. The SD pattern is not specific, however; it has also been observed in patients with mixed connective tissue disease and dermatomyositis.

A skin biopsy is performed rarely, primarily in patients with less severe sclerodermatous skin involvement or in the early stages of disease in which systemic involvement is not characteristic. *Scleroderma sine scleroderma* is a rare presentation, in which the patient has Raynaud's phenomenon and systemic disease without skin involvement. This condition can only be recognized by the characteristics of the systemic disease (eg, esophageal involvement) and the results of immunofluorescent ANA screening and specific autoantibody detection.

Mixed Connective Tissue Disease and Other Overlap Syndromes

Patients often present with symptoms caused by the joint occurrence of more than one diffuse connective tissue disease.[111–115] Terms such as RUPUS (rheumatoid arthritis and systemic lupus erythematosus), LUPODERMA (systemic lupus erythematosus and scleroderma), and mixed connective tissue disease are used to diagnose such conditions. In the latter disease, patients characteristically have signs and symptoms of at least 2 different diffuse connective tissue diseases, as well as high titers of U_1RNP antibodies.[4] These autoantibodies elicit a coarse granular nucleoplasmic pattern in HEp-2 cells and may be further and specifically tested using ELISA, immunoblot, or double immunodiffusion.

The diagnostic workup for patients with mixed connective tissue disease is entirely dependent on the clinical presentation. For example, if clinical findings of SLE are present, one must order tests for dsDNA and Sm antibodies and serum complement factors, and look for systemic disease. If sicca symptoms are a concern, the diagnostic workup should include tests for Sjögren's syndrome as delineated earlier. When chronic synovitis is seen, a workup for rheumatoid arthritis would include hand and feet radiographs, testing for rheumatoid factor of IgM or other isotypes, and a test for the antiperinuclear factor.[116] Associated proximal weakness signals polymyositis, and tests should be ordered accordingly.

Some autoantibodies have been characteristically described in subgroups of patients with overlapping syndromes. PM-Scl antibodies give a characteristic pattern of strong homogeneous nucleolar fluorescence on a weak homogeneous nucleoplasmic staining in HEp-2 cells. They typically occur in the overlap syndrome of polymyositis and scleroderma (25% of patients) but also in polymyositis (8% to 12% of patients) and scleroderma alone (2% to 5% of patients).[8,9,11,117] In Japanese patients, Ku antibodies (p70/p80) are considered markers for the PM-Scl overlap (sensitivity = 26%; specificity = 99%).[83,118] In the authors' experience, autoantibody to Ku was found in 10% of sera from more than 200 SLE sera, but in 0% of 100 scleroderma and overlap syndrome patients. Ki and U_1RNP are other autoantibodies that may be detected in patients with an overlap syndrome of polymyositis and scleroderma (up to 19% and 13%, respectively).

Autoantibodies With Cytoplasmic Patterns and Their Clinical Associations

Electron microscopy distinguishes 3 major classes of cytoplasmic fibers:

- Microtubules (25 nm in diameter; represented by tubulin, mitotic-associated proteins, and Tau protein)
- Intermediate filaments (10 nm in diameter; with proteins such as cytokeratins, neurofilaments, desmin, vimentin, and lamins)
- Microfilaments (6 nm in diameter; eg, actin)

The dense network of these fibers is resistant to standard detergent treatment used to extract the membrane and soluble cytoplasmic components and is therefore referred to as the cytoskeleton. The functions of these filaments are manifold; they play roles in structural support, cell division, force generation and movement, and uptake of materials from outside the cell.[119]

Anticytoskeletal antibodies in human sera have been described in a variety of conditions, carrying no clinical specificity. The following is a partial list of recognized specificities:

- Actin in long-term hemodialysis (18%), chronic active hepatitis (52%), primary biliary cirrhosis (44%), normal human sera (5%), myasthenia gravis, viral infections, cardiovascular diseases, and Crohn's disease (48%)[48,120–129]
- α-Actinin in some patients with myasthenia gravis[123]
- Desmin in long-term hemodialysis (28%), primary biliary cirrhosis (41%), Waldenström's macroglobulinemia, Crohn's disease (15%), cardiomyopathy in *Trypanosoma cruzi*–infected mice, and chronic active hepatitis (43%)[122,127,130]
- Keratin in alcoholic liver disease (69%), rheumatoid arthritis (18% to 46%, associated with high-titer rheumatoid factor), Sjögren's syndrome (64%), SLE (50%), Waldenström's macroglobulinemia, schistosomiasis, long-term hemodialysis (51%), chronic active hepatitis, squamous cell carcinoma of the esophagus, and Crohn's disease (20%)[126,127,131–133]
- Neurofilaments (205 kd and 160 kd) in SLE associated with neuropsychiatric manifestations [43,119,134]
- Tropomyosin in long-term hemodialysis (13%), chronic active hepatitis (34%), primary biliary cirrhosis (35%), Crohn's disease (5%), ulcerative colitis (95%), and normal human sera (5%)
- Troponin in chronic active hepatitis (11%), primary biliary cirrhosis (18%), and normal human sera (5%)[122,135]
- Tubulin in chronic active hepatitis (35%), primary biliary cirrhosis (55%), and normal human sera (5%)[47,121,127]
- Myosin (nonmuscle isoform) in myasthenia gravis and hepatitis C virus–associated chronic active hepatitis; skeletal muscle isoform in primary biliary cirrhosis (56%), myasthenia gravis, and chronic active hepatitis (31%); and cardiac muscle isoform in coxsackie viral pericarditis [123–126,136–147]
- Vinculin (140 kd) in normal human sera[49]
- Vimentin in normal human sera (9%), long-term hemodialysis (15%), Crohn's disease (17%), Sjögren's syndrome (43%), rheumatoid arthritis, scleroderma, mixed connective tissue disease, angioimmunoblastic lymphadenopathy, human immunodeficiency virus infection, schistosomiasis, Waldenström's macroglobulinemia, SLE (53%), primary biliary cirrhosis (35%), and chronic active hepatitis (23%)[42,122,127,148]

Table 13-2 shows the classification of cytoplasmic patterns currently used in reporting results, as well as the antigens recognized by autoantibodies and their clinical associations.

Summary

Systemic rheumatic diseases have distinct profiles of autoantibodies, which include the presence or absence of certain specificities, as well as differences in their mean titers.[12] The presence of autoantibodies may confirm the suspected disease; allow clinicians to monitor disease activity, severity, and response to therapy; and classify a patient in a better or worse prognostic subgroup.

Immunofluorescence microscopy is the standard screening test used for detecting ANAs in diffuse connective tissue diseases. The selection of further tests depends heavily on clinical findings and immunofluorescence results. Methods such as immunoblot, ELISA, counterimmune electrophoresis, double immunodiffusion, and immunoprecipitation should be used to confirm positive ANA findings.

Multiple autoantibodies are frequently seen in SLE; an average of 3 different specificities is typical. Sm and dsDNA autoantibodies are considered specific for diagnosing SLE, whereas drug-induced SLE characteristically presents histone or chromatin antibodies. Antibodies to U_1RNP are not specific; they may be detected in several rheumatic diseases in different average titers and frequencies. They are marker antibodies for mixed connective tissue disease. Sjögren's syndrome is serologically characterized by the presence of SS-A/Ro and SS-B/La autoantibodies, which are associated with more severe clinical manifestations. The 2 subgroups of scleroderma patients have distinct autoantibody profiles: centromere/kinetochore antibodies are typical for the more protracted and benign CREST

Table 13-2. Cytoplasmic Patterns in Indirect Immunofluorescence[15]

Cytoplasmic Patterns in Immunofluorescence (Cell Substrate)	Representative Antigens	Disease and Clinical Associations
Fibrous		
Stress fibers: linear cytoskeletal fibers, sometimes with small, discontinuous granular deposits (HEp-2, fibroblasts)	Actin Nonmuscle myosin	Both present in chronic active hepatitis, liver cirrhosis, and myasthenia gravis; actin present in autoimmune hepatitis, Crohn's disease, PEC, long-term hemodialysis, NHS, and DCTD (rare)
Filamentous: filaments and fibrils spreading out from the nuclear rim (HEp-2, PtK2 epithelial cells)	Vimentin Keratin	Antivimentin (often caused by cross-reaction with anti-α helix antibodies) detected in many infectious/inflammatory conditions, long-term hemodialysis, and DCTD (rare); both seen in NHS; keratin is major system in ALD (69%), also common in DCTD and psoriasis
Segmental: fluorescence of small fiber segments (periodic dense bodies) (HEp-2, fibroblasts)	α-Actinin, vinculin, tropomyosin	Present in myasthenia gravis, Crohn's disease, and ulcerative colitis
Speckled		
Fine speckled: scattered small speckles, mostly with homogeneous or dense fine speckled background (HEp-2)	Many aminoacyl-tRNA synthetases, mainly Jo-1	Detected in PM; "Jo-1 syndrome" (myositis and interstitial lung disease)
Dense fine speckled: cloudy, almost homogeneous throughout the cytoplasm (HEp-2)	rRNP, ribosomal phosphoproteins	Seen in neuropsychiatric SLE
Granular pole: perinuclear, arrow-shaped, coarse granular, corresponding to the lamellar stacks of the Golgi complex (HEp-2)	Golgi apparatus	Rare in SLE, Sjögren's syndrome, and other systemic rheumatic diseases; reported in idiopathic cerebellar ataxia, paraneoplastic cerebellar degeneration, and viral infections (including EBV and HIV)
Coarse reticular: coarse diffuse reticular and granular (HEp-2)	Proteins in the inner mitochondrial membrane	Found in PBC and scleroderma (43%); rare in other DCTDs; frequently associated with centromere antibodies
Scattered small speckled: countable cytoplasmic speckles irregularly distributed (HEp-2)	Lysosomes or peroxisomes	None recognized
Fine reticular: fine diffuse reticular and granular (HEp-2)	Endoplasmic reticulum and unknown proteins	CLD; detected in all types of (chronic) inflammatory conditions

Abbreviations: PBC = primary biliary cirrhosis; NHS = normal human serum; DCTD = diffuse connective tissue diseases; ALD = alcoholic liver disease; PM = polymyositis; rRNP = ribosomal ribonucleoprotein; SLE = systemic lupus erythematosus; EBV = Epstein-Barr virus; HIV = human immunodeficiency virus; CLD = chronic liver diseases.

syndrome, and topoisomerase I/Scl-70 antibodies are indicative of the more severe diffuse form. Anticytoskeletal antibodies have been described in a variety of conditions, ranging from acute infections to autoimmune diseases and cancer, but carry no clinical specificity.

References

1. Vitali C, Bombardieri S, Moutsopoulos HM, et al. Preliminary criteria for the classification of Sjögren's syndrome: Results of a prospective concerted action supported by the European Community. *Arthritis Rheum.* 1993;36:340–347.

2. Masi AT, Rodnan GP, Medsger TA, et al. Preliminary criteria for the classification of systemic sclerosis (scleroderma). *Arthritis Rheum*. 1980;23:581–590.

3. Alarcón-Segovia D, Cardiel MH. Comparison between 3 diagnostic criteria for mixed connective tissue disease: Study of 593 patients. *J Rheumatol*. 1989;16:328–334.

4. Kasukawa R, Tojo T, Miyawaki S, et al. Preliminary diagnostic criteria for classification of mixed connective tissue disease. In: Kasukawa R, Sharp GC, eds. *Mixed Connective Tissue Disease and Anti-Nuclear Antibodies*. New York, NY: Excerpta Medica; 1987:41–47.

5. Weinstein A, Bordwell B, Stone B, et al. Antibodies to native DNA and serum complement (C3) levels: Application to diagnosis and classification of systemic lupus erythematosus. *Am J Med*. 1983;74:206–216.

6. Plotz P, Targoff I. Myositis-associated antigens: Aminoacyl-tRNA synthetases Jo-1, PL-7, PL-12, EJ and OJ. In: van Venrooij WJ, Maini RN, eds. *Manual of Biological Markers of Disease*. Dordrecht, the Netherlands: Kluwer Academic Publishers; 1994:B6.1/1–B6.1/18.

7. Targoff IN. Autoantibodies associated with polymyositis and dermatomyositis. *Clin Aspects Autoimmun*. 1993;5:5–18.

8. Oddis CV, Okano Y, Rudert WA, et al. Serum autoantibody to the nucleolar antigen PM-Scl: Clinical and immunogenetic associations. *Arthritis Rheum*. 1992;35:1211–1217.

9. Genth E, Mierau R, Genetzky P, et al. Immunogenetic associations of scleroderma-related antinuclear antibodies. *Arthritis Rheum*. 1990;33:657–665.

10. Fritzler MJ. Autoantibodies in scleroderma. *J Dermatol*. 1993;20:257–268.

11. Marguerie C, Bunn CC, Copier J, et al. The clinical and immunogenetic features of patients with autoantibodies to the nucleolar antigen PM-Scl. *Medicine*. 1992;71:327–336.

12. Nakamura RM, Tan EM. Recent advances in laboratory tests and the significance of autoantibodies to nuclear antigens in systemic rheumatic diseases. *Clin Lab Med*. 1986;6:41–53.

13. Hang LM, Nakamura RM. Current concepts and advances in clinical laboratory testing for autoimmune diseases. *Crit Rev Clin Lab Sci*. 1997;34:275–311.

14. Krapf A, von Mühlen CA, Krapf F, et al. *Atlas of Immunofluorescent Antibodies*. Munich, Germany: Urban & Schwarzenberg; 1996:1–286.

15. von Mühlen CA, Tan EM. Autoantibody specificities in autoimmune rheumatic diseases. *Rev Bras Rheumatol*. 1994;34:173–194.

16. von Mühlen CA, Tan EM. Autoantibodies in the diagnosis of systemic rheumatic diseases. *Semin Arthritis Rheum*. 1995;24:323–358.

17. Nakamura RM, Ivor L, Hannon WH, et al. *Quality Assurance for the Indirect Immunofluorescence Test for Autoantibodies to Nuclear Antigen (IF-ANA); Approved Guideline*. 1996;I/LA2-A:1–24. [Abstract]

18. Toolan HW. Transplantable human neoplasms maintained in cortisone-treated laboratory animals: H.S.#1; H.Ep.#1; H.Ep.#2; H.Ep.#3; and H.Emb.Rh.#1. *Cancer Res*. 1954;14:660–666.

19. Moore AE, Sabachewsky L, Toolan HW. Culture characteristics of four permanent lines of human cancer cells. *Cancer Res*. 1955;15:598–602.

20. Cavallaro JJ, McDuffie FC, Byrd MG. Indirect immunofluorescence antinuclear antibody test. In: Cavallaro JJ, McDuffie FC, Byrd MG, et al. *Laboratory Methods for the Detection of Antinuclear Antibodies*. Atlanta, GA: U.S. Department of Health and Human Services, Public Health Service, Centers for Disease Control, Training and Laboratory Program Office, Division of Training; 1987:7–31.

21. Oliver JM, Senecal J-L, Rothfield NL. Autoantibodies to the cytoskeleton in human sera. *Cell Muscle Motil*. 1985;6:55–74.

22. Senecal J, Oliver JM, Rothfield N. Anticytoskeletal autoantibodies in the connective tissue diseases. *Arthritis Rheum*. 1985;28:889–898.

23. Senecal J, Ichiki S, Girard D, et al. Autoantibodies to nuclear lamins and to intermediate filament proteins: Natural, pathologic or pathogenic? *J Rheumatol*. 1993;20:211–219.

24. Konstantinov KN, Halberg P, Wiik A, et al. Clinical manifestations in patients with autoantibodies specific for nuclear lamin proteins. *Clin Immunol Immunopathol*. 1992;62:112–118.

25. Lassoued K, Guilly M-N, Danon F, et al. Anti-nuclear autoantibodies specific for lamins: Characterization and clinical significance. *Ann Intern Med*. 1988;108:829–833.

26. Konstantinov KN, Galcheva-Gargova Z, Hoier-Madsen M, et al. Autoantibodies to lamins A and C in sera of patients showing peripheral fluorescent antinuclear antibody pattern on HEp-2 cells. *J Invest Dermatol*. 1990;95:304–308.

27. Nakamura RM, Bylund DJ. Diagnostic significance of autoantibodies in autoimmune chronic active hepatitis. *Clin Immunol News*. 1991;11:161–167.

28. Wesierska-Gadek J, Penner E, Hitchman E, et al. Antibodies to nuclear lamin proteins in liver disease. *Immunol Invest*. 1989;18:365–372.

29. Mackay IR, Rowley MJ, Whittingham SF. Nuclear autoantibodies in primary biliary cirrhosis. In: Meyer zum Büschenfelde K-H, Hoofnagle JH, Manns M, eds. *Immunology and Liver*. Dordrecht, the Netherlands: Kluwer Academic Publishers; 1993:397–409.

30. Nickowitz RE, Worman HJ. Autoantibodies from patients with primary biliary cirrhosis recognize a restricted region within the cytoplasmic tail of nuclear pore membrane glycoprotein Gp210. *J Exp Med.* 1993;178:2237–2242.

31. Courvalin J-C, Lassoued K, Bartnik E, et al. The 210-kD nuclear envelope polypeptide recognized by human autoantibodies in primary biliary cirrhosis is the major glycoprotein of the nuclear pore. *J Clin Invest.* 1990;86:279–285.

32. Evans J, Reuben A, Craft J. PBC 95K, a 95-kilodalton nuclear autoantigen in primary biliary cirrhosis. *Arthritis Rheum.* 1991;34:731–736.

33. Okano Y, Steen VD, Medsger TA Jr. Autoantibody to U3 nucleolar ribonucleoprotein (fibrillarin) in patients with systemic sclerosis. *Arthritis Rheum.* 1992;35:95–100.

34. Pollard KM, Reimer G, Tan EM. Autoantibodies in scleroderma. *Clin Exp Rheumatol.* 1989;7(suppl):57–62.

35. Rodrigues-Sanchez JL, Gelpi C, Juarez C, et al. Anti-NOR 90: A new autoantibody in scleroderma that recognizes a 90-kDa component of the nucleolus-organizing region of chromatin. *J Immunol.* 1987;139:2579–2584.

36. Reimer G, Steen VD, Penning CA, et al. Correlates between autoantibodies to nucleolar antigens and clinical features in patients with systemic sclerosis (scleroderma). *Arthritis Rheum.* 1988;31:525–532.

37. Moroi Y, Peebles C, Fritzler MJ, et al. Autoantibody to centromere (kinetochore) in scleroderma sera. *Proc Natl Acad Sci U S A.* 1980;77:1627–1631.

38. Tan EM. *Antibody Markers in Systemic Autoimmunity.* Summit, NJ: Ciba-Geigy Corporation; 1992:1–57.

39. Berg PA, Klein R. Autoantibodies in primary biliary cirrhosis. *Springer Semin Immunopathol.* 1990;12:85–99.

40. Deicher HRG, Holman HR, Kunkel HG. Anti-cytoplasmic factors in the sera of patients with systemic lupus erythematosus and certain other diseases. *Arthritis Rheum.* 1960;3:1–15.

41. Kurki P, Helve T, Virtanen I. Antibodies to cytoplasmic intermediate filaments in rheumatic diseases. *J Rheumatol.* 1983;10:558–562.

42. Alcover A, Molano J, Renart J, et al. Antibodies to vimentin intermediate filaments in sera from patients with systemic lupus erythematosus. *Arthritis Rheum.* 1984;27:922–928.

43. Senecal J, Rauch J. Hybridoma lupus autoantibodies can bind major cytoskeletal filaments in the absence of DNA-binding activity. *Arthritis Rheum.* 1988;31:864–875.

44. Robbins ML, Kornguth SE, Bell CL, et al. Antineurofilament antibody evaluation in neuropsychiatric systemic lupus erythematosus: Combination with anticardiolipin antibody assay and magnetic resonance imaging. *Arthritis Rheum.* 1988:31:623–631.

45. Jacobsson L, Hansen BU, Manthorpe R, et al. Association of dry eyes and dry mouth with anti-Ro/SS-A and anti-La/SS-B autoantibodies in normal adults. *Arthritis Rheum.* 1992;35:1492–1501.

46. Zarmbinski MA, Messner RP, Mandel JS. Anti-dsDNA antibodies in laboratory workers handling blood from patients with systemic lupus erythematosus. *J Rheumatol.* 1992;19:1380–1384.

47. Lee S-L, Tsay GJ, Tsai R-T. Anticentromere antibodies in subjects with no apparent connective tissue disease. *Ann Rheum Dis.* 1993;52:586–589.

48. Guilbert B, Dighiero G, Avrameas S. Naturally occurring antibodies against nine common antigens in human sera, I: Detection, isolation and characterization. *J Immunol.* 1982;128:2779–2787.

49. Pfueller SL, Logan D, Tran TT, et al. Naturally occurring human IgG antibodies to intracellular and cytoskeletal components of human platelets. *Clin Exp Immunol.* 1990;79:367–373.

50. Fritzler MJ, Pauls JD, Kinsella TD, et al. Antinuclear, anticytoplasmic, and anti-Sjögren's syndrome antigen A (SSA/Ro) antibodies in female blood donors. *Clin Immunol Immunopathol.* 1985;36:120–128.

51. Tan EM, Feltkamp TEW, Smolen JS, et al. Range of antinuclear antibodies in "healthy" individuals. *Arthritis Rheum.* 1997;40:1601–1611.

52. Tan EM. Antinuclear antibodies: Diagnostic markers for autoimmune diseases and probes for cell biology. *Adv Immunol.* 1989;44:93–151.

53. Nakamura RM, Tan EM. Update on autoantibodies to intracellular antigens in systemic rheumatic diseases. *Clin Lab Med.* 1992;12:1–23.

54. Imai H, Ochs RL, Kiyosawa K, et al. Nucleolar antigens and autoantibodies in hepatocellular carcinoma and other malignancies. *Am J Pathol.* 1992;140:859–870.

55. Imai H, Nakano Y, Kiyosawa K, et al. Increasing titers and changing specificities of antinuclear antibodies in patients with chronic liver disease who develop hepatocellular carcinoma. *Cancer.* 1993;71:26–35.

56. Aho K, Koskela P, Mäkitalo R, et al. Antinuclear antibodies heralding the onset of systemic lupus erythematosus. *J Rheumatol.* 1992;19:1377–1379.

57. Emlen W, O'Neill L. Clinical significance of antinuclear antibodies: Comparison of detection with immunofluorescence and enzyme-linked immunosorbent assays. *Arthritis Rheum.* 1997;40:1612–1618.

58. Chan EKL, Pollard KM. Autoantibodies to ribonucleoprotein particles by immunoblotting. In: Rose NR, de Macario EC, Fahey JL, et al, eds. *Manual of Clinical Laboratory Immunology.* 4th ed. Washington, DC: American Society for Microbiology; 1992:755–761.

59. Towbin H, Staehelin T, Gordon J. Electrophoretic transfer of proteins from polyacrylamide gels to nitrocellulose sheets: Procedure and some applications. *Proc Natl Acad Sci U S A.* 1979;76:4350–4354.

60. Kessler SW. Rapid isolation of antigens from cells with a staphylococcal protein A-antibody adsorbent: Parameters of the interaction of antibody-antigen complexes with protein A. *J Immunol.* 1975;115:1617–1624.

61. Voytas D. Commonly used biochemical techniques. In: Ausubel FM, Brent R, Kingston RE, et al, eds. *Current Protocols in Molecular Biology.* New York, NY: John Wiley & Sons; 1988:A.3.1.–A.3.3.

62. Thorpe GHG, Kricka LJ, Mosely SB, et al. Phenols as enhancers of the chemiluminescent horseradish peroxidase-luminol-hydrogen peroxide reaction: Application in luminescence-monitored enzyme immunoassays. *Clin Chem.* 1985;31:1335–1341.

63. Talal N. Sjögren's syndrome: Historical overview and clinical spectrum of disease. *Rheum Dis Clin North Am.* 1992;18:507–515.

64. Chan EKL, Andrade LEC. Antinuclear antibodies in Sjögren's syndrome. *Rheum Dis Clin North Am.* 1992;18:551–570.

65. Kater L, de Wilde PCM. New developments in Sjögren's syndrome. *Curr Opin Rheumatol.* 1992;4:657–665.

66. Tsuzaka K, Ogasawara T, Tojo T, et al. Relationship between autoantibodies and clinical parameters in Sjögren's syndrome. *Scand J Rheumatol.* 1993;22:1–9.

67. Andrade LEC, Chan EKL, Raska I, et al. Human autoantibody to a novel protein of the nuclear coiled body: Immunological characterization and cDNA cloning of p80-coilin. *J Exp Med.* 1991;173:1407–1419.

68. Carmo-Fonseca M, Bohmann K, Carvalho MT, et al. P80 coilin. In: van Venrooij WJ, Maini RN, eds. *Manual of Biological Markers of Disease.* Dordrecht, the Netherlands: Kluwer Academic Publishers; 1994:B8.2/1–B8.2/11.

69. Coll J, Porta M, Rubiés-Prat J, et al. Sjögren's syndrome: A stepwise approach to the use of diagnostic tests. *Ann Rheum Dis.* 1992;51:607–610.

70. Daniels TE, Fox PC. Salivary and oral components of Sjögren's syndrome. *Rheum Dis Clin North Am.* 1992;18:571–589.

71. Gerli R, Muscat C, Giansanti M, et al. Quantitative assessment of salivary gland inflammatory infiltration in primary Sjögren's syndrome: Its relationship to different demographic, clinical and serological features of the disorder. *Br J Rheumatol.* 1997;36:969–975.

72. Schall GL, Anderson LG, Wolf RO. Xerostomia in Sjögren's syndrome: Evaluation by sequential salivary scintigraphy. *JAMA.* 1972;216:2109–2116.

73. Fossaluzza V, de Vita S, Geatti O. Sequential salivary scintigraphy in Sjögren's syndrome: Proposal for a new method of evaluation. *Clin Exp Rheumatol.* 1990;8:469–474.

74. Pennec YL, Leroy JP, Jouquan J, et al. Comparison of labial and sublingual salivary gland biopsies in the diagnosis of Sjögren's syndrome. *Ann Rheum Dis.* 1990;49:37–39.

75. Kohler PF, Winter ME. A quantitative test for xerostomia: The Saxon test, an oral equivalent of Schirmer's test. *Arthritis Rheum.* 1985;28:1128–1132.

76. Laroche M, Arlet P, Authier JP, et al. Le test à la compresse, un examen facile pour diagnostiquer et évaluer la xérostomie. *Presse Med.* 1987;16:1704.

77. Moschner L, Genth E, Genth A, et al. Der Saxon-test: eine einfache Methode zur Messung der Speichelsekretion. *Med Welt.* 1990;41:325–331.

78. Trentin Filho FJ, Staub HL, von Mühlen CA, et al. Avaliaçao da secreçao salivar nao-estimulada em pacientes reumáticos com xerostomia pelo teste de Saxon. *Rev Bras Reumatol.* 1993;33:165–168.

79. Friedlaender MH. Ocular manifestations of Sjögren's syndrome: Keratoconjunctivitis sicca. *Rheum Dis Clin North Am.* 1992;18:591–608.

80. Bohan A, Peter JB. Polymyositis and dermatomyositis (second of two parts). *N Engl J Med.* 1975;292:403–407.

81. Bohan A, Peter JB. Polymyositis and dermatomyositis (first of two parts). *N Engl J Med.* 1975;292:344–347.

82. Heffner RR Jr. Inflammatory myopathies: A review. *J Neuropathol Exp Neurol.* 1993;52:339–350.

83. Hirakata M, Mimori T, Akizuki M, et al. Autoantibodies to small nuclear and cytoplasmic ribonucleoproteins in Japanese patients with inflammatory muscle disease. *Arthritis Rheum.* 1992;35:449–456.

84. Jenkins EA, Hull RG, Thomas AL. D-Penicillamine and polymyositis: The significance of the anti-Jo-1 antibody. *Br J Rheumatol.* 1993;32:1109–1110.

85. Mathews MB, Bernstein RM. Myositis autoantibody inhibits histidyl-tRNA synthetase. *Nature.* 1983;304:177–179.

86. Nishikai M, Reichlin M. Heterogeneity of precipitating antibodies in polymyositis: Characterization of the Jo-1 antibody system. *Arthritis Rheum.* 1980;23:881–888.

87. Okada N, Mukai R, Harada F, et al. Isolation of a novel antibody, which precipitates ribonucleoprotein complex containing threonine tRNA from a patient with polymyositis. *Eur J Biochem.* 1984;139:425–429.

88. Targoff IN, Arnett FC, Berman L, et al. Anti-KJ: A new antibody associated with the syndrome of polymyositis and interstitial lung disease. *J Clin Invest.* 1989;84:162–172.

89. Yoshida S, Akizuki M, Mimori T, et al. The precipitating antibody to an acidic nuclear protein antigen, the Jo-1, in connective tissue disease: A marker for a subset of polymyositis with interstitial pulmonary fibrosis. *Arthritis Rheum.* 1983;26:604–611.

90. Targoff IN, Johnson AE, Miller FW. Antibody to signal recognition particle in polymyositis. *Arthritis Rheum.* 1990;33:1361–1370.

91. Targoff IN, Reichlin M. The association between Mi-2 antibodies and dermatomyositis. *Arthritis Rheum.* 1985;28:796–803.

92. Mierau R, Dick T, Bartz-Bazzanella P, et al. Strong association of dermatomyositis-specific Mi-2 autoantibodies with a tryptophan at position 9 of the HLA-DR beta chain. *Arthritis Rheum.* 1996;39:868–876.

93. Targoff IN, Nilasena DS, Trieu EP, et al. Clinical features and immunologic testing of patients with anti-Mi-2 antibodies. *Arthritis Rheum.* 1990;33:S72. [Abstract]

94. Plotz PH, Dalakas M, Leff RL, et al. Current concepts in the idiopathic inflammatory myopathies: Polymyositis, dermatomyositis, and related disorders. *Ann Intern Med.* 1989:111:143–157.

95. Elliot DL, Buist NRM, Goldberg L, et al. Metabolic myopathies: Evaluation by graded exercise testing. *Medicine (Baltimore).* 1989;68:163–172.

96. Schapira AHV, Cooper JM, Morgan-Hughes JA, et al. Mitochondrial myopathy with a defect of mitochondrial-protein transport. *N Engl J Med.* 1990;323:37–42.

97. Hug G, Bove KE, Soukup S. Lethal neonatal multiorgan deficiency of carnitine palmitoyltransferase II. *N Engl J Med.* 1991;325:1862–1864.

98. Okano Y. Antinuclear antibodies in systemic sclerosis (scleroderma). *Rheum Dis Clin North Am.* 1996;22:709–735.

99. Belch JJF. The clinical assessment of the scleroderma spectrum disorders. *Br J Rheumatol.* 1993;32:353–356.

100. Reveille JD, Arnett FC. Frequencies of scleroderma-related autoantibodies in patients meeting the American College of Rheumatology criteria for systemic sclerosis: Reply. *Arthritis Rheum.* 1993;36: 1333–1334.

101. Vlachoyiannopoulos PG, Drosos AA, Wiik A, et al. Patients with anticentromere antibodies, clinical features, diagnoses and evolution. *Br J Rheumatol.* 1993;32:297–301.

102. Nishioka M. Nuclear antigens in autoimmune hepatitis. In: Meyer zum Büchenfelde K-H, Hoofnagle JH, Manns M, eds. *Immunology and Liver*. Dordrecht, the Netherlands: Kluwer Academic Publishers; 1993:193–205.

103. Weiner ES, Earnshaw WC, Senécal J-L, et al. Clinical associations of anticentromere antibodies and antibodies to topoisomerase I: A study of 355 patients. *Arthritis Rheum.* 1988;31:378–385.

104. Aeschlimann A, Meyer O, Bourgeois P, et al. Anti-Scl-70 antibodies detected by immunoblotting in progressive systemic sclerosis: Specificity and clinical correlations. *Ann Rheum Dis.* 1989;48:992–997.

105. Ochs RL, Lischwe MA, Spohn WH, et al. Fibrillarin: A new protein of the nucleolus identified by autoimmune sera. *Biol Cell.* 1985;54:123–134.

106. Kurzhals G, Meurer M, Krieg T, et al. Clinical association of autoantibodies to fibrillarin with diffuse scleroderma and disseminated telangiectasia. *J Am Acad Dermatol.* 1990;23:832–836.

107. Hirakata M, Okano Y, Pati U, et al. Identification of autoantibodies to RNA polymerase II: Occurrence in systemic sclerosis and association with autoantibodies to RNA polymerases I and III. *J Clin Invest.* 1993;91:2665–2672.

108. von Mühlen CA, Anselmi OE, Ludwig EB, et al. Szintigraphische Diagnostik der Ösophagusbeteiligung bei systemischer Sklerose (Sklerodermie). *Z Rheumatol.* 1989;48:167–174.

109. Rozboril MB, Maricq HR, Rodnan GP, et al. Capillary microscopy in eosinophilic fasciitis: A comparison with systemic sclerosis. *Arthritis Rheum.* 1983;26:617–622.

110. Maricq HR, Harper FE, Kahn MM, et al. Microvascular abnormalities as possible predictors of disease subsets in Raynaud's phenomenon and early connective tissue disease. *Clin Exp Rheumatol.* 1983;1:195–205.

111. Reichlin M, Maddison PJ, Targoff IN, et al. Antibodies to a nuclear/nucleolar antigen in patients with polymyositis-overlap syndrome. *J Clin Immunol.* 1984;4:40–44.

112. Lazaro MA, Cocco JAM, Catoggio LJ, et al. Clinical and serologic characteristics of patients with overlap syndrome: Is mixed connective tissue disease a distinct clinical entity? *Medicine (Baltimore).* 1989;68:58–65.

113. Maddison PJ. Mixed connective tissue disease, overlap syndromes, and eosinophilic fasciitis. *Ann Rheum Dis.* 1991;50:887–893.

114. Kallenberg CGM. Overlapping syndromes, undifferentiated connective tissue disease, and other fibrosing conditions. *Curr Opin Rheumatol.* 1993;5:809–815.

115. Sharp GC, Irvin WS, Tan EM, et al. Mixed connective tissue disease—An apparently distinct rheumatic disease syndrome associated with a specific antibody to an extractable nuclear antigen (ENA). *Am J Med.* 1972;52:148–159.

116. Feltkamp TEW, Berthelot JM, Boerbooms AMT, et al. Interlaboratory variability of the antiperinuclear factor (APF) test for rheumatoid arthritis. *Clin Exp Rheumatol.* 1993;11:57–59.

117. Wolfe JF, Adelstein E, Sharp GC. Antinuclear antibody with distinct specificity for polymyositis. *J Clin Invest.* 1977;59:176–178.

118. Mimori T, Akizuki M, Yamagata H, et al. Characterization of a high molecular weight acidic nuclear protein recognized by autoantibodies in sera from patients with polymyositis-scleroderma overlap. *J Clin Invest.* 1981;68:611–620.

119. Nagle RB. A review of intermediate filament biology and their use in pathologic diagnosis. *Mol Biol Rep.* 1994;19:3–21.

120. Farrow LJ, Holborow EJ, Brighton WD. Reaction of human smooth muscle antibody with liver cells. *Nat New Biol.* 1971;232:186–187.

121. Dighiero G, Guilbert B, Avrameas S. Naturally occurring antibodies against nine common antigens in human sera, II: High incidence of monoclonal Ig exhibiting antibody activity against actin and tubulin and sharing antibody specificities with natural antibodies. *J Immunol.* 1982;128:2788–2792.

122. Mayet WJ, Press AG, Hermann E, et al. Antibodies to cytoskeletal proteins in patients with Crohn's disease. *Eur J Clin Invest.* 1990;20:516–524.

123. Williams CL, Lennon VA. Thymic B lymphocyte clones from patients with myasthenia gravis secrete monoclonal striational autoantibodies reacting with myosin, alfa-actinin, or actin. *J Exp Med.* 1986;164:1043–1059.

124. de Scheerder I, Vandekerckhove J, Robbrecht J, et al. Post-cardiac injury syndrome and an increased humoral immune response against the major contractile proteins (actin and myosin). *Am J Cardiol.* 1985;56:631–633.

125. de Scheerder IK, de Buyzere M, de Langhe J, et al. Humoral immune response against contractile proteins (actin and myosin) during cardiovascular disease. *Eur Heart J.* 1991;12(suppl D):88–94.

126. Toh B-H. Anti-cytoskeletal autoantibodies: Diagnostic significance for liver diseases, infections and systemic autoimmune diseases. *Autoimmunity.* 1991;11:119–125.

127. Kurki P, Virtanen I. The detection of human antibodies against cytoskeletal components. *J Immunol Methods.* 1984;67:209–223.

128. Kurki P. Cytoskeleton antibodies in chronic active hepatitis. In: Meyer zum Büschenfelde K-H, Hoofnagle JH, Manns M, eds. *Immunology and Liver.* Dordrecht, the Netherlands: Kluwer Academic Publishers; 1993:206–214.

129. Williams CL, Lennon VA. Striational autoantibodies: Paraneoplastic antibodies associated with thymoma and myasthenia gravis. *Clin Immunol News.* 1991;11:161–170.

130. Tibbetts RS, McCormick TS, Rowland EC, et al. Cardiac antigen-specific autoantibody production is associated with cardiomyopathy in *Trypanosoma cruzi*-infected mice. *J Immunol.* 1994;152:1493–1499.

131. Boki KA, Kurki P, Holthofer H, et al. Prevalence of antikeratin antibodies in Greek patients with rheumatoid arthritis: A clinical, serologic and immunogenetic study. *J Rheumatol.* 1995;22:2046–2048.

132. Gabay C, Prieur A-M, Meyer O. Occurrence of antiperinuclear, antikeratin, and anti-RA 33 antibodies in juvenile chronic arthritis. *Ann Rheum Dis.* 1993;52:785–789.

133. Montecucco C, Caporali R, Negri C, et al. Antibodies from patients with rheumatoid arthritis and systemic lupus erythematosus recognize different epitopes of a single heterogeneous nuclear RNP core protein: Possible role of cross-reacting antikeratin antibodies. *Arthritis Rheum.* 1990;33:180–186.

134. Virtanen I, Lehto V-P, Lehtonen E, et al. Expression of intermediate filaments in cultured cells. *J Cell Sci.* 1981;50:45–63.

135. Das KM, Dasgupta A, Mandal A, et al. Autoimmunity to cytoskeletal protein tropomyosin: A clue to the pathogenetic mechanism for ulcerative colitis. *J Immunol.* 1993;150:2487–2493.

136. Cunningham MW, McCormack JM, Fenderson PG, et al. Human and murine antibodies cross-reactive with streptococcal M protein and myosin recognize the sequence GLN-LYS-SER-LYS-GLN in M protein. *J Immunol.* 1989;143:2677–2683.

137. Weber K, Groeschel-Stewart U. Antibody to myosin: The specific visualization of myosin-containing filaments in nonmuscle cells. *Proc Natl Acad Sci U S A.* 1974;71:4561–4564.

138. Penn AS, Schotland DL, Rowland LP. Antibody to human myosin in man. *Trans Am Neurol Assoc.* 1969;94:48–53.

139. Fairfax AJ, Gröschel-Stewart U. Myosin autoantibodies detected by immunofluorescence. *Clin Exp Immunol.* 1977;28:27–34.

140. Williams CL, Lennon VA, Momoi MY, et al. Serum antibodies and monoclonal antibodies secreted by thymic B-cell clones from patients with myasthenia gravis define striational antigens. *Ann N Y Acad Sci.* 1987;505:168–179.

141. Neu N, Craig SW, Rose NR, et al. Coxsackie virus induced myocarditis in mice: Cardiac myosin autoantibodies do not cross-react with the virus. *Clin Exp Immunol.* 1987;69:566–574.

142. Wada K, Ueno S, Hazama T, et al. Radioimmunoassay for antibodies to human skeletal muscle myosin in serum from patients with polymyositis. *Clin Exp Immunol.* 1983;52:297–304.

143. McDonald BL, Dawkins RL, Robinson J. Myosin autoantibodies reacting with selective muscle fiber types. *Muscle Nerve.* 1979;2:37–43.

144. McCormack JM, Crossley CA, Ayoub EM, et al. Poststreptococcal anti-myosin antibody idiotype associated with systemic lupus erythematosus and Sjögren's syndrome. *J Infect Dis.* 1993;168:915–921.

145. Michels VV, Moll PP, Rodeheffer RJ, et al. Circulating heart autoantibodies in familial as compared with nonfamilial idiopathic dilated cardiomyopathy. *Mayo Clin Proc.* 1994;69:24–27.

146. Rizzo LV, Cunha-Neto E, Teixeira ARL. Autoimmunity in Chagas' disease: Specific inhibition of reactivity of CD4+ T cells against myosin in mice chronically infected with *Trypanosoma cruzi. Infect Immun.* 1989;57:2640–2644.

147. von Mühlen CA, Chan EKL, Peebles CL, et al. Nonmuscle myosin as target antigen for human autoantibodies in patients with hepatitis C virus-associated chronic liver diseases. *Clin Exp Immunol.* 1995;100:67–74.

148. Huidbüchel E, Blaschek M, Seigneurin JM, et al. Antiorganelle and anti-cytoskeletal autoantibodies in the serum of Epstein-Barr virus-infected patients. *Ann Med Interne.* 1991;142:343–346.

CHAPTER 14

Antiphospholipid-Protein Antibodies: Clinical and Laboratory Correlation

Douglas A. Triplett, MD

Antiphospholipid-protein antibodies (APAs) are a family of autoimmune and alloimmune immunoglobulins (IgG, IgM, IgA, or mixtures) that recognize protein-phospholipid (PL) complexes using in vitro laboratory tests.[1–3] A variety of laboratory tests, including complement fixation tests (eg, serologic tests for syphilis), various coagulation tests, radioimmunoassays, enzyme-linked immunosorbent assays (ELISAs), and flow cytometry, have been used to identify APAs.[4–11] Originally, it was believed the antibodies recognized anionic or neutral phospholipids as primary antigenic targets. However, later studies implicated a variety of PL-binding plasma proteins as antigenic targets.[12–15] Presumably, these proteins bind to perturbed or damaged cellular membranes that expose anionic phospholipids (eg, phosphatidylserine, phosphatidylcholine). The binding of proteins to the injured cellular membranes results in exposure of neoepitope(s) in the proteins.

A number of plasma proteins have been suggested as possible antigenic targets (**Table 14-1**).[1,2] Among these proteins, β_2 glycoprotein I (β_2 GPI) and prothrombin have received the most attention.[1,2,11,12,16–20] However, antibodies to protein C and protein S appear to be the most plausible explanation for the pathophysiology of venous thromboembolic events in affected patients.[1,2] Other potential mechanisms related to thrombosis include the ability of APAs to enhance platelet adhesion to collagen and the subendothelial matrix of damaged vessels.[21] It has also been suggested that APAs may play a role in the pathogenesis of atherosclerosis.[22,23]

Antiphospholipid-protein antibodies may be classified as either autoimmune or alloimmune (**Table 14-2**).[1] The presence of APAs in patients with well-defined connective tissue diseases by definition is classified as secondary autoimmune APA. In the absence of well-defined criteria for an underlying connective tissue disease, the presence of clinical findings (eg, venous or arterial thrombosis, recurrent fetal loss) together with demonstrable APAs indicate primary antiphospholipid syndrome (PAPS).[24] Alloimmune APAs are seen in a variety of different conditions, including infections, underlying malignancies (often hematologic), and drug reactions.[1,25,26] A few cases of well-defined familial APAs have been identified (**Table 14-3**).[27,28]

As already noted, APAs may interact with platelets. Autoantibodies to platelet glycoproteins IIb/IIIa and Ib/IX have been described in patients with both PAPS and secondary APS (antiphospholipid

Table 14-1. Potential Protein Targets of Antiphospholipid-Protein Antibodies

Vitamin K-dependent proteins
Prothrombin
Protein C
Protein S
Factor X
Others
β_2 glycoprotein I
Annexins
Coagulation proteins
Factor XI
High-molecular-weight kininogen
Low-molecular-weight kininogen
Factor H

Table 14-2. Classification of Antiphospholipid-Protein Antibodies

Autoimmune
Primary (do not fulfill criteria for systemic lupus erythematosus)
Secondary
Systemic lupus erythematosus
Other connective tissue diseases
Drug-induced (eg, by quinine, quinidine, procainamide, thorazine)
Alloimmune
Infections
Viral
Bacterial
Protozoal
Fungal
Malignancies
Hairy cell leukemia
Lymphoproliferative disorders

Table 14-3. The Antiphospholipid-Protein Antibody Family

Lupus anticoagulants
Anticardiolipin antibodies
Reagin
Specific antibodies to anionic phospholipids
Antiphosphatidylserine
Antiphosphatidic acid
Antiphosphatidylinositol
Specific antibodies to neutral phospholipids
Antiphosphatidylethanolamine (eg, hexagonal phase)

Table 14-4. Characteristics of Autoimmune and Alloimmune Infection-Related Antiphospholipid-Protein Antibodies*

	Autoimmune	Alloimmune Infection Related
Predominant isotype	IgG	IgM
Avidity	High	Low
Lupus anticoagulant	Yes (≈ 40%)	No
Persistence	Yes	No
Titer	High	Low
Cofactor dependent (β_2 GPI)	Yes	No
Cofactor enhancers (β_2 GPI)	Yes	No (inhibitory)
Antiphospholipid antibody syndrome	Yes	No

Abbreviations: Ig = immunoglobulin; β_2 GPI = β_2 glycoprotein I.
**Many patients do not fit these patterns of clinical and laboratory findings.*

syndrome).[29,30] An association between APAs and major histocompatibility complex class II molecules (HLA-DQB1*06) has been de-scribed.[31] Autoantibodies to GP-IV (CD36) have also been described with lupus anticoagulants (LAs).[21]

Relevant Clinical Parameters Useful to the Laboratory Scientist

The identification of APAs is based on laboratory testing for the presence of LAs (coagulation tests) and ELISAs for anticardiolipin antibodies (ACAs). Enzyme-linked immunosorbent assays, besides those for ACAs, have been introduced to detect antibodies to β_2 GPI and to phosphatidylserine.[32–34] Tests for APAs are requested by a wide variety of clinicians, including rheumatologists, cardiologists, obstetricians, internists, pediatricians, neurologists, and vascular surgeons. This reflects the underlying diversity of clinical presentations that may be seen in patients with APS. The availability of a clinical history for the interpretation of APA test results is invaluable. Often, the history allows the laboratorian to classify the antibodies as either alloimmune or autoimmune (**Table 14-4**).

Alloimmune antibodies are often seen following various types of infections (eg, viral, bacterial, protozoal).[25,26,35] They are typically transient and are rarely associated with clinical complications. A very important aspect in establishing the diagnosis of true autoimmune APS is to repeat a positive laboratory test approximately 6 to 8 weeks following the initial identification of an abnormal result. Persistent positivity of tests for APAs suggests an underlying autoimmune pathogenesis. Alloimmune APAs may represent a common mechanism of response to cellular injury in all individuals. These antibodies react with PL-binding proteins localized on damaged cells or membrane fragments. The APA immune complexes are then cleared by the reticuloendothelial system. Consequently, alloimmune APAs may be a protective response designed to clear damaged cells and PL microparticles from the circulation. Supporting this hypothesis is the fact that lymphocytes cultured from normal individuals often yield monoclonal antibodies with APA activity. Antiphospholipid-protein antibodies may also play a role in cell apoptosis.[36]

Autoimmune APAs are associated with a wide variety of clinical manifestations.[1,2] The underlying pathophysiologic mechanisms are thrombosis or ischemia (eg, placental). Typically, the isotype is IgG (frequently subclass IgG2).[34] The pathophysiology of thrombosis in the presence of autoimmune APAs appears to be multifactorial. In the case of arterial thrombosis, the model of heparin-induced thrombocytopenia (HIT) appears to be similar to that of APS (**Table 14-5**).[37] The formation of a complex of immunoglobulin and protein (eg, IgG–β_2 GPI, IgG-prothrombin) results in binding of the complex to an Fc γ-RIIA receptor on platelets.[38] Subsequently, there is platelet activation and generation of platelet microparticles. In patients with HIT, the complex is composed of IgG and platelet factor 4, whereas in patients with APS, the complex may be IgG and β_2 GPI, prothrombin, or other plasma proteins.[39]

Antiphospholipid syndrome is defined by the presence of clinical findings (venous or arterial

Table 14-5. Similarities of Antiphospholipid Syndrome and Heparin-Induced Thrombocytopenia

	Antiphospholipid Syndrome	Heparin-Induced Thrombocytopenia
Immunoglobulin	IgG2	IgG2
Epitope (complexes)	PL-II	PF4-H
Receptor	Fc γ-RIIA	Fc γ-RIIA
Cellular activation	Yes	Yes
Clinical	Venous and arterial thrombosis	Venous and arterial thrombosis

Abbreviations: PL-II = phospholipid-prothrombin complex; PF4-H = platelet factor 4-heparin complex.

Table 14-6. Criteria for Antiphospholipid Antibody Syndrome[40]

Clinical	Laboratory
Venous thrombosis	IgG anticardiolipin antibody (10 GPL units)*
Arterial thrombosis	Positive lupus anticoagulant test†
Recurrent fetal loss	IgM anticardiolipin antibody (>10 MPL units)*
Thrombocytopenia	

**GPL and MPL refer to IgG and IgM phospholipid antibodies. The units refer to the standards proposed by Harris et al.[42]*

†The diagnosis of lupus anticoagulant should be established using the criteria outlined by the International Society of Thrombosis and Haemostasis Scientific Standardization Committee Subcommittee on Lupus Anticoagulants/Antiphospholipid Antibodies.[41]

thrombosis, recurrent fetal loss, thrombocytopenia) and persistent positive laboratory tests for APAs[40–42] (**Table 14-6**). Patients with APS should have at least one clinical and one laboratory finding during disease progression. The APA test(s) should be positive on at least 2 occasions more than 8 weeks apart.

The Role of Coagulation and Immunology Laboratories in Diagnosis and Prognosis of APA

Lupus Anticoagulants

Definition

Lupus anticoagulants are immunoglobulins (IgG, IgM, IgA, or mixtures) that interfere with or inhibit one or more of the in vitro PL-dependent coagulation tests, including activated partial thromboplastin time (APTT), kaolin clotting time (KCT or KPTT), dilute Russell's viper venom time (dRVVT), dilute prothrombin time (dPT), and textarin time.[1] Paradoxically, despite prolonged in vitro coagulation tests, the vast majority of patients with LAs do not bleed.[1–3] The name is also something of a misnomer because the majority of patients in whom LAs are identified do not have underlying systemic lupus erythematosus (SLE). Ironically, the presence of LAs is often associated with both venous and arterial thromboembolic disease.[42,43]

Lupus anticoagulants may be encountered in any population group (**Table 14-7**). The vast majority of LAs seen in the pediatric population are caused by intercurrent infections (viral or bacterial). In the pediatric population, boys and girls are equally affected.[44] This is in contrast to LAs or ACAs encountered in young adult to middle-aged patients. The majority of cases in these age groups are seen in women and reflect the increased incidence of autoimmune disease in women compared with men.[44,45] In the geriatric population, the presence of LAs and/or ACAs is often associated with the use of various medications, including procainamide, quinidine, quinine, hydralazine, various antibiotics, and interferon alfa.[1,2,46,47] The frequency of APS in the geriatric population may also reflect a loss of regulatory aspects of the immunologic response associated with the appearance of various autoantibodies (eg, rheumatoid factor, ACAs).[48] Consequently, the interpretation of APA test results must include consideration of patient age, medications, and related disease states. The appearance of LAs or ACAs in the convalescent phase after infections is very common.[25,26,35] However, in such convalescent patients, the LAs and ACAs tend to be transient; consequently, it is important to obtain a second series of test results approximately 6 to 8 weeks following the initial identification of these antibodies. Persistence of LAs and ACAs is one of the criteria required to establish the diagnosis of APS.

Table 14-7. Lupus Anticoagulants: Demographics

	Pediatric	Adult	Geriatric
Sex predominance	M = F	F > M	F > M
Thrombosis	+	+++	–1 or absent
Antigen			
Prothrombin	++	++	+?
β_2 glycoprotein I	+	+	+
Association	Infections	Autoimmune	↑Frequency of autoantibodies; drugs

Abbreviations: M = male; F = female.

Requirements for Laboratory Diagnosis

The laboratory diagnosis of LAs remains one of the more challenging problems encountered in the coagulation laboratory. This is due in part to the protean clinical/laboratory situations in which they may be encountered.[1,2] By definition, LAs are circulating anticoagulants, or inhibitors, of blood coagulation.[1,49] Circulating anticoagulants may be classified into 3 general groups: specific inhibitors (antibodies that recognize individual coagulation factors, eg, factor VIII), nonspecific (eg, LAs), and global (eg, heparin) (**Table 14-8**).[50] It is important to accurately diagnose inhibitors of blood coagulation. There are situations in which patients may be misdiagnosed with LAs when, in fact, they may have factor VIII inhibitor.[51,52] An acquired factor VIII inhibitor is a medical emergency necessitating appropriate treatment and replacement therapy when indicated.[53] The simultaneous presence of LA and a factor VIII inhibitor may be seen in the hemophilia A population, particularly in patients who have tested positive for the human immunodeficiency virus.[54]

The Subcommittee on Lupus Anticoagulant/Phospholipid-dependent Antibodies of the Scientific and Standardization Committee (SSC) of the International Society of Thrombosis and Haemostasis has published guidelines for the diagnosis of LA.[41] The subcommittee recommended 4 criteria:

- Prolongation of a PL-dependent coagulation test(s)
- Evidence of inhibition demonstrated by mixing studies
- Evidence of PL dependence of the inhibitor
- Ruling out other coagulopathies

Laboratory Testing

Step 1: Screening

Screening patient plasmas for identification of LA requires a careful selection of tests. Based on a number of studies, more than one screening test is necessary to identify LA in a given sample.[55–58] Because of the marked heterogeneity of LA, the combination of screening tests used should evaluate different components of the coagulation system (**Table 14-9**).[55] An example of such a strategy includes a sensitive APTT test system (evaluation of the intrinsic pathway), a dPT (extrinsic system), and dRVVT (final common pathway). Using multiple screening tests enhances the overall sensitivity for LA detection.[55] Failure to incorporate multiple screening tests significantly impairs the laboratory's ability to identify LA.

Table 14-8. Classification of Circulating Inhibitors

Specific
Neutralizing
Factor VIII
Factor IX
Factor XI
Factor XIII
Fibrinogen
von Willebrand's factor
Nonneutralizing
Factor VIII
von Willebrand's factor
Prothrombin
Factor X
Nonspecific
Lupus anticoagulants
Paraproteins
Fibrin split products
Global
Heparin-like activity

Table 14-9. Lupus Anticoagulants: Screening Tests

Intrinsic Pathway	Extrinsic Pathway	Final Common Pathway
Activated partial thromboplastin time	Dilute prothrombin time	Dilute Russell's viper venom time
Kaolin clotting time		Textarin time
Colloidal slica clotting time		Taipan snake venom time

Step 2: Mixing Studies

If one or more of the screening tests are prolonged, the next step involves mixing studies to demonstrate the presence of an inhibitor as the cause of an abnormal screening test.[59] Comparative individual sensitivity and specificity of various screening tests was reported by Capel and colleagues.[60] In the presence of an inhibitor, a mixture of normal plasma and patient plasma has a persistent abnormal clotting time. Many different mixing study protocols are used. Various ratios of patient-to-normal plasma include 1:1, 4:1, and 1:4. Various sources of normal plasma, including pooled normal plasma and commercially available lyophilized normal plasma, have been used. In the case of the commercially available plasma, the residual PL concentration of the plasma is unknown. In addition, buffers and stabilizers are added to commercially prepared plasmas. It is important to have truly platelet-poor plasma for patient testing. By definition, the residual platelet count should be less than 5,000/µL. Plasmas that are LA positive may yield false-negative mixing study results if there is a significant number of residual platelets in the normal plasma used in the mixing study. It is well recognized that factor VIII inhibitors are time dependent (the inhibitory activity may be absent on initial testing but appears with incubation at 1 to 2 hours).[61] Typically, LAs are immediate inhibitors (ie, inhibitory activity is present on initial testing of the mixture). However, approximately 30% of LAs may be time dependent.[62] Testing for time-dependent inhibition is unnecessary if the immediate mixing study shows the presence of an inhibitor.

Step 3: Demonstration of PL Dependence

The third step requires demonstration of PL dependence by relative correction of the prolonged clotting time following the addition of phospholipids or platelets (freeze-thawed platelets or platelet vesicles).[63,64] In addition to the conventional approach using 3 discrete steps to establish the presence of PL-dependent inhibitors, integrated test systems have been introduced. These systems combine a screening assay, mixing study, and confirmatory procedure into a single test sequence. Commercially available samples of these tests include Staclot LA (Diagnostica Stago, Inc., Paris, France) and dRVVT systems.[1,65] The advantages of these combined approaches are ease of use and continuity of testing. The reagents include a source of normal plasma to correct for factor deficiencies in patient plasma and a heparin-neutralizing substance (polybrene) to neutralize heparin effect. A summary of LA confirmatory studies is included in **Table 14-10**.

By using the criteria recommended by the SSC, it is possible to achieve a sensitivity of 95% with a specificity approaching 100%. The presence of LAs when compared with ACAs has a stronger predictive value for clinical thromboembolic events.[66–68] In patients with SLE, the presence of LAs is associated with a risk for venous thrombosis that is approximately 6 times greater than that of patients without LAs.[69] In the same study, ACA-positive patients had twice the risk of venous thrombosis. Although ACA testing is more sensitive in broad patient population studies for the presence of APAs, it is considerably less specific than LA testing.

Anticardiolipin Antibodies

Definition

In 1983, Harris and colleagues[8] described a solid-phase radioimmunoassay that used cardiolipin as the antigen. They found this assay system to be 200 to 400 times more sensitive than traditional serologic tests for syphilis that employed an antigen composed of cardiolipin, phosphatidylcholine, and cholesterol (eg, Venereal Disease Reference Laboratory). The impetus behind the development of this test was the long-standing clinical recognition of an association between a chronic biologic false-positive serologic test for syphilis and a variety of clinical complications, including thrombocytopenia, thrombosis, and recurrent spontaneous abortion.[4,5] Subsequently, an ELISA system was described.[70]

In the vast majority of laboratories, ACA testing is done using an ELISA system. Recent studies have demonstrated that the antigenic target in the ACA assay in most cases is the plasma protein β_2 GPI.[71,72] This physiologic plasma protein has the ability to inhibit components of the coagulation system, including adenosine diphosphate–induced platelet aggregation, contact activation, and the prothrombinase reaction.[72] β_2 Glycoprotein I is a member of the short consensus repeat superfamily. Structurally, it contains 5 contiguous "sushi domains" (which resemble sushi). Other members of this superfamily include factor XIII, factor B, C4 binding protein, factor H, and haptoglobin.[72] In addition to antibodies to β_2 GPI detected in ACA testing, other proteins have been suggested as antigenic targets, including factor H, annexin V, and human prothrombin.[73–76]

Table 14-10. Confirmatory Studies of Lupus Anticoagulants*

Screening Assay	Confirmatory Procedures
APTT-based assays	PNP
	Hexagonal phase phospholipid
	Phospholipid dilutions
Dilute Russell viper venom time	DVV Confirm®
	Platelet vesicles
	Frozen-thawed platelets (PNP)
Taipan snake venom time	Frozen-thawed platelets (PNP)
Dilute prothrombin time	Phospholipid dilutions
Kaolin clotting time	Platelet vesicles
Silica clotting time	Inosithin
	Bovine phospholipids

Abbreviations: APTT = activated partial thromboplastin time; PNP = platelet neutralization procedure.
**Modified from Brandt et al.[41]*

Laboratory Testing

Many variables have been identified in the laboratory detection of ACAs. Among these are the blocking agent used (the source of β_2 GPI), type of microtiter plate (high sensitivity/conventional) and labeling of detector antibodies. Some commercially available kits use a screening step consisting of polyvalent antisera (anti-IgG, anti-IgM, anti-IgA) with confirmatory testing involving isotype-specific antisera. Commercially available reference plasmas are also employed to prepare a reference curve for semiquantitative expression of positive results.[42] Arbitrarily, GPL (IgG) and MPL (IgM) units (1 unit represents the binding activity of 1 μg/mL of affinity-purified ACA) have been used. Levels of IgG-positive ACA of greater than 40 GPL units have correlated with clinical thromboembolic complications.[77–79] An alternative means of expressing ACA results is as negative, low positive, positive, and high positive.

One of the most important aspects in establishing an ACA assay is to determine a cut-off point between normal and abnormal results. Various statistical approaches have been used, including standard deviation (3 to 5 SD above the mean [ACA results do not have a Gaussian distribution]) and multiples of the mean. If standard deviations are used to determine the normal range, the upper limit of normal is too low. A normal range using multiples of the mean is more accurate. Interlaboratory performance of ACA assays indicates a lack of agreement in the majority of cases. This is particularly true when comparing results expressed as ACA units. There is better correlation if laboratories express results as positive, high positive, low positive, or negative.

Other procedural aspects of ACA testing influence test results. Among these are the patient sample (plasma or serum), processing and handling of the sample (centrifugation, freezing, and thawing), the diluent used in the test, the blocking reagent (bovine serum albumin, human sera), the presence of nonanionic detergents, and the source of cardiolipin. The commercial source of microtiter plates plays an important role in the test system; the use of "highly sensitive" plates is recommended. Antibodies to β_2 GPI are more readily detected using such plates. β_2 Glycoprotein I binds to irradiated plates through a specific sequence (Glu 274 → CYS 288) in the fifth domain. Once β_2 GPI is bound, there is exposure of a "neoepitope" in the fourth domain.[72] This epitope is apparently the antigenic target in conventional ACA tests.

Anti–β_2 Glycoprotein I

A number of investigators have shown that β_2 GPI is required for the binding of ACAs to cardiolipin.[80] This is the case in patients with underlying autoimmune disease. In contrast, ACAs in patients with syphilis do not require the presence of β_2 GPI

Table 14-11. Antiphospholipid-Protein Antibodies: Controls/Reference

	Lupus Anticoagulants	Anticardiolipin Antibodies
Standards	No	No
Reference materials	No	Yes (Harris et al[8])
Positive controls	Yes	Yes
Quantify (titer)	No	Yes
Reproducible	—	Variable
Clinical correlation	—	Variable
Proficiency testing	Yes	Yes
Performance	Poor	Poor/variable

for such binding (**Table 14-11**). A number of reports have documented the presence of anti–β_2 GPI using microtiter plates coated with β_2 GPI. Some discrepancies in the literature with respect to the detection of anti–β_2 GPI may be explained by the type of microtiter plate used. Routine microtiter plates may not detect antibodies to β_2 GPI; highly sensitive or irradiated microtiter plates are required for optimal detection.

Viard and colleagues[81] were the first to demonstrate an association of anti–β_2 GPI and the presence of thrombosis in SLE patients. Subsequent studies confirmed an association of anti–β_2 GPI and clinical thromboembolic events.[16,18,19] In a report by Sanmarco and Soler,[82] IgG antibodies to β_2 GPI were found almost exclusively in patients with autoimmune disease. Furthermore, the presence of IgG anti–β_2 GPI was highly specific (98%) with a positive predictive value (87.5%) for APS. These antibodies were significantly associated with venous thrombosis ($P = .0025$). However, they had relatively low sensitivity (54%). Using a standard ACA assay, the sensitivity is significantly higher. It is recommended that laboratories use both ACA and anti–β_2 GPI assays. The ACA test should be used as a screen and, if positive, a follow-up anti–β_2 GPI may be indicated.

In any given patient, anti–β_2 GPI is heterogeneous.[83] Anti–β_2 GPI enhances the binding of proteins to surfaces (ie, in vivo damaged PL membranes or in vitro microtiter plates, which are negatively charged). In addition to enhancing the surface binding of β_2 GPI, the APAs also organize and/or optimize the arrangement of β_2 GPI on negatively charged surfaces. There have been reports of patients with APS and only anti–β_2 GPI positivity.[84,85] Consequently, in a patient presenting with symptoms consistent with APS for whom ACA testing is negative, tests for anti–β_2 GPI are indicated.

Prognostic Correlation

The demonstration of LAs in a patient sample correlates strongly with clinical venous thromboembolic events. Among the various laboratory tests used to demonstrate APAs, those for LAs appear to be most specific for clinical complications. Perhaps this reflects the relative quantity of antibodies present in a given patient. In detecting LAs in patient plasma, it is assumed there is a significant amount of antibody present. In contrast to ACA testing, lower levels of antibodies are detected, giving a higher frequency of positivity. Many ACA tests give low-positive results and reflect "transient" alloimmune antibodies, which are unrelated to clinical complications.

In the ACA assay, IgG positivity correlates with venous and arterial thromboembolic complications. In 2 prospective studies (the Physicians Health Study[77] and the Italian Registry of Antiphospholipid Antibodies[78]), a correlation between IgG ACA levels greater than 40 GPL units was demonstrated in venous thromboembolic events. Unfortunately, LA testing was not performed in the Physicians Health Study. The presence of IgM antibodies detected in ACA tests are less specific for thrombotic complications. Immunoglobulin M ACAs frequently may be seen in patients who have had recent infections. Once again, this emphasizes the need to repeat the test in approximately 6 to 8 weeks. Such IgM-positive ACA results are also seen in association with certain drugs (eg, chlorpromazine, quinidine, quinine, procainamide).[1]

Anti–β_2 GPI antibodies have a high degree of specificity and positive predictive value when detected in patients with APS. As already noted, however, the sensitivity of anti–β_2 GPI is significantly less than that of ACA. Consequently, both test systems should be used in the appropriate clinical setting.

Laboratory Monitoring of Anticoagulant Therapy

Because thromboembolic events are a major complication associated with APS, many affected patients are placed on therapeutic as well as prophylactic anticoagulant therapy. For long-term therapy, warfarin is the treatment of choice. Because there is a high frequency of recurrent thromboembolic events, a relatively higher intensity of oral anticoagulation is recommended (international normalized ratio [INR], 2.5 to 3.5).[86,87]

Moll and Ortel[88] reported on the ability of LAs to influence prothrombin times and INRs. Consequently, the accuracy of the INR in the monitoring of LA-positive patients has been questioned.[89–91] In these patients, it may be necessary to use other forms of monitoring, including assays of factor X activity, prothrombin-proconvertin times, or native prothrombin antigen.[88]

During the acute phase of anticoagulant therapy, the presence of LAs may also create difficulties in monitoring heparin. Alternative approaches to heparin monitoring include anti-Xa assay, thrombin time, and the use of an APTT reagent that is LA insensitive.

Problems often arise in monitoring patients who are being treated with heparin or low-molecular-weight heparin (LMWH) during the course of pregnancy. Because of the pharmacologic advantages of LMWH (predictable in vivo biologic recovery and long half-life), this drug is recommended for anticoagulation in pregnant patients.[92] It does not cross the placenta and requires little laboratory monitoring.

Specific Quality Assurance Recommendations

Because of the marked heterogeneity of LAs and ACAs, no standards are available (see Table 14-11). The reference plasmas that are commercially available to express ACA results in GPL and MPL units are helpful in day-to-day laboratory practice, but they are not standards. Commercially available positive controls for LA and ACA testing represent either frozen or lyophilized plasmas/sera obtained from patients with well-characterized APS. The performance of these controls in the laboratory varies somewhat depending on the choice of reagents used to detect LAs as well as the nature of the ACA ELISA.

Various external quality assessment schemes have been used to evaluate laboratory performance in the detection of LAs and ACAs. Among these are the National External Quality Assessment Scheme in the United Kingdom; the International Survey on Lupus Anticoagulants, which has been provided through the SSC; and the College of American Pathologists Survey Program.[60,93] All of these proficiency testing studies have demonstrated the marked variability of laboratory performance in LA and ACA testing.[94] In LA testing, the marked variability is due to the choice of screening tests (with their variable sensitivities) and the appropriate performance of confirmatory testing. In ACA testing, a significant portion of the variability is attributable to inappropriate definition of a normal reference interval (ie, not establishing a reference interval based on multiples of standard deviation).

Pathophysiology of Antiphospholipid-Protein Antibodies

In many respects, APAs represent an excellent paradigm of antibody-mediated thrombosis. The role of antibodies in the pathogenesis of thromboembolic disease has gained a great deal of attention due to HIT and APS models. A number of reports have correlated antibodies to endothelial cells with clinical thrombosis.[95]

Antiphospholipid syndrome is characterized by both venous and arterial thromboembolic events,[96,97] and there is remarkable fidelity of recurrent events in affected patients. If the initial event is a venous thrombosis, there is an extremely high probability that a subsequent event also will be venous.[86] This is also true with arterial thrombosis. This consistency suggests underlying differences in the pathophysiologies of venous and arterial thrombosis. The most probable pathophysiologic explanation for venous thrombosis is the ability of APAs to interfere with the protein C–protein S system.[98,99] Activated protein C is instrumental in down-regulating factors Va and VIIIa. The impaired generation or the inhibition of activated protein C activity results in a predilection to thrombosis. Antiphospholipid-protein antibodies have been demonstrated to inhibit protein C activation and the ability of activated protein C to downregulate factors Va and VIIIa.[100] In the latter case, laboratory test results are similar to those seen in patients with activated protein C resistance.

Antiphospholipid-protein antibodies also may be involved in arterial events through their interaction with platelets. In the presence of damaged endothelium, APAs accelerate the deposition of platelets by adhesion and aggregation at the site of injury. Subsequent microembolic events result in clinical stroke. Antiphospholipid-protein antibodies have been linked to accelerated atherosclerosis. There is significant concordance with APAs and antibodies to oxidized low-density lipoproteins.

Summary

Antiphospholipid-protein antibodies are a common cause of both venous and arterial thromboembolic events. Approximately 15% of venous thromboembolic events are related to APAs. Antiphospholipid-protein antibodies are associated with approximately 40% of strokes in patients younger than 50 years. Virtually every physician regardless of specialty or subspecialty will encounter patients with APAs. Clinicians are becoming increasingly more vigilant in identifying APAs as underlying causes of thrombosis. In addition, laboratories are more proactive in testing for the presence of APAs. In any case of unexplained thromboembolic events (venous or arterial), it is important to test for the presence of APAs.

References

1. Triplett DA. Antiphospholipid-protein antibodies: Laboratory detection and clinical relevance. *Thromb Res.* 1995;78:1–31.
2. Love PE, Santoro SA. Antiphospholipid antibodies: Anticardiolipin and the lupus anticoagulant in systemic lupus erythematosus (SLE) and in non-SLE disorders. *Ann Intern Med.* 1990;112:692–698.
3. Shapiro SS. The lupus anticoagulant/antiphospholipid syndrome. *Annu Rev Med.* 1995;47:533–553.
4. Moore JE, Mohr CF. Biologically false positive serologic tests for syphilis. *JAMA.* 1952;150:467–473.
5. Moore JE, Lutz WB. The natural history of systemic lupus erythematosus: An approach to its study through chronic biologic false positive reactors. *J Chronic Dis.* 1955;1:297–316.
6. Conley CL, Hartmann RC. A hemorrhagic disorder caused by circulating anticoagulant in patients with disseminated lupus erythematosus. *J Clin Invest.* 1952;31:621–622.
7. Brandt JT, Barna LK, Triplett DA. Laboratory identification of lupus anticoagulants: Results of the second international workshop for identification of lupus anticoagulants. *Thromb Haemost.* 1995;74: 1597–1603.
8. Harris EN, Gharavi AE, Boey ML, et al. Anticardiolipin antibodies: Detection by radioimmunoassay and association with thrombosis in systemic lupus erythematosus. *Lancet.* 1983;2:1211–1214.
9. Stewart MW, Etches WS, Russeu AS, et al. Detection of antiphospholipid antibodies by flow cytometry: Rapid detection of antibody isotype and phospholipid specificity. *Thromb Haemost.* 1993;70:603–607.
10. Frost SJ, Chakraborty J, Firth GB. Novel homogeneous liposomal immunoassay for colorimetric estimation of serum IgG anticardiolipin antibodies. *Clin Chem.* 1996;42:874–876.
11. Schultz DR. Antiphospholipid antibodies: Basic immunology and assays. *Semin Arthritis Rheum.* 1997:26:724–739.
12. McNeil HP, Simpson RJ, Chesterman CN, et al. Antiphospholipid antibodies are directed against a complex antigen that includes a lipid binding inhibitor of coagulation: β_2 glycoprotein I (apolipoprotein H). *Proc Natl Acad Sci U S A.* 1990;87:4120–4124.
13. Galli M, Comfurius P, Maassen C, et al. Anticardiolipin antibodies (ACA) directed not to cardiolipin but to a plasma cofactor. *Lancet.* 1990;335:1544–1547.
14. Bevers EM, Galli M, Barbui T, et al. Lupus anticoagulant IgG's (LA) are not directed to phospholipids only but to a complex of lipid bound prothrombin. *Thromb Haemost.* 1991;66:629–632.
15. Oosting JD, Derksen RHWM, Bobbink IWG, et al. Antiphospholipid antibodies directed against a combination of phospholipids with prothrombin, protein C, or protein S: An explanation for their pathogenic mechanism? *Blood.* 1993;81:2618–2625.
16. Forastiero RR, Martinuzzo ME, Cerrato GC, et al. Relationship of anti-β_2 glycoprotein I and antiprothrombin antibodies to thrombosis and pregnancy loss in patients with antiphospholipid antibodies. *Thromb Haemost.* 1997;78:1008–1014.
17. Fleck RA, Rapaport SI, Rao LVM. Antiprothrombin antibodies and the lupus anticoagulant. *Blood.* 1988;72:512–519.
18. Najmey SS, Keil LB, Adib DR, et al. The association of antibodies to β_2 glycoprotein I with the antiphospholipid syndrome: A meta-analysis. *Ann Clin Lab Sci.* 1997;27:41–46.

19. Pengo V, Biasolo A, Fior MG. Autoimmune antiphospholipid antibodies are directed against a cryptic epitope expressed when β_2 glycoprotein I is bound to a suitable surface. *Thromb Haemost.* 1995;73:29–34.

20. Arvieux J, Darnige L, Sarrot-Reynuuld F. Les nouvelles cibles des anticorps "antiphospholipides." *Rev Med Interne.* 1997;18:292–302.

21. Rock G, Chauhan K, Jamieson GA, et al. Anti CD36 antibodies in patients with lupus anticoagulant and thrombotic complications. *Br J Haematol.* 1994;88:878–880.

22. Vaarala O. Atherosclerosis in SLE and Hughes syndrome. *Lupus.* 1997;6:489–490.

23. Vaarala O, Puurunen M, Mantari M, et al. Antibodies to prothrombin imply a risk of myocardial infarction in middle-aged men. *Thromb Haemost.* 1996;75:456–459.

24. Hughes GRV. The antiphospholipid syndrome: Ten years on. *Lancet.* 1993;342:341–344.

25. Faler CA, Agiostratidou G. High levels of anti-phospholipid antibodies in uncomplicated and several plasmodium falciparum and *P. vivax malaris. Clin Exp Immunol.* 1994;95:304–309.

26. Prieto J, Yuste JR, Beloqui O, et al. Anticardiolipin antibodies in chronic hepatitis C; implication of hepatitis C virus as the cause of the antiphospholipid syndrome. *Hepatology.* 1996;23:199–204.

27. Ford PM, Brunet D, Lillicrap DP, et al. Premature stroke in a family with lupus anticoagulant and antiphospholipid antibodies. *Stroke.* 1990;21:66–71.

28. Mackie IJ, Colaco CB, Machin SJ. Familial lupus anticoagulants. *Br J Haematol.* 1987;67:359–363.

29. Macchi L, Rispal P, Clofent-Sanchez G, et al. Antiplatelet antibodies in patients with systemic lupus erythematosus and primary antiphospholipid antibody syndrome: Their relationship with the obscured thrombocytopenia. *Br J Haematol.* 1997;98:342–345.

30. Godeau B, Piette JC, Fromont P, et al. Specific antiplatelet glycoprotein autoantibodies are associated with the thrombocytopenia of primary antiphospholipid syndrome. *Br J Haematol.* 1997;98:873–879.

31. Panzer S, Pabinger I, Gschwandtner ME, et al. Lupus anticoagulants: Strong association with the major histocompatibility complex class II and platelet antibodies. *Br J Haematol.* 1997;98:342–345.

32. Roubey RAS, Eisenberg RA, Harper MF, et al. "Anticardiolipin" autoantibodies recognize β_2-glycoprotein I in the absence of phospholipid. *J Immunol.* 1995;154:954–960.

33. Sanmarco M, Soler C, Christides C, et al. Prevalence and clinical significance of IgG isotypes anti-β_2 glycoprotein I antibodies in antiphospholipid syndrome: A comparative study with anticardiolipin antibodies. *J Lab Clin Med.* 1997;129:499–506.

34. Arvieux J, Roussel B, Ponard D, et al. IgG2 subclass restriction of anti-β_2 glycoprotein I antibodies in autoimmune patients. *Clin Exp Immunol.* 1994;95:310–315.

35. Abuaf N, Laperche S, Rajoely B, et al. Autoantibodies to phospholipids and to the coagulation proteins in AIDS. *Thromb Haemost.* 1997;77:856–861.

36. Lafer EM, Rauch J, Andrzejewski C Jr, et al. Polyspecific monoclonal lupus autoantibodies reactive with both polynucleotide and phospholipids. *J Exp Med.* 1981;153:897–909.

37. Vermylen J, Hoylaerts MF, Arnout J. Antibody mediated thrombosis. *Thromb Haemost.* 1997;78:420–426.

38. Burgess JK, Lindeman R, Chesterman CN, et al. Single amino acid mutation of Fc γ receptor is associated with the development of heparin-induced thrombocytopenia. *Br J Haematol.* 1995;91:761–766.

39. Amiral J, Peynaud-Debayle E, Wolf M, et al. Generation of antibodies to heparin PF4 complexes without thrombocytopenia in patients treated with unfractionated or low molecular weight heparin. *Am J Hematol.* 1996;52:90–95.

40. Harris EN. Syndrome of the black swan. *Br J Rheumatol.* 1987;26:324–326.

41. Brandt JT, Triplett DA, Alving B, et al. Criteria for the diagnosis of lupus anticoagulants: An update. *Thromb Haemost.* 1996;74:1185–1190.

42. Harris EN, Gharavi AE, Patel SP, et al. Evaluation of the anti-cardiolipin test: Report of a standardized workshop held 4 April 1986. *Clin Exp Immunol.* 1987;68:215–222.

43. Khamashta MA, Asherson RA. Hughes syndrome: Antiphospholipid antibodies move closer to thrombosis in 1994. *Br J Rheumatol.* 1995;34:493–494.

44. Jude B, Goudemand J, Dolle I, et al. Lupus anticoagulant: A clinical and laboratory study of 100 cases. *Clin Lab Haematol.* 1988;10:41–51.

45. Horellou MH, Aurousseau MH, Buff MC, et al. Biological and clinical heterogeneity of lupus and lupus-like anticoagulant in fifty-seven patients. *J Med.* 1987;18;199–217.

46. Becker JC, Winkler B, Klingers S, et al. Antiphospholipid syndrome associated with immunotherapy for patients with melanoma. *Cancer.* 1994;73:1621–1624.

47. Morris LF, Lemak NA, Arnett FC, et al. Systemic lupus erythematosus diagnosed during interferon alpha therapy. *South Med J.* 1996;89:810–814.

48. Manoussakis MN, Tzioufas AG, Silis MP, et al. High prevalence of anticardiolipin and other autoantibodies in a healthy elderly population. *Clin Exp Immunol.* 1987;69:557–565.

49. Sallah S. Inhibitors of clotting factors. *Ann Hematol.* 1997;75:1–7.

50. Hoyer LW. Factor VIII inhibitors. *Curr Opin Hematol.* 1995;2:365–371.

51. Biron C, Durand L, Lemkecher T, et al. Simultaneous occurrence of lupus anticoagulant, factor VIII inhibitor and localized pemphigoid. *Am J Hematol.* 1996;51:250–251.

52. Ballard HS, Nyamuswa G. Life-threatening haemorrhage in a patient with rheumatoid arthritis and a lupus anticoagulant coexisting with acquired autoantibodies against factor VIII. *Br J Rheumatol.* 1993;32:515–517.

53. Hutlin MB. Acquired inhibitors in malignant and non malignant disease states. *Am J Med.* 1994;91:9–13.

54. Blanco AN, Cardozo MA, Candela M, et al. Antifactor VIII inhibitors and lupus anticoagulants in haemophilia patients. *Thromb Haemost.* 1997;77:656–659.

55. Johns AS, Chamley L, Ockelford PA, et al. Comparison of tests for the lupus anticoagulant and antiphospholipid antibodies in systemic lupus erythematosus. *Clin Exp Rheumatol.* 1994;12:523–526.

56. Denis-Magdelaine A, Flahaut A, Verdy E. Sensitivity of sixteen APTT reagents for the presence of lupus anticoagulants. *Haemostasis.* 1995;25:98–105.

57. Exner T. Comparison of two simple tests for the lupus anticoagulant. *Am J Clin Pathol.* 1985;83:215–218.

58. Triplett DA. Frequent difficulties encountered in the laboratory diagnosis of antiphospholipid-protein antibodies. *Ann Med Interne.* 1996;147:5–9.

59. Kaczor DA, Bickford NM, Triplett DA. Evaluation of different mixing study reagents and dilution effect in lupus anticoagulant testing. *Am J Clin Pathol.* 1991;95:408–411.

60. Capel P, Arnout J, Cauchie P, et al. Comparative study of antiphospholipid antibody detection in eleven Belgian laboratories. *Acta Clin Belg.* 1997;52:84–91.

61. Kasper CK. Laboratory tests for factor VIII inhibitors, their variation, significance and interpretation. *Blood Coagul Fibrinolysis.* 1991;2:7–10.

62. Clyne LP, White PF. Time dependency of lupus-like anticoagulants. *Arch Intern Med.* 1988;148:1060–1063.

63. Triplett DA, Brandt JT, Kaczor D, et al. Laboratory diagnosis of lupus inhibitors: A comparison of the tissue thromboplastin inhibition procedure with a new platelet neutralization procedure. *Am J Clin Pathol.* 1983;79:678–682.

64. Arnout J, Huybrechts E, Vanrusselt E, et al. A new lupus anticoagulant neutralization test based on platelet-derived vesicles. *Br J Haematol.* 1992;80:341–346.

65. Triplett DA, Barna LK, Unger GA. A hexagonal (II) phase phospholipid neutralization assay for lupus anticoagulant identification. *Thromb Haemost.* 1993;70:787–793.

66. Simioni P, Prandoni P, Zanon E, et al. Deep venous thrombosis and lupus anticoagulant: A case-control study. *Thromb Haemost.* 1996;76:187–189.

67. Jouhikainen T, Stephansson E, Leirisalo-Repo M. Lupus anticoagulant as a prognostic marker in systemic lupus erythematosus. *Br J Rheumatol.* 1993;32:568–573.

68. Horbach DA, Oort EV, Donders RCJM, et al. Lupus anticoagulant is the strongest risk factor for both venous and arterial thrombosis in patients with systemic lupus erythematosus. *Thromb Haemost.* 1996;76:916–924.

69. Wahl DG, Guillemi F, de Maistre E, et al. Risk for venous thrombosis related to antiphospholipid antibodies in systemic lupus erythematosus—a meta-analysis. *Lupus.* 1997;6:467–473.

70. Loizou S, McCrea JD, Rudge AC, et al. Measurement of anticardiolipin antibodies by an enzyme linked immunosorbent assay (ELISA): Standardization and quantitation of results. *Clin Exp Immunol.* 1985;62:738–745.

71. Roubey RAS. Antigenic specificities of antiphospholipid autoantibodies: Implications for clinical laboratory testing and diagnosis of the antiphospholipid syndrome. *Lupus.* 1996;5:425–430.

72. Amiral J, Adam M, Cluzeau D, et al. Different target specificities of phospholipid-dependent antibodies. *Ann Med Interne.* 1996;147:18–71.

73. Rand JH, Wu XX, Andree HAM, et al. Pregnancy loss in the antiphospholipid antibody syndrome: A possible thrombogenic mechanism. *N Engl J Med.* 1997;337:154–160.

74. Bajaj SP, Rapaport SI, Barclay S, et al. Acquired hypoprothrombinemia due to nonneutralizing antibodies to prothrombin: Mechanisms and management. *Blood.* 1985;65:1538–1543.

75. Galli M, Beretta G, Daldossi M, et al. Different anticoagulant and immunological properties of anti-prothrombin antibodies in patients with antiphospholipid antibodies. *Thromb Haemost.* 1997;77:486–491.

76. Eberhard A, Sparling C, Sudbury S, et al. Hypoprothrombinemia in childhood systemic lupus erythematosus. *Semin Arthritis Rheum.* 1994;24:12–18.

77. Ginsburg KS, Liang MH, Newcomer L, et al. Anticardiolipin antibodies and the risk for ischemic stroke and venous thrombosis. *Ann Intern Med.* 1992;117:997–1002.

78. Italian Registry of Antiphospholipid Antibodies (IR-APA). Thrombosis and thrombocytopenia in antiphospholipid syndrome (idiopathic and secondary to SLE): First report from the Italian Registry. *Haematologica.* 1993;78:313–318.

79. Excalante A, Brey RL, Mitchell BD, et al. Accuracy of anticardiolipin antibodies in identifying a history of thrombosis among patients with systemic lupus erythematosus. *Am J Med.* 1995;98:559–565.

80. Roubey RAS. Autoantibodies to phospholipid-binding plasma proteins: A new view of lupus anticoagulants and other "antiphospholipid" autoantibodies. *Blood*. 1994;84:2854–2867.

81. Viard JP, Amoura Z, Bach JF. Association of anti-β_2 glycoprotein-I antibodies with lupus-type circulating anticoagulant and thrombosis in systemic lupus erythematosus. *Am J Med*. 1992;93:181–186.

82. Sanmarco M, Soler C. Heterogeneity of anti-β_2 glycoprotein I antibodies. *Nouv Rev Fr Hematol*. 1995;37: S57–S60.

83. Amiral J, Larrivaz I, Cluzeau D, et al. Standardization of immunoassays for antiphospholipid antibodies with β_2 GPI and role of other phospholipid cofactors. *Haemostasis*. 1994;24:191–203.

84. Cabral AR, Amigo MC, Cabiedes J, et al. The antiphospholipid/cofactor syndromes: A primary variant with antibodies to β_2 glycoprotein I but no antibodies detectable in standard antiphospholipid assays. *Am J Med*. 1996;101:472–481.

85. Guerin V, Coachouron A, Vergnes C, et al. Antiphospholipid syndromes with anti-human β_2 glycoprotein I antibodies despite negative reactivity in conventional aPL and LA assays. *Thromb Haemost*. 1997;77:1037–1038.

86. Rosove MH, Brewer PMC. Antiphospholipid thrombosis clinical course after the first thrombotic event in 70 patients. *Ann Intern Med*. 1992;117:303–308.

87. Khamashta MA, Cuadrado MJ, Mujic F, et al. The management of thrombosis in the antiphospholipid antibody syndrome. *N Engl J Med*. 1995;332:993–997.

88. Moll S, Ortel TL. Monitoring warfarin therapy in patients with lupus anticoagulants. *Ann Intern Med*. 1997;127:177–185.

89. Lawrie AS, Purdy G, Mackie IJ, et al. Monitoring of oral anticoagulant therapy in lupus anticoagulant positive patients with the anti-phospholipid syndrome. *Br J Haematol*. 1997;98:887–892.

90. Della-Valle P, Crippa L, Safa O, et al. Potential failure of the international normalized ratio (INR) system in the monitoring of oral anticoagulation in patients with lupus anticoagulants. *Ann Med Interne*. 1996;147:10–14.

91. McCrae KR. Antiphospholipid antibody associated thrombosis: A consensus for treatment? *Lupus*. 1996;5:560–570.

92. Rivier G, Herranz MT, Khamashta MA, et al. Thrombosis and antiphospholipid syndrome: A preliminary assessment of three antithrombotic treatments. *Lupus*. 1994;3:85–90.

93. Jennings I, Kitchen S, Woods TAL, et al (on behalf of UK NEQAS for Blood Coagulation). Potentially clinically important inaccuracies in testing for the lupus anticoagulant: An analysis of results from three surveys of the UK National External Quality Assessment Scheme (NEQAS) for blood coagulation. *Thromb Haemost*. 1997;77:934–937.

94. Haemostasis Committee of the "Societe Francaise de Biologic Clinique." Laboratory heterogeneity of the lupus anticoagulant: A multicentre study using differing clotting assays of a panel of 78 samples. *Thromb Res*. 1992;66:349–364.

95. Navarro M, Cervera R, Font J, et al. Anti-endothelial cell antibodies in systemic autoimmune diseases: Prevalence and clinical significance. *Lupus*. 1997;6:521–526.

96. Triplett DA. Antiphospholipid antibodies and thrombosis: A consequence, coincidence, or cause? *Arch Pathol Lab Med*. 1993;117:77–88.

97. Lockshin MD. Why do patients with antiphospholipid antibody clot? *Lupus*. 1997;6:351–352.

98. Potzsch B, Kawamura H, Friessner KT, et al. Acquired protein C dysfunction but not decreased activity of thrombomodulin is a possible marker of thrombophilia in patients with lupus anticoagulant. *J Lab Clin Med*. 1995;125:56–65.

99. Nguyen P, Reynaud J, Pouzol P, et al. Vericella and thrombotic complications associated with transient protein C and protein S deficiencies in children. *Eur J Pediatr*. 1994;153:646–649.

100. Carreras LO, Forastiero RR. Pathogenic role of antiprotein-phospholipid antibodies. *Haemostasis*. 1996;26:340–357.

CHAPTER 15

Idiopathic Vasculitis and Antineutrophilic Cytoplasmic Antibodies

David J. Bylund, MD, and Rex M. McCallum, MD

Vasculitis is defined as inflammation causing vascular lesions, including necrosis, thrombosis, and fibrosis. These lesions may cause either ischemia or infarction of anatomic structures distal to the lesions. Alternatively, necrotizing inflammation may weaken a vessel wall until an aneurysm forms or the vessel ruptures.

Idiopathic (primary) vasculitis, the focus of this chapter, occurs when vascular inflammatory damage is the principal clinicopathologic finding but there is no other underlying illness (**Table 15-1**). In secondary vasculitis, an underlying disorder causes the vascular lesions (**Table 15-2**). Methods of diagnosis and management for secondary vasculitis depend on the underlying disorders; thus, they are discussed in the appropriate chapters of this book.

The clinical expressions of systemic necrotizing vasculitis are highly variable and can occur anywhere in the body. A patient often presents with a wide array of confusing and conflicting symptoms and signs, which can be exceedingly difficult to evaluate. However, specific diagnosis is important because treatment and prognosis depend on the sites and patterns of organ involvement.[1]

Accurate diagnosis is possible only after correlation of the patient's history and physical examination with ancillary radiographic and laboratory data. This chapter describes those clinical laboratory tests useful for the diagnosis and management of idiopathic vasculitis, as well as laboratory evaluation of related end-organ damage, which also may be relevant to secondary vasculitis.

Table 15-1. Idiopathic (Primary) Vasculitis

Churg-Strauss syndrome
Cutaneous leukocytoclastic vasculitis
Giant cell (temporal) arteritis
Henoch-Schönlein purpura
Isolated central nervous system vasculitis
Kawasaki's disease
Polyangiitis overlap syndrome
Polyarteritis nodosa
Takayasu's arteritis
Wegener's granulomatosis

Table 15-2. Secondary Vasculitis[1]

Behçet's disease
Connective tissue disease-associated vasculitis
Polymyositis/dermatomyositis
Rheumatoid arthritis
Scleroderma
Sjögren's syndrome
Systemic lupus erythematosus
Cryoglobulinemic vasculitis
Drug-related vasculitis
Foreign protein-related vasculitis
Hypergammaglobulinemic purpura
Hypocomplementemic urticarial vasculitis
Lymphomatoid granulomatosis
Radiation vasculitis
Relapsing polychondritis
Sarcoidosis
Transplant vasculitis (vascular rejection)
Vasculitis associated with infection
Vasculitis in malignancies

Classification

No standard classification system for idiopathic vasculitis is universally accepted. Historically, this group of disorders has been subtyped according to various combinations of clinical and pathologic findings.[2–4] In recent years, efforts at standardizing classification criteria have added some improvements,[5,6] although use of classification criteria for the diagnosis of vasculitis remains problematic.[7,8] Ultimately, the clinician's goal is an accurate diagnosis that defines proper treatment.

Pathogenesis of Vasculitis

Neither the etiology nor the pathogenesis of idiopathic vasculitis is proven except in instances of direct blood vessel injury from vascular infection. Although etiology remains elusive, there is emerging information that links infections and environmental toxins to vasculitis in some individuals with a genetic predisposition.[9,10]

Most cases of vasculitis are attributed to immune-mediated vascular injury induced by any of several mechanisms, including (1) immune-complex deposits; (2) direct autoantibody binding to vascular endothelium or basement membrane antigens; (3) antineutrophil cytoplasmic antibodies (ANCAs); and (4) T-cell–mediated inflammation.[11]

The pathogenic effects of these different mechanisms all unite in a final common pathway of vascular injury that activates humoral and cellular mediators of inflammation. These mediators initiate infiltration of inflammatory cells, activation of complement and coagulation cascades, and production of other molecules, such as cytokines or leukocyte adhesion molecules.[9,12]

Perspective on the Use of Clinical Laboratory Tests

Because no pathognomonic clinical or laboratory features of vasculitis have been defined, a physician must use clinical and laboratory findings to recognize patterns of disease. This may allow specific diagnosis or, more commonly, classification of a patient's disease as one in a group of vasculitic disorders with similar treatment, even when no specific entity in that group is identifiable.

The differential diagnosis of vasculitis is lengthy (**Table 15-3**), so deciding a patient has vasculitis strictly on the basis of clinical symptoms is risky. Consequently, histologic confirmation of vasculitis should be obtained from tissue biopsy for definitive diagnosis prior to therapy in most forms of the disease.[13]

Clinical laboratory tests alone are of limited value in establishing a specific diagnosis of vasculitis.[13] Clinicians use laboratory tests to accomplish the following:

- Identify patterns of organ involvement characteristic of vasculitis
- Evaluate the extent and severity of end-organ damage
- Differentiate idiopathic vasculitis from alternative secondary forms
- Establish baseline values of tests that may change with disease management

Recognition of the presence of ANCAs in association with certain idiopathic vasculitides has been an important aid in diagnosis and management. Antineutrophil cytoplasmic antibodies are discussed in detail later in this chapter.

Routine Tests

Patients whose histories and physical examinations suggest idiopathic vasculitis often have a confusing array of multisystem complaints that have been present for some time. Routine first-order tests

Table 15-3. Some Diseases That Mimic Systemic Vasculitis

Infection
Endocarditis
Histoplasmosis
Lyme disease
Mycobacterial
Parasitic
Malaria
Strongyloides
Toxoplasmosis
Trichinella
Pneumonia
Legionella
Streptococcus pneumoniae
Syphilis
Viral infections
Cytomegalovirus
Hepatitis (A, B, and C)
Human immunodeficiency virus
Occlusive Vascular Disease
Activated protein C resistance
Antiphospholipid syndrome
Disseminated intravascular coagulation
Protein C or S deficiency
Sickle cell anemia
Thromboangiitis obliterans
Thrombotic thrombocytopenic purpura
Neoplasms
Atrial myxoma
Carcinoma (disseminated, renal cell, colon, lung)
Hairy cell leukemia
Lymphoma
Myelogenous leukemias/myelodysplasia
Drugs
Amphetamines
Cocaine
Ergotamine
Phencyclidine
Warfarin-induced skin necrosis

Table 15-4. Antibodies Associated With Vasculitis

Antibodies	Disease Association	Assay Method
c-ANCA (rarely p-ANCA)	Wegener's granulomatosis	IIFM; ELISA
p-ANCA (rarely c-ANCA)	Microscopic polyarteritis	IIFM; ELISA
ANA	Connective tissue disease	IIFM; ELISA
C1q	Hypocomplementemic urticarial vasculitis	C1q binding
GBM	Anti-GBM disease	ELISA
Endothelial	Kawasaki's disease	ELISA
Hepatitis B	Hepatitis B-associated PAN	ELISA
Mixed cryoglobulins	HCV; cryoglobulin vasculitis	PROEL; IEP; IF
Rheumatoid factor	Rheumatoid vasculitis	Ne; LA; ELISA

Abbreviations: c-ANCA = cytoplasmic antineutrophil cytoplasmic antibodies; p-ANCA = perinuclear antineutrophil cytoplasmic antibodies; IIFM = indirect immunofluorescence microscopy; ELISA = enzyme-linked immunosorbent assay; ANA = antinuclear autoantibodies; GBM = glomerular basement membrane; PAN = polyarteritis nodosa; HCV = hepatitis C virus; PROEL = protein electrophoresis; IEP = immunoelectrophoresis; IF = immunofixation; Ne = nephelometry; LA = latex agglutination.

include the following: cultures for infectious agents, especially if the patient has fever; complete blood cell (CBC) count with differential count; erythrocyte sedimentation rate (ESR); urinalysis; blood chemistry panel; and tests for specific organ function, such as the liver. These tests help a clinician narrow the list of differential diagnoses, provide evidence of or confirm related organ involvement, and establish baseline data for management.

Special Tests

Special tests help to differentiate idiopathic vasculitis from alternative diagnoses. Relevant laboratory tests include those to identify the circulating antibodies listed in **Table 15-4**. Directed tissue biopsy for histologic confirmation of vasculitis and angiography revealing characteristic abnormalities are considered the definitive tests for idiopathic vasculitis.

Some Useful Laboratory Test Patterns in Suspected Vasculitis

Certain patterns of clinical laboratory test results are particularly helpful when vasculitis is a serious diagnostic consideration:

- The ESR is typically elevated in idiopathic vasculitis. If the ESR is not elevated, the diagnosis is probably not giant cell (temporal) arteritis or Wegener's granulomatosis (WG).
- Leukopenia and thrombocytopenia in idiopathic vasculitis are rare and suggest alternative diagnoses, such as systemic lupus erythematosus, neoplasm, bone marrow disorders, or hypersplenism.[13]
- Anemia with hemoglobin of less than 9 mg/dL usually results from conditions other than anemia of chronic disease, such as hemolysis, occult bleeding, or renal disease.[13]
- Elevated serum creatine kinase may indicate myositis or muscle ischemia.[13]
- Testing for antinuclear antibodies (ANAs) and rheumatoid factor (RF) is useful only if connective tissue disease is suspected.
- Peripheral blood eosinophilia occurs in a wide variety of inflammatory disorders. About 15% to 20% of patients with polyarteritis nodosa (PAN) or WG may have eosinophilia, but not to the high levels seen in Churg-Strauss syndrome (CSS).
- First morning urine, both before and after centrifugation, should be examined carefully for protein, hematuria, cells, and casts that accompany glomerulonephritis, which may occur in vasculitis. In renal amyloidosis, there is typically proteinuria without cells.
- Identification of cytoplasmic ANCAs (c-ANCAs) supports a diagnosis of WG in patients with the proper clinical features.[13]
- Untreated patients with WG do not have leukopenia.
- Polyarteritis nodosa associated with pancytopenia can be seen in patients with hairy cell leukemia.[13]

- When PAN is suspected, serologic tests for liver function and for hepatitis B virus, hepatitis C virus, or cytomegalovirus[13,14] should be obtained. Similarly, tests for hepatitis B and C are in order when a patient has cryoglobulins, leukocytoclastic vasculitis on cutaneous biopsy, and/or renal disease.
- Rheumatoid vasculitis is associated with high-titer RF.

Antineutrophil Cytoplasmic Antibodies

The availability of tests to detect ANCAs has proven to be an important laboratory aid in resolving the differential diagnosis of systemic necrotizing vasculitis. In recent years, the possible role of ANCAs in the pathogenesis of WG and other systemic necrotizing vasculitis has generated considerable interest.[2,15,16]

Antineutrophil cytoplasmic antibodies are heterogeneous autoantibodies that react with multiple different cytoplasmic antigens in primary azurophilic granules of neutrophils and in lysosomes of monocytes.[17] Using isolated normal human neutrophils, indirect immunofluorescence microscopy (IIFM) has revealed 2 distinct types of staining patterns associated with idiopathic vasculitis. The c-ANCA pattern has a 29-kd serine proteinase (PR3) as its major target antigen.[17–23] A perinuclear ANCA (p-ANCA) pattern is caused by autoantibodies against myeloperoxidase (MPO).[23,24]

Detection Methods

Currently, IIFM and antigen-specific enzyme-linked immunosorbent assays (ELISAs) are the 2 laboratory methods most commonly used to detect c-ANCA/PR3 and p-ANCA/MPO autoantibodies. Other specialized techniques, including radioimmunoassay, Western blot, dot blot, flow cytometry, and immunoprecipitation are currently impractical for routine use in most clinical laboratories.[17,25]

Indirect Immunofluorescence

Indirect immunofluorescence is the method most commonly used to screen for clinically significant ANCAs. A recommended immunofluorescence protocol is available to laboratories with the special equipment and technical expertise necessary to provide consistent ANCA results.[26]

The differential patterns of ethanol- and formalin-fixed human neutrophils are used to classify 3 types of ANCA patterns. Ethanol fixation of neutrophils allows redistribution of positively charged granules from the cytoplasm to the negatively charged nuclear membrane. The use of formalin rather than ethanol to fix neutrophils prevents redistribution of charged cytoplasmic granules to the nuclear membrane zone.[27]

The c-ANCA pattern, evident on both ethanol- and formalin-fixed neutrophils, indicates granular cytoplasmic immunofluorescence that is centrally accentuated between segmented nuclear lobes of neutrophils (**Image 15-1a,b**). The nucleus itself does not stain unless ANAs are present.

The p-ANCA pattern due to anti-MPO autoantibodies is identified when a perinuclear immunofluorescent pattern on ethanol-fixed neutrophils becomes diffuse and granular with cytoplasmic immunofluorescence on formalin-fixed neutrophils (**Image 15-2a,b**).[27] The fact that p-ANCAs due to anti-MPO are fixative dependent is helpful in separating this diagnosis from atypical p-ANCAs and ANAs.

An atypical p-ANCA pattern due to autoantibodies other than anti-MPO has a perinuclear appearance on ethanol-fixed neutrophils but, unlike p-ANCAs from anti-MPO, has either no or very weak smudgy, cytoplasmic fluorescence on formalin-fixed neutrophils (**Image 15-3a,b,c**).[28]

Antinuclear antibodies, including granulocyte-specific ANAs (GS-ANA), may be confused with p-ANCAs. However, ANAs are typically seen on ethanol- rather than formalin-fixed neutrophils (**Image 15-4a,b,c**). Indirect immunofluorescence microscopy using only HEp-2 cells to separate these antibodies is problematic, because they may occur concurrently and because granulocyte-specific ANAs often are not detected on HEp-2 cells.[17,29]

A protocol for identifying the various autoantibodies is provided in **Figure 15-1a,b**. Because identification of either c-ANCAs or p-ANCAs may have clinical significance, it is generally recommended that presumptive IIFM identification of ANCAs be confirmed with an appropriate antigen-specific ELISA for either PR3 or MPO.[17,30]

Criteria for differentiating ANCAs from nonspecific staining due to other autoantibodies include[17,25]

- A lack of central accentuation if c-ANCAs are considered
- Cytoplasmic staining in fewer than 95% of neutrophils

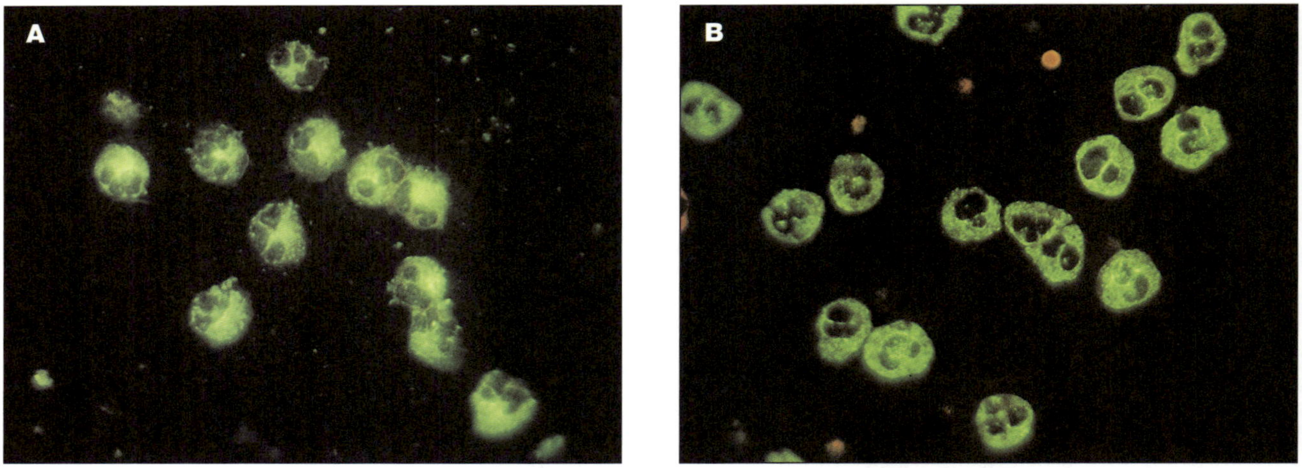

Image 15-1. A cytoplasmic antineutrophil cytoplasmic antibody pattern on indirect immunofluorescence microscopy. Finely granular cytoplasmic immunofluorescence is centrally accentuated between segmented nuclear lobes on both ethanol-fixed (**A**) and formalin-fixed human neutrophils (**B**).

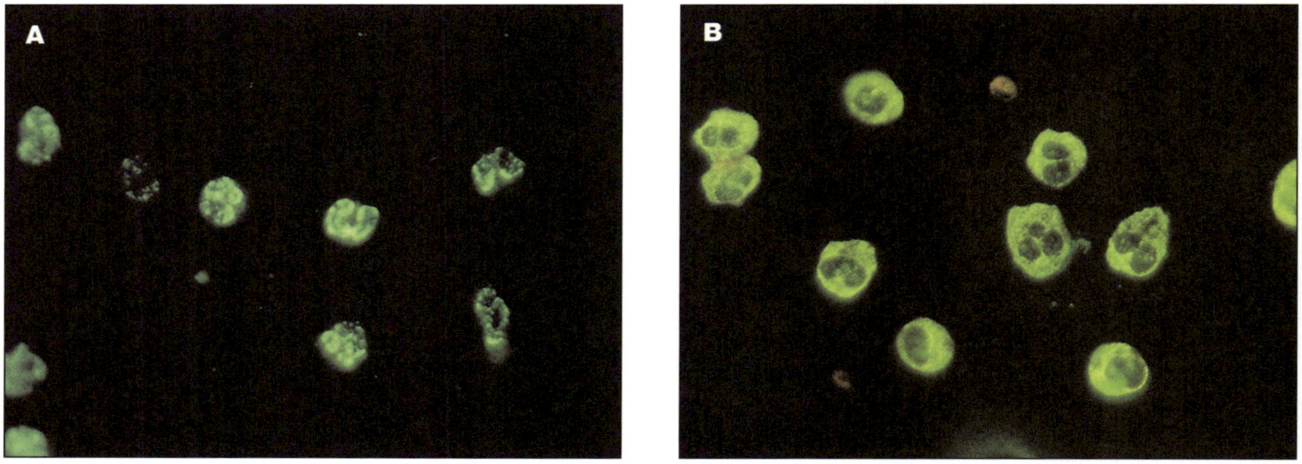

Image 15-2. A perinuclear antineutrophil cytoplasmic antibody pattern on indirect immunofluorescence microscopy. Perinuclear immunofluorescence on ethanol-fixed human neutrophils (**A**) becomes finely granular cytoplasmic immunofluorescence on formalin-fixed neutrophils (**B**).

- Nonneutrophil specificity (eg, cytoplasmic staining is also present in lymphocytes or on HEp-2 cells)
- Heterogeneous cytoplasmic granularity

Enzyme-Linked Immunosorbent Assay

Indirect immunofluorescence cannot distinguish among multiple antibody-antigen reactions that produce similar immunofluorescent patterns. Typically, semiquantitative antigen-specific ELISAs are used to confirm ANCA reactivity using IIFM. Efforts to standardize solid-phase ELISAs are being made in Europe.[30,31]

Licensed commercial ELISAs are available for both PR3 and MPO. Most use standard direct antigen coating of polystyrene microwell plates, so antigen purity is of critical importance in defining analytic sensitivity and specificity.[17,23] Attempts to preserve native antigen conformation are important because ANCAs to PR3 are directed against conformational epitopes.[16] Enzyme-linked immunosorbent assays to detect PR3 have shown results that generally correlate well with the presence of c-ANCAs visible by IIFM when used by technically experienced examiners.[17,23]

Atypical p-ANCAs not associated with idiopathic vasculitis are due to a variety of autoantibodies

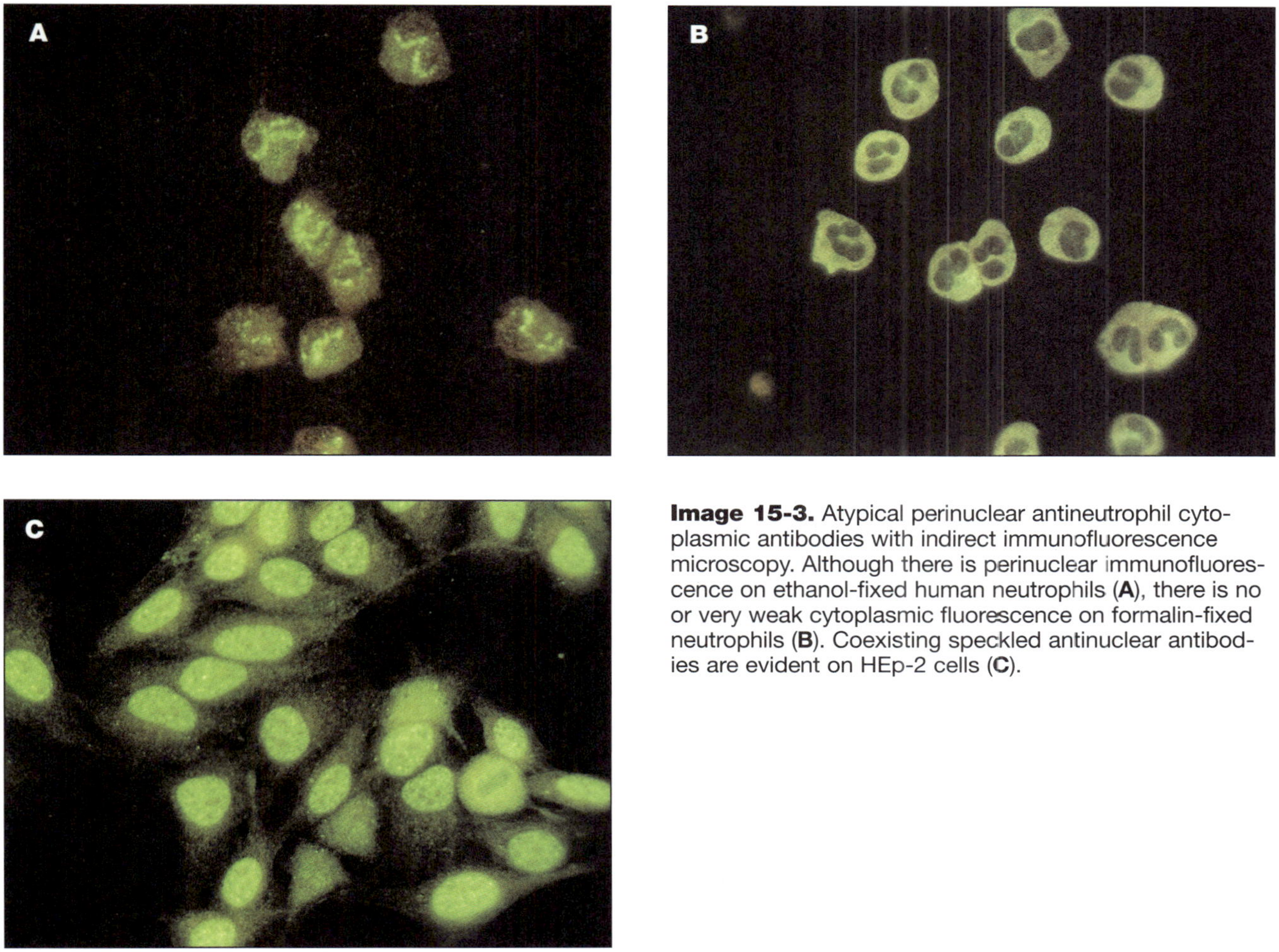

Image 15-3. Atypical perinuclear antineutrophil cytoplasmic antibodies with indirect immunofluorescence microscopy. Although there is perinuclear immunofluorescence on ethanol-fixed human neutrophils (**A**), there is no or very weak cytoplasmic fluorescence on formalin-fixed neutrophils (**B**). Coexisting speckled antinuclear antibodies are evident on HEp-2 cells (**C**).

against neutrophil cytoplasmic antigens other than PR3 and MPO, including elastase, lactoferrin, lactoperoxidase, cathepsin G, lysozyme, bactericidal/permeability-increasing (BPI) protein, and azurocidin.[23,27,32–37] Many of the target antigens have not yet been characterized.

Enzyme-linked immunosorbent assays have limitations; ultimately, each laboratory must carefully verify a manufacturer's claims so the clinician can receive information on performance characteristics. This proves especially important in confusing clinical situations where there may be discrepancies between clinical presentation and laboratory results and/or discordant results between IIFM and ELISA tests.

Disease Associations

As summarized in **Table 15-5**, ANCAs are associated with several pathologic conditions, including systemic vasculitis and inflammatory disease of the gastrointestinal and hepatobiliary tracts.

Systemic Vasculitis

Antineutrophil cytoplasmic antibodies are found in patients with WG, CSS, polyarteritis nodosa, idiopathic crescentic glomerulonephritis, and polyangiitis overlap syndromes.[23,38] About 90% of patients with active WG have c-ANCAs directed against PR3, whereas p-ANCA/MPO is identified in fewer than 10% of such patients. About 80% of those with PAN affecting small vessels (microscopic polyangiitis/polyarteritis) have about the same frequency of c-ANCAs and p-ANCAs.

Although p-ANCA/MPO accompanies CSS or idiopathic crescentic glomerulonephritis in 70% to 80% of patients with active disease, the latter group of diseases is rarely marked by c-ANCA/PR3 rather than p-ANCA.

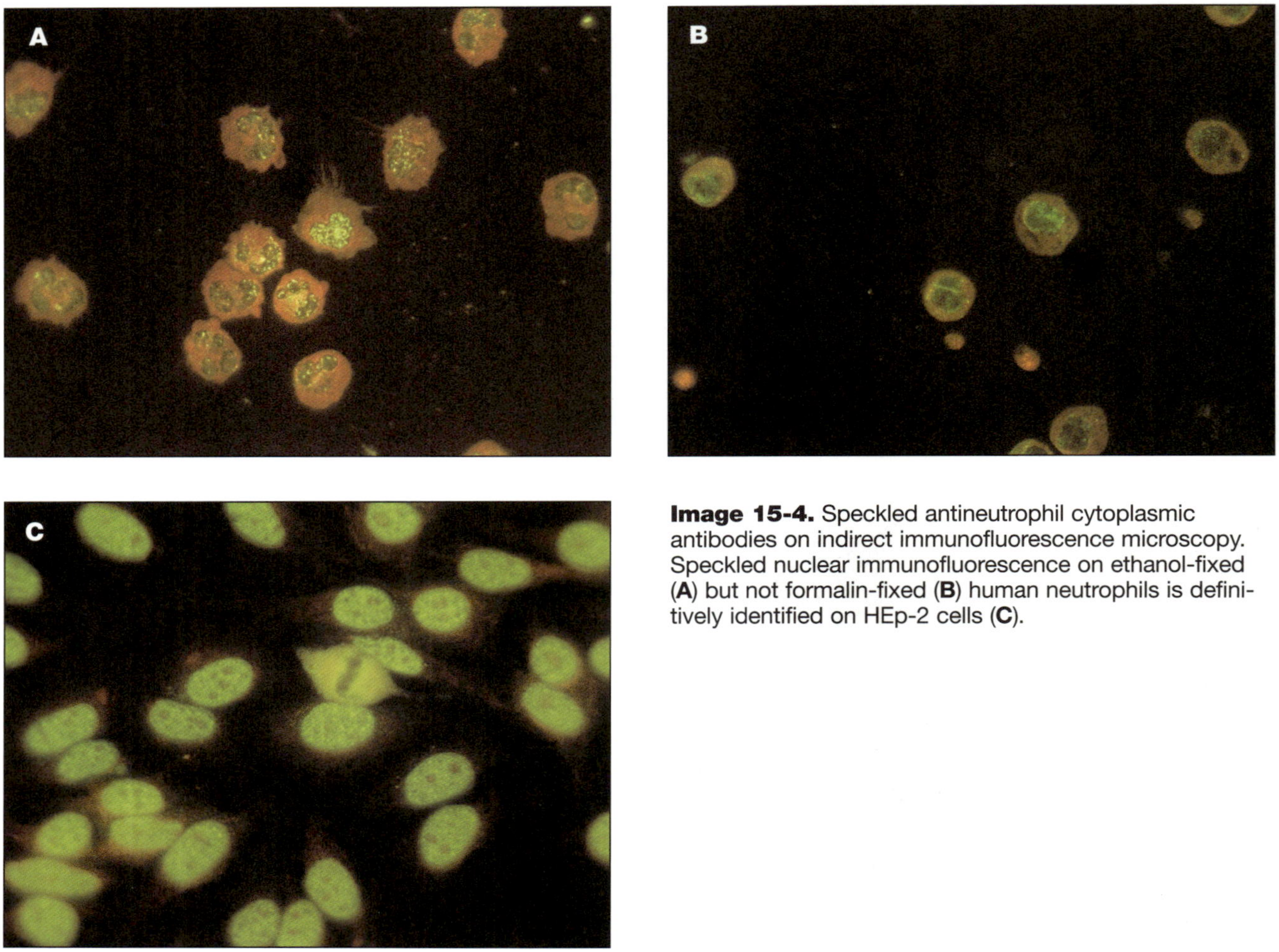

Image 15-4. Speckled antineutrophil cytoplasmic antibodies on indirect immunofluorescence microscopy. Speckled nuclear immunofluorescence on ethanol-fixed (**A**) but not formalin-fixed (**B**) human neutrophils is definitively identified on HEp-2 cells (**C**).

The coexistence of ANCAs and anti–glomerular basement membrane zone (anti-GBM) antibody has been reported.[23,39] Affected patients may have clinical manifestations of ANCA-associated vasculitis that would not be expected in anti-GBM disease alone.[15]

Inflammatory Disease of the Gastrointestinal and Hepatobiliary Tracts

Several reports link ANCAs with inflammatory diseases of the gastrointestinal and hepatobiliary tracts.[27,28] Atypical p-ANCAs are identified in 50% to 90% of patients with active ulcerative colitis or primary sclerosing cholangitis and in 15% to 30% of patients with Crohn's disease.

The target antigen specificities of p-ANCAs in inflammatory bowel disease are not fully defined, although MPO is not a dominant target antigen. Autoantibodies against lactoperoxidase, lactoferrin,[40] or cathepsin G have been documented.[27]

Other Diseases

Antineutrophil cytoplasmic antibodies have been associated with drugs and recorded for many diseases other than systemic vasculitis. Those associated with drugs include hydralazine-induced lupus erythematosus with anti-MPO and antielastase antibodies, hydralazine-associated vasculitis with anti-MPO, and minocycline-induced arthritis.[16,17]

Antineutrophil cytoplasmic antibodies also have been reported in several other diseases, including systemic lupus erythematosus, rheumatoid arthritis, Felty's syndrome, Sjögren's syndrome, human immunodeficiency virus infection, other infections, cystic fibrosis, and certain neoplasms.[27,41] Generally, these conditions have atypical p-ANCAs directed to a variety of target antigens, many of which have yet to be defined. Cytoplasmic ANCAs directed against PR3 very rarely occur in these conditions.

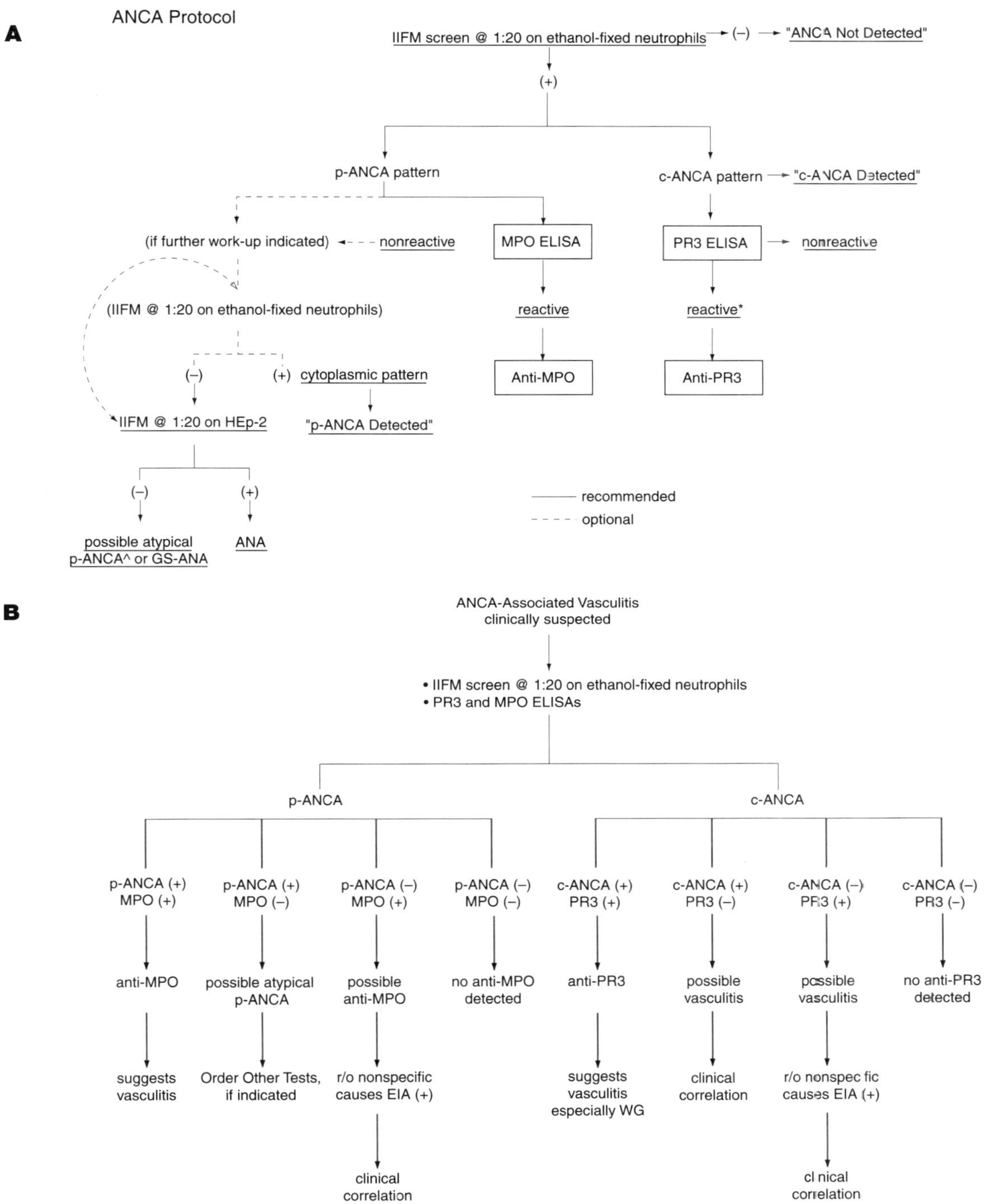

Figure 15-1. Protocol for antineutrophil cytoplasmic antibody identification. Abbreviations: IIFM = indirect immunofluorescence microscopy; ANCA = antineutrophil cytoplasmic antibody; p-ANCA = perinuclear antineutrophil cytoplasmic antibody; c-ANCA = cytoplasmic antineutrophil cytoplasmic antibody; MPO = myeloperoxidase; ELISA = enzyme-linked immunosorbent assay; GS-ANA = granulocyte-specific antinuclear antibody. *In rare instances, some c-ANCA-positive sera may be due to autoantibodies other than PR3, such as BPI (bactericidal/permeability-increasing protein), or ELISAs may not detect some anti-PR3 due to technical factors such as denaturation of conformational epitopes. †Occasionally, c-ANCA-negative sera may be PR3 positive. Clinical confirmation is necessary. ‡An atypical p-ANCA pattern is caused by antibodies other than MPO, such as lactoferrin, elastase, or cathepsin G.

Table 15-5. Antineutrophil Cytoplasmic Antibodies (ANCA)-Associated Disorders[16]

c-ANCA/Proteinase-3
- Systemic necrotizing vasculitis
  - Common
    - Wegener's granulomatosis
    - Churg-Strauss syndrome
  - Uncommon
    - Microscopic polyarteritis
- Drug
  - Propylthiouracil

p-ANCA/Myeloperoxidase
- Systemic necrotizing vasculitis
  - Common
    - Microscopic polyarteritis
    - Churg-Strauss syndrome
  - Uncommon
    - Wegener's granulomatosis
- Drugs
  - Hydralazine
  - Minocycline
  - Propylthiouracil

p-ANCA to various antigens, not myeloperoxidase
- Connective tissue disease
  - Antiphospholipid antibody syndrome
  - Juvenile chronic arthritis
  - Polymyositis/dermatomyositis
  - Relapsing polychondritis
  - Rheumatoid arthritis
  - Sjögren's syndrome
  - Systemic lupus erythematosus
- Inflammatory bowel disease
  - Ulcerative colitis (40% to 80%)
  - Crohn's disease (10% to 40%)
  - Bacterial enteritis (rare)
- Autoimmune liver disease
  - Primary sclerosing cholangitis
  - Autoimmune hepatitis
- Infections
  - Chromomycosis
  - Human immunodeficiency virus, type 1
  - Acute malaria

Test Interpretation

Interpretation of ANCA tests should consider the following factors:

- These tests should not be used to screen nonselected patient groups where the prevalence of vasculitis is low.
- Tests are most valuable when selectively ordered in clinical situations where some form of ANCA-associated vasculitis is seriously considered.
- A c-ANCA immunofluorescence pattern should be confirmed using PR3 ELISA.
- Anti-PR3 reactivity is most often seen in active WG or PAN, but also may be seen in idiopathic crescentic glomerulonephritis or CSS.
- A c-ANCA test for patients with WG is considered highly sensitive (67% to 97%) in signaling active systemic disease with renal involvement but of only moderate sensitivity (60% to 70%) in spotting limited or localized disease.[23] The sensitivity of this test for patients in complete remission is only about 30%.[29]
- The predictive value of an increased c-ANCA titer as a harbinger of WG relapse is controversial, because not all increases in c-ANCA titer are followed by worsening of the disease.[29]
- A p-ANCA pattern with IIFM is diagnostically nonspecific.
- Perinuclear ANCAs due to anti-MPO antibodies are most often seen in PAN, idiopathic crescentic glomerulonephritis, or CSS; however, they may be seen in WG.
- Neither a diagnosis of systemic necrotizing vasculitis nor a decision to treat should be based solely on a positive ANCA test result.
- A negative ANCA result should not be used to exclude disease.

The present authors regard a positive c-ANCA result as suggestive of WG and a signal for further evaluation. Ultimately, the interpretation of an ANCA test depends on the philosophy and experience of the individual clinician treating vasculitis.

Synopses of Major Idiopathic Vasculitic Syndromes

Polyarteritis Nodosa

Epidemiology

Polyarteritis nodosa, like all idiopathic vasculitis, is an uncommon disease. Estimates of the annual incidence rate vary from 4.6 per 100,000 in England and 9.0 per 1 million in Olmsted County, Minnesota, to 77 per 100,000 in an Alaskan Eskimo population hyperendemic for hepatitis B.[1,42] Polyarteritis nodosa may occur in either gender and at any age, but is most common in men (male-female ratio = 2:1) between 40 and 60 years old.[1] There is no observed racial predilection.[42]

Clinical Features

The clinical manifestations of classic PAN vary widely. Patients often present with nonspecific symptoms, such as fever, weight loss, malaise, and commonly hypertension. The disease may afflict virtually any organ system, and symptomatic involvement of the skin, joints, peripheral nerves, gastrointestinal tract, and kidneys usually dominate the clinical picture.[42] Tests indicating abnormal liver function suggest the possibility of concurrent hepatitis B infection.[1] Pulmonary involvement in classic PAN is rare and even controversial. Some investigators designate pulmonary PAN as a stand-alone entity,[4] whereas others believe that such patients probably have CSS or WG, both of which commonly include pulmonary disease.[1,43] Polyarteritis nodosa follows a course of remissions and relapses that, when untreated, ends in death.[43]

Clinical Laboratory Findings

Results of clinical laboratory tests, although diagnostically nonspecific, reflect the systemic inflammatory nature of PAN. Typical findings include normocytic normochromic anemia, neutrophilic leukocytosis, hypoalbuminemia, hypergammaglobulinemia, and a markedly elevated ESR. Abnormalities in serum creatinine and blood urea nitrogen or in the results of urinalysis to check for proteinuria, hematuria, and abnormal sediment may indicate impaired renal function. Positivity for ANA or RF found in 10% to 40% of these patients may be associated with decreased levels of complement components C3 and C4. Additionally, all patients with PAN should undergo serologic testing for hepatitis B surface antigen and antibody.[1,42] Peripheral blood eosinophilia is rare in this patient population, but when present at a high level, may be an indicator of CSS.[43]

Diagnosis

Polyarteritis nodosa can be difficult to diagnose given its nonspecific presentation, potential for diverse organ involvement, and low prevalence. However, once suspected, it is diagnosed based on angiography and, whenever possible, histologic demonstration of the lesions on biopsy of tissue from symptomatic sites. Pathologically, PAN is a focal but panmural necrotizing arteritis of small- and medium-size muscular arteries, preferentially occurring at vessel branch points. Necrotizing mixed cell inflammation with fibrinoid necrosis, either circumferential or segmental in the vessel wall, is the hallmark lesion of active PAN. Microaneurysm or aneurysmal dilatation also is characteristic of acute phase PAN. The inflammatory process halts and healing follows when fibroblastic proliferation leads to proliferative endarteritis. Typically, active and/or healing lesions lie adjacent to normal blood vessel segments.[1]

Sites that should be considered for biopsy include muscle, skin, sural nerve, kidney, rectum, and testis. Angiography may be especially valuable when none of these sites is available for biopsy or when probing for gastrointestinal abnormalities is warranted. In particular, angiography should be considered before attempting a closed-needle biopsy of the liver or kidney in patients thought to have PAN, because the predilection for aneurysms at these sites increases the risk of severe bleeding.[1]

Treatment and Prognosis

Patients with PAN are treated with glucocorticoids, optimally under a protocol that controls the disease but does not induce significant complications from the drug itself. Cyclophosphamide should be used for patients with severe PAN; however, treatment of all patients with PAN using both cyclophosphamide and glucocorticoid remains controversial.[1]

The prognosis for PAN patients has greatly improved with the use of glucocorticoids, extending the 5-year survival rate from 13% to 60%. The majority of deaths are within the first year after diagnosis, but, whether before or after 1 year of disease, mortality most often results from either infection as a complication of treatment or sequelae of vessel obliteration, such as myocardial infarction or stroke.[1]

Churg-Strauss Syndrome

Epidemiology

Churg-Strauss syndrome is a rare clinical condition, but no extensive epidemiologic data are available.[42] It can begin when patients are 15 to 69 years old, with 38 years as the median age for onset of vasculitis.[1] The male-female ratio is about 2:1.

Clinical Features

Churg-Strauss syndrome, also called allergic angiitis and granulomatosis, is a systemic necrotizing vasculitis recognizable by patients' vascular and extravascular granulomatous inflammation, multiple organ involvement, and often allergic rhinitis, severe asthma, and hypereosinophilia.[1,43] Clinical manifestations of CSS may resemble those of PAN in many respects, but they differ in that, although lung disease is typical in patients with CSS, renal disease is uncommon and, even when present, is usually less severe than in patients with PAN.[43]

The clinical course of CSS is often divided into 3 distinct phases, although in reality these phases are not always distinct and may overlap[1]:

1. Prodromal phase characterized by allergic respiratory disease
2. Eosinophilic phase with peripheral blood and tissue hypereosinophilia
3. Vasculitic phase

Cardiac involvement, either transmural eosinophilic carditis or coronary vasculitis, occurs in 25% to 62% of patients with CSS and is the major cause of death.[1]

Clinical Laboratory Findings

A hallmark of CSS is obvious peripheral blood eosinophilia, which, despite the demarcation of phases, may develop at any point in the disease. The peripheral blood eosinophil count reaches 1,000 eosinophils/mL in 80% or more of CSS patients[42]; however, eosinophilia may be absent in patients undergoing either steroid treatment for asthma or the wide and rapid fluctuation in eosinophil count common to this disorder. Normalization of the eosinophil count in response to steroid treatment is a feature of CSS and helps distinguish it from the hypereosinophilic syndrome in which eosinophilia is frequently steroid resistant. The degree of eosinophilia may correlate with the activity of vasculitic disease in some patients.

Other laboratory findings in CSS are nonspecific. Anemia, leukocytosis, and increased ESR frequently accompany the vasculitic phase. Serum immunoglobulin (Ig) E levels may be elevated, and serum RF has been identified, usually at low titer. Serum complement is reported to be normal.[42] In contrast to PAN, no association between CSS and hepatitis B has been described.[1]

Diagnosis

Historically, the diagnosis of CSS has been made solely on histologic demonstration of necrotizing eosinophilic vasculitis, eosinophilic tissue infiltration, and extravascular granuloma. In practice, however, few biopsy specimens contain all these findings. To increase the likelihood of identifying and diagnosing CSS, the emphasis can be shifted from these diagnostic indicators to include clinical features. One study[42] has recommended the following criteria:

- Asthma
- Peripheral blood eosinophilia in excess of 1.5 cells/mL
- Systemic vasculitis involving 2 or more extrapulmonary organs

Without question, however, definitive diagnosis requires biopsy-derived proof of vasculitis. Open-lung biopsy frequently does not confirm all histologic features of CSS but must be considered before the institution of therapy if there is any concern over possible infection. When clinical symptoms so indicate, the best biopsy specimens are most often from skin, muscle, sural nerve, prostate, and kidney. The differential diagnosis of CSS generally includes PAN, WG, and the hypereosinophilic syndrome.[1]

Treatment and Prognosis

Corticosteroids are the basis for treatment of CSS. The usefulness of immunosuppression with azathioprine or cyclophosphamide therapy is unproven.[1]

Early diagnosis of CSS and corticosteroid treatment has put affected patients' 5-year survival rate at around 62%. In 48% of patients, death is caused by congestive heart failure and myocardial infarction. Other potential causes include cerebral hemorrhage, renal failure, gastrointestinal perforation or hemorrhage, status asthmaticus, and respiratory failure. A short interval between the onset of asthma and the onset of vasculitis is considered an unfavorable prognostic sign.

Polyangiitis Overlap Syndrome

The term *polyangiitis overlap syndrome* is applied to a heterogeneous group of patients who have systemic necrotizing vasculitis but in whom the disease does not manifest in such a way that they can be placed clearly in a specific diagnostic category. Patients with polyangiitis overlap syndrome may have combined features of several vasculitic diseases, similarly mixed pathologic findings, or atypical symptoms that do not fit one specific disease or syndrome.[1]

Like well-defined vasculitic syndromes, polyangiitis overlap syndrome is a true systemic vasculitis with the potential to affect multiple organ systems. Although no prognosis is established for this syndrome, serious organ damage and life-threatening disease are risks. Both diagnostically and therapeutically, the management of affected patients should be approached as for those with a well-defined vasculitic syndrome. A careful history, physical examination, and laboratory evaluation are necessary to define the extent of systemic defects. Ultimately, a diagnosis of polyangiitis overlap syndrome requires the demonstration of vasculitis, which should be aggressively pursued through either biopsy or angiography. Once the presence of a systemic necrotizing vasculitis has been confirmed and other diagnoses, specifically infection, have been ruled out, treatment with corticosteroids should begin and the addition of immunosuppressive agents (eg, cyclophosphamide) should be considered.[1]

Wegener's Granulomatosis

Epidemiology

No data are available regarding the annual incidence or prevalence of WG, which is believed to be less common than PAN. Wegener's granulomatosis can arise in people of any age, race, or gender, although it affects predominantly whites and has a slight male predominance.[42] The mean age at onset is 41 years.[1]

Clinical Features

Wegener's granulomatosis is a clinicopathologic syndrome of unknown etiology characterized pathologically by necrotizing granulomatous inflammation of upper and lower respiratory tracts, focal segmental glomerulonephritis, and necrotizing vasculitis involving predominantly medium and small arteries. It presents in the ear, nose, and throat regions with sinusitis, nasal obstruction or ulceration, otitis media, or hearing loss. At the time of diagnosis, 45% of patients have some pulmonary abnormality, and 85% eventually manifest lung disease. Commonly these manifestations include pulmonary infiltrates, pulmonary nodules, hemoptysis, or pleuritis. Although renal disease initially afflicts only about 18% of affected patients, glomerulonephritis develops in 80% at some time during the course of WG. Other usual signs of systemic illness are skin rash, arthralgias, fever, eye disorders, and weight loss. Although patients with WG limited to the respiratory tract without renal involvement have been described ("limited WG"), more than 50% of patients who initially present with limited disease later develop the more generalized form.[1,4,43]

Clinical Laboratory Findings[1,42,43]

Clinical laboratory findings typical of WG include moderate leukocytosis without striking eosinophilia, mild normochromic anemia, and thrombocytosis. Because untreated patients do not have leukopenia, this finding distinguishes WG from other disorders. The presence of c-ANCAs supports the diagnosis. Circulating immune complexes, measurable by C1q binding, may be found together with normal complement levels. Hypergammaglobulinemia is noted, and often the IgA level is elevated. Indicators of glomerular involvement include microscopic or gross hematuria, proteinuria, red blood cell casts, and/or elevations of serum creatinine and blood urea nitrogen. More than 50% of these patients are RF positive, but ANAs are usually absent. Additionally, serologic tests for anti-GBM antibodies are negative. Preceding treatment, 80% of patients have elevated ESRs.

Diagnosis

Although clinical and laboratory findings may be suggestive, a diagnosis of WG should be made only after tissue biopsy confirmation. Pulmonary tissue obtained through open-lung biopsy offers the best opportunity for an accurate diagnosis,[1] whereas, in more than 90% of patients, transbronchial biopsy does not yield adequate tissue for diagnosis. Although head and neck tissue is more directly accessible, fewer than 23% of such biopsy specimens contain the characteristic pathologic features. Diagnostically useful tissue from the head and neck regions are best obtained (in decreasing order of frequency) from paranasal sinuses, nasal tissue, and the subglottic region. Glomerular changes in renal biopsy tissue may suggest WG but are rarely diagnostic.[1]

Although the morphologic spectrum of WG is broad, the hallmark pathologic lesion in this disease is necrotizing granulomatous vasculitis. Affected vessels undergo fibrinoid necrosis with early infiltration by polymorphonuclear leukocytes followed by mononuclear cells. Pulmonary tissue may reveal some combination of necrosis, vasculitis, and granulomatous inflammation, although biopsy specimens often do not include all these characteristic features. The best signal of WG in a renal biopsy is segmental necrotizing glomerulonephritis, found at varying degrees of severity in 80% of specimens.

Renal vasculitis at sites other than glomeruli is unusual enough that only 8% of biopsies are positive. Skin biopsies most commonly show leukocytoclastic vasculitis, although dermal necrotizing granuloma or necrotizing vasculitis of the larger dermal arteries or veins has been noted.[1]

Many disorders, including infectious or noninfectious granulomatous diseases, CSS, Goodpasture's syndrome, idiopathic midline granuloma, lymphomatoid granulomatosis, and neoplasms of the upper airway or lungs, can mimic WG.[43] Regardless of the disorder, infection is a critical consideration, because misdiagnosis can have fatal consequences if an immunosuppressive drug is used for treatment. Therefore, aggressive pursuit of tissue diagnosis is of extreme importance, both to confirm WG and to rule out other diagnostic possibilities.[1]

Treatment and Prognosis

A regimen of daily oral cyclophosphamide and corticosteroids is the therapy of choice for WG. Using this regimen, the National Institutes of Health reported marked improvement or partial remission in 91% of patients and complete remission in 75%, compared with 100% mortality for untreated patients. With treatment, the overall mortality rate was 20%, 13% of which could be completely or partially attributed to WG. Despite the greatly improved rates of survival and remission attributed to the drugs, half of the complete remissions were followed by one or more relapses, which occurred 3 months to 16 years after achieving remission.[1] During the first year of WG, the extent of renal disease is the factor most closely related to prognosis. Thereafter, lung involvement becomes the most important prognostic indicator, but glomerulonephritis does not appear to significantly affect prognosis.

Lymphomatoid Granulomatosis

Lymphomatoid granulomatosis is an unusual lymphoproliferative disorder that may evolve into malignant lymphoma in approximately 50% of patients. It mainly affects the lungs, where it clinically mimics WG. The histologic markers are prominent angiocentric infiltration and destruction of blood vessels, much like the lesions of vasculitis, but the cellular morphology is more suggestive of lymphoma or lymphoproliferative disorder.[1] There are no specific clinical laboratory tests for lymphomatoid granulomatosis.

Henoch-Schönlein Purpura

Epidemiology

Henoch-Schönlein purpura (HSP) is primarily a disease found in children between the ages of 4 and 11 years,[42] but it also afflicts some adults. In both groups, males predominate at a ratio of 3:2.[1] The disease most commonly presents in the spring and classically follows an upper respiratory tract infection.[42]

Clinical Features

Henoch-Schönlein purpura, sometimes referred to as anaphylactoid purpura, is a systemic small-vessel vasculitis classified as a subgroup of hypersensitivity vasculitis. Its etiology is unknown. Typical clinical findings in persons with HSP include nonthrombocytopenic palpable purpura, arthralgias, renal disease, and gastrointestinal tract abnormalities.[1] Seventy percent of patients with HSP manifest gastrointestinal signs and symptoms that include colicky abdominal pain associated with nausea and vomiting, blood or mucus in the stool, life-threatening gastrointestinal hemorrhage, and intussusception.[1] The related renal disease appears as focal proliferative glomerulonephritis, the expression of which varies from isolated hematuria with red blood cell casts, to acute renal failure, and rarely to chronic renal failure.[1,4,43]

Clinical Laboratory Findings

Clinical laboratory studies for HSP are nonspecific, so their primary use is in excluding other disorders and assessing the state of kidney function. Leukocytosis and elevated ESR may be seen. A CBC with platelet count and coagulation screening tests are important in the evaluation of cutaneous purpura, because the associated lesions do not stem from thrombocytopenia. Intermittent stool guaiacs should be performed to check for occult blood loss. Serum complement levels are usually normal, although HSP has been linked to the congenital absence of complement component C2.[42] Urinalysis and serum creatinine measurements are performed at the onset of illness and twice weekly until the systemic signs of the disease disappear.[1] Direct immunofluorescence studies, when available, characteristically reveal granular deposits of IgA and complement in cutaneous vessels and renal glomeruli.[42]

Diagnosis

Diagnosing HSP is fairly straightforward, except when major sites other than cutaneous vessels are involved before palpable purpura appears. Unlike other systemic necrotizing vasculitis, diagnosis is clinical. Laboratory studies are used mostly as an adjunct to rule out other disorders. Renal biopsy (to identify proliferative glomerulonephritis) is usually unnecessary for diagnosis but is a good way to assess the severity of disease and estimate prognosis. Disorders to be considered in the differential diagnosis of HSP include those that cause acute abdominal pain, nephritis, or purpura.[1]

Treatment and Prognosis

Treatment of HSP is supportive, because no specific regimen has proven beneficial for HSP nephritis. Although glucocorticoids may successfully decrease edema, joint pain, and abdominal discomfort, sustained glucocorticoid therapy is not helpful, because it does not decrease the risk of recurrent disease or improve the outlook for kidney function.[1] Nonsalicylate pain relievers for analgesia may soothe joint and soft-tissue discomfort. Therapy for adults is similar to that for children, although in adults, hypertension must be controlled carefully.[1]

The prognosis is good for patients with this generally self-limited disease, which lasts from 6 to 16 weeks.[42] The mortality rate is about 1% to 3%, and renal disease is the major cause of death.[1] Patients with an acute nephritic condition, particularly with nephrotic syndrome, have the worst outcome, with fewer than 50% returning to normal renal function in 2 years. Another prognostic indicator may be the percentage of glomeruli with crescents.

However, an important disclaimer is that the course of HSP can be extremely variable. Affected patients with severe clinical or histologic abnormalities may recover fully, and those with relatively mild symptoms may progress to renal insufficiency. The disease recurs largely with skin manifestations in 25% to 40% of patients. Deterioration or improvement may be most notable during the first 2 to 3 years after resolution of the acute episode, although marked changes in outcome may develop later. Regular follow-up with blood pressure measurement and urinalysis is extremely important for at least the first 5 years after an episode of HSP.[1]

Giant Cell (Temporal) Arteritis

Epidemiology

Giant cell (GC) arteritis is a relatively common vasculitic disorder, the incidence of which increases with age. One study[42] that included biopsy-proven GC arteritis asserted that the annual incidence was 23.3 per 100,000 persons older than 50 years. Nearly all cases of GC arteritis begin after patients reach the age of 50.

Clinical Features

Giant cell arteritis is a systemic disease in which granulomatous inflammation affects medium to large arteries. Although these arteries may be in numerous sites, the temporal artery and/or other branches of the carotid artery are the classic targets of GC arteritis.[43] Clinical manifestations include fever, headache, anemia, and jaw claudication. Moreover, ischemic optic neuritis can lead to sudden blindness, particularly in untreated patients.[43] Giant cell arteritis is closely associated with polymyalgia rheumatica—stiffness and pain of the neck, shoulders, lower back, hips, and thighs—that is worst in the morning and lessens with normal daily activity.[43]

Clinical Laboratory Findings

Characteristic laboratory findings include normochromic anemia and elevations in ESR and serum alkaline phosphatase. Hypergammaglobulinemia and increased levels of complement and immune complexes have been reported.[43]

Diagnosis

Diagnosis is based on identifying the typical clinical manifestations and a high ESR in middle-aged to elderly patients who may or may not also have symptoms of polymyalgia rheumatica.[43] Diagnosis is confirmed by biopsy of the temporal artery.

Treatment and Prognosis

Giant cell arteritis is treated with glucocorticoids, usually followed by a dramatically positive response. The prognosis is good because most patients achieve and maintain complete remission after receiving the glucocorticoid regimen.[43] Unfortunately, when blindness develops secondary to GC arteritis, the recovery of sight is rare, even with rapid and high-dose corticosteroid therapy.

Takayasu's Arteritis

Epidemiology

Like all idiopathic vasculitis, Takayasu's arteritis is uncommon, and the epidemiology is not accurately documented. Most (80% to 90%) cases occur in women, and this disorder is most prevalent in adolescent girls and young women from 10 to 30 years in age. Although more common in Japan, this disease has no proven racial or geographic restrictions.[42,43]

Clinical Features

Takayasu's arteritis is a granulomatous vasculitis of medium to large elastic arteries that causes stenosis or occlusion. This condition has a strong predilection for the aortic arch and its large branches, including pulmonary arteries. Accordingly, the disorder is sometimes called aortic arch syndrome or pulseless disease. Patients present with acute systemic symptoms, including fever, malaise, night sweats, and weight loss. Ischemia in organs receiving their blood supply through the affected vessel(s) causes organ-specific symptoms and signs. The term "pulseless" refers to the chronic obliterative phase of the disease, during which pulses decrease or stop completely in affected arteries, most commonly in the subclavian artery. Vascular bruits and hypertension are frequent. Other findings include aortic regurgitation, cardiomegaly secondary to aortic or pulmonary hypertension, and stroke. Takayasu's arteritis may progress slowly, stabilize, or rapidly cause death.[1,43]

Clinical Laboratory Findings

Laboratory study of blood samples from patients with Takayasu's arteritis uncovers a systemic inflammatory disorder.[1] The ESR is elevated in 75% to 100% of patients with active disease but tends to return to normal over time. The ESR is believed to be a reliable index of inflammatory activity and has been used as a test to monitor the effectiveness of therapy. Resolution of the disease, both symptomatically and angiographically, has been found to correlate with a decline in ESR.

Hematologic studies often show mild to moderate normochromic anemia and/or mild leukocytosis. Rheumatoid factor and ANA tests are usually negative. Hypergammaglobulinemia, hyperfibrinogenemia, and hypoalbuminemia may become evident.[42] Although up to 50% of affected patients have circulating immune complexes, these complexes do not coincide with disease activity.

Diagnosis

Takayasu's arteritis is diagnosed by correlating data from the history, physical examination, and angiography. The disease should be considered as a diagnostic possibility in any girl or young woman who lacks or has a markedly diminished peripheral pulse rate or who has blood pressure discrepancies and/or arterial bruits.[43] Characteristic angiographic findings help confirm the clinical diagnosis. Tissue biopsy for confirmation of diagnosis is seldom required or done.[43] The important feature that often separates this syndrome from other diagnostic considerations, particularly GC arteritis, is its predominance in girls and young women.[1]

Treatment and Prognosis[1]

Corticosteroid therapy is the initial treatment of choice for patients with active Takayasu's arteritis. When the disease remains active despite corticosteroids, cyclophosphamide or methotrexate may be administered. Vasodilators, anticoagulants, and nonsteroidal anti-inflammatory agents are used for symptomatic relief. At the other end of the treatment spectrum, surgical intervention may be necessary for vascular stenosis or occlusion.

The clinical course of Takayasu's arteritis varies. Although spontaneous remissions occur, most patients require treatment. Prognosis appears to be related to the presence and severity of complications. Major complications include Takayasu's retinopathy, secondary hypertension, aortic valve insufficiency, and aortic/arterial aneurysm. The overall survival rate declines from 97% to 72% at 5 years and is 59% at 10 years after diagnosis as the number and/or severity of complications increase. Related deaths usually occur from vascular defects, such as congestive heart failure, stroke, myocardial infarction, and aneurysm rupture.

Isolated Central Nervous System Vasculitis

Epidemiology

Isolated central nervous system vasculitis (ICNSV) is a rare condition that is so difficult to diagnose that it hinders epidemiologic studies. Slightly more men than women (4:3) suffer from ICNSV, which begins in midlife at a mean age of 43 years.[1]

Clinical Features

Patients with ICNSV complain of headaches, focal neurologic deficits, and altered mental status.[43] Their initial symptoms are generalized, and more specific neurologic symptoms and signs do not develop until later in the course of the disease.[1] The subsequent course may be rapidly progressive or wax and wane over an extended period.

Clinical Laboratory Findings

Laboratory studies are helpful in excluding other disease processes. The ESR is elevated in many, but not all, patients. Anemia has been seen in only 17%, and other hematologic parameters are usually normal. Rheumatoid factor, ANAs, and ANCAs typically are absent. However, the cerebrospinal fluid is usually abnormal as manifested by increased opening pressure, elevated protein, and lymphocytic pleocytosis. Because the cerebrospinal fluid also can be completely normal, such testing does not always rule out the possibility of vasculitis.[1]

Diagnosis

The diagnosis of ICNSV remains one of exclusion. Proposed diagnostic criteria include

- Central nervous system dysfunction that is not explained by clinical, laboratory, or neurologic investigation
- Arteritis within the central nervous system, documented by angiogram and/or biopsy
- No evidence of systemic vasculitis or other conditions to which angiographic or pathologic features could be secondary

Given the difficulty of establishing the absence of systemic vasculitis or related conditions with any degree of certainty and the occurrence of noninflammatory lesions, central nervous system biopsies are probably underused.

Even so, the use of brain biopsy to evaluate potential ICNSV remains controversial, although some advocates state that such biopsy is essential for a definitive diagnosis. Factors precluding greater use of brain biopsy are not only its invasive nature but also the unreliability of demonstrating histologic vasculitis even in a patient with active disease. No one has established the optimal location for taking such a biopsy. Nevertheless, when performed, the yield from this procedure may be increased by obtaining samples of both parenchyma and leptomeningeal vessels. Considering the obstacles to confirming a diagnosis of ICNSV, the clear-cut importance of a biopsy is to rule out other possibilities. Histologically, the brain tissue of affected patients may contain segmental mixed inflammation with necrosis involving predominantly small and medium-size cranial arteries. Granulomatosis inflammation may be present. Thrombosis is often noted, but extracranial arteries are rarely involved.[1,44] Therefore, differential diagnoses must be considered carefully in all cases and used in deciding appropriate tests both to support a diagnosis of ICNSV and to exclude other processes.

Treatment and Prognosis

Aggressive treatment is indicated for patients after other disorders are ruled out and the diagnosis of ICNSV is supported. The treatment advocated is a combination of corticosteroids and daily cyclophosphamide; however, prognosis is poor, for 60% to 70% of patients with ICNSV die of their disease within 1 year of diagnosis.[1]

Kawasaki's Disease

Kawasaki's disease, or mucocutaneous lymph node syndrome, is a form of vasculitis involving small and medium-size arteries. This disease typically occurs in children, and the symptoms are cervical lymphadenitis and alterations in skin and mucous membranes. The disease is usually self-limited, but arteritis causes coronary aneurysms in 25% of affected patients. The 3% who die usually succumb from coronary vasculitis. Antiendothelial cell autoantibodies have been demonstrated in patients with Kawasaki's disease.[43]

Summary

Diagnosis of idiopathic systemic autoimmune vasculitis requires a high degree of suspicion and can be troublesome because of the numerous alternatives to consider. There are no pathognomonic laboratory test results in patients with systemic necrotizing vasculitis; even so, laboratory tests are highly useful for defining the extent and pattern of organ involvement. Testing for ANCAs is useful in the workup of suspected systemic vasculitis. The predictive value of a positive ANCA result is increased if it is due to either anti-PR3 or anti-MPO autoantibodies.

Despite the availability of tests to detect ANCAs, tissue biopsy of symptomatic sites, with histologic confirmation of disease and careful consideration of disease patterns on history and physical examination, remains the most important procedure for confident diagnosis of systemic vasculitis. In this context, the authors regard a positive ANCA result as a signal for further evaluation.

References

1. Langford CA, McCallum RM. Idiopathic vasculitis. In: Belch JJF, Zurier RB, eds. *Connective Tissue Diseases.* London, England: Chapman and Hall; 1995:179.
2. Jennette JC, Falk RJ. Small-vessel vasculitis. *N Engl J Med.* 1997;337:1512–1523.
3. Lie JT. Nomenclature and classification of vasculitis: Plus ça change, plus c'est la même chose. *Arthritis Rheum.* 1994;37:181.
4. Lie JT. Systemic and isolated vasculitis: A rational approach to classification and pathologic diagnosis. In: Rosen PP, Fechner RE, eds. *Pathology Annual, Part 1.* Norwalk, CT: Appleton & Lange; 1989:25.
5. Hunder GG, Arend WP, Bloch DA, et al. The American College of Rheumatology 1990 criteria for the classification of vasculitis. *Arthritis Rheum.* 1990;33:1065.
6. Jennette JC, Falk RJ, Andrassy K, et al. Nomenclature of systemic vasculitides. Proposal of an international consensus conference. *Arthritis Rheum.* 1994;37:187.
7. Rao JK, Allen NB, Pincus T. Limitations of the 1990 American College of Rheumatology classification criteria in the diagnosis of vasculitis. *Ann Intern Med.* 1998;129:345–352.
8. Hunder GG. The use and misuse of classification and diagnostic criteria for complex diseases. *Ann Intern Med.* 1998;129:417–418. [Editorial]
9. Nowack R, Flores-Suárez LF, van der Woude FJ. New developments in pathogenesis of systemic vasculitis. *Curr Opin Rheumatol.* 1998;10:3–11.
10. Cohen Tervaert JW, Stegeman CA, Kallenberg CGM. Silicon exposure and vasculitis. *Curr Opin Rheumatol.* 1998;10:12–17.
11. Sundy JS, Haynes BF. Pathogenic mechanisms of vessel damage in vasculitis syndromes. *Rheum Dis Clin North Am.* 1995;21:861–881.
12. Sneller MC, Fauci AS. Pathogenesis of vasculitis syndromes. *Med Clin North Am.* 1997;81:221–242.
13. Mandell BF, Hoffman GS. Differentiating the vasculitides. *Rheum Dis Clin North Am.* 1994;20:409.
14. Golden MP, Hammer SM, Wanke CA, et al. Cytomegalovirus vasculitis. Case reports and review of the literature. *Medicine (Baltimore).* 1994;73:246.
15. Jennette JC, Falk RJ. Vasculitis. In: Rose NR, Mackay IR, eds. *The Autoimmune Diseases.* 3d ed. San Diego, CA: Academic Press; 1998:705–724.
16. Hoffman GS, Specks U. Antineutrophil cytoplasmic antibodies. *Arthritis Rheum.* 1998;41:1521–1537.
17. Roberts DE. Antineutrophil cytoplasmic autoantibodies. *Clin Lab Med.* 1992;12:85.
18. Davies DJ, Moran JE, Niall JF, et al. Segmental necrotising glomerulonephritis with antineutrophil antibody: Possible arbovirus aetiology? *Br Med J.* 1982;2:606.
19. Goldschmeding R, van der Schoot CE, ten Bokkel Huinink D, et al. Wegener's granulomatosis autoantibodies identify a novel diisopropyl fluorophosphate-binding protein in the lysosomes of normal human neutrophils. *J Clin Invest.* 1989;84:1577–1587.
20. Niles JL, McCluskey RT, Ahmad MF, et al. Wegener's granulomatosis autoantigen is a novel serine proteinase. *Blood.* 1989;74:1888–1893.
21. Tan EM, Chan EKL, Sullivan KF, et al. Antinuclear antibodies (ANAs): Diagnostically specific immune markers and clues toward the understanding of systemic autoimmunity. *Clin Immunol Immunopathol.* 1988;47:121–141.
22. Bruyn GAW, Zegers BJM, van Furth R. Mechanisms of host defense against infection with *Streptococcus pneumoniae. Clin Infect Dis.* 1992;14:251–262.
23. Niles JL. Value of tests for antineutrophil cytoplasmic autoantibodies in the diagnosis and treatment of vasculitis. *Curr Opin Rheumatol.* 1993;5:18.
24. Falk RJ, Jennette JC. Anti-neutrophil cytoplasmic autoantibodies with specificity for myeloperoxidase in patients with systemic vasculitis and idiopathic necrotizing and crescentic glomerulonephritis. *N Engl J Med.* 1988;318:1651–1657.
25. Wieslander J. How are antineutrophil cytoplasmic autoantibodies detected? *Am J Kidney Dis.* 1991;18:154.
26. Wiik A. Antineutrophil cytoplasmic antibodies. In: Rose NR, Conway de Macario E, Folds JD, et al, eds. *Manual of Clinical Laboratory Immunology.* 5th ed. Washington, DC: ASM Press; 1997:954–959.
27. Jennette JC, Falk RJ. Antineutrophil cytoplasmic autoantibodies in inflammatory bowel disease. *Am J Clin Pathol.* 1993;99:221.
28. Keren DF, Goeken JA. Autoimmune reactivity in inflammatory bowel disease. In: Keren DF, Nakamura RM, eds. *Clinics in Laboratory Medicine.* Philadelphia, PA: WB Saunders Co; 1997:465–481.
29. Specks U, Homburger HA. Laboratory medicine and pathology: Anti-neutrophil cytoplasmic antibodies. *Mayo Clin Proc.* 1994;69:1197.
30. Hagen EC, Daha MR, Hermans J, et al. Diagnostic value of standardized assays for anti-neutrophil cytoplasmic antibodies in idiopathic systemic vasculitis. EC/BCR project for ANCA assay standardization. *Kidney Int.* 1998;53:743–753.
31. Hagen EC, Andrassy K, Csernok E, et al. Development and standardization of solid phase assays for the detection of anti-neutrophil cytoplasmic antibodies (ANCA): A report on the second phase of an international cooperative study on the standardization of ANCA assays. *J Immunol Methods.* 1996;196:1–15.
32. Murphy LK, Targan SR. Antineutrophil cytoplasmic antibodies in inflammatory bowel diseases. In: Peter JB, Shoenfeld Y, eds. *Autoantibodies.* Amsterdam, the Netherlands: Elsevier Biomedical; 1996:47–52.

33. Zhao M-H, Lockwood CH. Antineutrophil cytoplasmic autoantibodies with specificity other than PR3 and MPO (X-ANCA). In: Peter JB, Shoenfeld Y, eds. *Autoantibodies*. Amsterdam, the Netherlands: Elsevier Biomedical; 1996:68–73.

34. Yang JJ, Tuttle R, Falk RJ, et al. Frequency of anti-bactericidal/permeability-increasing protein (BPI) and anti-azurocidin in patients with renal disease. *Clin Exp Immunol*. 1996;105:125–131.

35. Zhao MH, Lockwood CM. Azurocidin is a novel antigen for anti-neutrophil cytoplasmic autoantibodies (ANCA) in systemic vasculitis. *Clin Exp Immunol.* 1996;103:397–402.

36. Stoffel MP, Csernok E, Herzberg C, et al. Anti-neutrophil cytoplasmic antibodies (ANCA) directed against bactericidal/permeability increasing protein (BPI): A new seromarker for inflammatory bowel disease and associated disorders. *Clin Exp Immunol.* 1996;104:54–59.

37. Schultz H, Csernok E, Johnston TW, et al. Use of native and recombinant bactericidal/permeability-increasing proteins (BPI) as antigens for detection of BPI-ANCA. *J Immunol Methods*. 1997;205:127–133.

38. Tervaert JWC, Limburg PC, Elema JD, et al. Detection of autoantibodies against myeloid lysosomal enzymes: A useful adjunct to classification of patients with biopsy-proven necrotizing arteritis. *Am J Med*. 1991;91:59.

39. Bonsib SM, Goeken JA, Kemp JD, et al. Coexistent anti-neutrophil cytoplasmic antibody and antiglomerular basement membrane antibody associated disease: Report of six cases. *Mod Pathol.* 1993;6:526.

40. Peen E, Almer S, Bodemar G, et al. Anti-lactoferrin antibodies and other types of ANCA in ulcerative colitis, primary sclerosing cholangitis, and Crohn's disease. *Gut*. 1993;34:56.

41. Peter HH, Metzger D, Rump A, et al. ANCA in diseases other than systemic vasculitis. In: *Proceedings of the 5th International ANCA Workshop*. Cambridge, UK: St. John's College; 1993:12.

42. Conn DL, Hunder GG, O'Duffy JD. Vasculitis and related disorders. In: Kelley WN, Harris ED Jr, Ruddy S, et al, eds. *Textbook of Rheumatology*. 4th ed. Philadelphia, PA: WB Saunders Co; 1993:1077.

43. Fauci AS. The vasculitis syndromes. In: Fauci AS, Braunwald E, Isselbacher KJ, et al, eds. *Harrison's Principles of Internal Medicine.* 14th ed. New York, NY: McGraw-Hill; 1998:1910–1922.

44. Rhodes RH, Madelaire C, Petrelli M, et al. Primary angiitis and angiopathy of the central nervous system and their relationship to systemic giant cell arteritis. *Arch Pathol Lab Med*. 1995;119:334.

SECTION III

Organ-Directed Autoimmune Diseases

CHAPTER 16

Autoimmune Skin Diseases

David J. Bylund, MD, and Gene T. Izuno, MD

Classification of Autoimmune Skin Diseases

The diagnosis of autoimmune diseases affecting skin, mucous membranes, or both is based on the correlation of clinical, histologic, and immunologic findings. In this chapter, these conditions are collectively referred to as autoimmune skin disorders, and this label includes those immune-mediated diseases that affect skin, mucous membranes, or both. The major autoimmune skin diseases are listed in **Table 16-1**.

Often the diagnosis of an autoimmune skin disease is suspected when a patient's clinical presentation is correlated with pathologic findings noted on light microscopic study of a tissue biopsy. Immunologic studies are then essential or highly useful for confirming the diagnosis through identification of cutaneous antigen-autoantibody reactions and/or detection of autoantibodies in the circulation.

Numerous dermatology and dermatopathology textbooks discuss clinical and histologic findings in autoimmune skin diseases. This chapter describes immunofluorescent findings that characterize the major autoimmune skin disorders encountered in clinical practice.

Table 16-1. Autoimmune Skin Diseases

Intraepidermal vesicular, bullous, or pustular dermatoses
Suprabasal
Pemphigus vulgaris and vegetans
Subcorneal or intraspinous
Pemphigus foliaceus
IgA pemphigus/intercellular IgA dermatitis
Pemphigus erythematosus
Paraneoplastic pemphigus
Subepidermal bullous disorders
Pemphigoid
Benign mucous membrane pemphigoid
Herpes gestationis
Epidermolysis bullosa acquisita
Bullous lupus erythematosus
Dermatitis herpetiformis
Linear IgA dermatosis
Chronic bullous dermatosis of childhood

Abbreviation: Ig = immunoglobulin.

Detection Methods

Direct Immunofluorescence Microscopy

Direct immunofluorescence microscopy (DIFM) is used to detect autoantibodies bound directly to the patient's skin. To avoid potentially misleading changes, an early lesion that includes perilesional skin should be biopsied.

If a fresh biopsy specimen can be submitted immediately, it is covered with saline-soaked gauze and transported to the laboratory. If the specimen cannot be submitted promptly, or if it must be sent some distance to a reference laboratory, it must be placed in a suitable transport medium that allows tissues to be stored at room temperature for up to several months while retaining antigenic reactivity. The specimen should not be placed in formalin fixative.

Either a punch or shave biopsy is usually sent to the laboratory. Specimens in transport medium are washed in phosphate-buffered saline solution. Shave biopsies are embedded intact on edge. Punch biopsies with diameters of 4 mm or less are embedded on a side, and then sectioned into the center after freezing. Larger punch biopsies are bisected unless a gross blister is evident, in which case the biopsy is either sectioned off center to preserve the blister or submitted intact and step-sectioned into the lesion.

Biopsy specimens are embedded in optimal cutting temperature compound, snap frozen using isopentane/dry ice, and kept frozen at –20°C or –70°C until use. Unfixed frozen sections of the specimen are cut and incubated with fluorescein isothiocyanate–labeled conjugates directed against human immunoglobulins (Igs) G, A, and M; complement components C1q and C3; and fibrinogen. A fluorescent microscope is used to look for immunoreactants.

Stained sections from each biopsy are first studied without knowledge of clinical information or suspected diagnosis. This practice encourages orderly and unbiased study of the specimen and should generate a differential diagnosis based only on morphologic findings. Careful clinicopathologic correlation then usually allows specific diagnosis or limits diagnostic alternatives to a few disorders.

Fluorescent Patterns

Immunofluorescent patterns can be classified in terms of morphology of the specific immunoreactants observed and their location(s). In many instances, immunoreactants are an admixture of immunoglobulins and complement components. In selected diseases, either a single immunoglobulin, such as IgA, or a single complement component is observed.

The morphology of immunoreactants can be classified as focal or diffuse (continuous) and as linear or granular. A linear pattern appears smooth and homogeneous without easily discernible granularity. A granular pattern is composed of immunoreactants that may vary from fine to coarse.

The common locations of immunoreactants in autoimmune skin diseases are the basement membrane zone (BMZ), epidermal/epithelial intercellular spaces (ICS), and dermal blood vessels. **Figure 16-1** offers an algorithm for using DIFM pattern analysis based on location of the immunoreactants. In all cases, correlation of DIFM findings with the clinical presentation is necessary.

Normal skin shows minimal background immunofluorescence, which is helpful in visualizing cutaneous architecture. However, the clinician should be aware of several nonspecific patterns when interpreting DIFM results[1]:

- Autofluorescence of normal structures such as sweat gland acini or dermal collagen fibers (**Image 16-1**)
- Granular fluorescent aggregates over the entire slide, usually implying immunoglobulin clumps that should be removed by ultracentrifugation of the fluoresceinated antiserum
- Heterophile antibodies that produce fluorescence in the superficial epidermis, typically in the stratum granulosum
- Antinuclear autoantibodies staining epidermal nuclei
- Epidermal cytoplasmic staining of uncertain clinical significance

Indirect Immunofluorescence Microscopy

Indirect immunofluorescence microscopy (IIFM)[2] is a semiquantitative procedure used to detect and titer circulating autoantibodies. A patient's blood is drawn into a red-top tube without anticoagulant and processed to obtain serum. Test serum is serially diluted with phosphate-buffered saline, initially at 1:10, and usually doubling the dilutions thereafter. Serum is layered over tissue substrate and allowed to incubate with the tissue for 30 minutes. After washing, bound autoantibodies are detected using fluorescein isothiocyanate–labeled conjugates similar to those used in DIFM.

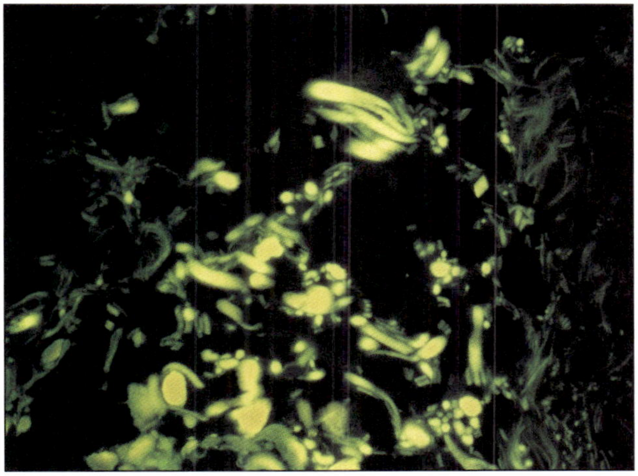

Image 16-1. Orange autofluorescence of dermal collagen fibers.

The choice of tissue substrate may vary among laboratories. Monkey esophagus is probably the best substrate for routine indirect studies. Guinea pig esophagus or lip is a good substrate that works best for BMZ immunofluorescence or when pemphigus foliaceous is suspected. These substrates are available from commercial suppliers. The use of normal human skin has been described, but it is generally used only for salt-split skin studies.

Salt-Split Skin

The use of frozen sections of salt-split normal human skin is critical to differentiate bullous pemphigoid (BP) from epidermolysis bullosa acquisita (EBA) and bullous lupus erythematosus (BLE). In this method, dermal tissue is trimmed from 4-mm squares of normal human skin that is then incubated with 1 mol/L sodium chloride for 48 to 72 hours at 4°C. After washing in phosphate-buffered saline to remove excess salt, the epidermis is first manually separated from the dermis, then layered back over the dermis and snap frozen in isopentane/dry ice.[2,3]

Fluorescent Patterns

Patterns seen in IIFM studies are identical to those described for DIFM.

Pemphigus

Pemphigus refers to a group of disorders characterized clinically by blisters and histologically by acantholysis. There are 3 major types of pemphigus:

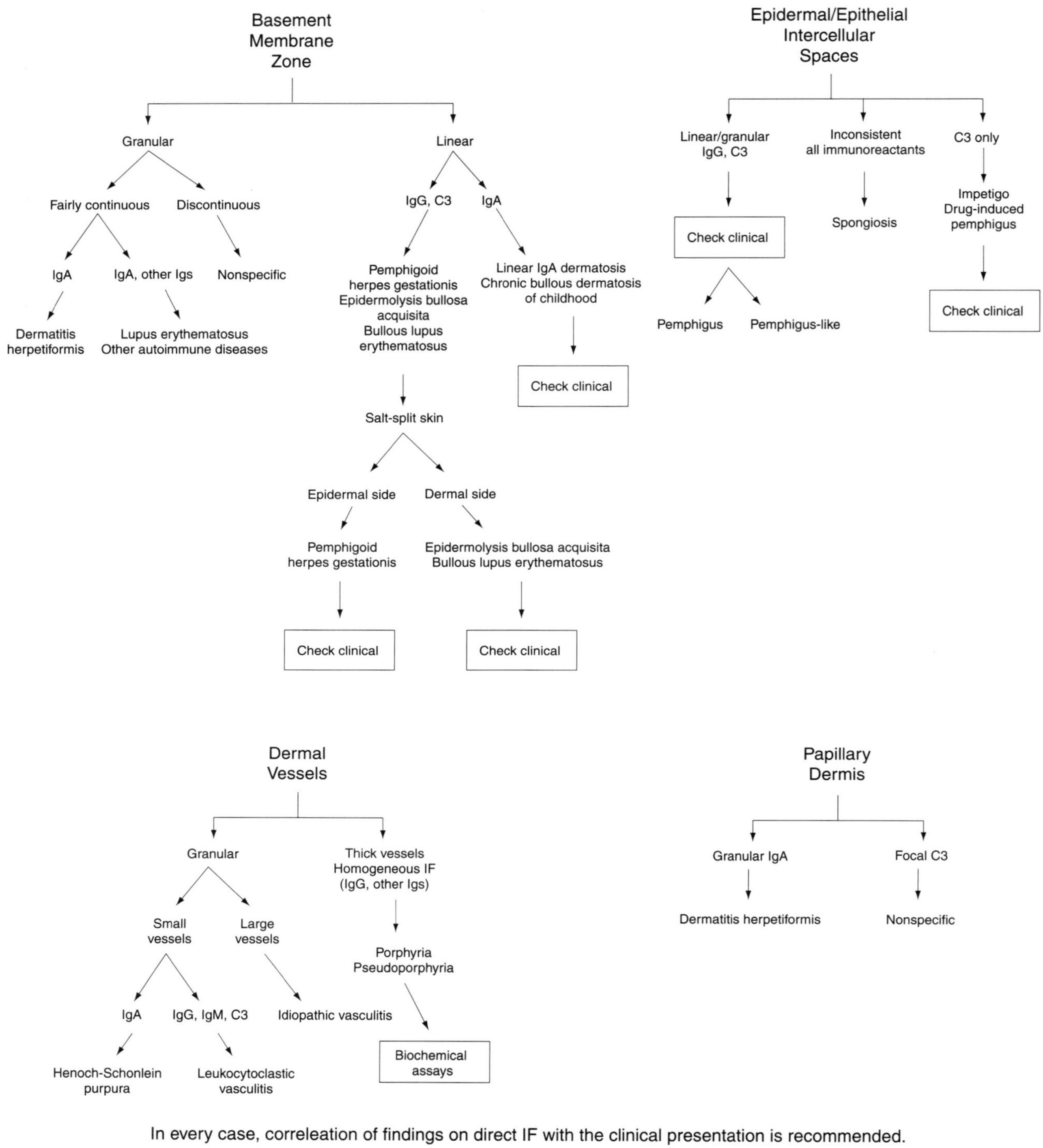

Figure 16-1. Algorithm for direct skin immunofluorescence.

pemphigus vulgaris (PV), pemphigus foliaceus (PF), and paraneoplastic pemphigus (PNP). Each is characterized by autoantibodies to desmosomal adhesion molecules.

Both IIFM (to detect circulating autoantibodies) and the more informative DIFM (to identify tissue-bound autoantibodies) are used for initial evaluations to maximize diagnostic sensitivity.

Pemphigus Vulgaris

Pemphigus vulgaris is a rare disorder that occurs in all racial and ethnic groups, although the incidence is slightly increased in the Jewish population. The disease affects either gender and most commonly occurs in individuals between 40 and 60 years of age.[4] The major antigen in PV is desmoglein 3.[5,6]

Direct Immunofluorescence

Direct immunofluorescence of perilesional skin shows linear-granular IgG and C3 ICS immunofluorescence without BMZ staining. The pattern is often said to have a "chicken wire" appearance that preferentially stains the lower half of the epidermis (**Images 16-2** to **16-4**). Immunoglobulin G, especially the subclass IgG4, is present in nearly 100% of affected patients; C3 is present in 50% to 100% of patients, often in acantholytic areas.[4,5,7] Immunoglobulin A or M immunoreactants are seen 30% to 50% of patients.[8] C3 immunofluorescence alone, without IgG, is described in drug-induced pemphigus and in impetigo.[2]

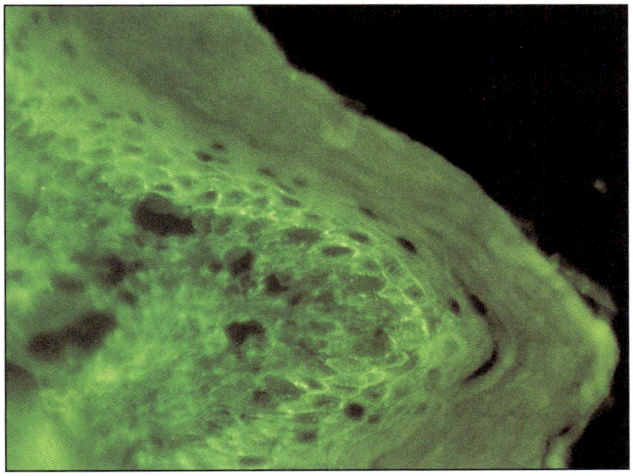

Image 16-2. Direct intercellular space pattern in pemphigus vulgaris. Intact epidermis demonstrates IgG immunofluorescence of epidermal intercellular spaces located predominantly in the basal cell layer.

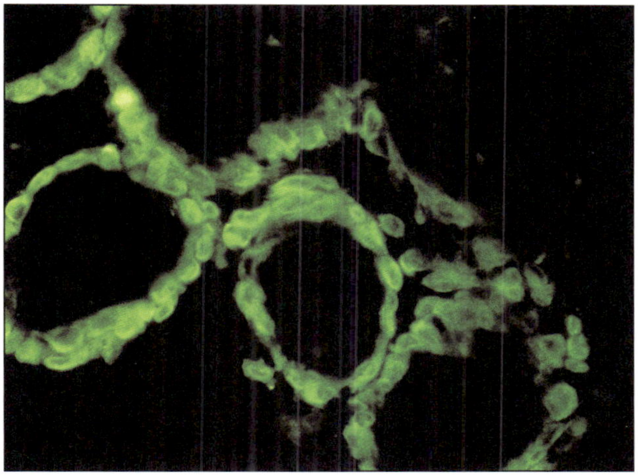

Image 16-3. Direct intercellular space pattern in pemphigus vulgaris. Immunoglobulin G immunofluorescence of epidermal intercellular spaces is seen in basal keratinocytes lining preserved dermal papillae in a suprabasal acantholytic blister.

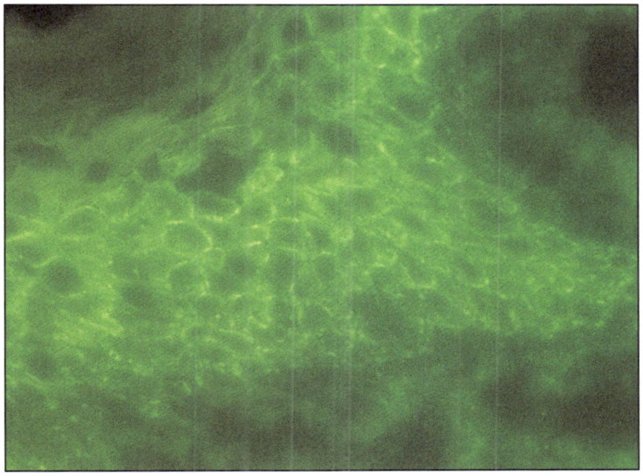

Image 16-4. Direct intercellular space pattern in pemphigus vulgaris. In some cases, the immunofluorescence has a linear to finely granular appearance.

Indirect Immunofluorescence

Indirect immunofluorescence should detect circulating IgG autoantibodies to the surfaces of squamous epithelial cells in 100% of patients with active disease (**Image 16-5**).[2] Monkey esophagus is the best tissue substrate.

The presence of PV autoantibodies is abnormal at any titer. The titer generally correlates with disease activity, and increasing titers may be predictive of relapse.[4,9] Exceptions to this correlation do occur, so

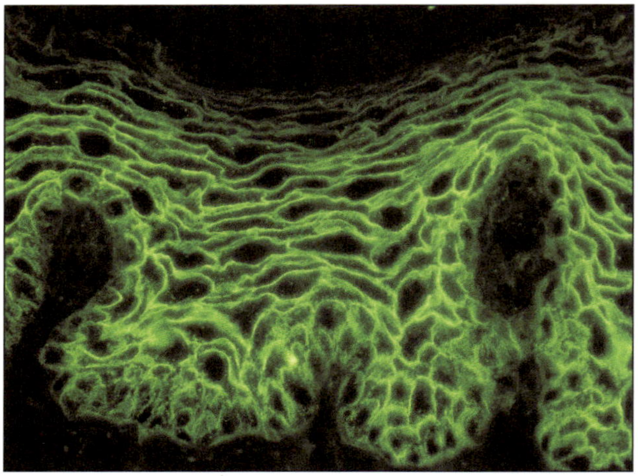

Image 16-5. Indirect intercellular space pattern in pemphigus vulgaris. Full-thickness linear IgG immunofluorescence of epithelial intercellular spaces is evident. This pattern is variably described as "chicken wire" or "fishnet."

serial testing of IgG titers to monitor patients must be carefully correlated with the clinical findings.

Patients with only oral mucosal lesions may not have detectable circulating PV autoantibodies. In these patients, diagnosis is made using DIFM.[8]

Low titers of ICS-like autoantibodies may be detected infrequently in diverse conditions, such as skin burns, penicillin or other drug allergy, toxic epidermal necrolysis, systemic lupus erythematosus (SLE), myasthenia gravis, pemphigoid, and lichen planus. They are rarely seen in healthy individuals (<1%).[2,4,10]

Pemphigus Foliaceus

The subsets of PF include idiopathic PF, endemic PF (fogo selvagem), drug-induced PF, and pemphigus erythematosus (PE). The major antigen in PF is desmoglein 1.[5,6]

Direct Immunofluorescence

For all forms of PF except PE, the DIFM pattern is similar to that for PV. In some cases, the staining predominates in the superficial epidermis at the level of the stratum granulosum (**Image 16-6**). In PE, there is linear IgG staining of epidermal intercellular spaces combined with granular immunoreactants along the BMZ.

Indirect Immunofluorescence

Indirect immunofluorescence should detect circulating IgG ICS autoantibodies in virtually 100% of PF patients with active disease.[2] About 90% of these patients have detectable autoantibodies when monkey esophagus is used for indirect studies. Guinea pig esophagus is somewhat more sensitive in that it detects autoantibodies in the remaining 10% of patients, and the indirect titers tend to be higher than those obtained when using monkey esophagus.[11]

Paraneoplastic Pemphigus

Paraneoplastic pemphigus, an uncommon disorder characterized by painful blisters or erosions of mucous membranes and skin, is a condition of patients with neoplasms. The blisters or erosions usually erupt in the mouth, but they have been reported in other mucosal sites. Malignant neoplasms that have been associated with PNP include malignant lymphoma, chronic lymphocytic leukemia, thymoma, bronchogenic squamous cell carcinoma, and sarcoma. In rare cases, PNP is associated with benign neoplasms.[7,12,13]

Mutasim et al[12] have proposed the following criteria to define PNP:

- Painful mucosal erosions and a polymorphous skin eruption, with papular lesions progressing to blisters and erosive lesions affecting trunk, extremities, and palms and soles, associated with an occult or clinically known neoplasm
- Suprabasilar acantholysis, keratinocyte necrosis, and vacuolar interface changes on light microscopic tissue sections
- Immunoglobulin G in ICS combined with linear-granular complement and IgG BMZ

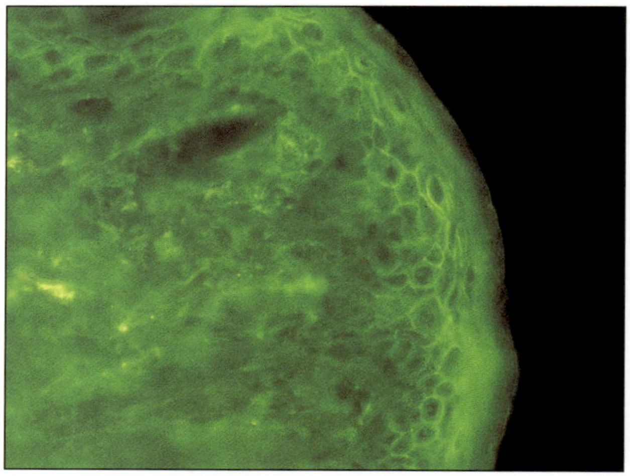

Image 16-6. Direct intercellular space pattern in pemphigus foliaceus. The IgG immunofluorescence of epidermal intercellular spaces predominates in the upper half of the epidermis.

- Circulating ICS autoantibodies that bind to monkey and guinea pig esophagus, as in pemphigus, and also to rodent bladder epithelium
- When needed, immunoprecipitation of a complex of 4 proteins from keratinocytes bound by the autoantibodies

Paraneoplastic pemphigus associated with malignant neoplasms signals an extremely poor prognosis. Although clinical improvement or remission of mucocutaneous lesions after tumor resection has been reported, treatment for malignancy-associated PNP is supportive. The disease associated with a benign neoplasm remitted after tumor resection.[12]

Direct Immunofluorescence

Direct immunofluorescence of perilesional skin and/or mucosa from patients with PNP detects IgG ICS immunoreactant with or without complement. Granular or, less commonly, linear BMZ deposits of complement also are present in addition to IgG ICS immunofluorescence.[12]

Indirect Immunofluorescence

Equally valuable, IIFM using monkey esophagus and rodent bladder transitional epithelium demonstrates IgG autoantibodies that yield both ICS and BMZ immunofluorescence. Paraneoplastic pemphigus differs from other types of pemphigus in that autoantibodies in patient sera bind to rodent (rat or mouse) bladder epithelium.[12,14]

Immunoglobulin A Pemphigus/ Intercellular Immunoglobulin A Dermatosis

Intercellular IgA dermatosis is a rare intraepidermal vesiculobullous disorder. Direct studies show linear ICS immunofluorescence for IgA that is suprabasilar and particularly accentuated in the upper epidermis. Indirect immunofluorescence detects circulating IgA anti-ICS autoantibodies.[7,15]

Pemphigoid

Bullous pemphigoid is a subepidermal bullous disease of unknown cause. It can occur in patients of any age but mainly affects adults older than 60 years. Bullous pemphigoid typically involves flexor surfaces of the arms, legs, groin, axilla, and lower abdomen. The oral mucous membranes may be affected, but such lesions are rarely the presenting or predominant sign, a point that differentiates BP from PV.

Two hemidesmosomal proteins of keratinocytes are the major antigens in BP: the intracellular 230-kd protein (BP Ag1) and the transmembrane 180-kd protein (BP Ag2).[2,5]

Direct Immunofluorescence

Direct immunofluorescence of unblistered, perilesional skin from the edge of a fresh blister is diagnostically sensitive and typically enables the demonstration of linear BMZ immunofluorescence in nearly 100% of patients (**Images 16-7** and **16-8**). C3 and IgG, or C3 alone, are the predominant immunoreactants. Also, IgA and/or IgM may be present in up to approximately 25% of patients, usually in weaker intensity and in combination with IgG.[8,9,16]

A linear epidermal BMZ pattern can be identified in several disparate clinical disorders, including cicatricial pemphigoid, EBA, herpes gestationis (gestational pemphigoid), and BLE.

Salt-split direct skin biopsies are useful to distinguish these disorders.[17] In BP and herpes gestationis, linear IgG is localized to the epidermal side, or roof, of the split. Linear C3 immunoreactant, however, may be seen in epidermal and dermal locations. In EBA and bullous SLE, immunoreactants are seen along the dermal side of the split.[2] Clinical correlation then becomes important in resolving the differential diagnosis.

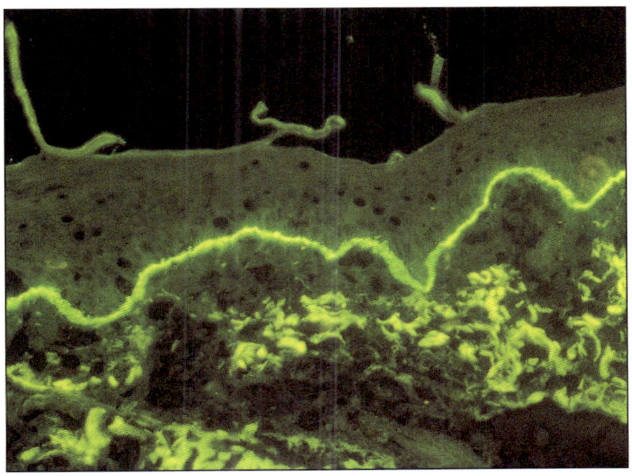

Image 16-7. Direct linear basement membrane zone pattern in bullous pemphigoid. Immunoglobulin G and C3 immunofluorescence is intense and continuous along the basement membrane zone.

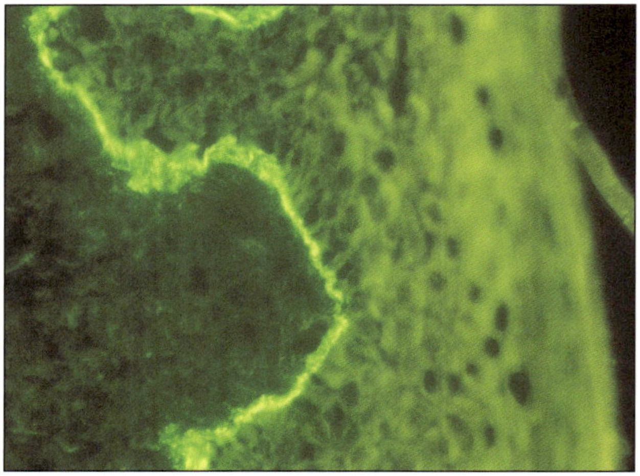

Image 16-8. Direct linear basement membrane zone pattern, with IgG and C3 immunoreactants. Although this image is from a case of bullous pemphigoid, a similar pattern may be seen in epidermolysis bullosa acquisita. If intense IgA alone were seen in this pattern, the diagnosis would be linear IgA dermatosis.

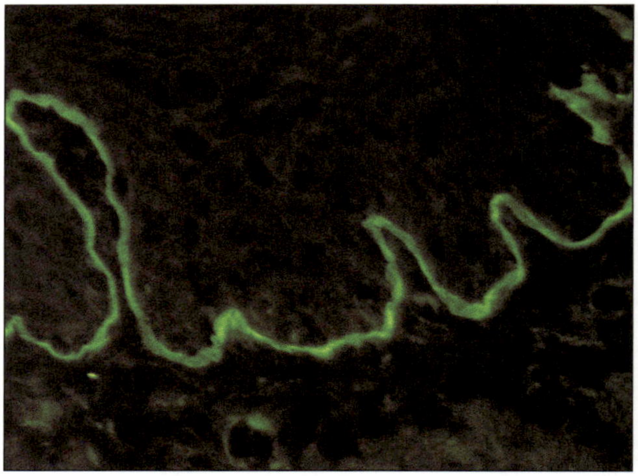

Image 16-9. Indirect basement membrane zone pattern in bullous pemphigoid. Linear basement membrane zone immunofluorescence for IgG using monkey (or guinea pig) substrate.

Indirect Immunofluorescence

Bullous pemphigoid is characterized serologically by the presence of circulating autoantibodies to cutaneous or oral mucosa BMZ (**Image 16-9**). Although IIFM detects circulating IgG anti-BMZ autoantibodies in about 50% of patients with BP, sensitivity increases to 70% to 80% if normal human salt-split skin is used as substrate.[2,8,17]

Autoantibodies bind only to the roof of salt-split skin in 80% of patients with BP. Autoantibodies bind to the dermal base, or floor, of the split in 50% of patients with EBA and bullous SLE.[9,16,17]

Benign Mucous Membrane Pemphigoid

Benign mucous membrane pemphigoid (BMMP), or cicatricial pemphigoid, consistently affects oral and ocular mucosa. Other possible mucosal sites of these lesions are the nasopharynx, larynx, genitalia, rectum, and esophagus.[18] Scarring follows the healing of lesions, and blindness is the most feared complication.

Direct Immunofluorescence

The DIFM pattern is similar to that seen in BP (**Image 16-10**). Sensitivity is 90%, but this increases if additional biopsies are taken. Chronic localized scarring pemphigoid, also known as cicatricial pemphigoid of Brunsting-Perry, is a variant of BMMP that is localized to the head and neck region.[19] In this variant, DIFM demonstrates IgG only along the BMZ without IgA or IgM; circulating anti-BMZ autoantibodies are rare.[8]

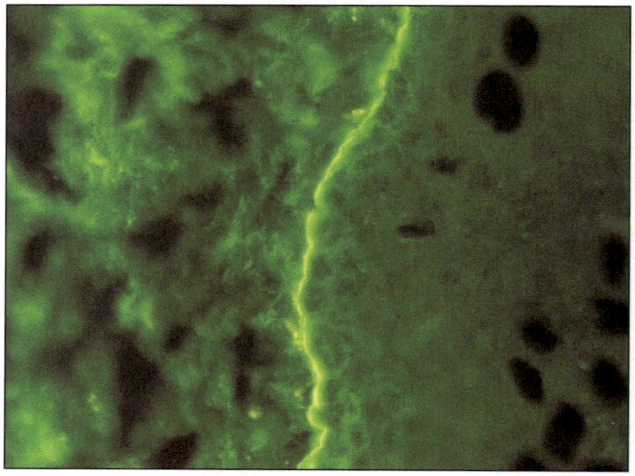

Image 16-10. Direct basement membrane zone pattern in benign mucous membrane (cicatricial) pemphigoid. The pattern is identical to that seen in bullous pemphigoid. The squamous mucosa lacks a rete pattern, and there are no adnexal structures.

Indirect Immunofluorescence

Indirect immunofluorescence detects circulating IgG autoantibodies in fewer than 33% of patients with BMMP when oral mucosal substrate is used and in 5% to 15% of patients when standard substrates are used.[2,9,19] Salt-split human skin studies may reveal deposits of IgA, IgG, or both in about 80% of affected patients.[19] There is no correlation between the presence and titer of autoantibodies and disease activity.

Herpes Gestationis

Infrequently, the subepidermal bullous disease herpes gestationis (gestational pemphigoid) develops during or soon after pregnancy.[8] Lesions typically are pruritic and located predominantly on the abdomen and/or extremities.

Direct Immunofluorescence

With DIFM, linear C3 deposits are typically found along the cutaneous BMZ. Associated IgG deposits are detected in 30% to 40% of patients, but IgA and IgM are rare.[8]

Indirect Immunofluorescence

Linear C3 deposits may be visualized only along the BMZ, but often autoantibody titers are too low to be seen using standard IIFM substrates. Complement may be detected if complement immunofixation using normal human salt-split skin is used as substrate.[2,8]

Epidermolysis Bullosa Acquisita and Bullous Lupus Erythematosus

These acquired subepidermal blistering diseases are characterized by the presence of autoantibodies to type VII collagen in BMZ protein.[20]

Epidermolysis bullosa acquisita can occur at any age but most commonly presents in adults between the ages of 40 and 50 years. There is no ethnic or gender predominance. All patients are afflicted with a combination of blisters, erosions, scars, milia, and dyspigmentation of skin, most often located on trauma-susceptible extensor skin surfaces, such as knees, elbows, and dorsa of the hands and feet.[20] Bullous lupus erythematosus occurs in patients with lupus erythematosus.

Direct Immunofluorescence

Using DIFM, patients with EBA and BSLE have linear BMZ immunoreactants that most commonly consist of IgG and C3. Using direct salt-split skin biopsy tissue, the linear immunoreactants are localized at the dermal aspect of the induced blister.

Indirect Immunofluorescence

Only about 40% of patients with EBA have demonstrable autoantibodies when human skin without salt treatment is used as substrate. Using indirect salt-split skin technique, circulating autoantibodies can be identified in about 50% to 85% of patients.[2,21]

Dermatitis Herpetiformis

A pruritic subepidermal bullous disease, dermatitis herpetiformis (DH) is associated with gluten-sensitive enteropathy, as well as with HLA-B8, HLA-DR3 histocompatibility types.[9]

Direct Immunofluorescence

The direct biopsy specimen should be perilesional skin, because lesional skin biopsy may be negative. Direct immunofluorescence detects granular IgA in the tips of dermal papillae in approximately 80% to 100% of affected patients (**Images 16-11** and **16-12**).[7] There may be concomitant IgA deposits along the BMZ. C3 deposits are found often with IgA, but IgG and/or IgM are detected infrequently.[8]

Indirect Immunofluorescence

Patients with DH do not have detectable anti-BMZ autoantibodies. However, antiendomysial IgA autoantibodies are detected in 30% of patients (**Image 16-13**). These autoantibodies are identified by their characteristic immunofluorescence pattern in the subepithelial muscularis mucosa of monkey esophagus.[22]

Linear Immunoglobulin A Dermatosis

Linear IgA dermatosis is an uncommon subepidermal blistering condition that is considered a distinct clinical entity rather than a variant of DH

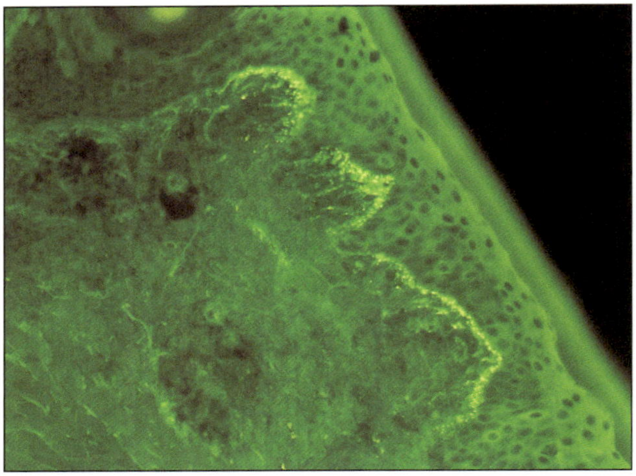

Image 16-11. Direct study in dermatitis herpetiformis. Granular IgA is evident in the tips of dermal papillae and focally along the basement membrane zone.

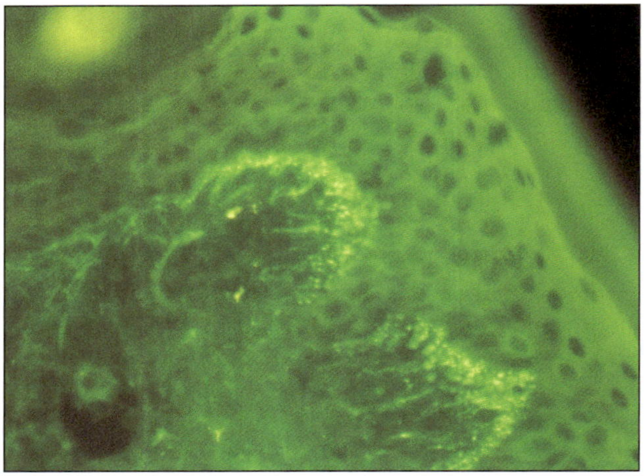

Image 16-12. Direct study in dermatitis herpetiformis.

as was once thought.[8,9] Most cases are idiopathic, but some are associated with drugs.[23,24] Chronic bullous dermatosis of childhood is similar to linear IgA dermatosis both clinically and immunopathologically.[25]

Direct Immunofluorescence

In nearly 100% of patients, DIFM demonstrates intense linear IgA deposits along the BMZ but none in dermal papillae.[8] Although concomitant weak C3 BMZ staining may occur occasionally, immunoreactants other than IgA usually are not present.

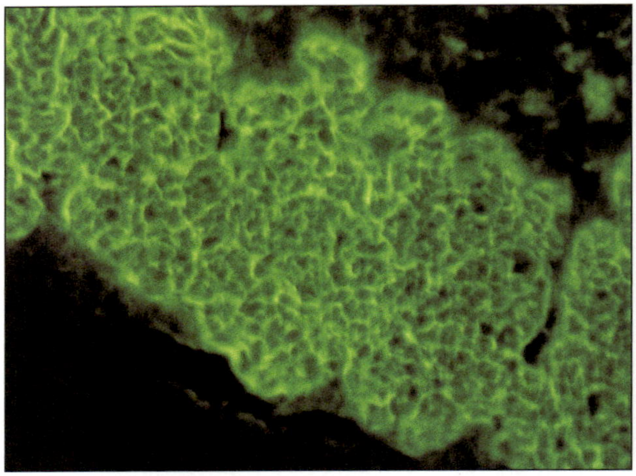

Image 16-13. Indirect assay for antiendomysial IgA autoantibodies using monkey esophagus substrate. These autoantibodies are detected in individuals with dermatitis herpetiformis and/or gluten-sensitive enteropathy.

Indirect Immunofluorescence

Circulating IgA anti-BMZ autoantibodies can be detected with IIFM in about 10% to 30% of patients.[7,9]

Lupus Erythematosus

This disorder is characterized serologically by the presence of multiple autoantibodies, including antinuclear antibodies, anti-native DNA, antihistones, and anti-Sm. Autoantibodies typically identified in this and other systemic autoimmune diseases are described in Chapter 9.

Direct Immunofluorescence

Characteristic coarse and granular continuous deposits of immunoglobulins and complement are seen along the epidermal BMZ in 50% to 95% of patients with SLE (**Images 16-14** and **16-15**).[8] Basement membrane zone deposits of the complement membrane attack complex C5b-9 in lesional skin may be a marker for SLE.[26]

Affected patients commonly have IgG, IgM, and C3 deposits, but immunoglobulins of all classes may be identified. When nonlesional skin concurrently contains IgG, IgA, and/or IgM in the typical pattern, a diagnosis of SLE is highly likely. Although characteristic, this reaction pattern also can be seen in other

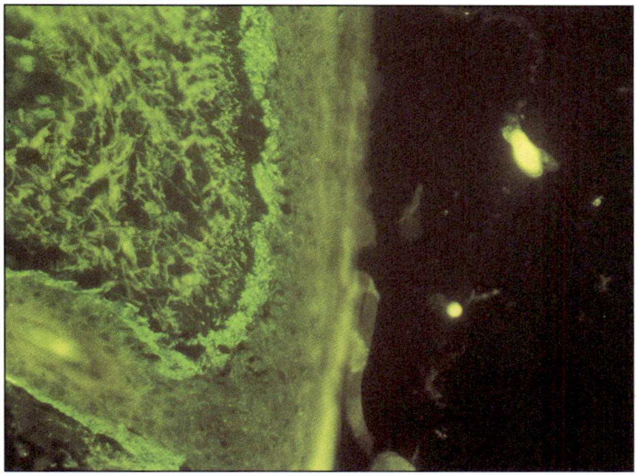

Image 16-14. Direct study in lupus erythematosus. There is continuous, granular basement membrane zone immunofluorescence for immunoglobulins and complement.

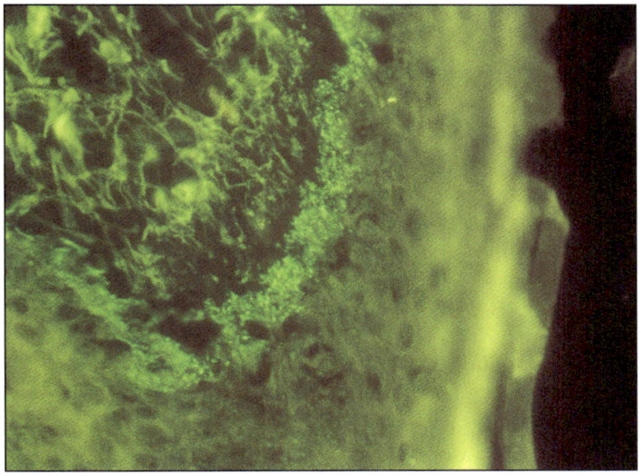

Image 16-15. Direct study in lupus erythematosus. The granular nature of immunoreactants along a thickened BMZ is highlighted.

disorders, such as mixed connective tissue disease, dermatomyositis, graft-versus-host reaction, drug eruptions, and vasculitis.[8] Therefore, it is mandatory to correlate direct results with both the clinical presentation and the results of light microscopic study of a skin biopsy. This information is then interpreted in the context of the clinician's direct findings to categorize the clinical type of lupus erythematosus.

A great many publications cite the utility of DIFM for diagnosing SLE from biopsied skin, with or without lesions, and from sun-exposed or sun-protected sites. In patients diagnosed with SLE, normal sun-exposed skin proves positive about 70% of the time, whereas normal sun-protected skin is positive in about 40% of patients. However, the potential for predicting disease activity or renal involvement in this way remains controversial.[8]

Perhaps the most practical clinical application of laboratory testing comes in the differential diagnosis of SLE from discoid lupus erythematosus (DLE). Up to 95% of individuals with DLE have coarse, granular, continuous BMZ deposits similar to those seen in SLE. However, positive DIFM findings in DLE are confined to lesional skin, whereas skin with or without lesions can give positive DIFM findings that denote SLE.[8]

Subacute cutaneous lupus erythematosus (SCLE) is characterized clinically by arthritis, mild systemic manifestations, and anti–Sjögren's syndrome-A/Ro autoantibody. Direct immunofluorescence of skin biopsies from affected patients detects BMZ immunoglobulin and/or complement deposits in only 50% of lesional skin biopsies and 30% of uninvolved skin biopsies.[8] Indirect immunofluorescence is positive in 50% to 70% of patients with SCLE.

Other major systemic autoimmune diseases do not offer diagnostically specific findings by either DIFM or IIFM. Although some patients have granular IgM deposits along the BMZ, this immunopathologic finding is considered a completely nonspecific marker that may be detected in any autoimmune disease, in a large number of inflammatory dermatitides, or in sun-exposed skin of clinically normal individuals.[8]

Vasculitis

Vasculitis in the skin has a number of synonyms, including leukocytoclastic vasculitis, allergic vasculitis, and hypersensitivity angiitis/vasculitis. Histologically, small blood vessels of the dermis show endothelial cell swelling, neutrophilic exocytosis and nuclear debris ("leukocytoclasis"), and thrombi in conjunction with extravasated red blood cells.

Biopsy of a vasculitic lesion within 24 hours of onset may display vascular deposits of IgM, C3, fibrinogen, and sometimes IgG. A negative result does not exclude vasculitis; biopsies of lesions older than 24 hours may not be helpful, because nonspecific fibrinogen staining may be the only finding. Histologic confirmation of the diagnosis is therefore essential.

Henoch-Schönlein purpura is diagnosed when granular IgA vascular immunofluorescence, with or without C3, is seen (**Images 16-16** to **16-18**).

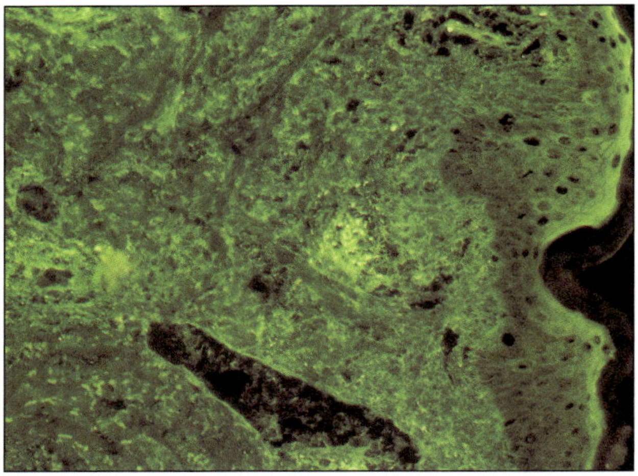

Image 16-16. Direct IgA immunofluorescence involving vessels of the superficial capillary plexus in Henoch-Schönlein purpura.

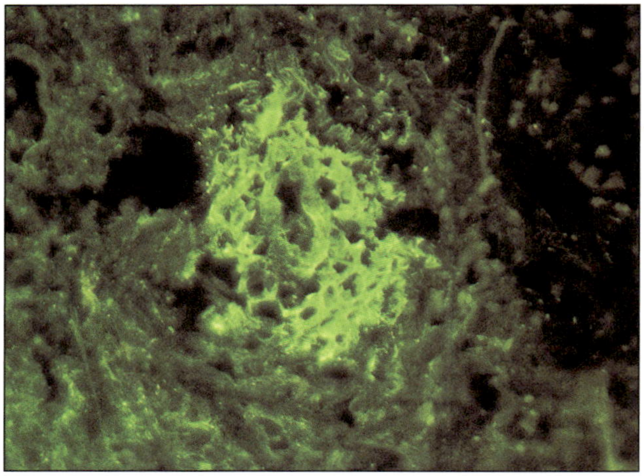

Image 16-17. Direct IgA immunofluorescence in Henoch-Schönlein purpura. Granular IgA vascular mural and perivascular immunoreactant are evident.

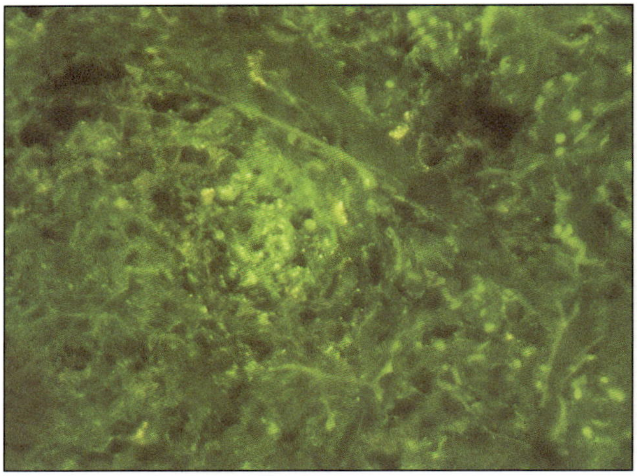

Image 16-18. Direct fibrinogen immunofluorescence in Henoch-Schönlein purpura. Fibrinogen has a smudgy appearance, especially in the perivascular tissue. Although compatible with vasculitis, this finding by itself is completely nonspecific. It may be due to trauma from the biopsy procedure.

Acknowledgment

The author thanks Dr. Gene Izuno for his helpful review of this manuscript. Thanks also to Carol Peebles for her expert assistance with the immunofluorescence images.

References

1. Valenzuela R, Bergfeld WF, Deodhar SD. *Interpretation of Immunofluorescent Patterns in Skin Diseases*. Chicago, IL: ASCP Press; 1984.
2. Nousari HC, Anhalt GJ. Skin diseases. In: Rose NR, Conway de Macario E, Folds JD, et al, eds. *Manual of Clinical Laboratory Immunology*. 5th ed. Washington, DC: ASM Press; 1997:997–1004.
3. Gammon WR, Fine J-D, Forbes M, et al. Immunofluorescence on split skin for the detection and differentiation of basement membrane zone autoantibodies. *J Am Acad Dermatol*. 1992;27:79–87.
4. Becker BA, Gaspari AA. Pemphigus vulgaris and vegetans. In: Thiers BH, Crosby DL, Diaz LA, eds. *Dermatologic Clinics. Bullous Diseases*. Philadelphia, PA: WB Saunders Co; 1993:429–452.
5. Lin M-S, Liu Z, Drolet BA, et al. Cutaneous autoimmune diseases. In: Rose NR, Mackay IR, eds. *The Autoimmune Diseases*. 3rd ed. San Diego, CA: Academic Press; 1998:545–570.
6. Naparstek Y, Plotz PH. The role of autoantibodies in autoimmune disease. *Annu Rev Immunol*. 1993;11:79.
7. Flotte TJ, Margolis RJ, Mihm MC Jr. Skin. In: Colvin RB, Bhan AK, McCluskey RT, eds. *Diagnostic Immunopathology*. 2nd ed. New York, NY: Raven Press; 1995:123.
8. Izuno GT. Cutaneous immunofluorescence. *Clin Lab Med*. 1986;6:85.
9. Crosby DL, Diaz LA. Autoimmune diseases of the skin. In: Altman LC, ed. *Immunology and Allergy Clinics of North America: Autoimmune Diseases*. Philadelphia, PA: WB Saunders Co; 1993:395.
10. Mutasim DF, Pelc NJ, Anhalt GJ. Drug-induced pemphigus. In: Thiers BH, Crosby DL, Diaz LA, eds. *Dermatologic Clinics. Bullous Diseases*. Philadelphia, PA: WB Saunders Co; 1993:463–471.

11. Jiao D, Bystryn J-C. Sensitivity of indirect immunofluorescence, substrate specificity, and immunoblotting in the diagnosis of pemphigus. *J Am Acad Dermatol.* 1997;37:211–216.

12. Mutasim DF, Pelc NJ, Anhalt GJ. Paraneoplastic pemphigus. In: Thiers BH, Crosby DL, Diaz LA, eds. *Dermatologic Clinics. Bullous Diseases*. Philadelphia, PA: WB Saunders Co; 1993:473–481.

13. Camisa C, Helm TN. Paraneoplastic pemphigus is a distinct neoplasia-induced autoimmune disease. *Arch Dermatol.* 1993;129:883.

14. Liu AY, Valenzuela R, Helm TN, et al. Indirect immunofluorescence on rat bladder transitional epithelium: A test with high specificity for paraneoplastic pemphigus. *J Am Acad Dermatol.* 1993;28:696.

15. Teraki Y, Amagai N, Hashimoto T, et al. Intercellular IgA dermatosis of childhood. Selective deposition of monomer IgA1 in the intercellular space of the epidermis. *Arch Dermatol.* 1991;127:221.

16. Korman NJ. Bullous pemphigoid. In: Thiers BH, Crosby DL, Diaz LA, eds. *Dermatologic Clinics. Bullous Diseases*. Philadelphia, PA: WB Saunders Co; 1993:483–498.

17. Domloge-Hultsch N, Bisalbutra P, Gammon WR, et al. Direct immunofluorescence microscopy of 1 mol/L sodium chloride-treated patient skin. *J Am Acad Dermatol.* 1991;24:946.

18. Mutasim DF, Pelc NJ, Anhalt GJ. Cicatricial pemphigoid. In: Thiers BH, Crosby DL, Diaz LA, eds. *Dermatologic Clinics. Bullous Diseases*. Philadelphia, PA: WB Saunders Co; 1993:499–510.

19. Sarret Y, Hall R, Cobo LM, et al. Salt-split human skin substrate for the immunofluorescent screening of serum from patients with cicatricial pemphigoid and a new method of immunoprecipitation with IgA antibodies. *J Am Acad Dermatol.* 1991;24:952.

20. Gammon WR, Briggaman RA. Epidermolysis bullosa acquisita and bullous systemic lupus erythematosus. Diseases of autoimmunity to Type VII collagen. In: Thiers BH, Crosby DL, Diaz LA, eds. *Dermatologic Clinics. Bullous Diseases*. Philadelphia, PA: WB Saunders Co; 1993:535–547.

21. Fine J-D. Laboratory tests for epidermolysis bullosa. In: Thiers BH, Rapini RP, eds. *Dermatologic Clinics. Use of the Laboratory in Dermatology*. Philadelphia, PA: WB Saunders Co; 1994:123–132.

22. Peters MS, McEvoy MT. IgA antiendomysial antibodies in dermatitis herpetiformis. *J Am Acad Dermatol.* 1989;21:1225.

23. Nousari HC, Anhalt GJ. Bullous skin diseases. *Curr Opin Immunol.* 1995;7:844–852.

24. Kuechle MK, Stegemeir E, Maynard B, et al. Drug-induced linear IgA bullous dermatosis: Report of six cases and review of the literature. *J Am Acad Dermatol.* 1994;30:187–192.

25. Elenitsas R, Jaworsky C, Murphy GF. Diagnostic methodology: Immunofluorescence. In: Murphy GF, ed. *Dermatopathology. A Practical Guide to Common Disorders*. Philadelphia, PA: WB Saunders Co; 1995:29–45.

26. Helm KF, Peters MS. Deposition of membrane attack complex in cutaneous lesions of lupus erythematosus. *J Am Acad Dermatol.* 1993;28:687–691.

CHAPTER 17

Autoimmune Kidney Disease

Jonathan L. Myles, MD, and Raymond R. Tubbs, DO

Few pathologists are involved in interpretation of a medical renal biopsy. This is due to a variety of factors: the need for ancillary studies, such as immunofluorescence and electron microscopy; small numbers of specimens such that it is difficult to maintain expertise in interpretation; and lack of sufficient exposure to renal pathology during residency training. This chapter serves as a guide to the interpretation of medical renal biopsies in regard to autoimmune renal disease and to appropriate specimen processing.

Two major autoimmune diseases affect the kidney: antiglomerular basement membrane disease and systemic lupus erythematosus (SLE). Most patients with antiglomerular basement membrane disease present with rapidly progressive glomerulonephritis and have a crescentic glomerulonephritis. This chapter will discuss the differential diagnosis of crescentic glomerulonephritis and will emphasize the diagnostic features of antiglomerular basement membrane disease. Systemic lupus erythematosus may take on a variety of morphologic forms in the kidney, and this chapter will present the differential diagnosis of the World Health Organization (WHO) subtypes of SLE. A brief discussion of tubulointerstitial disease and renal transplantation also follows; although these entities are not necessarily autoimmune in etiology, they represent manifestations of an altered immune system.

Processing of the Biopsy Specimen

Evaluation of the renal biopsy specimen begins when it is received by the surgical pathology laboratory. It is preferable for specimens to be sent on saline-soaked gauze. The specimen should be evaluated under a dissecting microscope to determine the number of glomeruli present. Glomeruli are small round structures that sometimes protrude above the surrounding renal parenchyma (**Image 17-1**). Generally, at least 10 glomeruli are needed for the biopsy to be considered adequate; however, this number is not absolute. For example, 5 glomeruli may be all that is necessary to establish antiglomerular basement membrane disease if a linear anti-immunoglobulin (Ig) G staining pattern is present by immunofluorescence and all glomeruli contain cellular crescents. Conversely, 15 glomeruli may not be enough to establish a focal segmental glomerulosclerosis-type pattern of injury if only a few glomeruli contain the diagnostic lesion and these are not present in the biopsy specimen.

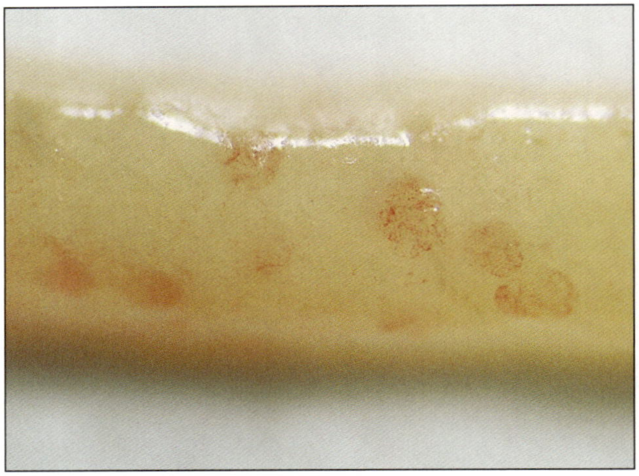

Image 17-1. Gross photograph of a core needle biopsy specimen. Small red dots represent glomeruli.

The specimen next may be divided for light, immunofluorescence, and electron microscopy. In most cases, tissue should be processed for all 3 types of microscopy; however, in cases of suspected transplant rejection, electron microscopy is performed only when disease other than acute rejection is suspected or when there is an unexplained etiology for graft failure. In cases where insufficient glomeruli are available for study, the traditional paraffin-embedded tissue for light microscopy is generally forgone and the tissue is processed for immunofluorescence and electron microscopy, because "light microscopic" data may also be obtained from frozen tissue and plastic sections.

Tissue for light microscopy may be fixed successfully in a variety of fixatives, including buffered formalin. The authors prefer Hollande's fixative, in which we fix most of our surgical pathology biopsy specimens. At the minimum, hematoxylin and eosin (H&E) and periodic acid–Schiff (PAS) stains should be performed. The PAS stain highlights the basement membranes and is useful in evaluating foci of sclerosis. The normal glomerular basement membranes should approximate the thickness of the normal renal tubular basement membranes. In renal amyloidosis the expanded mesangial regions are PAS negative, whereas in a focal segmental glomerulosclerosis-type pattern of injury they are positive.

Other special stains may be performed as indicated. For example, Congo red stain may be used in cases of suspected amyloid. Jones and trichrome stains are useful but not essential in most cases. Jones stain is useful in evaluating basement membranes and is particularly useful in identifying the collapsing variant of focal segmental glomerulosclerosis. Masson trichrome stain is useful in highlighting interstitial connective tissue; however, this usually can be evaluated with H&E. Normally, the renal tubular basement membranes in the cortex should touch each other. If they do not, the expanded interstitium is usually caused by fibrosis, a cellular infiltrate, or edema.

Immunomicroscopy, whether by immunoperoxidase or immunofluorescence, is essential in subcategorizing renal disease. Although immunofluorescence is fast and generally preferable technically, the use of immunoperoxidase is also an option.[1] One advantage of immunoperoxidase is that the slides are available in the file for review; these stains fade much more slowly than immunofluorescent stains. However, immunofluorescent stains tend to be much crisper and easier to interpret.

A routine immunofluorescent panel should include IgG, IgA, IgM, complement C3c, and albumin stains. The albumin stain is important because it detects nonspecific protein binding and is useful in avoiding misinterpretation. In patients with heavy proteinuria, particularly those with diabetes mellitus, there is often linear staining for IgG along the glomerular basement membranes. If a similar or more intense staining pattern is present for albumin, the staining is most likely nonspecific. A lack of crescents also supports the determination of nonspecific linear staining. Kappa and lambda immunostains are performed in selected cases, especially when amyloid or light chain nephropathy is suspected. In amyloid nephropathy, an infiltrative process is evident by light microscopy; in light-chain nephropathy, the glomerular basement membranes are thickened and an abnormal tubular basement membrane is evident by electron microscopy (**Images 17-2** and **17-3**). An interesting new process is the use of fluorescence microscopy with H&E stains. Preliminary evidence suggests that this method may be useful in identifying immune complexes; however, its clinical usefulness has not yet been determined.[2]

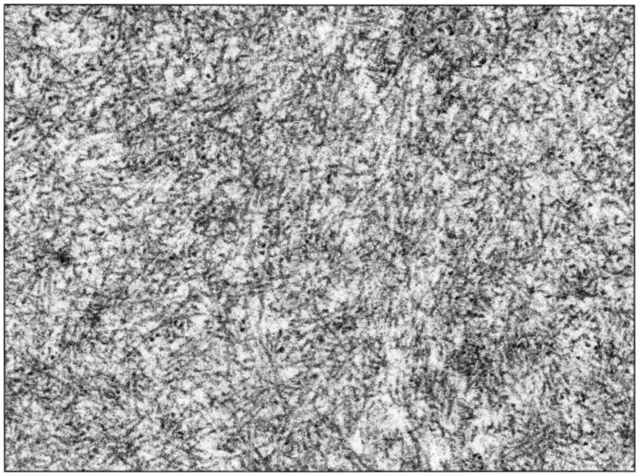

Image 17-2. Electron micrograph of amyloid fibrils. The fibrils are straight and nonbranching; they measure about 10 nm in diameter (×24,000).

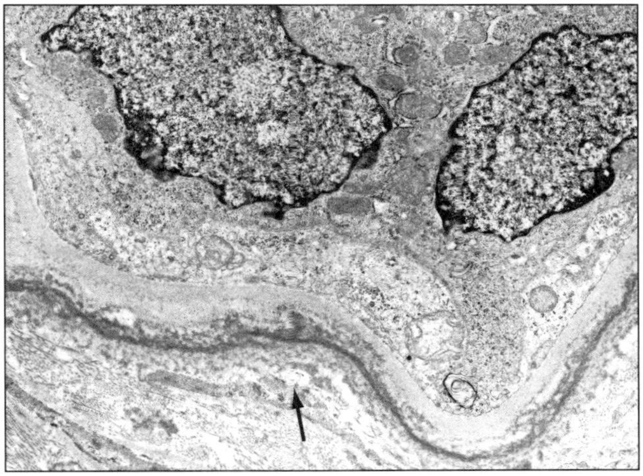

Image 17-3. Electron micrograph of light chain nephropathy. Arrow denotes electron dense material adjacent to the tubular basement membrane (×3,600).

Electron microscopy often provides information not obtainable by light or immunomicroscopy.[3] Tissue for electron microscopy is generally fixed in glutaraldehyde. Whether or not this tissue is examined ultrastructurally, if limited glomeruli are present for evaluation, examination of thick toluidine blue sections provides additional light microscopic information. If tissue is submitted for electron microscopy, toluidine blue–stained sections should always be examined in renal transplant biopsies. In selecting glomeruli for thin sections that will be examined ultrastructurally, it is important to avoid globally sclerotic areas. Electron-dense deposits are often trapped in foci of sclerosis, and their presence in these locations is not indicative of an immune complex disease. Fusion of epithelial foot processes is not pathognomonic of minimal change disease and may be seen in several renal disorders.

The renal biopsy report must contain more information than just the final diagnosis. For example, a type I membranoproliferative–type pattern of injury may be present, with multiple positive immunoglobulins. A comment should be added to the report addressing possible etiologies for this anatomic abnormality, including lupus, hepatitis, or infectious endocarditis as diagnostic possibilities. The light microscopic description should include the total number of glomeruli, numbers and type of crescents, and the number of globally sclerotic glomeruli. A description of the interstitium and small blood vessels should follow. Immunofluorescent findings should be described for each antibody. Staining should be described as focal or diffuse (some or many glomeruli) and segmental or generalized (a portion or all of a glomerulus affected). In focal segmental glomerulosclerosis, the focal segmental nature of the process is often accentuated with IgM staining in the sclerotic areas. Staining in structures other than glomeruli should be noted. In antiglomerular basement membrane disease and light-chain nephropathy, there may be staining in the tubular basement membranes as well as in the glomeruli. Staining in blood vessels may or may not be significant. Granular staining in vessel walls for C3c is usually nonspecific; however, linear staining is associated with acute vascular rejection in renal transplants (**Image 17-4**). The report of the ultrastructural analysis describes electron-dense deposits, epithelial foot processes, fibrillar deposits, and basement membrane abnormalities. If electron-dense deposits are identified, high magnification views should be obtained in an attempt to identify any substructure, such as that associated with cryoglobulinemia (**Image 17-5**).

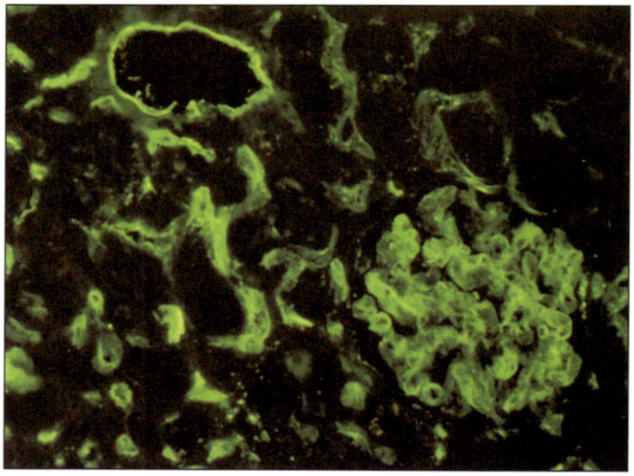

Image 17-4. Immunofluorescence of acute vascular rejection in a renal transplant. There is linear staining for C3c in capillary loops and arterioles.

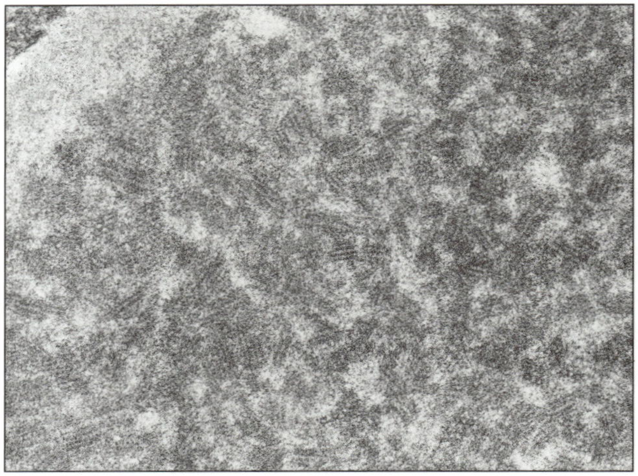

Image 17-5. Electron micrograph in cryoglobulinemia. There is a substructure to the electron dense deposits composed of aggregates of tubules, which are slightly curved (×24,000).

Crescentic Glomerulonephritis and Antiglomerular Basement Membrane Disease

Perhaps the most important function a general pathologist is asked to perform in regard to renal pathology is the evaluation of a biopsy for the presence of crescentic glomerulonephritis. This is important because cellular crescentic lesions are potentially reversible. Treatment options vary depending on the classification of the crescentic lesion.

The definition of a crescent varies. Crescentic lesions are defined as a proliferation of epithelial and monocytoid cells in Bowman's space, often accompanied by fibrin.[4] Although there may be some proliferation of epithelial cells present, if obliteration of Bowman's space is greater than 25%, the lesion is classified as a crescent. Crescents are subclassified into cellular, fibrous, and fibrocellular types. The number of cellular crescents generally is reported as a percentage of total glomeruli (**Image 17-6**). Ultrastructurally, there are often breaks in the glomerular basement membrane. As the crescent ages, there may be resolution or scarring. Fibrocellular crescents contain some fibrous tissue, although epithelial cells are easily identified. Fibrous crescents contain a paucity of epithelial cells and are irreversible lesions. The number of crescents necessary to classify a lesion as crescentic glomerulonephritis varies. Generally, if more than 20% of the glomeruli contain crescents, the lesion is classified as crescentic glomerulonephritis. If fewer than 20% of

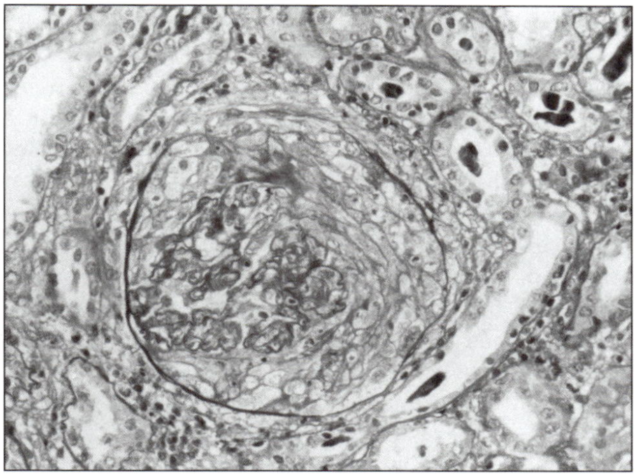

Image 17-6. Cellular crescent. Bowman's space is obliterated by a proliferation of epithelial and monocytoid cells (periodic acid–Schiff).

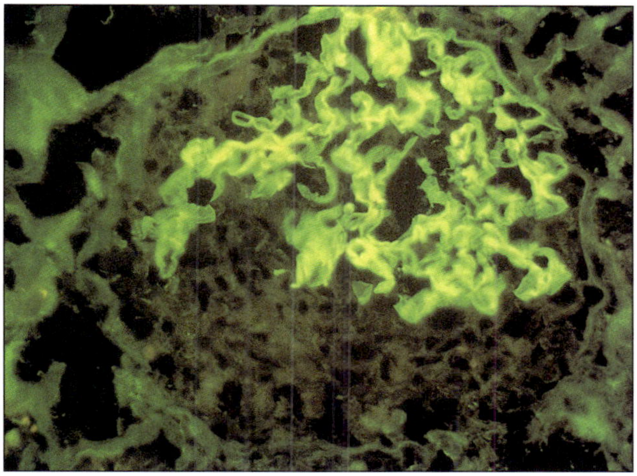

Image 17-7. Immunofluorescence in anti-glomerular basement membrane disease. Linear staining along the glomerular basement membrane for IgG.

crescents are present, "with crescents" is noted in the diagnostic line and the percentage of crescents is specified in the microscopic description.

Once a crescentic lesion is identified, subclassification is important. Crescentic glomerulonephritis is divided into 3 categories: antiglomerular basement membrane disease, immune complex-mediated disease, and pauci-immune disease.[5,6] This major subclassification is generally resolved by immunofluorescence and may be performed within hours of receiving a biopsy.

Antiglomerular basement membrane disease is caused by an autoantibody directed against the noncollagenous domain of type IV collagen. Patients may present with pulmonary hemorrhage and nephritis.[7,8] Susceptibility is related to HLA-DRB1 genes.[9] Antiglomerular basement membrane antibodies may be present, although antineutrophilic cytoplasmic antibodies (ANCAs) also may be present.[10]

Antiglomerular basement membrane lesions are identified by linear staining with IgG and/or C3c (**Image 17-7**). Linear staining with IgG along the glomerular basement membrane is present in antiglomerular basement membrane disease. This staining is generally diffuse and global. Staining with C3c is variable, although an interrupted linear pattern or finely granular pattern often may be present. Linear staining with IgG also may be seen in diabetes mellitus and light-chain deposition disease. However, crescents are not typically present in diabetes, and a similar staining pattern is present for albumin. In light-chain deposition disease, there is generally more intense staining around the tubules, and, ultrastructurally, finely granular electron-dense deposits are seen along the tubular and glomerular basement membranes. Light-chain deposition disease demonstrates kappa or lambda light-chain restriction; however, in antiglomerular basement membrane disease, the antibody deposition demonstrates a mixture of kappa and lambda staining. Electron-dense deposits are not an ultrastructural feature of antiglomerular basement membrane disease.

A granular staining pattern is usually present along the glomerular basement membranes and mesangia for immune complex-mediated lesions. Such lesions include lupus erythematosus, hepatitis, postinfectious nephropathy, and IgA nephropathy.

Pauci-immune lesions have negative immunofluorescence and are often associated with systemic vasculitis, although the vasculitis often is not identified in the biopsy specimen. Antineutrophilic cytoplasmic antibodies are often present. Cytoplasmic-ANCA (c-ANCA) is directed against proteinase 3, and perinuclear-ANCA (p-ANCA) is directed against myeloperoxidase.[11] Cytoplasmic-ANCA is most commonly associated with Wegener's granulomatosis, and p-ANCA may be positive in other vasculitides. The presence of c-ANCA has the greatest specificity for Wegener's granulomatosis. The presence of ANCA is usually determined by indirect immunofluorescence. A strong cytoplasmic staining pattern is seen in c-ANCA when patient serum is mixed with alcohol-fixed reagent neutrophil cells. A perinuclear staining pattern is seen in p-ANCA. When formalin-fixed cells are used, an identical cytoplasmic staining pattern is seen for c-ANCA and p-ANCA. Antinuclear antibodies may mimic p-ANCA when alcohol-fixed cells are used. In equivocal cases, formalin-fixed cells can be used as a confirmatory test.

In crescentic glomerulonephritis, some component of active interstitial nephritis is usually present. This is usually secondary to the crescentic lesion and not a primary process.

Lupus Nephritis

Systemic lupus erythematosus affects multiple organs, including the kidney. Renal failure has been described as the most frequent cause of death in patients with systemic lupus nephritis. Renal involvement may demonstrate various morphologic patterns[12] that are useful in predicting prognosis.[13,14] Although lupus nephritis is commonly diagnosed clinically prior to renal biopsy, the presence of multiple immunoglobulins (IgG, IgA, and IgM) is commonly seen in the biopsy specimen by immunofluorescence. If such a "full house" pattern is identified by immunofluorescence, lupus should be excluded clinically if this has not already been done. Other diseases in which all 3 immunoglobulins may be present include hepatitis and infectious endocarditis. IgG in association with IgM may be seen in cryoglobulinemia, and IgG is often associated with IgA in IgA nephropathy.

A classification commonly used for the morphologic lesions of lupus nephritis is the original WHO classification.[12] Glomeruli that are normal by light microscopy, immunofluorescence, and electron microscopy are considered class I lesions. Class II lesions are composed purely of mesangial disease. In class IIa, the abnormalities are detected only by immunofluorescence or electron microscopy. In class IIb, mesangial hypercellularity is also present. Class II lupus may be confused with IgA nephropathy. In IgA nephropathy, the dominant immunoglobulin is IgA. Although IgG is usually present, a "full house" pattern is rarely evident. Histologically, IgA nephropathy is indistinguishable from Henoch-Schönlein purpura, but clinical features are useful in distinguishing it from lupus nephritis. Focal segmental lesions are considered class III, diffuse proliferative glomerulonephritis is class IV, and membranous glomerulonephritis is class V.

In the modified WHO classification, classes III, IV, and V are subdivided further. In class III, the lesions are subcategorized as active necrotizing lesions, sclerosing lesions, or a combination of both. A sclerosing class III lupus nephritis demonstrates a focal segmental glomerulosclerosis (FSGS)–type pattern of injury. This pattern may be seen in numerous diseases (hypertension, IgA nephropathy, lupus, human immunodeficiency virus nephropathy, chronic transplant rejection, hyperfiltration injury, and so forth) and is not necessarily indicative of idiopathic FSGS. In lupus, electron-dense deposits are identified in nonsclerotic areas; in idiopathic FSGS, such deposits are present only in sclerotic areas.

The most common type of lupus nephritis seen in a biopsy specimen is class IV. Subcategories of class IV lupus nephritis include nephritis without segmental lesions, with active necrosing lesions, with sclerosing lesions, or with active and sclerosing lesions. Subcategories of class V lupus are nephritis with pure membranous lesions (nephritis associated with lesions of class II). If evident, proliferative changes should be noted.

In a non-lupus type of membranous nephropathy usually only IgG and C3 are typically present. Although most cases of membranous nephropathy are obvious by ultrastructural analysis, electron-dense deposits may be subtle in some cases.

A summary of the WHO classification for lupus nephritis is presented in **Table 17-1**. Perhaps the most important thing a surgical pathologist must recognize is the class IV lesions, because these lesions are most associated with a poor prognosis. Class IV lesions tend to be treated more aggressively than other lesions. Many researchers consider class III to be a stage of class IV. If significant proliferative changes are present, class V lesions are generally lumped into the class IV subtype. Patients with class V lesions have a variable clinical course, depending on the degree of glomerulonephritis.[15] Patients with class IV lesions have the worst prognosis; among class IV patients, those with chronic lesions have a worse prognosis.[16,17] It is important to note that lupus nephritis may recur in renal transplants.[18]

Ultrastructurally, electron-dense deposits are identified in classes II through V. Although there is no specific substructure to the deposits, a fingerprint deposit is highly suggestive of lupus nephritis (**Image 17-8**). Mesangial deposits are typically present in class II lupus nephritis. In class IV, the predominant deposit is subendothelial. In class III, both subendothelial and mesangial deposits are present, although the deposits in class III are typically focal and segmental. Focal segmental lesions are also char-

Table 17-1. World Health Organization Classification of Lupus Nephritis

Class	Light Microscopy	Immunofluorescence	Electron Microscopy
I	Normal	Negative	No deposits
II	Normal or mesangial hypercellularity	Positive in mesangium	Mesangial
III	Focal segmental and necrosis or sclerosis	Focal segmental and mesangial	BM Subendothelial and mesangial
IV	Diffuse proliferative	Granular BM and mesangial	Subendothelial and mesangial
V	Diffuse membranous	Granular BM and mesangial	Subepithelial and mesangial

Abbreviation: BM = basement membrane.

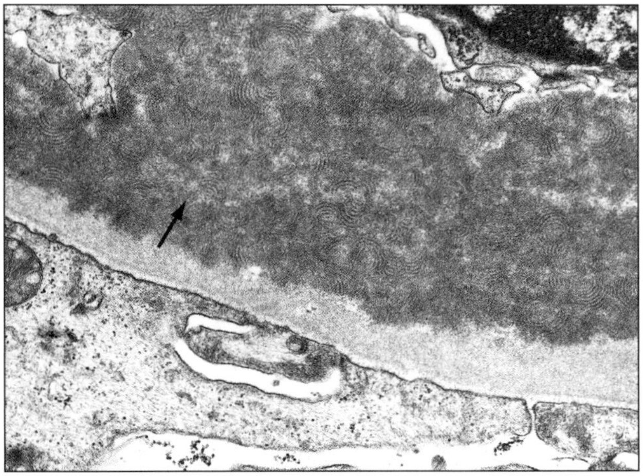

Image 17-8. Systemic lupus erythematosus. Electron microscopy demonstrates electron dense deposits with "fingerprint" substructure (arrow) (×13,000).

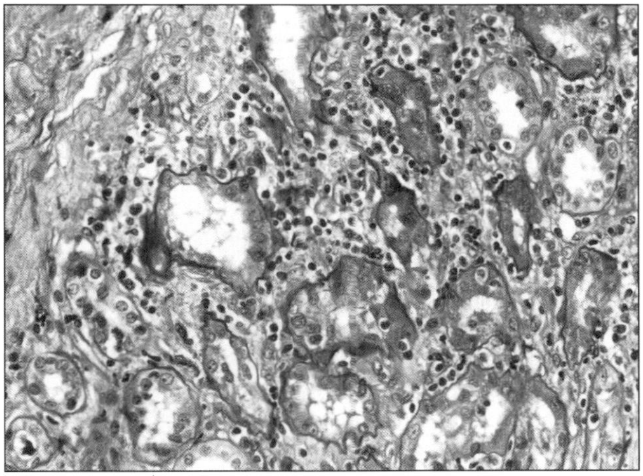

Image 17-9. Acute tubulointerstitial nephritis. An inflammatory infiltrate predominantly composed of lymphocytes without fibrosis is expanding the interstitium. (periodic acid–Schiff).

acterized by light microscopy in class III lesions. Subepithelial deposits predominate in class V disease.

In the modified WHO classification, the additional category of class VI was described. In this category, the predominant pattern is glomerulosclerosis. Generally, at least 80% of the glomeruli must be globally sclerotic to be considered class VI.

Interstitial nephritis is a common component of lupus nephritis, although it is predominantly associated with class IV lesions. The glomerular changes tend to overshadow the interstitial lesions, and the classification of lupus nephritis is based on the glomerular lesion.

The inflammatory infiltrate is composed predominantly of T cells. There is some evidence that the cells are oligoclonal and may be directed against nephritogenic antigens.[19]

Tubulointerstitial Nephritis

As stated previously, tubulointerstitial nephritis is commonly seen in crescentic lesions. Usually the infiltrate is composed mostly of lymphocytes (**Image 17-9**). The presence of eosinophils raises the possibility of a hypersensitivity reaction, although this finding is not specific. The presence of neutrophils, particularly in aggregates and tubular lumina, raises the possibility of an infectious etiology. Interstitial nephritis is seen as a complication of drug therapy (most notably with nonsteroidal anti-inflammatory agents and antibiotics).[20–25] It is also seen as a component of systemic diseases, such as sarcoidosis. The lymphocytes present are predominantly composed of T cells.

Chronic tubulointerstitial nephritis may also be due to a variety of etiologies, and one subclass is idiopathic. Immunofluorescent studies may demonstrate granular deposits of immunoglobulins and complement in the tubular basement membrane. In rare instances, linear deposits may be present, but these deposits are of uncertain clinical significance outside of antiglomerular basement membrane disease. Histologically, interstitial fibrosis is present in addition to chronic inflammation. The fibrosis is often present in periglomerular locations; interstitial fibrosis is an adverse prognostic indicator. Tubular atrophy is present. Some tubules become dilated and contain eosinophilic proteinaceous material in the tubular lumen, so-called thyroidization (**Image 17-10**). As fibrosis becomes more widespread, the glomeruli become ischemic. There is a widening of Bowman's space, and the glomeruli eventually become sclerotic.

Renal Transplantation

A discussion of renal transplantation rejection is included here because it is an immune-mediated process directed against an internal organ. Even if a pathologist is practicing in a center that does not do renal transplants, these patients are ubiquitous and the pathologist may have to interpret a biopsy on an urgent basis.

Not all pathologic processes in a renal transplant biopsy are indicative of rejection. In the early posttransplant period, the most common reason for graft dysfunction is acute tubular necrosis. Rejection is possible, although a fine scattering of lymphocytes in the interstitium is often present immediately following transplant. In addition, there are often small collections of lymphocytes present in the capsular region as the graft acclimates to its new environment. Renal cortical necrosis is possible due to arterial thrombosis, venous thrombosis, and hyperacute rejection. In the late posttransplant period, acute rejection is also possible, although chronic rejection may be seen as well as de novo, recurrent, or transplant glomerulopathies.

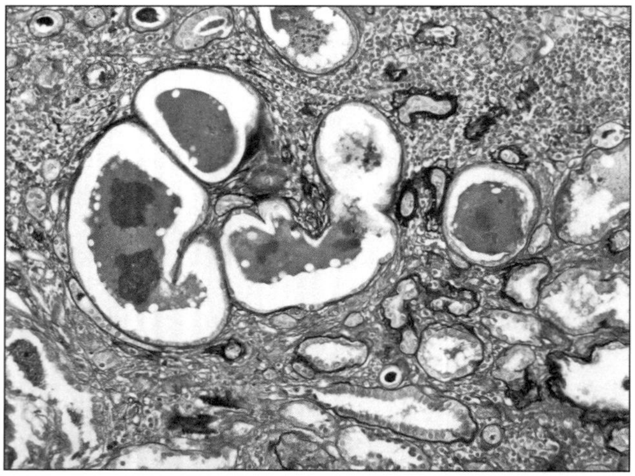

Image 17-10. Chronic tubulointerstitial nephritis. There are dilated tubules with eosinophilic material within the lumen, a condition called "thyroidization." Interstitial fibrosis is present (periodic acid–Schiff).

Several criteria have been described to diagnose acute rejection in the transplant. Most grading schemes rely on some quantitation of interstitial inflammation. To standardize grading of rejection for renal transplant patients, the Banff Working Classification of kidney transplant pathology was proposed in 1993.[26] It was developed by a group of individuals who first met in Banff, Canada, in 1991 to establish some international standardization of nomenclature and criteria for the classification of renal allograft rejection. The Banff classification of acute rejection relies on 2 major criteria: tubulitis and endotheliitis (**Table 17-2**). Tubulitis is defined as the presence of lymphocytes within the renal tubular epithelia (**Image 17-11**). A PAS stain is often useful in delineating these lymphocytes because they often have a clear halo around them. Endotheliitis is defined as lymphocytes present in the subendothelial region of arterioles (**Image 17-12**). Lymphocytes in venules do not count as endotheliitis in the Banff classification scheme.

Several studies have demonstrated that the presence of interstitial inflammation alone does not necessarily indicate acute rejection, particularly in the early posttransplant period, when interstitial inflammation is present. In the Banff schema, tubulitis must be present for a diagnosis of acute cellular rejection.

Very mild acute rejection is also known as borderline changes in the Banff schema. No endotheliitis is present, but some tubulitis may be seen. If present, tubulitis is mild, and 1 to 4 mononuclear inflammatory cells may be seen per tubular cross section.

Mild acute rejection is also known as grade 1 acute rejection. Moderate tubulitis is present (5 to 10 mononuclear cells per tubular cross section or group of 10 tubular cells), and more than 25% of the renal parenchyma must have some interstitial inflammation. No endotheliitis is present. In moderate acute rejection (grade 2) endotheliitis or intense tubulitis is present.

Grade 3, or severe acute rejection, is rarely seen. It is defined as patients with severe intimal arteritis or

Table 17-2. Banff Criteria

Diagnostic Category	Features
Normal	
Hyperacute rejection	Humoral (antibody-mediated) rejection
Borderline	No arteritis
	1-4 mononuclear cells/tubule cross section
Mild acute rejection	No arteritis
	5-10 mononuclear cells/tubule cross section
Moderate acute rejection	Arteritis or
	>10 mononuclear cells/tubule cross section
Severe acute rejection	Transmural arteritis: fibrinoid necrosis, focal infarction, and interstitial hemorrhage often present

Adapted from Solez et al.[26]

transmural arteritis with fibrinoid change and necrosis of medial smooth muscle cells. Often, some degree of infarction and interstitial hemorrhage are present.

This section refers to acute cellular rejection, which is the most common type of acute rejection seen in the renal transplant patient. Rejection may also be mediated by antibodies; this is referred to as humoral rejection. In the Banff schema, hyperacute rejection is caused by preformed donor antibodies. Within 1 hour of transplant, there is endothelial damage in the glomerular capillaries, capillary thrombosis, and neutrophil accumulation. Any cellular infiltrate is usually sparse. This type of rejection is extremely unusual in the transplant population.

Although not described in the Banff schema, there is a more delayed type of humoral rejection, generally referred to as acute vascular rejection. The light microscopic features are similar to those of hyperacute rejection. Because it usually occurs in the first few months following transplant rather than immediately, immunofluorescent studies are useful in identifying this lesion. By immunofluorescence, there is usually linear staining for IgG and C3 in the glomerular capillaries and in the small blood vessels. This same immunofluorescent pattern is seen in hyperacute rejection.

Rejection may be present histologically in acute vascular rejection, although clinical signs and symptoms may not be present.[27] There is some

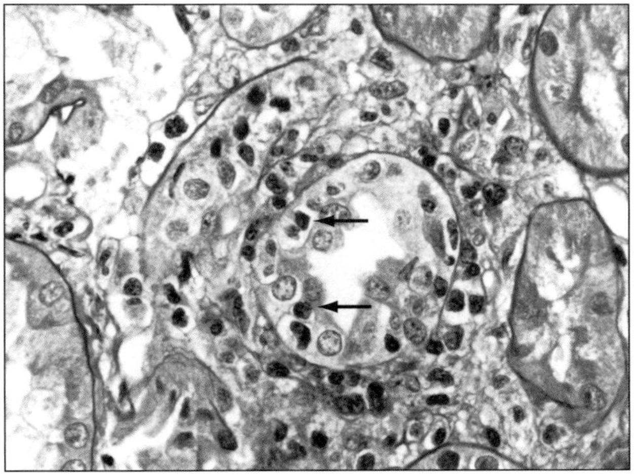

Image 17-11. Tubulitis in acute transplant rejection. Lymphocytes (arrows) are infiltrating tubular epithelium (periodic acid–Schiff).

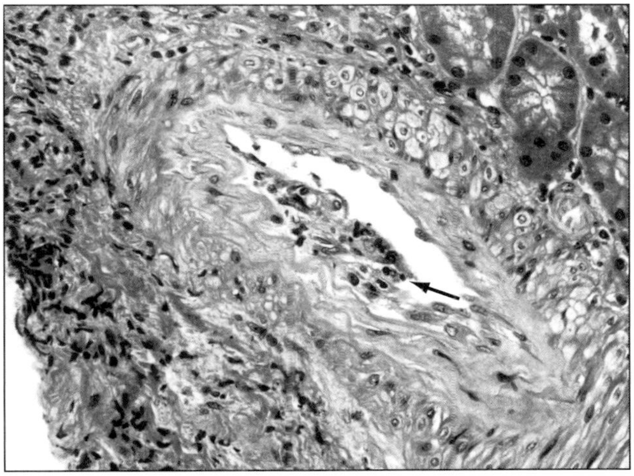

Image 17-12. Endotheliitis in acute transplant region. Lymphocytes (arrow) are infiltrating blood vessels in subendothelial locations (periodic acid–Schiff).

evidence that this is associated with later impaired graft function.[28] The number of acute rejection episodes is a predictor of long-term graft survival.[29]

There is overlap between the histologic features of chronic rejection, chronic cyclosporine toxicity, hypertensive vascular disease, and chronic infection and reflux.[30,31] Because of this, the Banff classification groups all these diseases under chronic allograft nephropathy. For example, vascular thickening from chronic rejection may be difficult to distinguish from that of chronic cyclosporine toxicity (**Image 17-13**). In chronic rejection, there is new-onset arterial fibrous intimal thickening. In chronic cyclosporine toxicity, the vessel wall appears to be more uniformly hyalinized, and the hyaline is often asymmetrically distributed. In chronic rejection, the intimal proliferation is more uniformly circumferential. Interstitial fibrosis may be present in both chronic rejection and chronic cyclosporine toxicity. Interstitial fibrosis is irreversible; however, there is some evidence that the vascular lesion of cyclosporine toxicity may be at least partially reversible. Global glomerular sclerosis is also seen in chronic rejection. The term *transplant glomerulopathy* refers to a characteristic lesion, visible by electron microscopy, in which the glomerular basement membranes are thickened and a subendothelial lucent zone is present (**Image 17-14**). This change may be seen in chronic rejection and/or cyclosporine toxicity. A focal segmental glomerular sclerosis–type pattern of injury is commonly seen in chronic allograft nephropathy. This may be a manifestation of chronic rejection, chronic cyclosporine toxicity, hypertensive vascular disease, or recurrent or de novo glomerulopathy.

The Banff criteria also address specimen adequacy. If no glomeruli or arteries are present, the specimen is referred to as unsatisfactory. Marginal specimens contain 1 to 6 glomeruli with an artery present. Adequate specimens are considered to contain 7 or more glomeruli with arteries present. The Banff schema recommends that 7 histologic slides be made, including 3 H&E-stained sections, 3 PAS stains, and 1 trichrome. Although this full panel may be useful in some centers, 1 ribbon of an H&E-stained section, 1 ribbon of a PAS-stained section, and 1 ribbon of an H&E stain of the frozen section for immunofluorescence are usually adequate for evaluation.

The original Banff criteria have been updated (revised Banff criteria or Banff 97 working classification).[32] Acute rejection is divided into three types: Type I is tubulitis without endarteritis, Type II contains endarteritis, and Type III is arteritis with transmural changes. If there is no arteritis and there are fewer than 4 lymphocytes in a tubular cross section or less than 25% of the parenchyma is affected, the biopsy is classified as borderline/suspicious for rejection. Banff 97 also grades chronic/sclerosing allograft nephropathy and has a separate category for antibody-mediated rejection.

In conclusion, the pathologist provides essential diagnostic and prognostic information when evaluating a patient with autoimmune renal disease. Proper specimen processing and triage for conventional light

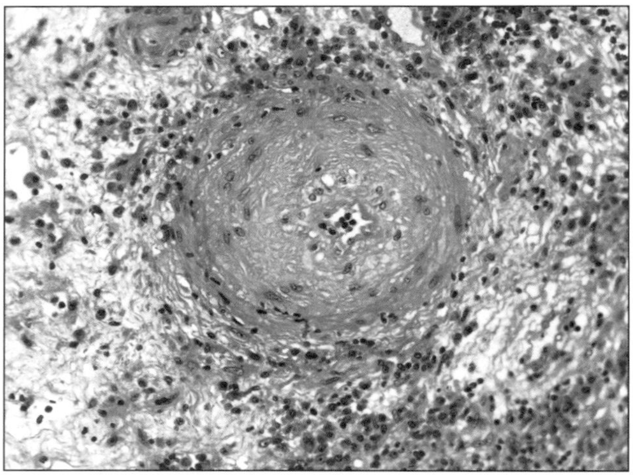

Image 17-13. Chronic rejection. There is marked thickening of the vascular wall (H&E).

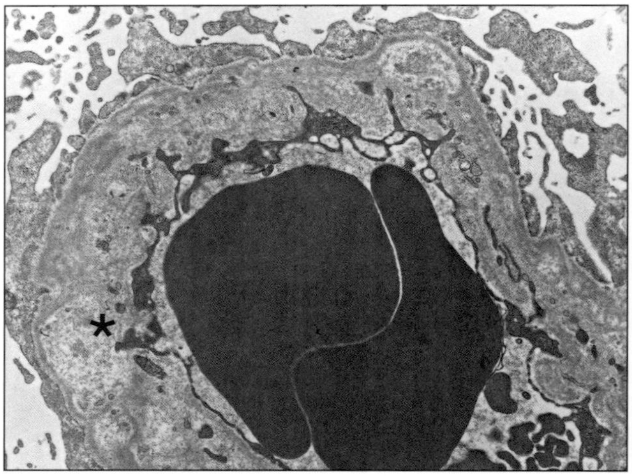

Image 17-14. Chronic transplant glomerulopathy. This electron micrograph shows subendothelial lucencies(*) (×6,000).

microscopy, immunofluorescence, and electron microscopy will allow for proper classification of disease.[33] Classification of cresentic glomerulonephritis will allow for optimum treatment to be initiated. Lupus nephritis may involve the kidney in many forms, and morphologic findings have prognostic and therapeutic implications. Various abnormalities may occur in the transplanted kidney. The biopsy is essential to determining the optimum course of treatment.

References

1. Tubbs R, Gephardt G, Valenzuela R, et al. An approach to immunomicroscopy of renal disease with immunoperoxidase and periodic acid Schiff counterstain (IMPAS stain). *Am J Clin Pathol*. 1980;73:240–246.
2. McMahon JT, Myles JL, Tubbs RR. A novel use of fluorescence microscopy in evaluation of renal biopsies. *Proc Microscopy Microanalysis*. 1997;3:355–356.
3. Haas M. A reevaluation of routine electron microscopy in the examination of native renal biopsies. *J Am Soc Nephrol*. 1997;8:70–76.
4. Lan HY, Nikolic-Paterson DJ, Mu W, et al. Local macrophage proliferation in the pathogenesis of glomerular crescent formation in rat antiglomerular basement membrane (GBM) glomerulonephritis. *Clin Exp Immunol*. 1997;110:223–240.
5. Ambrus JL Jr, Sridhar NR. Immunologic aspects of renal disease. *JAMA*. 1997;278:1938–1945.
6. Grcevska L, Polenakovic M. Crescentic glomerulonephritis as renal cause of acute renal failure. *Ren Fail*. 1995;17:595–604.
7. Daly C, Conlon PJ, Medwar W, et al. Characteristics and outcome of antiglomerular basement membrane disease: A single-center experience. *Ren Fail*. 1996;18:105–112.
8. Niles JL, Bottinger EP, Saurina GR, et al. The syndrome of lung hemorrhage and nephritis is usually an ANCA-associated condition. *Arch Intern Med*. 1996;156:440–445.
9. Fisher M, Pusey CD, Vaughan RW, et al. Susceptibility to antiglomerular basement membrane disease is strongly associated with HLA-DRB1 genes. *Kidney Int*. 1997;51:222–229.
10. Hellmark T, Niles JL, Collins AB, et al. Comparison of anti-GBM antibodies in sera with or without ANCA. *J Am Soc Nephrol*. 1997;8:376–385.
11. Jennette JC, Falk RJ. Antineutrophil cytoplasmic autoantibodies: Discovery, specificity, disease associations and pathogenic potential. *Adv Pathol Lab Med*. 1995;8:363–378.
12. Schwartz ML. The renal biopsy in lupus nephritis: Lessons from clinicopathologic studies. *Adv Pathol Lab Med*. 1993;6:423–444.
13. Baqi N, Moazami S, Singh A, et al. Lupus nephritis in children: A longitudinal study of prognostic factors and therapy. *J Am Soc Nephrol*. 1996;6:924–929.
14. Kashgarian M. The role of the kidney biopsy in the treatment of lupus nephritis. *Ren Fail*. 1996;18:765–773.
15. Sloan RP, Schwartz MM, Korbet SM, et al. Long-term outcome in systemic lupus erythematosus membranous glomerulonephritis. Lupus nephritis collaborative study group. *J Am Soc Nephrol*. 1996;7:299–305.
16. Mitjavila F, Pac V, Moga I, et al. Clinicopathological correlations and prognostic factors in lupus nephritis. *Clin Exp Rheumatol*. 1997;15:625–631.
17. Mosca M, Pasquariello A, Tavoni A, et al. Predictors of renal outcome in diffuse proliferative glomerulonephritis in systemic lupus erythematosus. *Lupus*. 1997;6:371–378.
18. Stone JH, Millward CL, Olson JL, et al. Frequency of recurrent lupus nephritis among ninety-seven renal transplant patients during the cyclosporine era. *Arthritis Rheum*. 1998;41:678–686.
19. Massengill SF, Goodenow MM, Sleasman JW. SLE nephritis is associated with an oligoclonal expansion of intrarenal T cells. *Am J Kidney Dis*. 1998;31:418–426.
20. Ivanyi B, Marcussen N, Olsen S. Tubulitis in primary vascular and glomerular renal disease. *Pathol Res Pract*. 1995;191:1245–1257.
21. Bennett WM, Henrich WL, Stoff JS. The renal effects of nonsteroidal anti-inflammatory drugs: Summary and recommendations. *Am J Kidney Dis*. 1996;28:S56–S62.
22. Dhillon S, Higgins RM. Interstitial nephritis. *Postgrad Med J*. 1997;73:151–155.
23. Schwarz A, Perez-Canto A. Nephrotoxicity of anti-infective drugs. *Int J Clin Pharmacol Ther Toxicol*. 1998;36:164–167.
24. Bhaumik SK, Kher V, Arora P, et al. Evaluation of clinical and histological prognostic markers in drug-induced acute interstitial nephritis. *Ren Fail*. 1996;18:97–104.
25. Ivanyi B, Hamilton-Dutoit SJ, Hansen HE, et al. Acute tubulointerstitial nephritis; phenotype of infiltrating cells and prognostic impact of tubulitis. *Virchows Arch*. 1996;428:5–12.
26. Solez K, Axelse R, Hallgrimur B, et al. International standardization of criteria for the histologic diagnosis of renal allograft rejection: The Banff working classification of kidney transplant pathology. *Kidney Int*. 1993;44:411–422.
27. Rush DN, Henry SF, Jeffery JR, et al. Histological findings in early routine biopsies of stable renal allograft recipients. *Transplantation*. 1994;57:208–211.
28. Rush DN, Jeffery JR, Gough J. Sequential protocol biopsies in renal transplant patients. Clinicopathological correlations using the Banff schema. *Transplantation*. 1995;59:511–514.

29. Ferguson R. Acute rejection episodes—best predictor of long-term primary cadaveric renal transplant survival. *Clin Transpl*. 1994;8:328–331.

30. Drachenberg CB, Steinberger E, Hoehn-Saric E, et al. Specificity of intertubular capillary changes: Comparative ultrastructural studies in renal allografts and native kidneys. *Ultrastruct Pathol*. 1997;21:227–233.

31. Seron D, Moreso F, Bover J, et al. Early protocol renal allograft biopsies and graft outcome. *Kidney Int*. 1997;51:310–316.

32. Racusen LC, Sulez K, Colvin RB, et al. The Banff 97 working classification of renal allograft pathology. *Kidney Int*. 1999;55:713–723.

33. Striker G, Striker LJ, D'Agati V. *The Renal Biopsy*. 3rd ed. Philadelphia, PA: WB Saunders; 1997.

CHAPTER 18

Autoimmune Diseases of the Liver

David J. Bylund, MD, and John G. McHutchison, MD

Primary biliary cirrhosis (PBC) and PBC-like syndromes, autoimmune hepatitis (AiH), primary sclerosing cholangitis (PSC), and drug-induced immune hepatitis are generally cited as the most clinically important autoimmune liver diseases. Despite evidence that autoimmune mechanisms contribute to tissue injury in these diseases, specific causes are presently unknown except in drug-related cases.[1–3] Apparently autoimmune mechanisms also contribute to the pathogenesis of other liver disorders, including viral hepatitis A, B, and C; possibly alcohol-related liver disease; and Wilson's disease.[4]

For the purpose of clinical management, autoimmune liver disease must be considered as a possible diagnosis whenever a patient presents with chronic inflammation of the liver. At the point when differential diagnoses include autoimmune liver diseases, the choices among common disorders include alcohol-related liver disease, drug-induced hepatitis, chronic viral hepatitis, and nonalcoholic fatty liver disease (nonalcoholic steatohepatitis). Less common diagnostic alternatives are hemochromatosis, Wilson's disease, α_1-antitrypsin deficiency, and hepatic involvement in systemic diseases.

A clinical laboratory helps characterize autoimmune liver disease by identifying certain distinct autoantibodies. This chapter concentrates on describing autoantibodies that characterize the major autoimmune liver diseases and on presenting synopses of these disorders, excluding drug-related immune hepatitis.

Useful Laboratory Tests

Routine Tests

Serum assays for transaminases, alkaline phosphatase, bilirubin, albumin, and prothrombin are first-order tests for the evaluation of hepatobiliary disease. The patient's history, a physical examination, and results of first-order tests generally point toward either an obstructive or a parenchymal disorder, and the subsequent workup is then individualized. A general outline of steps in the initial workup for suspected chronic liver disease is shown in **Figure 18-1**.

Second-Order Tests

If the initial workup generates serious consideration of autoimmune liver disease, the availability of tests to identify autoantibodies helps the clinician resolve the differential diagnosis of chronic liver disease and classify the various autoimmune liver diseases. Although numerous autoantibodies have been reported in autoimmune liver disease, five distinct types of autoantibodies are currently most relevant to clinical practice: liver-kidney-microsomal autoantibodies (LKMs), smooth muscle autoantibodies (SMAs), antinuclear autoantibodies (ANAs), antimitochondrial autoantibodies (AMAs), and antineutrophil cytoplasmic autoantibodies. Antineutrophil cytoplasmic autoantibodies are discussed in detail in Chapter 15.

Indicated tests and expected result profiles for each autoimmune liver disease are shown in **Tables 18-1** and **18-2**.

Detection Methods

Indirect Immunofluorescence Microscopy

Indirect immunofluorescence microscopy (IIFM) remains the method most commonly used in medical laboratories to screen for LKMs, ANAs, SMAs, and AMAs. This method requires capital investment in a high-quality fluorescent microscope and a staff of experienced technicians who can identify clinically significant fluorescent patterns, although there is always the possibility for interlaboratory and/or interobserver variation, especially when the antibody of interest is present in low titer.[5]

The technical procedure itself is fairly rapid and straightforward.[6,7] Liver-kidney-microsomal autoantibodies, SMAs, and AMAs can be identified presumptively using mouse or rat stomach-kidney-liver (MSKL or RSKL) combined tissue blocks. These tissue substrates are available from several commercial sources. Alternatively, frozen sections can be prepared in the laboratory using unfixed tissue that has been snap frozen in isopentane cooled in dry ice.

Human epithelial (HEp-2) cells on glass slides purchased from commercial suppliers are now used in most laboratories to screen for ANAs. Antinuclear antibodies also are detected on both MSKL and RSKL.

Indirect immunofluorescence microscopy has the advantage of detecting many autoantibodies, whether or not their specific antigen is known. In a reference laboratory setting, it is not uncommon to identify autoantibodies that cannot be further defined because the specific target antigen has not yet been

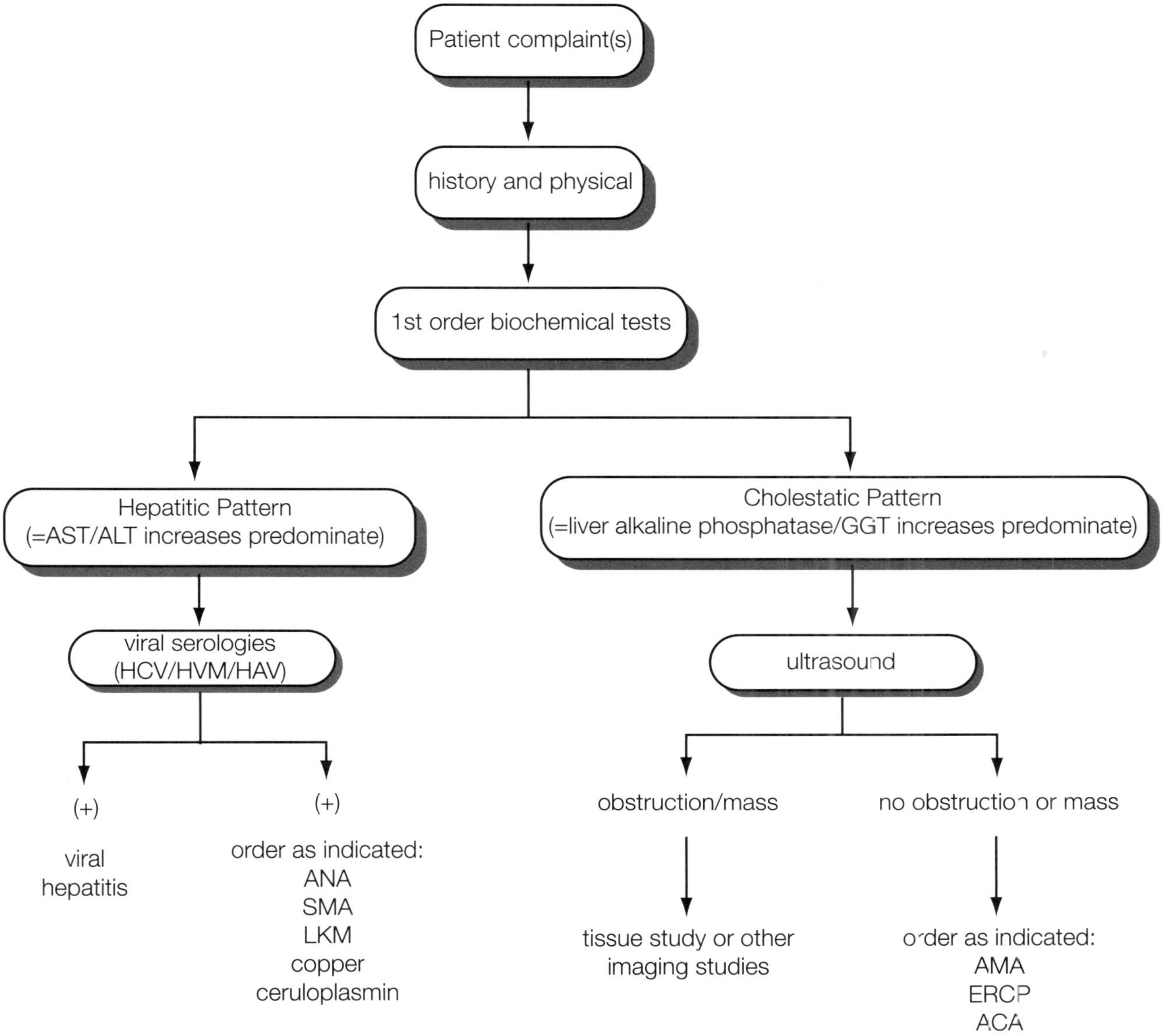

Consider liver biopsy, as clinically indicated.

ACA = anticarbonic anhydrase
ALT = alanine transaminase
AMA = antimitochondrial autoantiodies
ANA = antinuclear autoantibodies
AST = aspartate transaminase
ERCP = endoscopic retrograde cholangiography
GGT = gamma glutamyl transaminase
HAV = hepatitis A virus
HBV = hepatitis B virus
HCV = hepatitis C virus
LKM = liver-kidney-microsomal autoantibodies
SMA = smooth muscle autoantibodies

Figure 18-1. Summary of a diagnostic algorithm for chronic hepatitis.

Table 18-1. Useful Tests in Autoimmune Liver Diseases

Disease	Clinical Tests	Biochemical Tests	Serologic Tests		Research Tests
			First Order	Second Order	
PBC		AP↑, IgM↑	AMA	ANA	
AiH		AST↑, ALT, IgG↑	ANA, SMA, LKM	ANCA	See Table 18-5
AiC		AP↑	AMA, ANA		CA
"Overlap"		AP↑, AST↑, ALT↑	AMA, ANA		
PSC	ERCP	AP-	AMA	ANCA	

Abbreviations: PBC = primary biliary cirrhosis; AP = alkaline phosphatase; IgM = immunoglobulin M; AMA = antimitochondrial autoantibodies; ANA = antinuclear autoantibodies; AiH = autoimmune hepatitis; AST = aspartate transaminase; ALT = alanine transaminase; IgG = immunoglobulin G; SMA = smooth muscle autoantibodies; LKM = liver-kidney-microsomal autoantibodies; AiC = autoimmune cholangitis; CA = carbonic anhydrase antibodies; PSC = primary sclerosing cholangitis; ERCP = endoscopic retrograde cholangiography; ANCA = antineutrophil cytoplasmic antibodies.

Table 18-2. Typical Immunoserologic Profiles in Autoimmune Diseases of Liver

	AMA	ACA	ANA	SMA	LKM1	Atypical p-ANCA
Primary biliary cirrhosis	+		+/–			
Overlap syndrome	+		+			
Autoimmune cholangitis		+				
Autoimmune hepatitis						
Type 1			+	+		+
Type 2					+	
Primary sclerosing cholangitis			+/–			+

Abbreviations: AMA = antimitochondrial autoantibodies; ACA = carbonic anhydrase antibodies; ANA = antinuclear autoantibodies; SMA = smooth muscle autoantibodies; LKM1 = liver-kidney-microsomal autoantibodies; ANCA = antineutrophil cytoplasmic autoantibodies.

characterized. However, the presence of an autoantibody of unknown specificity, especially at high titer, is often abnormal, so its detection may help the clinician resolve alternative diagnoses in a given clinical situation.

A limitation of IIFM is its inability to differentiate heterogeneous antigen-antibody systems that produce similar fluorescent patterns. Consequently, antigen-specific assays, such as enzyme-linked immunosorbent assay (ELISA), are necessary to identify specific autoantibodies.

Enzyme-Linked Immunosorbent Assay

Antigen-specific ELISAs allow identification of specific autoantibodies. Because many of the clinically relevant autoantibodies are defined using IIFM, antigen-specific ELISAs must be validated carefully to establish appropriate levels of analytic and diagnostic sensitivity and specificity. If such clinically relevant criteria are met, ELISAs provide for other considerations, such as objective assay results, automation, and faster high-volume turnaround times. The availability of ELISAs also obviates the need for a fluorescent microscope and for personnel trained in IIFM pattern recognition. For example, the US Food and Drug Administration has approved for clinical use commercial ELISA kits that use specific mitochondrial autoantigens to detect AMAs that are almost PBC-specific.

Liver-Kidney-Microsomal Autoantibodies

Molecular studies have identified at least 3 LKM subtypes. Their corresponding autoantigens and disease associations are summarized in **Table 18-3**.[8–12]

Detection Methods

Indirect Immunofluorescence

For routine clinical purposes, IIFM is the standard method used to presumptively identify LKM.

Table 18-3. Microsomal Autoantibodies in Autoimmune Liver Diseases[13]

Autoantibody	Autoantigen	MW (kd)	Disease Association(s)
LKM1	P450IID6	50	Autoimmune hepatitis, type 2; HCV disease; halothane hepatitis (rare)
LKM2	P450IIC9	50	Tienilic acid-induced hepatitis
LKM3	UGT1	55	Chronic hepatitis delta
LM	P450IA2	52	Autoimmune polyendocrine syndrome, type 1; dihydralazine-induced hepatitis

Abbreviations: HCV = hepatitis C virus; LKM = liver-kidney-microsomal autoantibodies; LM = liver-microsomal autoantibodies; UGT = UDP-glucuronosyl-transferases family 1.

Cryostat sections of RSKL or MSKL are used as substrates. It is important that tissue sections include sampling of distal renal tubules to allow distinction of LKMs from AMAs. Adult sera are screened at 1:40 dilutions and children's at 1:10 dilutions.

The characteristic LKM pattern in AiH is diffuse and homogeneous cytoplasmic fluorescence of proximal tubules (P3 portion) in kidney and hepatocytes throughout the liver acini, but no staining of stomach parietal cells. Liver-kidney-microsomal autoantibodies typically do not stain distal renal tubules, although in rare instances there may be weak immunofluorescence in this region (**Image 18-1**). In autoimmunity associated with hepatitis C virus, IIFM shows an LKM pattern in kidney with or without concomitant staining of the stomach parietal cells.

Liver-kidney-microsomal autoantibodies may be confused with AMAs. Unlike LKMs, AMAs in PBC characteristically show intense granular staining of distal renal tubules and gastric parietal cells with less intense staining of proximal kidney tubules. Concomitant serologic detection of AMAs and LKMs, although theoretically possible, is apparently rare based on the absence of published reports in the literature.

Liver microsomal autoantibodies (LMs) stain hepatocytes in liver but do not stain either kidney or stomach.

Differential immunofluorescent patterns for LKMs and AMAs are shown in **Table 18-4**.

Enzyme-Linked Immunosorbent Assay and Immunoblot

Although there are reports that both ELISA and immunoblot using recombinant proteins can detect LKM subtypes and LMs, these assays are currently available only from specialized laboratories. Because the autoantigens are known, it is anticipated that ELISAs from commercial suppliers will be forthcoming. Immunoblot using recombinant P450IID6 is reported to be the most sensitive and specific method available for detection of LKM1.[14]

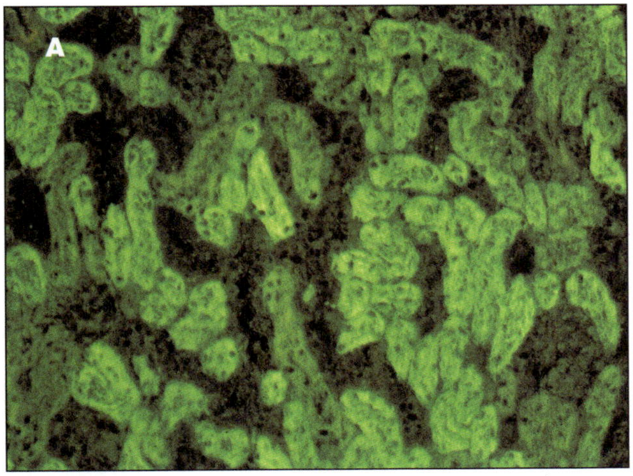

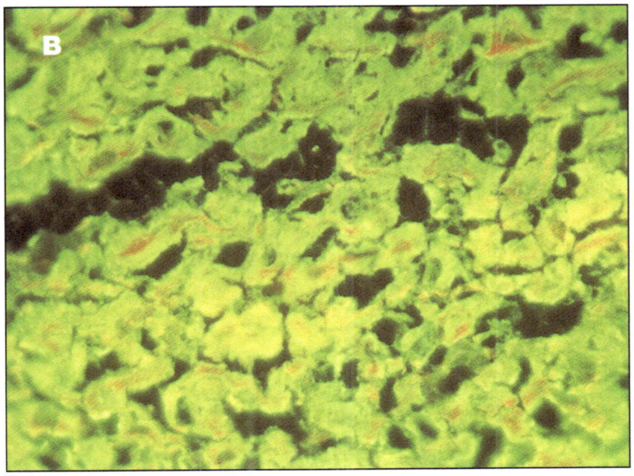

Image 18-1. Liver-kidney-microsomal autoantibodies. (A) Homogeneous cytoplasmic immunofluorescence of variable intensity is limited to the proximal renal tubules on mouse stomach-kidney substrate. (B) There is strong homogeneous immunofluorescence of hepatocytes throughout the acini on rat liver.

Table 18-4. Typical Antimitochondrial and Liver-Kidney-Microsomal Autoantibody Patterns With Indirect Immunofluorescence

Rodent Tissue Substrates	M2 AMA	M1 AMA	M3 AMA	M5 AMA	LKM
Kidney					
Distal tubules	++++ (granular)	++ (diffuse)	++	+/–	–
Proximal tubules	+	+	++	++	+++ (selective)
Stomach					
Parietal cells	+++	Weak	+++	–	–
Liver					
Hepatocytes	+++ (granular)	++ (diffuse)	++ (granular)	+ (granular)	+++ (homogeneous)

Abbreviations: AMA = antimitochondrial autoantibodies; LKM = liver-kidney-microsomal autoantibodies.
Adapted from Meek et al.[13]

Test Interpretation

The presence of LKMs supports a diagnosis of AiH when viral serologies are negative and other criteria for a diagnosis of AiH are met; LKMs can be seen in patients with hepatitis C virus. If LKMs are detected when neither AiH nor hepatitis C virus are concerns, the possibility of drug-associated antibodies should be considered.

Antinuclear Autoantibodies

Specific Antinuclear Autoantibodies and Detection Methods

Antinuclear autoantibodies are discussed in detail in Chapters 9 through 13, but relevant points are summarized here.

Indirect Immunofluorescence

Human epithelial cells are most commonly used to detect ANAs, but also are seen on rodent tissue substrates used to screen for AMAs, LKMs, and SMAs. Patient sera are screened at 1:40 dilutions and positive samples are titered to end point. Homogeneous or speckled immunofluorescent patterns are the most common patterns seen in patients with AiH (**Images 18-2** to **18-4**).

Nuclear membrane ANAs (M-ANAs) that recognize nuclear pore membrane glycoprotein gp210 have been reported as highly specific ANA in 10% to 25% of patients with PBC (**Image 18-5**). A second ANA producing a pattern of multiple nuclear dots (MND-ANA) that react with nuclear protein Sp100 have been reported as highly specific in 27% of patients with PBC (**Image 18-6**).[15] Anticentromere ANAs are detected in about 10% of these patients (**Image 18-7**).[16]

Test Interpretation

- Antinuclear autoantibodies are sensitive but not specific markers of AiH.[8,17]
- Antinuclear autoantibodies in AiH are generally high titer and exceed 1:80 in about 80% of patients with this disease (type 1).[18]
- Antinuclear autoantibodies may be detected in nonhepatic autoimmune diseases or in several hepatic disorders other than AiH, including PBC (60%), alcohol-related liver disease (50%), hepatitis B virus (40%), and hepatitis C virus

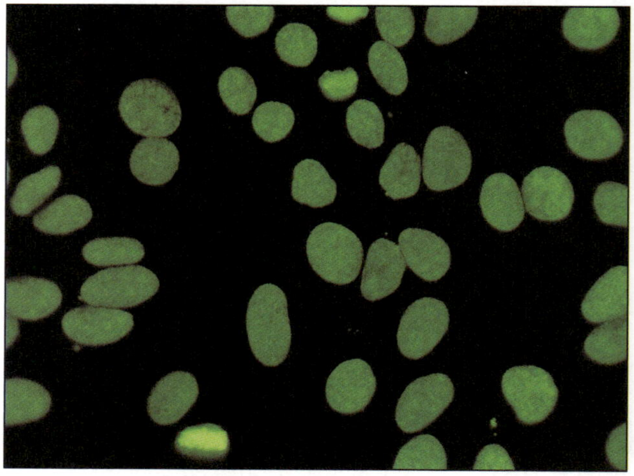

Image 18-2. Homogeneous antinuclear autoantibody pattern on HEp-2 cells.

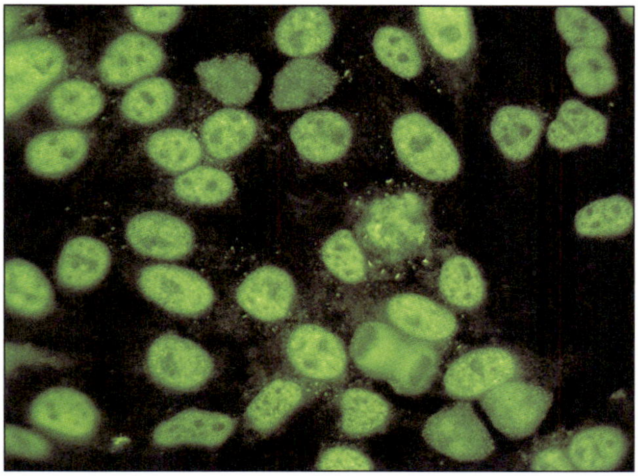

Image 18-3. Speckled antinuclear autoantibody pattern on HEp-2 cells.

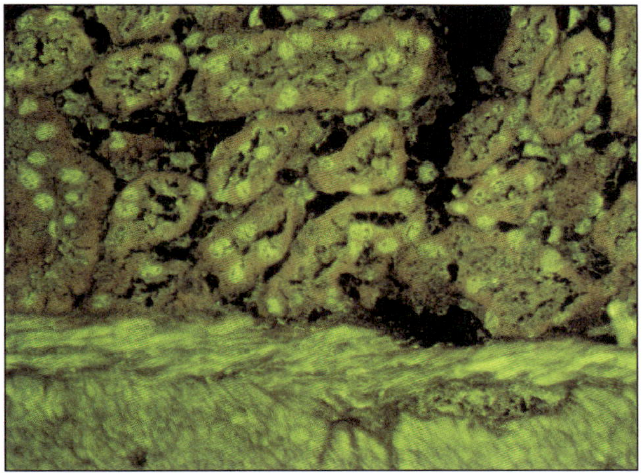

Image 18-4. Coexisting speckled antinuclear autoantibodies and smooth muscle autoantibodies on mouse stomach-kidney substrate. This pattern is often seen in patients with autoimmune hepatitis.

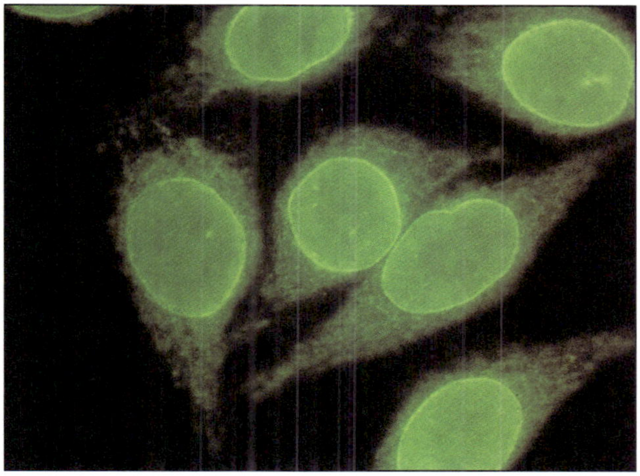

Image 18-5. Nuclear membrane antinuclear autoantibody pattern on HEp-2 cells.

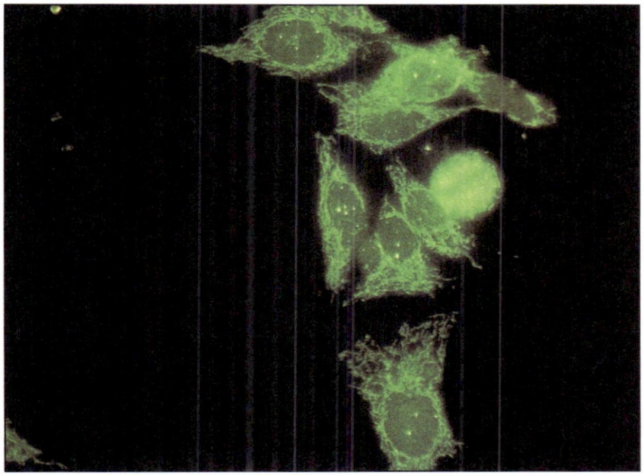

Image 18-6. Multiple nuclear dots and antimitochondrial autoantibodies on HEp-2 cells.

(20% to 30%).[18–20] In these disorders, titers are generally lower than in AiH.

- If either M-ANA or MND-ANA patterns are seen, PBC should be considered.

Smooth Muscle Autoantibodies

Smooth muscle autoantibodies were originally defined using IIFM as autoantibodies that react with smooth muscle components in tissue substrates. They are in fact a heterogeneous group of autoantibodies that target specific cytoskeletal filaments. These filaments include actin; intermediate filaments, such as vimentin and desmin; and microtubules containing tubulin.

Specific autoantibodies to F-actin (antiactin) are an SMA subset characteristic of AiH. F-actin is the biologically active polymeric form of actin found in eukaryotic cells, where it functions in muscle contraction and other cellular processes.[21]

Detection Methods

Indirect Immunofluorescence

Unfixed frozen sections of RSKL or MSKL are the usual tissue substrates. Unfixed substrates are

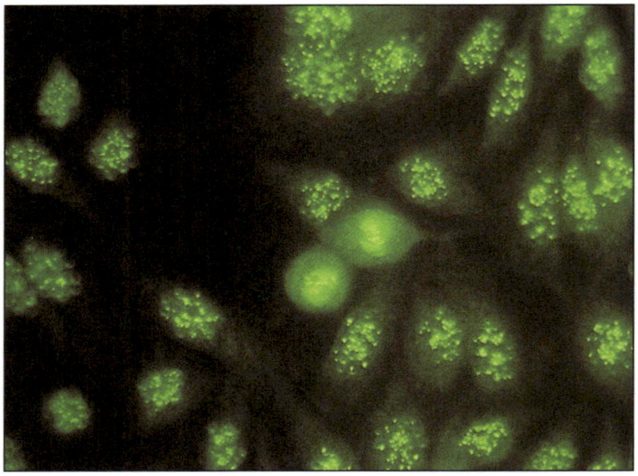

Image 18-7. Anticentromere antinuclear autoantibody pattern on HEp-2 cells.

preferable to preserve the reactivity of antiactin, which is reported to be highly dependent on the natural conformation of epitopes in F-actin.[21] Adult sera are screened at 1:40 dilutions and children's sera at 1:10.

The SMA pattern that correlates with the presence of antiactin is homogeneous immunofluorescence of stomach muscularis mucosa and intramucosal muscle fibers, mesangial cells in renal glomeruli, and media of blood vessels (**Image 18-8**).[21,22] Although antiactin can be identified specifically using either acetone-fixed fibroblasts treated with vinblastine or with ELISA, such assays for antiactin antibodies are not performed in most clinical laboratories.[9,21] Smooth muscle autoantibodies demonstrate "cable-like" cytoplasmic staining using HEp-2 cells.

Enzyme-Linked Immunosorbent Assay

Some ELISAs have been reported to detect antibodies to G-actin with 60% to 70% sensitivity and 94% specificity, but these assays are not widely used in clinical laboratories.[23] One report indicates that routine screening for antiactin alone may actually miss 5% of patients with AiH, so testing for SMAs using IIFM is still recommended.[24]

Test Interpretation[9,15,18,21,22,24,25]

- Smooth muscle autoantibodies are a sensitive but not specific marker of AiH.
- In autoimmune hepatitis, SMAs often coexist with ANAs.
- Smooth muscle autoantibody titers greater than 1:80 are identified most commonly in AiH, but may be seen in other chronic inflammatory liver diseases, including PSC, PBC, and alcohol-related liver disease.
- Smooth muscle autoantibody titers greater than 1:320 generally correlate with antiactin specificity, but specific antiactin assays are not widely available.
- Smooth muscle autoantibodies may be detected transiently in a variety of infectious diseases, including viral hepatitis and infectious mononucleosis. These SMAs are often low titer (<1:80) immunoglobulin (Ig) M autoantibodies.

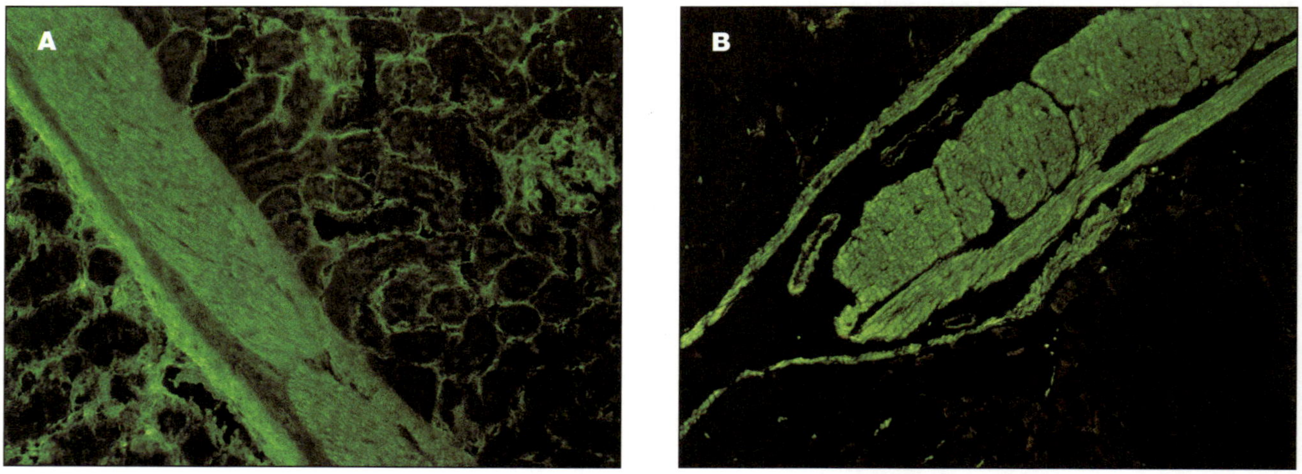

Image 18-8. Smooth muscle autoantibodies on mouse stomach-kidney substrate. There is homogeneous immunofluorescence of (**A**) stomach muscularis mucosa, intramucosal muscle fibers, and mesangial cells in renal glomeruli, and (**B**) muscularis mucosa and media of blood vessels.

- Smooth muscle autoantibodies are detected in fewer than 5% of apparently healthy individuals, but frequency may rise with advancing age.

Other Liver-Specific Autoantibodies

Numerous other liver autoantibodies have been described in AiH, and some of these are listed in **Table 18-5**.[4] Assays to measure these autoantibodies are neither routinely done in clinical laboratories nor widely available except in specialized research laboratories. Their identification may be useful in problematic cases.

Antimitochondrial Autoantibodies

Researchers using modern molecular methods have defined subunits of the three 2-oxo-acid dehydrogenase complexes as the principal autoantigens in PBC. These complexes, localized to the inner mitochondrial membrane of eukaryotic cells, participate in energy metabolism.[26] Antimitochondrial autoantibodies to these PBC-related antigens have been called M2. The dominant 2-oxo-acid dehydrogenase autoantigens in PBC are the E2 and E3BP subunits of pyruvate dehydrogenase, designated PDH-E2 and PDH-E3BP, respectively[10,15,26,27] (**Table 18-6**).

Antimitochondrial autoantibodies that are distinguished from M2 have been described on the basis of immunofluorescence pattern and/or disease association; these AMAs include M1 and M3 through M9 using M nomenclature; certain disease associations are listed in **Table 18-7**.[28] Although M1 and M2 autoantigens are known, the specific identities of other M autoantigens are still at issue.[15,29]

A group of serum autoantibodies called naturally occurring mitochondrial autoantibodies (NOMAs) has been identified among individuals who are in close contact with PBC patients and in laboratory personnel who process sera from such patients, but NOMAs are not directed to the same antigenic epitopes as are AMAs. Moreover, patients with PBC rarely produce NOMAs. Some individuals become NOMA positive after infection with the Epstein-Barr virus, cytomegalovirus, and other pathogens. Even though the clinical significance of NOMAs is both uncertain and controversial, their presence in persons closely associated with PBC patients or their sera has raised questions about possible infectious agents in serum.[10,30,31]

Detection Methods

Indirect Immunofluorescence

Patient sera are screened at 1:40 dilutions, and positive samples are titered to at least 1:160.

The characteristic AMA pattern in PBC is 3 to 4+ granular immunofluorescence of distal renal tubules, stomach parietal cells, and liver hepatocytes; proximal renal tubules also stain but the intensity may vary (**Images 18-9** to **18-11**).

M2 antimitochondrial autoantibodies characteristic of PBC can be confused with M1, M3, and

Table 18-5. Other Liver-Specific Autoantibodies

Anti-asialoglycoprotein receptor
Anti-GOR
Anti–liver cytosol 1 and 2
Anti–liver membrane
Anti–liver-pancreas protein
Anti–liver-specific membrane lipoprotein
Anti–soluble liver antigen

Table 18-6. M Nomenclature for Antimitochondrial Antibody Subtypes in Primary Biliary Cirrhosis[13,14,28]

M Designation	Autoantigen	Molecular Weight (kd)	Antibody Frequency (%)
M2a	PDH-E2 acetyltransferase	70-74	90-95
M2c	Protein X	50-52	90-95
M2d	PDH-E1α decarboxylase	41	40-60
M2c	OGDC-E2	48-52	65-85
M2c	BCOADC-E2	52-56	50-55
M2e	PDH-E1ß	36	1-7

Abbreviations: PDH = pyruvate dehydrogenase; OGDC = 2-oxo-glutarate dehydrogenase; BCOADC = branched-chain 2-oxo-acid dehydrogenase.

Table 18-7. Antimitochondrial Autoantibody M Subtypes in Non–Primary Biliary Cirrhosis Disorders

M Designation	Clinical Association	Antigen
M1	Syphilis	Cardiolipin
M3	Venocuran-induced pseudolupus	Unknown
M5	Connective tissue diseases	Unknown
M6	Iproniazid-induced hepatitis	Unknown
M7	Acute myocarditis and dilated cardiomyopathy	Unknown

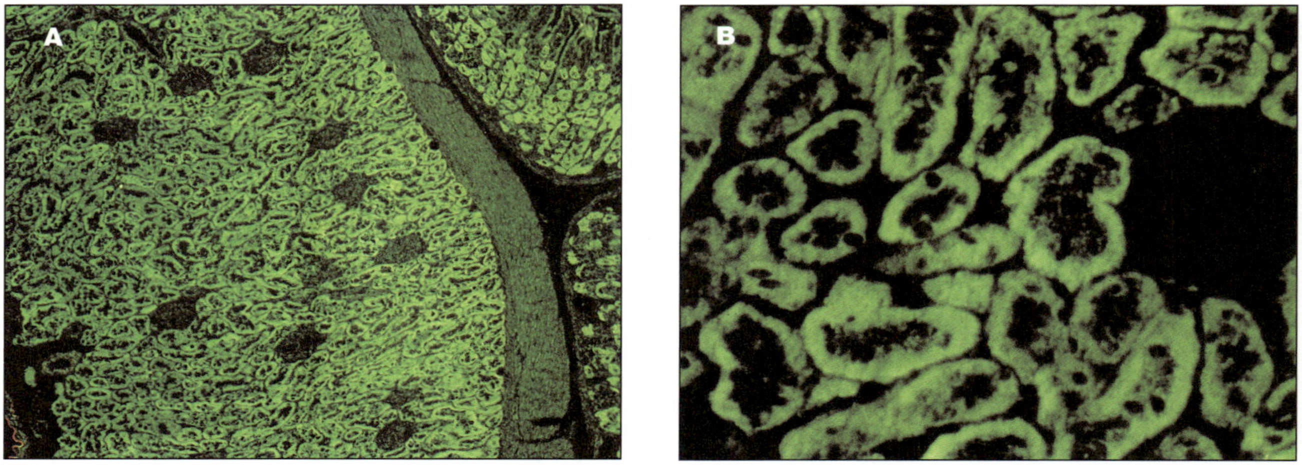

Image 18-9. Antimitochondrial autoantibodies in primary biliary cirrhosis using mouse stomach-kidney substrate. (**A**) A low-power view shows strong, finely granular immunofluorescence of renal tubules and stomach parietal cells. (**B**) A high-power view illustrates the diffuse, finely granular cytoplasmic immunofluorescence in distal renal tubules characteristic of antimitochondrial autoantibodies in primary biliary cirrhosis.

M5 AMAs, as shown in Table 18-4 (**Image 18-12**).[13] It may be useful to identify the M1 AMA pattern associated with secondary syphilis or anticardiolipin autoantibodies that may correlate with the antiphospholipid syndrome.

Another potential source of confusion is the presence of heterophil antibodies in human sera. Heterophil antibodies are present in about 3% of clinically normal individuals. Rat and (to a lesser extent) mouse tissue substrates may show heterophil binding in the brush borders of proximal renal tubular cells, renal tubular basement membranes, gastric parietal cells, and Kupffer's cells in liver.

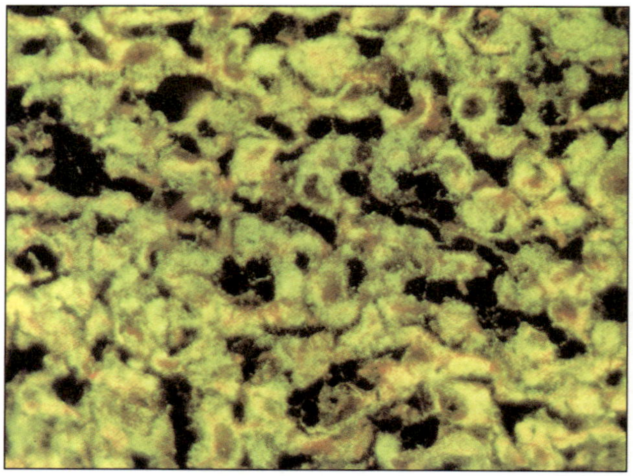

Image 18-10. Antimitochondrial autoantibodies in primary biliary cirrhosis using rat liver substrate. Note the diffuse, finely granular immunofluorescence of rat liver hepatocytes.

Enzyme-Linked Immunosorbent Assay

The availability of commercially prepared ELISA kits that have been approved by the Food and Drug Administration and that measure M2 AMAs should help with IIFM limitations. These ELISAs use either

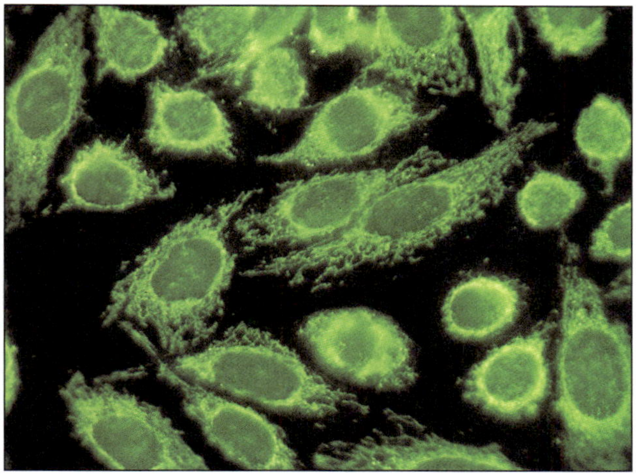

Image 18-11. Antimitochondrial autoantibody pattern in primary biliary cirrhosis using HEp-2 cells. There is diffuse cytoplasmic speckling.

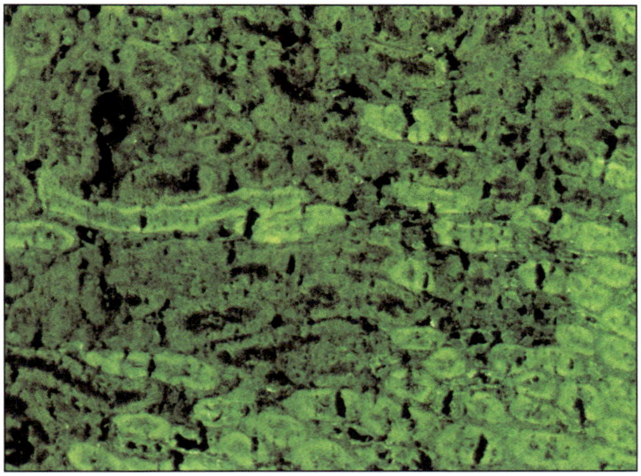

Image 18-12. Atypical antimitochondrial autoantibody pattern using mouse stomach-kidney substrate. In this example, it is difficult to distinguish M1 and M2b patterns; an M2 enzyme-linked immunosorbent assay would be helpful in this situation.

purified natural antigen—mainly PDH-E2 and PDH-E3BP—or recombinant proteins to identify M2 AMAs.

The availability of ELISAs should at least help standardize this test and add objectivity to identification of circulating AMAs in PBC. They may be limited in sensitivity, however, if conformational epitopes are denatured during antigen preparation. Each laboratory must therefore work to understand the performance characteristics and limitations of its particular ELISA to assist clinicians in interpreting test results when confusing situations inevitably arise.

Test Interpretation

- M2 antimitochondrial autoantibodies are the most sensitive and specific immunologic markers for PBC.
- Antimitochondrial autoantibody IIFM is about 95% sensitive for PBC.
- Definitive diagnosis of PBC is based on correlation of all available clinical, biochemical, and liver biopsy information.[32,33]
- As a useful guideline, titers equal to or greater than 1:160 are highly predictive of PBC, but about 10% of PBC patients have AMA titers less than 1:16.[31,34–37]
- Antimitochondrial autoantibody IIFM titers less than 1:160 are considered nondiagnostic.
- M2 antimitochondrial autoantibodies in PBC have ranged from 83% to 100% depending on the ELISA format.[15,32,38]

There are conflicting reports on the relationship between the AMA titer and disease activity in PBC,[15] but clinicians generally do not rely on either the presence or the titer of AMAs to predict duration, severity, or stage of the disorder. Despite dissenting opinion, about 5% of patients with the characteristic features of PBC do not have detectable AMAs. A clinician's diagnosis of AMA-negative PBC is based on the patient's presenting symptoms, liver biopsy findings, and cholangiography to rule out PSC.

The clinical course of patients with PBC who are AMA negative appears to be no different than that for AMA-positive patients.[32,39] Reevaluation of AMA-negative individuals over time or using newer laboratory procedures may amend the diagnostic picture by providing an M2 AMA–positive test result.

There are reports of positive AMA test results in diverse disorders, including AiH (8% to 28%) or connective tissue disease (2% to 29%). Chronic graft-versus-host disease also may include an AMA component, although the autoantigen is apparently different from that seen in PBC.[40] With respect to hepatitis, AMAs are present much less frequently in patients afflicted with AiH (20%) than in those with PBC (>95%). Also, the AMA titer in patients with AiH is rarely greater than 1:40.[34–37] Recently, AMAs have been reported in patients with chronic hepatitis C.[41]

Antimitochondrial autoantibodies are rarely identified in normal individuals (<1%) or within a general hospital population, mostly patients with autoimmune disorders (1%).[25] These individuals should be monitored over time to check for the development of liver disease. Available studies of AMA in patients with PBC who have undergone orthotopic liver transplantation indicate that AMA titers generally decline but remain detectable after surgery.[2,42]

Other Organ-Directed Autoantibodies

A significant number of patients with autoimmune liver disease have autoantibodies directed at other organs or tissues including antithyroid microsomal, antithyroglobulin, and anti–parietal cell autoantibodies.[35] Thus, there is some putative interrelationship between autoimmune liver disease and other human autoimmune diseases.

Synopses of Major Autoimmune Liver Diseases

Autoimmune Hepatitis

Autoimmune hepatitis classically occurs in women during their fourth decade of life. These patients present with high concentrations of serum transaminases, hypergammaglobulinemia, and circulating serum autoantibodies. Amenorrhea, arthralgia, cushingoid features, and acneiform rashes are normally present. Patients are not usually jaundiced.

Autoimmune hepatitis is a heterogeneous group of disorders of uncertain etiology. The International Autoimmune Hepatitis Group (IAHG) has integrated clinical and laboratory features at patient presentation into a scoring system for definitive or probable diagnosis of AiH. **Table 18-8** lists clinical laboratory parameters used as criteria to diagnose AiH; other criteria and scoring interpretations can be found in the references.[8,43] There are no pathognomonic features to AiH and, importantly, the absence of ANA, SMA, or LKM1 does not exclude this diagnosis.

Although AiH subtypes based on autoantibody patterns are presented in the medical literature, the clinical utility of such subtyping is uncertain and the IAHG does not recommend subdivision of AiH based on autoantibody profiles. From a clinical perspective, AiH can be viewed as a chronic liver disease characterized by the presence of a variety of autoantibodies. Most experts seem to agree that AiH types 1 and 2 are the major forms of this disease, whereas additional subtypes are still at issue.

Because the various AiH subtypes are widely quoted, they are provided here for reference:

- Antinuclear autoantibodies and SMAs characterize (classic) type 1 AiH.
- Type 2 AiH is marked by LKM1. Antibodies to liver cytosolic antigens 1 and 2 (anti–LC-1 and anti–LC-2) are rare but coincide with LKM1.[9,44]
- Autoantibodies to soluble-liver antigen (anti-SLA) or autoantibodies to liver-pancreas antigen (anti-LP) have been proposed to define type 3 AiH when ANAs, SMAs, and LKM1 are not detected.[8,10,45] Assays to reliably detect anti-SLA are technically difficult and as yet are not routinely available in clinical laboratories.
- Smooth muscle autoantibodies define a putative fourth AiH subtype that has been described most frequently in young children. This subgroup is characterized by high titers of antiactin autoantibodies without other detectable autoantibodies.[10]

Histologic study of the liver in patients with AiH shows chronic inflammation with lymphocytes and plasma cells in portal tracts, piecemeal necrosis, and a variable degree of lobular necroinflammatory changes.[46,47] Piecemeal necrosis is a nonspecific finding seen in patients with AiH and in those with chronic viral hepatitis, drug-related hepatitis, alcohol-related liver disease, PBC, Wilson's disease, and α_1-antitrypsin deficiency.[47–49] It may progress to fibrosis and eventually to irreversible cirrhosis. A prompt and rapid clinical response to corticosteroids is typical and an almost diagnostic feature of AiH.

Primary Biliary Cirrhosis

This disease usually affects women between the ages of 40 and 60 years; only about 10% of patients are men. The clinical hallmarks of PBC are those of chronic cholestatic liver disease.[10,31,32] That is, most patients present with pruritis and jaundice or a prominent elevation of serum alkaline phosphatase (with or without hyperbilirubinemia), an increase in polyclonal IgM, and serum AMA. Tests for chronic viral hepatitis and obstruction are negative.

A large number of affected patients initially seem to be asymptomatic, although this term is defined rather loosely. On closer questioning, about 50% of individuals initially diagnosed as having asymptomatic PBC actually have symptoms suggestive of either thyroid dysfunction or an autoimmune disease other than liver related. Recently, the true prevalence of

Table 18-8. Laboratory Parameters and Scores for Diagnosis of Autoimmune Hepatitis

Clinical Laboratory Parameters	Score
Biochemistry	
Ratio of increased alkaline phosphatase to aminotransferase	
>3.0	–2
<3.0	+2
Normal α_1-antitrypsin	
No increased urinary copper excretion after D-penicillamine	
Total serum globulin, globulin, or IgG (× upper normal limit)	
>2.0	+3
1.5-2.0	+2
1.0-1.5	+1
<1.0	0
Autoantibodies (IIFM on rodent tissues)	
Adults	
ANA, SMA, LKM1	
>1:80	+3
1:80	+2
1:40	+1
<1:40	0
Children	
ANA, LKM1	
>1:20	+3
1:10 or 1:20	+2
<1:10	0
SMA	
>1:20	+3
1:20	+2
<1:20	0
AMA	
Detected	–2
Not detected	0
Adults and children (if ANA, SMA, LKM1 not detected)	
Liver autoantibodies such as SLA, ASGP-R, LC-1	
Detected	+2
Not detected	0
Viral markers	
Acute HAV or HBV	–3
HCV by ELISA and/or RIBA	–2
HCV RNA by PCR	–3
Other active viral infection	–3
Seronegative for known viruses	+3
Genetic factors	
HLA B8-DR3 or DR4 allotype	+1

Abbreviations: IgG = immunoglobulin G; IIFM = indirect immunofluorescence; ANA = antinuclear autoantibodies; SMA = smooth muscle autoantibodies; LKM1 = liver-kidney-microsomal autoantibodies, type 1; AMA = antimitochondrial autoantibodies; SLA = soluble-liver antigen; ASGP-R = anti-asialoglycoprotein receptor; LC-1 = liver cytosolic antigen 1; HAV = hepatitis A virus; HBV = hepatitis B virus, HCV = hepatitis C virus; ELISA = enzyme-linked immunosorbent assay; RIBA = radioimmunobinding assay; RNA = ribonucleic acid; PCR = polymerase chain reaction; HLA = human leukocyte antigen.
Adapted from Johnson and McFarlane.[43]

PBC was increased on the basis of identifying patients with circulating AMAs without other findings.[5,32,50]

Clinical disorders associated with PBC include Raynaud's disease, sicca syndrome, thyroiditis, rheumatoid arthritis, gluten-sensitive enteropathy (celiac disease), and scleroderma. A variant of scleroderma that also occurs in PBC patients is termed CREST syndrome, an abbreviation for the characteristic subcutaneous calcinosis, Raynaud's phenomenon, esophageal dysfunction, sclerodactyly, and telangiectasia.

Histologic findings in the livers of patients with PBC have been categorized into 4 stages that often overlap, but the general picture is one of nonsuppurative destructive cholangitis. The distinguishing hallmark is destructive granulomatous cholangitis or the florid duct lesion affecting interlobular and septal bile ducts.[32,51]

The cause of PBC is unknown. Although this disease is classically associated with serum AMA, T-cell–mediated immune injury to intrahepatic interlobular bile ducts dominates tissue lesions.[2,32,33,51] The recent discovery of retroviral antibody in PBC patients has been ascribed to either an autoimmune response or immune reactivity to viral proteins that share antigenic determinants with retroviruses.[29]

Approximately 10% to 15% of PBC patients manifest an overlap syndrome that combines features of PBC and AiH.[52] These patients have evidence of cholestasis, as indicated by an elevated serum alkaline phosphatase, but they also have elevated levels of serum transaminases and high titers of AMAs and ANAs. Histologically, their liver biopsies show the features of both AiH and PBC.[22,29]

Orthotopic liver transplantation offers the only chance of survival for patients with end-stage PBC. Patients diagnosed with PBC/AiH overlap usually respond to immunosuppression.

Autoimmune Cholangitis

Autoimmune cholangitis (AiC) is a chronic cholestatic liver disease, which does not appear to be a variant of PSC.[53,54] The clinical presentation and histologic appearance of the liver resemble those seen in patients with PBC, but serologic findings mimic AiH type 1. Antimitochondrial autoantibodies are not detected. Additionally, an autoantibody to carbonic anhydrase has been detected in some AiC patients.[55]

Although the connection between AiC and PBC is not known, AiC may be the same as AMA-negative PBC. Generally, AiC patients respond to immunosuppression.

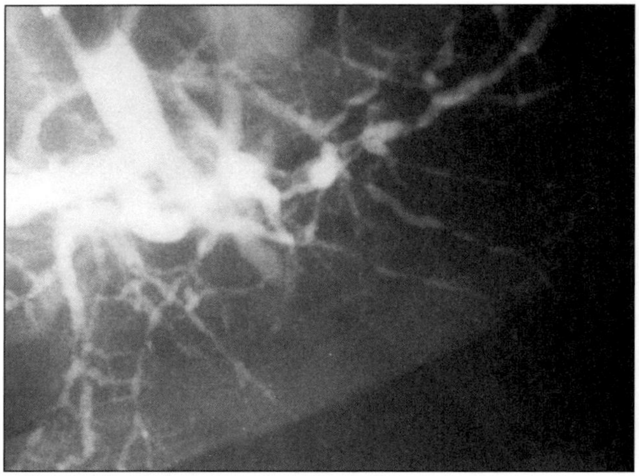

Image 18-13. Antimitochondrial autoantibodies in primary biliary cirrhosis using rat liver substrate. Note the diffuse, finely granular immunofluorescence of rat liver hepatocytes.

Primary Sclerosing Cholangitis

Primary sclerosing cholangitis typically occurs in men, and at least 50% also have inflammatory bowel disease, usually ulcerative colitis. Typically, a diagnosis of PSC is based on cholangiography, which reveals a characteristic beading pattern of bile ducts due to multifocal strictures at those sites (**Image 18-13**). The hallmark histologic lesion is fibrous cholangitis of large and/or small bile ducts, although in practice a wide spectrum of chronic inflammatory lesions is seen on liver biopsy.

Routine biochemical studies demonstrate an elevation in alkaline phosphatase and an increase of transaminases, with or without hyperbilirubinemia. Although ANAs may be present, AMAs are not. Furthermore, IIFM on ethanol- and formalin-fixed neutrophils displays a high prevalence of atypical perinuclear antineutrophil cytoplasmic antibodies, as described in Chapter 15.[10,56–58]

References

1. Krawitt EL, Wiesner RH. *Autoimmune Liver Disease*. New York, NY: Raven Press, 1991.
2. Manns MP, Nakamura RM. Autoimmune liver diseases. In: Deodhar S, ed. *Clinics in Laboratory Medicine*. Philadelphia, PA: WB Saunders Co; 1988:281–301.
3. Meyer zum Büschenfelde KH, Lohse AW, Manns M, et al. Autoimmunity and liver disease. *Hepatology*. 1990;12:354–363.

4. Geller SA. Autoimmune hepatitis. *Pathology (Phila).* 1994;3:57–76.

5. Munoz LE, Thomas HC, Scheuer PJ, et al. Is mitochondrial antibody diagnostic of primary biliary cirrhosis? *Gut*. 1981;22:136–140.

6. Leung PSC, Manns MP, Coppel RL, et al. Detection of antimitochondrial autoantibodies in primary biliary cirrhosis and liver-kidney microsomal antibodies in autoimmune hepatitis. In: Rose NR, Conway de Macario E, Folds JD, et al, eds. *Manual of Clinical Laboratory Immunology*. 5th ed. Washington, DC: ASM Press; 1997:989–996.

7. Cavallaro JJ, Palmer DF, Bigazzi PE. Indirect immunofluorescence (IIF) detection of mitochondrial and smooth muscle antibodies. Part 4. In: *Immunofluorescence Detection of Autoimmune Diseases*. Atlanta, GA: U.S. Department of Health, Education, and Welfare, Public Health Service, Centers for Disease Control; 1976:71–89.

8. Manns MP, Lüttig B, Obermayer-Straub P. Autoimmune diseases: The liver. In: Rose NR, Mackay IR, eds. *The Autoimmune Diseases*. 3d ed. San Diego, CA: Academic Press; 1998:511–544.

9. Krawitt EL. Autoimmune hepatitis. *N Engl J Med*. 1996;334:897–903. [Review article]

10. Manns MP. Autoimmune diseases of the liver. *Clin Lab Med*. 1992;12:25–40.

11. Manns M, Kyriatsoulis A, Amelizad Z, et al. Relationship between the target antigen of liver-kidney microsomal (LKM) autoantibodies and rat isoenzymes of cytochrome P-450. *J Clin Lab Anal*. 1988;2:245–248.

12. Strassburg CP, Manns MP. Autoimmune hepatitis versus viral hepatitis C. *Liver*. 1995;15:225–232. [Invited review]

13. Meek F, Khoury EL, Doniach D, et al. Mitochondrial antibodies in chronic liver diseases and connective tissue disorders: Further characterization of the autoantigen. *Clin Exp Immunol*. 1980;41:43–54.

14. Manns MP. Liver/kidney microsomal autoantibodies. In: Peter JB, Shoenfeld Y, eds. *Autoantibodies*. Amsterdam, the Netherlands: Elsevier Biomedical; 1996:462–466.

15. Bassendine MF, Jones DEJ. Antimitochondrial and other autoantibodies in primary biliary cirrhosis. In: Krawitt EL, Wiesner RH, Nishioka M, eds. *Autoimmune Liver Diseases*. 2nd ed. Amsterdam, the Netherlands: Elsevier Biomedical; 1998:287–304.

16. Bernstein RM, Callender ME, Neuberger JM, et al. Anticentromere antibody in primary biliary cirrhosis. *Ann Rheum Dis*. 1982;41:612–614.

17. Nishioka M, Morshed SA, Parveen S, et al. Heterogeneity of antinuclear antibodies in autoimmune liver diseases. In: Krawitt EL, Wiesner RH, Nishioka M, eds. *Autoimmune Liver Diseases*. 2nd ed. Amsterdam, the Netherlands: Elsevier Biomedical; 1998:179–216.

18. Nakamura RM, Bylund DJ. Diagnostic significance of autoantibodies in autoimmune chronic active hepatitis. *Clin Immunol Newsletter*. 1991;11:161–167.

19. Cassani F, Bianchi FB, Lenzi M, et al. Immunomorphological characterization of antinuclear antibodies in chronic liver disease. *J Clin Pathol*. 1985;38:801–805.

20. Penner E, Kindas-Mugge I, Hitchman E, et al. Nuclear antigens recognized by antibodies present in liver disease sera. *Clin Exp Immunol*. 1985;63:428–433.

21. Whittingham S, Mackay IR. Smooth muscle autoantibodies. In: Peter JB, Shoenfeld Y, eds. *Autoantibodies*. Amsterdam, the Netherlands: Elsevier Biomedical; 1996:767–773.

22. Abuaf N, Johanet C, Homberg J-C. Autoantibodies in autoimmune chronic active hepatitis. In: Krawitt EL, Wiesner RH, eds. *Autoimmune Liver Diseases*. New York, NY: Raven Press; 1991:93–109.

23. Morshed SA, Parveen S, Nishioka M. Antibodies to cytoskeleton antigens in autoimmune liver diseases. In: Krawitt EL, Wiesner RH, Nishioka M, eds. *Autoimmune Liver Diseases*. 2nd ed. Amsterdam, the Netherlands: Elsevier Biomedical; 1998:217–256.

24. Czaja AJ, Cassani F, Cataleta M, et al. Frequency and significance of antibodies to actin in type 1 autoimmune hepatitis. *Hepatology*. 1996;24:1068–1073.

25. Keren DF. Immunology and serology. In: Jacobs DS, DeMott WR, Finley PR, et al, eds. *Laboratory Test Handbook*. 3rd ed. Hudson, OH: Lexi-Comp Inc; 1994:627–766.

26. Leung PSC, Coppel RL, Gershwin ME. Mitochondrial autoantibodies. In: Peter JB, Shoenfeld Y, eds. *Autoantibodies*. Amsterdam, the Netherlands: Elsevier Biomedical; 1996:494–500.

27. Bassendine MF, Yeaman SJ. Primary biliary cirrhosis: Nature of autoantigens. *Springer Semin Immunopathol*. 1990;12:73–83.

28. Berg PA, Klein R. Mitochondrial antigen/antibody systems in primary biliary cirrhosis: Revisited. *Liver*. 1995;15:281–292. [Invited review]

29. Davis PA, Leung P, Manns M, et al. M4 and M9 antibodies in the overlap syndrome of primary biliary cirrhosis and chronic active hepatitis: Epitopes or epiphenomema? *Hepatology*. 1992;16:1128–1136.

30. Mason AL, Xu L, Guo L, et al. Detection of retroviral antibodies in primary biliary cirrhosis and other idiopathic biliary disorders. *Lancet*. 1998;351:1620–1624.

31. Bylund DJ, McHutchison J, Nakamura RM. Antimitochondrial antibodies in primary biliary cirrhosis. *Clin Immunol Newsletter*. 1992;12:1–5.

32. Poupon R, Poupon RE. Primary biliary cirrhosis. In: Zakim D, Boyer TD, eds. *Hepatology—A Textbook of Liver Disease*. 3rd ed. Philadelphia, PA: WB Saunders Co; 1996:1329–1365.

33. Manns MP. Cytoplasmic autoantigens in autoimmune hepatitis: Molecular analysis and clinical relevance. *Semin Liver Dis*. 1991;11:205–214.

34. Berg PA, Baum H. Serology of primary biliary cirrhosis. *Springer Semin Immunopathol*. 1980;3:355–373.

35. Doniach D, Roitt IM, Walker JG, et al. Tissue antibodies in primary biliary cirrhosis, active chronic (lupoid) hepatitis, cryptogenic cirrhosis, and other liver diseases and their clinical implications. *Clin Exp Immunol.* 1966;1:237–262.

36. Deodhar SD, Yazhek A, Achkar E, et al. Mitochondrial antibody test: A clue to diagnosis of primary biliary cirrhosis: Report of two interesting cases. *Cleve Clin Q.* 1971;38:105–109.

37. Doniach D, Walker G. Progress report: Mitochondrial antibodies. *Gut.* 1974;15:664–668.

38. Mackay IR, Gershwin ME. Primary biliary cirrhosis: Considerations on pathogenesis based on identification of the M2 autoantigens. *Springer Semin Immunopathol.* 1990;12:101–119.

39. Gershwin ME, Coppel RL, Mackay IR. Primary biliary cirrhosis and mitochondrial autoantigens—Insights from molecular biology. *Hepatology.* 1988;8:147–151.

40. Siegert W, Stemerowicz R, Hopf U. Antimitochondrial antibodies in patients with chronic graft-versus-host disease. *Bone Marrow Transplant.* 1992;10:221–227.

41. Grimbert S, Johanet C, Bendjaballah F, et al. Antimitochondrial antibodies in patients with chronic hepatitis C. *Liver.* 1996;16:161–165.

42. Gouw AS, Haagsma EB, Manns M, et al. Is there recurrence of primary biliary cirrhosis after liver transplantation? A clinicopathologic study in long-term survivors. *J Hepatol.* 1994;20:500–507.

43. Johnson PJ, McFarlane IG. Convenors on behalf of the panel. Meeting report: International autoimmune hepatitis group. *Hepatology.* 1993;18:998–1008.

44. McNeil HP, Simpson RJ, Chesterman CN, et al. Antiphospholipid antibodies are directed against a complex antigen that includes a lipid-binding inhibitor of coagulation: b2-glycoprotein I (apolipoprotein H). *Proc Natl Acad Sci U S A.* 1990;87:4120–4124.

45. Czaja AJ, Carpenter HA, Manns MP. Antibodies to soluble liver antigen, P450IID6, and mitochondrial complexes in chronic hepatitis. *Gastroenterology.* 1993;105:1522–1528.

46. Baggenstoss AH, Soloway RD, Summerskill WHJ, et al. Chronic active liver disease—The range of histologic lesions, their response to treatment and evolution. *Hum Pathol.* 1972;3:183–198.

47. Popper H, Geller SA. Pathogenetic considerations in the histologic diagnosis of drug-induced injury. In: Fenoglio CM, Wolff M, eds. *Progress in Surgical Pathology*. New York, NY: Masson; 1981:233–246.

48. Mackay IR. Pathogenesis of autoimmune chronic active hepatitis. In: Krawitt EL, Wiesner RH, eds. *Autoimmune Liver Diseases*. New York, NY: Raven Press; 1991:21–42.

49. Meyer zum Büschenfelde KH, Manns M. Immune response to liver membrane antigens in acute and chronic hepatitis. In: Chisari FV, ed. *Advances in Hepatitis Research*. New York, NY: Masson; 1984:152–162.

50. Mitchison HC, Bassendine MF, Hendrick A, et al. Positive antimitochondrial antibody but normal alkaline phosphatase: Is this primary biliary cirrhosis? *Hepatology.* 1986;6:1279–1284.

51. Batts KP, Ludwig J. Histopathology of autoimmune chronic active hepatitis, primary biliary cirrhosis, and primary sclerosing cholangitis. In: Krawitt EL, Wiesner RH, eds. *Autoimmune Liver Disease*. New York, NY: Raven Press; 1991:75–92.

52. Berg PA, Klein R. Autoantibody patterns in primary biliary cirrhosis. In: Krawitt EL, Wiesner RH, eds. *Autoimmune Liver Disease*. New York, NY: Raven Press; 1991:123–142.

53. Goodman ZD, McNally PR, Davis DR, et al. Autoimmune cholangitis: A variant of primary biliary cirrhosis. Clinicopathologic and serologic correlations in 200 cases. *Dig Dis Sci.* 1995;40:1232–1242.

54. Tsui WMS, Lam TW. The mystery of autoimmune cholangitis: A new entity or variant? [New entity]. *Adv Anat Pathol.* 1997;4:64–69.

55. Gordon SC, Quattrociocchi-Longe TM, Khan BA, et al. Antibodies to carbonic anhydrase in patients with immune cholangiopathies. *Gastroenterology.* 1995;108:1802–1809.

56. Bansi DS, Fleming KA, Chapman RW. Importance of antineutrophil cytoplasmic antibodies in primary sclerosing cholangitis and ulcerative colitis: Prevalence, titre, and IgG subclass. *Gut.* 1996;38:384–389.

57. Lo SK, Fleming KA, Chapman RW. A 2-year follow-up study of anti-neutrophil antibody in primary sclerosing cholangitis: Relationship to clinical activity, liver biochemistry and ursodeoxycholic acid treatment. *J Hepatol.* 1994;21:974–978.

58. Gur H, Shen G, Sutjita M, et al. Autoantibody profile of primary sclerosing cholangitis. *Pathobiology.* 1995;63:76–82.

CHAPTER 19

Autoimmune Disease of the Gastrointestinal Tract

David F. Keren, MD

Background

Many autoreactive phenomena have been described in gastrointestinal disease. The relationship between autoantibodies, self-reactive cell-mediated immunity, and gastrointestinal pathology in these conditions is not always clear-cut. The coexistence of autoantibodies against enterocytes and gastrointestinal pathology in some patients with inflammatory bowel disease, for instance, is not conclusive evidence that the autoantibodies are the causative agents of the pathology. The autoantibodies may be secondary to the damage or may be coincidental. This chapter reviews 3 gastrointestinal diseases in which autoantibodies are found and in which the study of serum for the presence of these autoantibodies may be a useful means of evaluating a patient for clinical or epidemiological purposes.

Stomach-Pernicious Anemia

Pathogenesis

Patients with pernicious anemia may have a variety of clinical problems, including neurologic, hematologic, and gastrointestinal symptoms. Diagnosis of this disease currently involves screening for the level of urinary methylmalonic acid (the Schilling test).[1] Because of its striking hematologic consequences, pernicious anemia is often not thought of as an autoimmune disease involving the stomach. However, the destruction of parietal cells in the stomach underlies the hematologic and systemic features of this disease.

The parietal cells, located in the main body of the stomach, synthesize and secrete a 114,000-dalton glycoprotein called *intrinsic factor* into the lumen of the stomach. In the stomach, the low pH of intrinsic factor facilitates separation of vitamin B_{12} (cobalamin) from nutrient sources.[2] Each molecule of intrinsic factor can combine with 2 molecules of nutrient cobalamin. In the terminal ileum, intrinsic factor attaches to the microvillous epithelium via specific receptors. The cobalamin-intrinsic factor complex is then absorbed by these epithelial cells. Within the epithelium, cobalamin binds to a protein called *transcobalamin II*. This complex then passes into the systemic circulation to fulfill its role in DNA synthesis. In the absence of intrinsic factor, cobalamin is not efficiently absorbed, which leads to the deranged cellular metabolism characteristic of pernicious anemia. All cells of the body are affected; the severity with which a cell is affected depends on its mitotic rate. Because the erythrocyte precursors proliferate so rapidly, anemia is a prominent feature, but affected patients also have pancytopenia and suffer from a variety of neuropsychiatric complaints due to demyelination.[3] Due to the loss of parietal cells, patients with pernicious anemia are achlorhydric or hypochlorhydric, in addition to producing insufficient quantities of intrinsic factor. Recently, a specific association has been reported between pernicious anemia and the presence of antithyroid peroxidase (antimicrosomal) antibodies.[4]

Due to the relatively large store of cobalamin in the body, depletion to the point of clinical manifestations takes years to develop. Pernicious anemia patients are typically middle-aged or older individuals, often of Scandinavian or Northern European origin. However, all ages and races may be affected by pernicious anemia. It should be noted that recent data indicate that HIV-positive individuals, in whom pernicious anemia might not be suspected, are at increased risk of developing pernicious anemia.[2] An association between pernicious anemia and thyroid autoimmune disease has been recognized for many years.

Nonimmunologic methods of diagnosis include recognizing the presence of megaloblasts and hypersegmented neutrophils on a peripheral blood sample, measurement of cobalamin levels and/or methylmalonic acid in the urine, and biopsy of the stomach to check for the presence of the mucosal lesions of atrophic gastritis.

Pathology

The histologic features of the stomach in pernicious anemia are similar to those of type A chronic atrophic gastritis.[5] Typically, the mucosa is markedly thinned. Grossly, submucosal blood vessels may be seen through the mucosal surface. Histologically, there is patchy intestinal metaplasia with prominent goblet cells (**Image 19-1**). In addition, there is often a prominent hyperplasia of gastric endocrine cells, including carcinoid tumors.[6] The lamina propria typically contains an infiltrate of lymphocytes, plasma cells, and monocytes. Some eosinophils may be seen, whereas neutrophils are usually infrequent. Nuclei are often large and may appear atypical due to the disturbance in DNA synthesis.

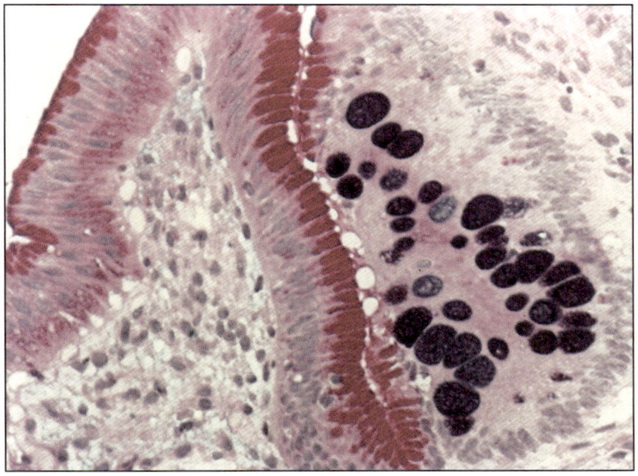

Image 19-1. Biopsy of body of stomach from patient with pernicious anemia. Note prominent goblet cells in the area involved, with intestinal metaplasia (PAS/alcian blue stain).

Role of Immune System

Both anti–parietal cell antibodies and anti–intrinsic factor antibodies are found in the serum of most, but not all, patients with pernicious anemia.[7,8] These autoantibodies have been linked to the pathologic features of this disease in experiments showing that the IgG fraction of sera from patients with anti–parietal cell activity correlates with the complement-mediated cytotoxicity of canine gastric mucosal cells.[9]

The fact that the chronic inflammatory infiltration in the deep gastric mucosa develops relatively early in the course of the disease suggests that it may play a role in epithelial damage.[10] The metaplasia in the stomach represents a host response to the now-alkaline environment of the stomach. Animal models, including neonatal thymectomies in mice, have produced similar histologic lesions to those of pernicious anemia, in addition to anti–parietal cell antibodies. The major molecules targeted by the parietal cell autoantibodies in this experimental model are the same as those targeted in humans with pernicious anemia.[11] It is still not clear, however, whether the autoantibodies result from damage to the surface epithelium or if they initiate the damage. Indeed, some recent data suggest that *Helicobacter pylori* may play a role in the pathogenesis of the morphologic features seen in pernicious anemia, but its role is not yet proven.[12]

Immunologic Testing

Antibodies to intrinsic factor exist in both the serum and the mucosal secretions of most patients with pernicious anemia.[13] Some of the antibodies that react with intrinsic factor attach to the site on the intrinsic factor molecule where cobalamin attaches (this class of antibodies is termed type I or blocking antibody), while other antibodies (termed type II) react with sites that do not interfere with cobalamin attachment.[14] The percentages of anti–parietal cell and anti–intrinsic factor antibodies detected in patients with pernicious anemia and in control subjects vary widely in reported studies. Typically, studies record the presence of anti–parietal cell antibodies in about 90% of pernicious anemia patients, whereas anti–intrinsic factor antibodies are seen in approximately 50% to 70% of patients.[15] In patients of some ethnic groups (particularly Latin Americans and African Americans), anti–intrinsic factor antibodies are almost universally present.[16] In type I diabetes, there is a high prevalence of anti–parietal cell antibodies associated with clinical autoimmune gastritis.[17]

This variability in the prevalence of autoantibodies may result from both technical and temporal factors. There are differences in the results of immunologic testing for intrinsic factor antibodies from one kit manufacturer to the next.[18,19] It is well-documented that there are temporal changes in the presence of these antibodies as the disease progresses. Davidson et al[20] noted that although 90.9% of their pernicious anemia patients had anti–parietal cell antibodies at time of diagnosis, the percentage fell to 82.8% after therapy with a mean follow-up of 70 months, whereas anti–intrinsic factor antibodies were present in only 39.1% of their patients at time of diagnosis, but in 58.7% of patients after 70 months. Although the researchers hypothesized that this shift may indicate a loss of parietal cells, (presumably because of less antigenic stimulation), they determined that there is no practical use in following either antibody once the diagnosis of pernicious anemia is secured.

Likewise, another problem in using anti–parietal cell antibodies to diagnose or monitor pernicious anemia patients is that most studies find these antibodies in a respectably large percentage of healthy control adults. One recent study reported that 18% of its control subjects had anti–parietal cell antibodies. Therefore, the presence of these antibodies alone does not provide evidence of pernicious anemia.[8] Typically, the percentage of these antibodies increases with age. Below the age of 20 years, only 2% of healthy people are found to be positive.[21] Unfortunately, the incidence of pernicious anemia also increases with age. Therefore, the population most likely to give a false-positive result is also the population in which one is most likely to find the disease. Anti–parietal cell antibodies are also commonly found in patients with endocrine disorders and gastric ulcers.

Fortunately, anti–intrinsic factor antibodies are uncommonly detected in control subjects. The presence of either or both of these autoantibodies in patients with cobalamin deficiency is useful diagnostic information. Therefore, with appropriate clinical information, anti–intrinsic factor assays can be useful in establishing a diagnosis of pernicious anemia. However, one does not need to follow these antibodies once the diagnosis is secured.

Assays for Autoantibodies

Indirect immunofluorescence is used to detect anti–parietal cell antibodies. This requires incubation of the patient's serum (usually diluted 1:20 in the kit wash buffer) on mouse stomach and kidney cells. Following incubation, the patient's serum is washed off the section and fluorescein-conjugated anti-human immunoglobulin is added to the tissue section. After another incubation-and-wash step, the slide is examined under a microscope equipped for detecting fluorescence. Granular cytoplasmic fluorescence in the parietal cells with a lack of such staining in kidney tubules is considered a positive result for anti–parietal cell antibodies (**Image 19-2**). The presence of antimitochondrial antibodies will also result in granular staining of the parietal cells; however, in this situation, the kidney tubules will also fluoresce.[21]

To detect anti–intrinsic factor, either enzyme-linked immunosorbent assay (ELISA) or radioimmunoassay techniques can be used. Several commercial kits are available for detecting these antibodies. Type I (blocking) antibodies against intrinsic factor can be measured separately from total antibodies (type I + type II). The method chosen should detect both type I and type II, because in making the clinical diagnosis, the presence of either is helpful.[13,14] Although anti–intrinsic factor antibodies are present within the lumen of the intestine, there is no diagnostic reason to measure antibodies in intestinal fluids; serum samples are perfectly adequate.

Small Intestine—Celiac Disease (Gluten-Sensitive Enteropathy)

Pathology

The surface of the small intestine is lined by finger-like villi that project into the lumen. These villi contain surface epithelial cells that have microvilli on their surface. Because a major function of these epithelial cells is to absorb nutrients from the gut lumen, the villi and microvilli serve to increase intestinal surface area and therefore the efficiency with which nutrients are taken up by the epithelial cells.

In celiac disease, the surface epithelial cells are damaged by an immune response to the dietary protein gluten. Histologically, there is marked atrophy of the villi, and often they may appear completely flattened. This villous atrophy has been related to an increased amount of small intestinal apoptosis in patients with celiac disease.[22] Furthermore, the surface epithelial cells over the remaining blunted villi exhibit a paucity of goblet cells.[23] In contrast, the small intestinal crypts are elongated due to the proliferation of cells required to replace the damaged surface epithelium. The increased mitotic rate in the crypts is typical, although not diagnostic, of celiac disease. In addition to the epithelial damage and proliferation in the crypts, there are increased numbers of plasma cells in the lamina propria and increased numbers of interepithelial lymphocytes.[24] Despite occasional reports of deposition of IgA in subepithelial locations,

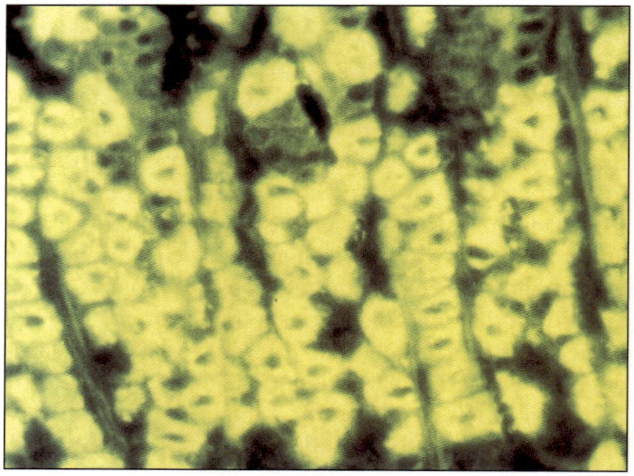

Image 19-2. Indirect immunofluorescence of serum from a patient with anti–parietal cell antibodies reacted on rat stomach epithelium (dark-field photomicrograph with fluorescein-conjugated anti-human IgG).

there is no practical reason to perform immunohistologic studies on small bowel biopsies when celiac disease is in the differential diagnosis.[25,26] The presence of such deposits is not diagnostic and their absence does not exclude the disease.

Diagnosis

Histopathologic examination of the small bowel is key to securing the diagnosis of celiac disease.[27] Although endoscopic biopsies are relatively small, the villous atrophy may be appreciated by studying the specimen with a dissecting microscope before histologic sections are made.[28] For the diagnosis, the initial small bowel biopsy, obtained while the patient is on a diet containing gluten, must demonstrate the atrophy of villi, hyperplasia of the crypts, and increased mitotic rate noted above. Involvement of the bowel in celiac disease may be patchy; therefore, it is desirable to examine biopsies from several sites. After the patient has recovered clinically while on a gluten-free diet, a second series of biopsies should be taken to evaluate the expected restoration of villous architecture and decrease in the length of the crypts and the mitotic rate. Rechallenge with gluten is then followed by a third biopsy documenting the renewed deterioration of the mucosa following this insult.[29]

Strict adherence to this schedule of biopsies prevents misdiagnoses of transient infections, sensitivities against other antigens, and autoimmune enteropathy as celiac disease. Autoimmune enteropathy is a rare condition that may cause severe diarrhea in children. Antiepithelial antibodies and anti–goblet cell antibodies have been described in the sera of these patients, but are not thought to play a primary role in the disease.[30] Like children with celiac disease, children with autoimmune enteropathy have a decrease in villous height and an increase in crypt depth. Unlike in celiac disease, however, in autoimmune enteropathy the plasma cells are not increased in the lamina propria and Paneth cells are often absent. Furthermore, endocrine cells are absent from the crypts.[30] Patients with autoimmune enteropathy do not respond to a gluten-free diet, but have had favorable responses to steroid therapy.[31]

Epidemiology and Dermatitis Herpetiformis

Older statistics suggest that celiac disease is a lifelong condition that occurs rarely (approximately 1 in 3,000 individuals) in the US. However, more recent data from the pediatric literature suggests that a large number of undiagnosed cases may exist.[32,33] In their study, Hill et al[33] used IgA antiendomysium to screen 1,200 children between the ages of 6 and 12 who presented with symptoms of celiac disease. They found that 21 cases with biopsy proven celiac disease out of these 1,200 children. The pathogenesis of celiac disease relates to a genetic proclivity toward forming a humoral and cellular immune response to the gliadin alcohol-soluble fraction of gluten.[34] Celiac disease has been described in association with many other diseases, including insulin-dependent diabetes mellitus (Type I diabetes), autoimmune thyroid disease, and even idiopathic hypoparathyroidism, but its strongest association has been with dermatitis herpetiformis.[35,36] Granular deposits of IgA at the dermal-epidermal junction help define the skin lesions of dermatitis herpetiformis. Patients with dermatitis herpetiformis also have the same atrophy of villi with hyperplasia of the crypts in the small intestine as that seen in celiac disease. In these patients, removal of gluten from the diet resolves both the mucosal and the dermatologic lesions.[37] Some researchers have noted a cross-reactivity between dietary gluten and dermal elastin and have hypothesized that this may be the basis of the skin lesions in patients with dermatitis herpetiformis.[38] Nonetheless, there is still no agreement as to why individuals with dermatitis herpetiformis develop lesions in both the skin and the mucosa.

Humoral and Cellular Immunity

Although study of humoral responses may be useful in the diagnosis of celiac disease, the pathologic lesions typical of the condition are more likely related to cellular immune responses. Following challenge by gluten, interepithelial T lymphocytes increase in the villi of patients with celiac disease.[39] The expression of HLA class II DR antigens by surface epithelial cells is increased due to the presence of cytokines that are probably released by activated T cells following stimulation by exposure to gluten.[40] Human intestinal epithelium usually expresses little HLA class II antigen, but individuals with conditions that involve inflammation of the intestine (eg, inflammatory bowel disease) also have a dramatic increase in expression of this antigen.[41] The strong expression of HLA-DR antigens after exposure to gluten suggests that these cells play a role in presenting the antigen to nearby lymphocytes.[40] HLA-DQ2– and HLA-DQ8–positive antigen-presenting cells in the lamina propria may present the gluten peptides, thereby promoting the immune response to gliaden (see below).[41] Jabri et al[42] have recently reported an increase in the number of intraepithelial lymphocytes expressing CD94 in active celiac disease. CD94 detects the HLA-E–specific natural killer receptor; its presence may indicate activation of T-cell receptors.[42]

Most lymphocytes present in the lamina propria of patients with celiac disease are activated T lymphocytes that express mainly an αβ T-cell receptor, although a larger number of lymphocytes possess the γ-δ T-cell receptor than are normally found among lymphocytes in the intestine.[43]

Indeed, an increased number of γ-δ–bearing lymphocytes in the epithelium may be a clue to the diagnosis of latent celiac disease.[44] Although it is not usually thought of as being affected by celiac disease, the rectal mucosa is also sensitized to gluten; challenge to rectal mucosa via local gluten administration results in an increase in the number of local lymphocytes.[45,46] Whereas some researchers have hypothesized that natural killer cells may play a role in this disease, the evidence supporting this hypothesis is meager.[47] While these cellular studies are of epidemiological interest, they are not needed to diagnose or follow individual patients. Therefore, flow cytometric studies are not relevant to the diagnosis of celiac disease.

Genetic Basis

The local hypersensitive immune reactivity of celiac disease probably has a genetic basis. There is an increased incidence (approximately 10% to 50%) of celiac disease among first-degree relatives of patients with this condition.[48] Among identical twins, celiac disease occurs in both individuals in 70%, and among siblings the concordance is 30% in HLA-identical individuals.[29,49-51] At the molecular level, an HLA DQw2 phenotype heterodimer encoded by DQ α 1*0501 and DQ β 1*0201 has been found in the vast majority of patients with celiac disease.[34,48,52] A smaller group of patients with celiac disease has been reported to express the DQ8 heterodimers DQ α 1*0301 and DQ β 1*0302.[53,54] T-cell clones specific for gluten have been isolated from the intestinal lesions of patients with celiac disease. These clones are largely restricted to the expression of HLA-DQ2 and DQ8 heterodimers and produce high levels of interferon gamma after stimulation by gluten.[55] These findings suggest that dysfunctional mucosal cellular immunity plays a role in the pathologic response to gluten.

Autoantibodies in Celiac Disease

The vast majority of patients with celiac disease have antibodies that react with gliaden, endomysium, and tissue transglutaminase (TTG). Some researchers suggest that tests for these antibodies may someday be able to replace biopsies as a means of diagnosing celiac disease. Because of the presence of these antibodies in the overwhelming majority of patients with celiac disease, serology can be used to identify patients at risk for this disease.[56] Tests for IgA antiendomysial antibody and IgA anti-TTG have a sensitivity above 95% and specificity that approaches 100%[56] (**Table 19-1**). Because false negatives occur in children with mild disease, and in IgA deficiency, the negative predictive value is lower. The use of serology has been extensively explored in patients with Down syndrome, who have an increased incidence of celiac disease.[57]

Trier[29] claims that the presence of circulating IgA antigliaden is more specific for celiac disease, but is less sensitive for it than is the presence of IgG antigliaden. Assays for antigliaden antibodies are not as effective as assays for IgA antiendomysium or IgA anti-TTG antibodies in detecting patients with celiac disease.[56] Another potential concern about using only IgA antiendomysium or IgA anti-TTG to screen for celiac disease is that congenital selective IgA deficiency is relatively common, occurring in 1 in 700 individuals. Obviously, celiac disease patients who have IgA deficiency would give a false-negative result with these tests. Indeed, IgA-deficient children have a considerable increase in the occurrence of celiac disease. Meini et al[58] report a 20-times-higher frequency of celiac disease among children with IgA deficiency than among the general population. Detection of IgG antigliaden has been useful in the identification of the 2% to 10% of celiac disease patients who also have IgA deficiency.[56] However, they are not as useful in monitoring compliance with diet.[58]

Monitoring the level of antigliadin or antiendomysial antibody reactivity can help determine whether an individual is following the gluten-free diet. Patients who remove gluten from the diet experience a decline in the level of antigliadin and antiendomysium in the serum.[60] Because the antiendomysium antibodies often persist longer than antigliadin when an individual is receiving a gluten-free diet, some authors feel that antigliadin antibody may be the most

Table 19-1. Sensitivity and Specificity and Positive and Negative Predictive Values of Serologic Tests for Untreated Celiac Sprue

Serologic Test	Sensitivity*	Specificity*	Positive Predictive Value	Negative Predictive Value
Test for IgA antiendomysial antibody				
Indirect immunofluorescence assay	85–98	97–100	98–100	80–95
ELISA that uses guinea pig tissue transglutaminase	95–98	94–95	91–95	96–98
Dot blot test that uses human tissue transglutaminase	93	99	99	93
Test for IgA antigliadin antibodies	75–90	82–95	28–100	65–100
Test for IgG antigliadin antibodies	69–85	73–90	20–95	41–88

*There are wide variations in the sensitivity and specificity of these tests among different laboratories.
†ELISA denotes enzyme-linked immunosorbent assay.
Table from Farrell and Kelly[56]. Used with Permission.

useful autoantibody to follow when determining a patient's compliance with the special diet.[61]

Technique for Autoantibody Detection

Detection of IgA antiendomysial antibodies is commonly performed on frozen sections of monkey esophagus or human umbilical cord tissue (**Image 19-3**). The tissue is frozen and cut into 5-µm sections. The unfixed tissue is dried on the slide and used to detect antiendomysial antibodies. Slides are incubated for 30 minutes with a 1:5 and 1:50 dilution of the patient's serum. Both dilutions are used because many individuals have anti–smooth muscle (anti-actin) antibodies that can obscure the presence of anti-endomysial antibodies when the higher concentration is used. At 1:50, the sera of most celiac disease patients will still have a positive reaction with antiendomysium. The 1:5 dilution provides better sensitivity if anti–smooth muscle antibodies are absent. Following a triple wash in buffered saline, the sections are then incubated with antihuman IgA for another 30 minutes, washed, and cover-slipped. Volta and colleagues[62] claimed a sensitivity of 95% and a specificity of 100% for these tests using either monkey esophagus or human umbilical cord as the substrate. IgG and IgA antigliaden and IgA anti-TTG are performed by enzyme-linked immunosorbent assay.[56]

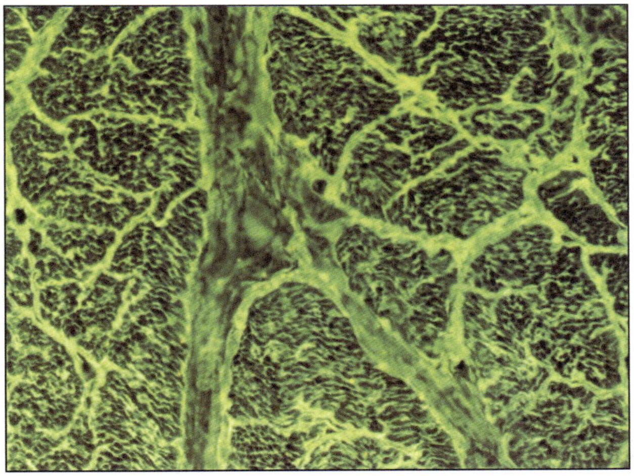

Image 19-3. Indirect immunofluorescence of serum from a patient with IgA antiendomysial antibodies reacted on monkey esophagus (dark-field photomicrograph with fluorescein-conjugated anti-human IgA). Photograph provided by Dr. Vijay Kumar at IMMCO Diagnostics.

Although testing for IgA antiendomysial antibodies and antigliaden antibodies is a useful adjunctive method in detecting celiac disease, these tests have not yet replaced biopsy in diagnosing this condition. Celiac disease is a lifelong condition in which patients must adhere to a difficult-to-follow diet to control the symptoms, so a correct diagnosis is very important. Cases of celiac disease that are negative for these antibodies occur in sufficient numbers that one cannot rule out the diagnosis by the lack of the appropriate antibody. Nonetheless, the presence of these autoantibodies may help select patients who would benefit from further histologic study to diagnose the celiac disease. Furthermore, by following the titers of these two antibodies, along with the patient's clinical response to the gluten-free diet, one may be able to avoid the second and third biopsies that are often needed to confirm the diagnosis and response to therapy. Of course, a biopsy should be performed in any patient in whom the response to the diet is not complete.

Colon—Ulcerative Colitis and Crohn's Disease

Pathology

Ulcerative colitis (UC) and Crohn's disease (CD) are the 2 diseases usually referred to when one speaks of inflammatory bowel disease (IBD). Although many papers have been written implicating a variety of inflammatory and immunologic dysfunctions in the pathogenesis of IBD, there is no definitive evidence that an abnormal immune system initiates IBD.

Diagnosis

The diagnosis of IBD depends upon the appropriate histologic findings in the appropriate clinical setting. Ulcerative colitis almost always involves the rectum and proceeds without interruption for varying distances through the colon. Some patients have only rectal involvement, but more severe cases may have involvement of the entire colon and occasionally even the terminal ileum. Histologically, UC involves the mucosa of the affected portion of bowel. During active UC, acute inflammatory cells are abundant. They gather in crypt lumina (where they form crypt abscesses), within the epithelial cells as cryptitis, and often in the lamina propria as well (**Image 19-4**). Occasionally in UC, the surface epithelium of the affected areas is denuded. In more chronic forms of the disease, increased numbers of plasma cells and lymphocytes occur within the lamina propria (**Image 19-5**).[63] Furthermore, the crypts appear distorted, forked, and sometimes shortened, or may be entirely absent due to prior acute damage. The location of plasma cells beneath the crypts is a histologic hallmark of the disease.

Crohn's disease is more variable in its clinical and histological presentations and is often more difficult to diagnose than UC. CD involves the entire thickness of the bowel wall, but tends to not involve the rectum and often does not involve the colon at all. Any portion of the bowel may be involved. When the colon is involved, histologically normal intervening segments of bowel may be found despite the presence of disease distally and proximally to the normal segments. CD patients may have acute lesions similar to those seen in UC, including crypt abscesses. However, in CD, the inflammation tends to be more patchy than in UC. Furthermore, granulomas may occur in the affected bowel. Because of the involvement of all layers of the bowel wall, fat wrapping, fistulas, and strictures are common features of CD that are not found in UC. Occasionally, immunohistochemistry may be required to help distinguish acute self-limited colitis from active IBD.[63,64] In active IBD, the number of IgG-containing plasma cells is considerably greater than that found in either normal bowel tissue or acute self-limited colitis.

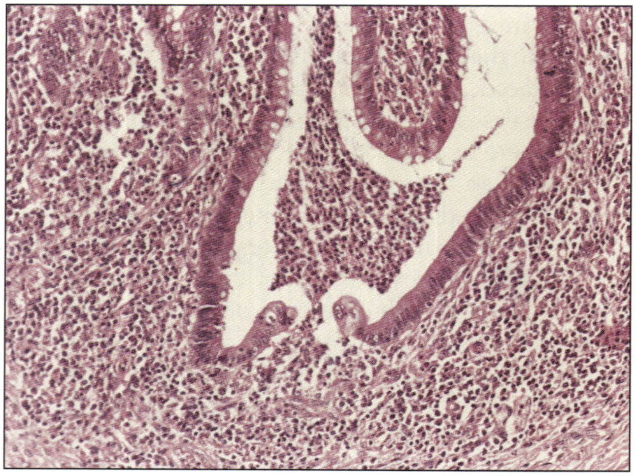

Image 19-4. Biopsy of rectum from patient with active ulcerative colitis. Note prominent crypt abscess with damage to the base of the crypt epithelium (hematoxylin and eosin).

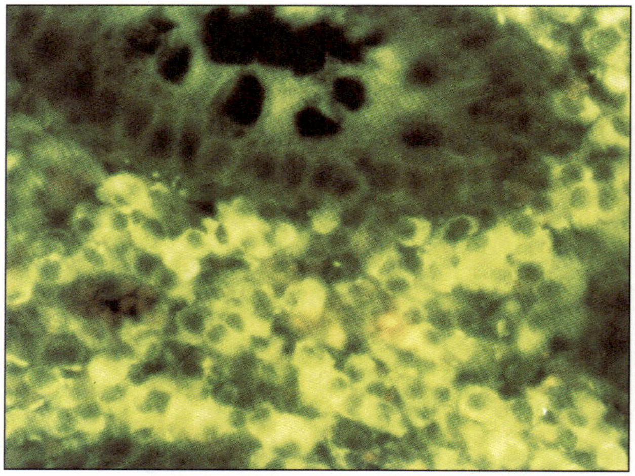

Image 19-5. Direct immunofluorescence on biopsy of colon from a patient with chronic ulcerative colitis. There is a marked increased in the number of IgA-containing plasma cells (dark-field photomicrograph with fluorescein-conjugated anti-human IgA).

A wide variety of autoantibodies and autoreactive phenomena have been described in patients with IBD. Over 30 years ago, Broberger and Perlmann[65] recorded the existence in the serum from patients with IBD of a cytotoxic activity against the intestinal epithelium. Furthermore, several animal and in vitro models have attempted to associate the cytotoxic immunologic phenomena with the etiology of the specific diseases, to no avail. Some recent researchers have concentrated on evaluating the possible roles of oxidative stress and cytokines in causing the damage seen in the bowels of patients with IBD.[66,67] Although these studies shed light on the immunologic and inflammatory events occuring within IBD-affected tissue, they cannot distinguish the events that initiate the injury from those that follow it. Therefore, this author has chosen to concentrate on recent studies that indicate that the presence of antineutrophil cytoplasmic antibodies in these patients could be used to further either diagnosis or estimation of disease activity.

Antineutrophil Cytoplasmic Antibodies (ANCA)

It would be extremely useful to have a serologic test that reliably detects one or both of these IBDs. Although no such test exists, a relationship has been found between a serologic test for vasculitis and IBD. Approximately a decade ago, it was discovered that patients with Wegener's granulomatosis and microscopic angiitis have antibodies in their sera that react with the cytoplasm of neutrophils.[68] On indirect immunofluorescence, 2 types of reaction patterns are typically seen. When sera from patients with Wegener's granulomatosis are placed on a substrate of human neutrophils that have been fixed with ethanol and then reacted with fluorescein-conjugated antihuman IgG, a granular cytoplasmic fluorescence is seen (**Image 19-6**). This effect is due to a reaction with serine protease 3 in the granules of these neutrophils. When sera from patients with various other forms of microscopic vasculitis are reacted with human neutrophils that have been fixed with ethanol, a perinuclear pattern of fluorescence is seen that resembles antinuclear antibody staining (**Image 19-7**). This pattern is usually due to a reaction with myeloperoxidase that is able to escape from the neutrophil granules after ethanol fixation and bind to the nuclear membrane. When neutrophils are fixed in formalin, reactions with both types of sera result in granular staining.[69,70]

These tests have proven to be among the most sensitive and specific of all autoantibody tests. The cytoplasmic (C)-ANCA pattern is highly specific and sensitive for detecting Wegener's granulomatosis. Unlike ANA reactivity, which is found in as many as 15% to 20% of control subjects in some studies, C-ANCA is almost never seen in a control serum.[70-73] Other antigens, including cathepsin G, elastase,

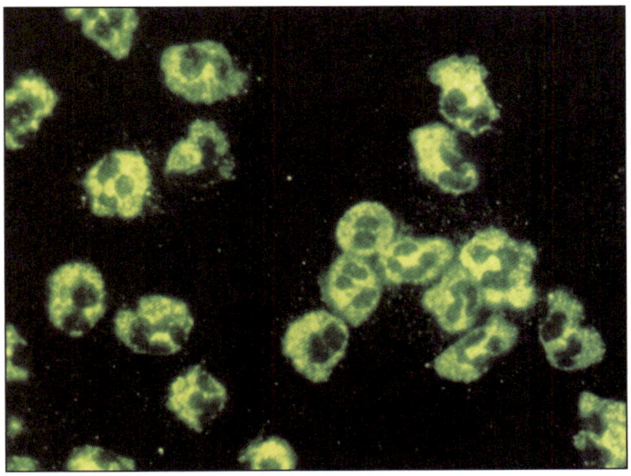

Image 19-6. Indirect immunofluorescence of serum from a patient with antiserine protease 3 reacted on human neutrophils fixed in ethanol. Note the presence of granular cytoplasmic staining (dark-field photomicrograph with fluorescein-conjugated antihuman IgG).

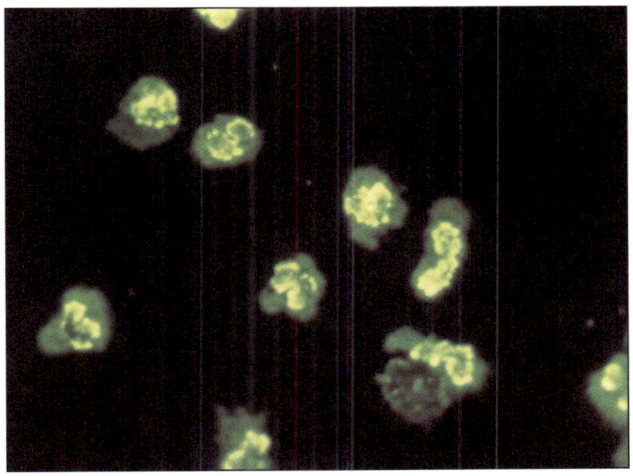

Image 19-7. Indirect immunofluorescence of serum from a patient with antimyeloperoxidase reacted on human neutrophils fixed in ethanol. Note the presence of perinuclear staining (dark-field photomicrograph with fluorescein-conjugated antihuman IgG).

CAP57, eosinophil peroxidase, bactericidal/permeability-increasing protein (BPI), and lactoferrin also have been found in a few patients with vasculitis.[74,75]

These tests have relevance for epidemiological investigations of individuals and the families of individuals with IBD. As many as 90% (in some studies) of patients with UC have serum antibodies that give a perinuclear (p-)ANCA-staining pattern on ethanol- (but not usually formalin-) fixed neutrophils.[72,76-81] The antigen responsible for this reaction has not been characterized; although some studies have found reactivity of the antibodies against cathepsin G,[82] another suggests that the antibodies recognize some antigen other than double-stranded DNA on the inner side of the nuclear membrane,[83] and yet another claims the use of a DNAse treatment provides a high level of specificity for detecting UC.[84,85] Indeed, Hoffenberg et al[86] reported that 60% of the p-ANCA staining was eliminated by pretreatment with DNAse in serum from children with UC. The antigens involved in IBD reactivity are different from those involved in vasculitis.[71] Stoffel et al[87] found that up to 44% of sera from patients with IBD had reactivity with a novel target antigen of neutrophils called bactericidal/permeability-increasing protein. Unfortunately, they also found such reactivity in 23% of CD sera. Clearly this is not useful for distinguishing between the 2 conditions in difficult cases. Walmsley et al[88] went on to note that the presence of anti-BPI seems to correlate with disease activity in UC. Unfortunately, the demonstration by this group that anti-BPI is also present in 23% of patients with infectious enteritis makes it probable that anti-BPI is a result of inflammation and damage rather than an initiating factor in IBD.

As many as 30% of patients with CD also have p-ANCA reactivity.[79,89] Unfortunately, an ANCA-reactivity test alone is not useful in distinguishing colonic UC from CD, because patients with colonic CD are more likely to be ANCA-positive than those with noncolonic CD.[76,88]

Because ANCA is also found in some asymptomatic relatives of patients with UC, it has little practical value as a diagnostic laboratory test for UC.[90] Although some researchers have suggested that evaluation of the presence of ANCA may be useful in evaluating the extent of the disease (eg, identifying left-sided colitis), the evidence has been highly variable, and biopsy and radiological studies are still required for workup of the individual patient.[76,91-93]

One possible diagnostic use of the test may be to help distinguish patients who have irritable bowel syndrome from those with true IBD, yet even in this situation, ANCA reactivity could not rule in or out either disease. Another possible association may lie in the presence of p-ANCA in most patients who are prone to develop pouchitis. However, the presence of p-ANCA again fails the test of specificity, because in one study, almost half of the patients who did not develop pouchitis also had p-ANCA.[94]

It has been reported that as many as 60% to 70% of patients with CD have been reported to have IgG and/or IgA antibodies against the yeast *Saccharomyces cervisiae* in their serum, whereas they are relatively uncommon in patients with UC.[86] In their study of 25 children with UC, Hoffenberg et al[86] reported that 20 had either c- or p-ANCA or both, while only 3 had anti-saccharomyces cerevisiae antibodies (ASCA) in their serum. In contrast, of 20 CD patients, 8 had ANCA, whereas 12 had ASCA; unfortunately, controls also demonstrated both ANCA (8 of 74) and ASCA (4 of 74) reactivity.[86] Furthermore, as many as 20% of healthy first-degree relatives of patients with IBD may have ASCA in their serum, further confounding the significance of its presence.[86,95] The level of antibody reactivity may have use. Vasiliauskas et al[96] noted that high levels of ASCA correlated with an early age of onset of CD, whereas high levels of ANCA are associated with later onset of CD and UC-like clinical behavior of CD. These intriguing reports provide ample background material for launching large epidemiological studies about the relevance of these antibodies to the initiation and propagation of these poorly understood conditions. Whether they are useful in the diagnostic process for individual patients is highly controversial. A recent independent review concluded that ANCA testing is not directly useful in either the diagnosis or prognosis for IBD.[97] Whereas several publications in the medical literature suggest the utility of this type of testing in clinical diagnosis, the reader is cautioned to note a possible conflict of interest of the authors, some of whom are related to a commercial laboratory that markets these tests to gastroenterologists. Yet, some independent information suggests that although ANCA and ASCA even together do not achieve sensitivity to use in population screening, serologic studies may be helpful in some cases to help with distinction between UC and CD.[86] Still, confirmation of the data by large studies by authors independent of commercial enterprises would help to clarify the potential use of these tests in the diagnosis and prognosis of IBD patients.[98]

IBD remains a tantalizing area of investigation for those of us interested in immunology and the gastrointestinal tract. Perhaps the newer studies of lymphocyte subsets and cytokines will help us understand this condition. Although new articles about the immunologic and inflammatory events surrounding IBD are of great interest, it is still not apparent that IBD is caused by autoimmunity. As a final note, even though this chapter appears in a text about autoimmune disease, the author must caution that we should not eliminate consideration of microorganisms as a possible cause of IBD.

References

1. Pruthi RK, Tefferi A. Pernicious anemia revisited. *Mayo Clin Proc*. 1994;69:144–150.
2. Markle HV. Cobalamin. *Crit Rev Clin Lab Sci*. 1996;33: 247–356.
3. Antony AC. Megaloblastic anemia. In: Stein, JH, ed. *Internal Medicine*. 4th ed. St. Louis, MO: Mosby; 1994:845–852.
4. Ottesen M, Feldt-Rasmussen U, Andersen J, et al. Thyroid function and autoimmunity in pernicious anemia before and during cyanocobalamin treatment. *J Endocrinol Invest*. 1995;18:91–97.
5. Appelman HD. Gastritis: Terminology, etiology, and clinicopathological correlations: Another biased view. *Hum Pathol*. 1994;25:1006–1019.
6. Spoelstra-de Man AM, Wagenaar SS, van der Sluys Veer A, et al. Relationship between pernicious anaemia and gastric neuroendocrine cell disorders. *Neth J Med*. 2000;56:56–62.
7. Carmel R. Reassessment of the relative prevalences of antibodies to gastric parietal cell and to intrinsic factor in patients with pernicious anaemia: influence of patient age and race. *Clin Exp Immunol*. 1992;89:74–77.
8. Ottesen M, Feldt-Rasmussen UF, Andersen J, et al. Pernicious anemia: A study of initial forms of the disease and diagnostic significance of determination of the intrinsic factor antibody and parietal cell antibody. *Ugeskr Laeger*. 1992;154:3758–3762.
9. De Aizpurua HJ, Cosgrove LJ, Ungar B, et al. Autoantibodies cytotoxic to gastric parietal cells in serum of patients with pernicious anemia. *N Engl J Med*. 1983;309:625–629.
10. Burman P, Kampe O, Kraaz W, et al. A study of autoimmune gastritis in the postpartum period and at a 5-year follow-up. *Gastroenterology*. 1992;103:934–942.
11. Jones CM, Callaghan JM, Gleeson PA, et al. The parietal cell autoantigens recognized in neonatal thymectomy-induced murine gastritis are the alpha and beta subunits of the gastric proton pump. *Gastroenterology*. 1991;101:287–294.
12. Varis O, Valle J, Siurala M. Is *Helicobacter pylori* involved in the pathogenesis of the gastritis characteristic of pernicious anaemia? Comparison between pernicious anaemia relatives and duodenal ulcer relatives. *Scand J Gastroenterol*. 1993;28:705–708.
13. Keren, DF. Pernicious anemia with atrophic gastritis. *ASCP Check Sample Immunopathol*. 1985;35-1:1–5.
14. Jeffries GH, Hoskins DW, Sleisenger MH. Antibody to intrinsic factor in serum from patients with pernicious anaemia. *J Clin Invest*. 1962;41:1106–1115.
15. Samhoff IM, et al. Blocking and binding antibodies to intrinsic factor and parietal cell antibody in pernicious anemia. *Gastroenterology*. 1968;55:575–581.
16. Carmel R. Reassessment of the relative prevalences of antibodies to gastric parietal cell and to intrinsic factor in patients with pernicious anaemia: Influence of patient age and race. *Clin Exp Immunol*. 1992;89:74–77.
17. De Block CE, De Leeuw IH, Van Gaal LF. High prevalence of manifestations of gastric autoimmunity in parietal cell antibody-positive type I (insulin-dependent) diabetic patients. *J Clin Endocrinol Metab*. 1999;84:4062–4067.
18. Waters HM, Dawson DW, Howarth JE, et al. High incidence of type II autoantibodies in pernicious anaemia. *J Clin Pathol*. 1993;46:45–47.
19. Shackleton PJ, Fish DI, Dawson DW. Intrinsic factor antibody tests. *J Clin Pathol*. 1989;42:210–212.
20. Davidson RJ, Atrah HI, Sewell HF. Longitudinal study of circulating gastric antibodies in pernicious anaemia. *J Clin Pathol*. 1989;42:1092–1095.
21. Cavallaro JJ, Palmer DF, Bigazzi PE, January 1976. Immunofluorescence Detection of Autoimmune Diseases, Immunology Series No. 7. Atlanta, GA: Centers for Disease Control.
22. Moss SF, Attia L, Scholes JV, et al. Increased small intestinal apoptosis in coeliac disease. *Gut*. 1996;39:811–814.
23. Yardley JH, Bayless TM, Norton JH. A study of the jejunal epithelium before and after a gluten-free diet. *N Engl J Med*. 1962;267:1173–1180.
24. Scott BB, Goodall A, Stephenson P, et al. Small intestinal plasma cells in coeliac disease. *Gut*. 1984;25:41–46.
25. Jos J, Labbe F, Geny B, et al. Immunoelectron-microscopic localization of immunoglobulin A and secretory component in jejunal mucosa from children with coeliac disease. *Scand J Immunol*. 1979;9:441–450.
26. Scott BB, Scott DG, Losowsky MS. Jejunal mucosal immunoglobulin A and secretory component in jejunal mucosa from children with coeliac disease. *J Pathol*. 1977;121:219–223.
27. Michalski JP, McCombs CC. Celiac disease: Clinical features and pathogenesis. *Am J Med Sci*. 1994;307: 204–211.
28. Stevens FM, McCarthy CF. The endoscopic demonstration of coeliac diseaes. *Endoscopy*. 1976;8:177–180.

29. Trier JS. Celiac sprue. *N Engl J Med*. 1991;325:1709–1719.

30. Moore L, Xu X, Davidson G, et al. Autoimmune enteropathy with anti-goblet cell antibodies. *Hum Pathol*. 1995;26:1162–1168.

31. Bousvaros A, Leichtner AM, Book L, et al. Treatment of pediatric autoimmune enteropathy with tacrolimus (FK506). *Gastroenterology*. 1996;111:237–243.

32. Chartrand LJ, Seidman EG. Celiac disease is a lifelong disorder. *Clin Invest Med*. 1996;19:357–361.

33. Hill I, Fasano A, Schwartz, et al. The prevalence of celiac disease in at-risk groups of children in the United States. *J Pediatr*. 2000;136:86–90.

34. Murray JA. Celiac disease: Pathogenesis and serologic tests. In: Keren DF, Nakamura R, eds. *Controversies in Autoimmune Disease*. Philadelphia, PA: WB Saunders; 1997:445–464.

35. Kumar V, Valeski JE, Wortsman J. Celiac disease and hypoparathyroidism: Cross-reaction of endomysial antibodies with parathyroid tissue. *Clin Diag Lab Immunol*. 1996;3:143–146.

36. Weinstein WM, Brow JR, Parker F, et al. The small intestinal mucosa in dermatitis herpetiformis, II: Relationship of the small intestinal lesion to gluten. *Gastroenterology*. 1971;60:362–369.

37. Otley C, Hall RP III. Dermatitis herpetiformis. *Clin Dermatol*. 1990;8:759–769.

38. Bodvarsson S, Jonsdottir I, Freysdottir J, et al. Dermatitis herpetiformis—an autoimmune disease due to cross-reaction between dietary glutenin and dermal elastin? *Scand J Immunol*. 1993;38:546–550.

39. Marsh MN. Studies of intestinal lymphoid tissue, IV: The predictive value of raised mitotic indices among jejunal epithelial lymphocytes in the diagnosis of gluten-sensitive enteropathy. *J Clin Pathol*. 1992;35:517–525.

40. Arato A, Savilahti E, Tainio VM, et al. HLA-DR expression, natural killer cells and IgE containing cells in the jejunal mucosa of coeliac children. *Gut*. 1987;28:988–994.

41. Shuppen D. Current concepts of celiac disease pathogenesis. *Gastroenterology*. 2000;119:234–242.

42. Jabri B, de Serre NP, Cellier C, et al. Selective expansion of intraepithelial lymphocytes expressing the HLA-E-specific natural killer receptor CD94 in celiac disease. *Gastroenterology*. 2000;118:867–879.

43. Russell GJ, Winter HS, Fox VL, et al. Lymphocytes bearing the gamma-delta T-cell receptor in normal human intestine and celiac disease. *Hum Pathol*. 1991;22:690–694.

44. Maki M, Holm K, Collin P, et al. Increase in gamma-delta T cell receptor bearing lymphocytes in normal small bowel mucosa in latent coeliac disease. *Gut*. 1991;32:1412–1414.

45. Austin LL, Dobbins WO. Studies of the rectal mucosa in coeliac sprue: The intraepithelial lymphocyte. *Gut*. 1988;29:200–205.

46. Loft DE, Marsh MN, Sandle GI, et al. Studies of intestinal lymphoid tissue, XII: Epithelial lymphocyte and mucosal responses to rectal gluten challenge in celiac sprue. *Gastroenterology*. 1989;97:29–37.

47. Nguyen HH, Farre MA, Tlaskalova H, et al. The interaction of gliadin with effector and target cells in NK cell activity of patients with celiac disease. In: Mestecky J, ed. *Advances in Mucosal Immunology*. New York, NY: Plenum Press; 1995:1359–1362.

48. Thurley CA, Kwan WC, Freeman HJ, et al. T cell receptor gene expression and genotypes in celiac disease. *Pathobiology*. 1994;62:311–318.

49. Polanco I, Biemond I, van Leeuwen A, et al. Gluten-sensitive enteropathy in Spain: Genetic and environmental factors. In: McConnell RD, ed. *Genetics of Coeliac Disease: Proceedings of International Symposium (1979)*. Lancaster, England: MTP Press; 1981:211–231.

50. Mearin ML, Pena AS. Clinical indications of HLA typing and measurement of gliadin antibodies in coeliac disease. *Neth J Med*. 1987;31:279–285.

51. Tighe MR, Ciclitira PJ. The implications of recent advances in coeliac disease. *Acta Paediatr*. 1993;82:805–810.

52. Sollid LM, Thorsby E. HLA susceptibility genes in celiac disease: Genetic mapping and role in pathogenesis. *Gastroenterology*. 1993;105:910–922.

53. Lundin KEA, Scott H, Fausa O, et al. T cells from the small intestinal mucosa of a DR4,DQ7/DR4,DQ8 celiac disease patient preferentially recognize gliadin when presented by DQ8. *Hum Immunol*. 1994;41:285–291.

54. Lundin KEA, Gjertsen HA, Scott H, et al. Functions of DQ2 and DQ8 as HLA susceptibility molecules in celiac disease. *Hum Immunol*. 1994;41:24–27.

55. Lundin KEA, Sollid LM, Anthonsen D, et al. Heterogeneous reactivity patterns of HLA-DQ-restricted, small intestinal T-cell clones from patients with celiac disease. *Gastroenterology*. 1997;112:752–759.

56. Farrell RJ, Kelly CP. Celiac sprue. *N Engl J Med*. 2002;346:180–188.

57. Papadatou B, Crino A, Giannotti A, et al. Antiendomysial and antigliadin antibodies in patients with Down syndrome. *Dev Brain Dysfunct*. 1996;9:129–132.

58. Meini A, Pillan NM, Villanacci V, et al. Prevalence and diagnosis of celiac disease in IgA-deficient children. *Ann Allergy Asthma Immunol*. 1996;77:333–336.

59. Cataldo F, Lio D, Marino V, et al. IgG(1) antiendomysium and IgG antitissue transglutaminase (anti-tTG) antibodies in coeliac patients with selective IgA deficiency. Working Groups on Celiac Disease of SIGEP and Club del Tenue. *Gut*. 2000;47:366–369.

60. Fotoulaki M, Nousia-Aryanitakis S, Augoustidou-Savvopoulou P, et al. Clinical application of immunological markers as monitoring tests in celiac disease. *Dig Dis Sci.* 1999;44:2133–2138.

61. Burgin-Wolff A, Gaze H, Hadzieselimovic F, et al. Antigliadin and antiendomysium antibody determination for celiac disease. *Arch Dis Child.* 1991;66:941–947.

62. Volta U, Molinaro N, De Franceschi L, et al. IgA antiendomysial antibodies on human umbilical cord tissue for celiac disease screening: Save both money and monkeys. *Dig Dis Sci.* 1995;40:1902–1905.

63. Keren DF, Kumar NB, Appelman HD. Quantification of IgA-containing plasma cells as an adjunct to histiopathology in distinguishing acute self-limited colitis from active idiopathic inflammatory bowel disease. *Pathol Immunopathol Res.* 1987;6:435–441.

64. Rosekrans PCM, Meijer CJ, Van der Val AM, et al. Immunoglobulin containing cells in inflammatory bowel disease of the colon: A morphometric and immunohistochemical study. *Gut.* 1980;21:941–947.

65. Broberger O, Perlmann P. Autoantibodies in human ulcerative colitis. *J Exp Med.* 1959;110:657–665.

66. Simpson SJ, Hollander GA, Mizoguchi E, et al. Expression of pro-inflammatory cytokines by TCR alpha-beta+ and TCR delta-gamma+ T cells in an experimental model of colitis. *Eur J Immunol.* 1997;27:17–25.

67. Nielsen OH, Rask-Madsen J. Mediators of inflammation in chronic inflammatory bowel disease. *Scand J Gastroenterol.* 1996;31(suppl 216):149–159.

68. Davies DJ, Moran JE, Niall JF, et al. Segmental necrotizing glomerulonephritis with antineutrophil antibody: Possible arbovirus aetiology? *BMJ.* 1982;285:606.

69. Casper FM, Coen F, Stegeman CA, et al. Anti-proteinase 3- and antimyeloperoxidase-associated vasculitis. *Kidney Int.* 2000;57;2195–2206.

70. Savige J, Davies D, Falk RJ, et al. Antineutrophil cytoplasmic antibodies and associated diseases: a review of the clinical and laboratory features. *Kidney Int.* 2000;57:846–862.

71. Jennette JC, Falk RJ. Antineutrophil cytoplasmic autoantibodies in inflammatory bowel disease. *Am J Clin Pathol.* 1993;99:221–223.

72. Kallenberg CGM, Mulder AHL, Tervaert JWC. Antineutrophil cytoplasmic antibodies: A still-growing class of autoantibodies in inflammatory disorders. *Am J Med.* 1992;93:675–682.

73. van der Woude FJ, Rasmussen N, Lobatto S, et al. Autoantibodies to neutrophils and monocytes: A new tool for diagnosis and marker of disease activity in Wegener's granulomatosis. *Lancet.* 1985;2:425–429.

74. Bosch X, Asherson RA. The antigenic significance and methods of detection of the anti-neutrophil cytoplsmic autoantibodies (ANCA). *Postgrad Med J.* 1992;68:707–713.

75. Stoffel MP, Csernok E, Herzberg C, et al. Anti-neutrophil cytoplasmic antibodies (ANCA) directed against bactericidal/permeability increasing protein (BPI): A new seromarker for inflammatory bowel disease and associated disorders. *Clin Exp Immunol.* 1996;104:54–59.

76. Hertervig E, Wieslander J, Johansson C, et al. Anti-neutrophil cytoplasmic antibodies in chronic inflammatory bowel disease: Prevalence and diagnostic role. *Scand J Gastroenteroly.* 1995;30:693–698.

77. Cambridge G, Rampton DS, Stevens TRJ. Antineutrophil antibodies in inflammatory bowel disease: Prevalence and diagnostic role. *Gut.* 1992;33:668–674.

78. Vidrich A, Lee J, James E, et al. Segregation of pANCA antigenic recognition by DNase treatment of neutrophils: Ulcerative colitis, Type 1 autoimmune hepatitis, and primary sclerosing cholangitis. *J Clin Immunol.* 1995;15:293–299.

79. Rump JA, Scholmerich J, Gross V, et al. A new type of perinuclear anti-neutrophil cytoplasmic antibody (p-ANCA) in active ulcerative colitis but not in Crohn's disease. *Immunobiology.* 1990;181:406–413.

80. Sung JY, Chan KL, Hsu R, et al. Ulcerative colitis and antineutrophil cytoplasmic antibodies in Hong Kong Chinese. *Am J Gastroenterology.* 1993;88:864–869.

81. Sung JY, Chan FKL, Lawton J, et al. Anti-neutrophil cytoplasmic antibodies (ANCA) and inflammatory bowel diseases in Chinese. *Dig Dis Sci.* 1994;39:886–892.

82. Sobajima J, Ozaki S, Okazaki T, et al. Anti-neutrophil cytoplasmic antibodies (ANCA) in ulcerative colitis: Anti-cathepsin G and a novel antibody correlate with a refractory type. *Clin Exp Immunol.* 1996;105:120–124.

83. Billing P, Tahir S, Calfin B, et al. Nuclear localization of the antigen detected by ulcerative colitis-associated perinuclear antineutrophil cytoplasmic antibodies. *Am J Pathol.* 1995;147:979–987.

84. Vidrich A, Lee J, James E, et al. Segregation of pANCA antigenic recognition by Dnase treatment of neutrophils: Ulcerative colitis, type I autoimmune hepatitis, and primary sclerosing cholangitis. *J Clin Immunol.* 1995;15:293–299.

85. Ruemmele FM, Targan SR, Levy G, et al. Diagnostic accuracy of serological assays in pediatric inflammatory bowel disease. *Gastroenterology.* 1998;115:822-829.

86. Hoffenberg EJ, Fidanz S, Sauaia A. Serologic testing for inflammatory bowel disease. *J Pediatr.* 1999;134: 447–452.

87. Stoffel MP, Csernok E, Gross WL. Target antigen for anti-neutrophil cytoplasmic antibodies in inflammatory bowel disease. *Scand J Gastroenterol.* 1996;31:943–944.

88. Walmsley RS, Zhao MH, Hamilton MI, et al. Antineutrophil cytoplasm autoantibodies against bactericidal/permeability-increasing protein in inflammatory bowel disease. *Gut.* 1997;40:105–109.

89. Schnabel A, Hauschild S, Gross W. Anti-neutrophil cytoplasmic antibodies in generalized autoimmune diseases. *Int Arch Allergy Immunol*. 1996;109:201–206.

90. Shanahan F, Duerr RH, Rotter JI, et al. Neutrophil autoantibodies in ulcerative colitis: Familial aggregation and genetic heterogeneity. *Gastroenterology*. 1992;103:456–461.

91. Broekroelofs J, Mulder AHL, Nelis GF, et al. Anti-neutrophil cytoplasmic antibodies (ANCA) in sera from patients with inflammatory bowel disease (IBD) relation to disease pattern and disease activity. *Dig Dis Sci*. 1994;39:545–549.

92. Kim WH, Choi PM, Landers CJ, et al. Role of anti-neutrophil cytoplasmic antibodies in an ethnically distinct population: Korean patients with ulcerative colitis. *Am J Gastroenterol*. 1995;90:1–6.

93. Sandborn WJ, Landers CJ, Tremaine WJ, et al. Association of antineutrophil cytoplasmic antibodies with resistance to treatment of left-sided ulcerative colitis: Results of a pilot study. *Mayo Clin Proc*. 1996;71:431–436.

94. Sandborn WJ, Landers CJ, Tremaine WJ, et al. Anti-neutrophil cytoplasmic antibody correlates with chronic pouchitis after ileal pouch-anal anastomosis. *Am J Gastroenterol*. 1995;90:740–747.

95. Sendid B, Quinton J-F, Charrier G, et al. Anti-Saccharomyces cerviciae mannan antibodies in familial Crohn's disease. *Am J Gastroenterol*. 1998;93:1755–1759.

96. Vasiliauskas EA, Kam LY, Karp LC, et al. Marker antibody expression stratifies Crohn's disease into immunologically homogeneous subgroups with distinct clinical characteristics. *Gut*. 2000;47:487–496.

97. Roozendaal C, Kallenberg CGM. Are anti-neutrophil cytoplasmic antibodies (ANCA) clinically useful in inflammatory bowel disease (IBD)? *Clin Exp Immunol*. 1999;116:206–213.

98. Keren DF, Goeken JA. Autoimmune reactivity in inflammatory bowel disease. *Clin Lab Med*. 1997;17:465–481.

CHAPTER 20

Autoimmune Diseases of Muscle: Myasthenia Gravis and Autoimmune Myositis

LeMing Hang, MD, and Robert M. Nakamura, MD

Immunologic injury to skeletal muscle can affect either the neuromuscular junction, causing impaired impulse transmission and motor dysfunction, or myocyte constituents, causing muscle inflammation and necrosis. The former is exemplified by myasthenia gravis (MG) and the latter by autoimmune myositis (also called idiopathic inflammatory myopathy).

The incidence of myasthenia gravis is 40 to 60 new cases per million people per year with a bimodal age distribution. The first peak is in the second to third decade of life, and the second peak is in the sixth decade of life. Symptoms of MG are often noticed first by the affected individuals after infection, stress, or exposure to certain antibiotics or neuroleptic drugs. The characteristic clinical symptoms are fatigability and weakness affecting muscles of swallowing, speech, eye movements, and facial expression.[1]

The incidence of autoimmune myositis is 5 to 10 new cases per million people per year, also with a bimodal age distribution. The first peak age is between 10 and 14 years, with a second larger peak at 45 to 64 years. Accurate diagnosis of this autoimmune disease can be a clinical challenge, because the presenting symptoms are often nonspecific, ranging from vague myalgia, fatigue, skin rash, dysphagia, or bowel dysfunction to fatal respiratory difficulties, cardiac arrhythmias, or congestive heart failure. This disease may mimic infectious, toxic, dystrophic, rheumatic, endocrine, neuropathic, and paraneoplastic myopathies. Timely recognition of this disease and institution of therapy are important because delay in treatment can adversely affect prognosis.[2–5]

The purpose of this chapter is to review (1) the current disease classifications and the clinicopathologic features of myasthenia gravis and autoimmune myositis, (2) the laboratory tests necessary for disease diagnosis and monitoring, (3) other conditions that can mimic these diseases, and (4) the implicated risk factors and mechanisms for disease pathogenesis.

Myasthenia Gravis

Disease Classification and Clinicopathologic Features

Myasthenia gravis is the prototype of antibody-mediated autoimmune disease of neuromuscular junction. Anti–acetylcholine receptor (anti-AChR) antibody, directed against alpha subunits of AChR along the postsynaptic membrane, is the associated pathogenic autoantibody. These autoantibodies can bind AChRs; block AChR activities; accelerate AChR degradation; and induce lytic destruction of postsynaptic membranes, causing decreased impulse transmission from motor nerve axons to muscle endplates. The characteristic clinical symptoms of MG are ocular and/or generalized muscle weakness that worsen with exercise but improve with rest. A positive edrophonium chloride (Tensilon) response is the most helpful clinical test for the diagnosis of MG. As listed in **Table 20-1**, myasthenia gravis can be classified into five distinct groups[1,6–8]:

- Early-onset disease (fewer than 40 years old) MG, associated with thymic hyperplasia
- Late-onset disease (more than 40 years old) MG, associated with thymic atrophy and often concurrent systemic or other organ-specific autoimmune diseases
- Thymoma-associated MG, most likely a paraneoplastic myasthenia syndrome
- Myasthenia gravis without detectable anti-AChR autoantibodies (seronegative MG)

Table 20-1. Classification of Myasthenia Gravis and Clinicopathologic Features[1,8,9]

Type and Incidence (%) in Each Disease Group	Thymic Pathology	Age at Onset	Anti-AChR	Weakness
Early onset (55%)	Hyperplasia	<40 years	High titer	Diffuse
Late onset (20%)	Atrophy	>40 years	Low titer	Diffuse/ocular
Thymoma associated (10%)	Thymoma	Any age	Intermediate titer	Diffuse
Seronegative* (15%)	Expanded T-cell "areas"	Any age	None detected	Diffuse/ocular
D-Penicillamine–induced MG (<1%)	Unknown	Any age	Variable titer	Diffuse/ocular

Abbreviations: AChR = acetylcholine receptor; MG = myasthenia gravis.

**No anti-AChR antibodies can be detected in sera from "seronegative" patients with myasthenia gravis by routine assays, but these patients have a similar disease course and response to plasmapheresis treatment as "seropositive" patients.*

- D-Penicillamine–induced MG occurring in 1% of rheumatoid arthritis or Wilson's disease patients receiving this drug (MG disease symptoms and anti-AChR titers usually regress after D-penicillamine is withdrawn)

Neonatal MG is a transient disease caused by passively transferred maternal anti-AChR antibodies. Congenital MG is not associated with anti-AChR and does not respond to anticholinesterase drugs or plasmapheresis; it is a rare hereditary neuromuscular disorder due to structural and functional defects of both AChR molecules and membrane synaptic vesicles.[7,8]

Diagnostic Laboratory Tests

The most useful laboratory test to confirm a diagnosis of MG is identification of anti-AChR antibodies in symptomatic patients. The overall diagnostic sensitivity of this test is over 88%, but anti-AChR antibodies can occur in 5% to 15% of lung cancer patients and 15% of patients with other organ-specific or systemic autoimmune diseases. Low-titer anti-AChR antibodies also have been detected in bone marrow transplant recipients.[6–12]

Assay methods for anti-AChR antibodies have traditionally employed immunoprecipitation procedures that require fresh skeletal muscle from human amputations as the source of AChRs. The isolated human AChRs are tagged with iodine 125 (^{125}I-labeled) α-bungarotoxin which binds irreversibly to active sites of AChR. The ^{125}I-tagged AChR-bungarotoxin preparation is then incubated with the suspected antibodies in patient sera, allowing immune complex formation. These immune complexes are then precipitated by antihuman immunoglobulin (Ig) G or staphylococcal A protein. The anti-AChR antibody titer is determined by the amount of ^{125}I activity in the immunoprecipitate.[9,10]

Types of Anti-AChR Antibodies and Their Clinical Significance

Three functionally different types of anti-AChR antibodies are detected in MG patients:

- AChR-binding antibody, present in 88% of MG patients, which binds randomly to AChR and induces conformational changes but does not correlate with disease severity
- AChR-blocking antibody, present in 35% to 88% of MG patients, which has specificity for AChR binding sites and correlates with disease activity
- AChR-modulating antibody, present in more than 80% of MG patients, which can cross-link AChR to accelerate its degradation and correlates closely to disease activity

Thus, the blocking and modulating antibodies are useful tests for patient management because they correlates closely with disease activity.[13–15]

Detection of these antibodies requires functional assays in which soluble AChRs are used to measure binding activity while intact muscle cells are needed to assess blocking and modulating activities. The AChR-binding and AChR-blocking antibody activities are determined by the amount of ^{125}I in the immunoprecipitate, whereas the modulating antibody activity is estimated by the amount of ^{125}I released into the supernatant from degraded AChRs (AChR loss). These assays have not been available as routine tests due to their technical complexity and requirement for fresh human muscle as the AChR source.

Recently, a human rhabdomyosarcoma (RD) cell line (TE671) has been developed for use, in place of fresh muscle from human amputations as the source of AChRs, for both quantitative and functional anti-AChR assays. These "RD-cell" test results have shown comparable sensitivity and specificity. More hospital laboratories may now consider including these functional assays in the MG test panel.[16–18]

Seronegative Myasthenia Gravis

Seronegative MG refers to the 10% to 15% of patients with clinical MG symptoms, but no detectable anti-AChR autoantibodies, who respond to anticholinesterase drugs and plasmapheresis in the same way as anti-AChR–positive patients.[1,6–8] There is evidence that such patients may have anti-AChR antibodies that react with other AChR antigenic epitopes not included in the currently available assays. One recent study[19] showed that plasma from seronegative MG patients can decrease AChR function. In addition, immunoblot tests have demonstrated that circulating lymphocytes from seronegative patients can produce anti-AChR antibodies. These tests are still in the investigational stage and are not yet available for clinical use.[20]

Specific Tests for Thymoma-Associated Myasthenia Gravis

Two additional autoantibodies are detected in patients with thymoma-associated MG. These are antistriational and anti–ryanodine receptor antibodies directed against skeletal muscle sarcomere titin, actin, and myosin proteins and ryanodine receptors.[21–24]

Antistriational antibodies (detected by indirect immunofluorescence or enzyme immunoassay) occur in 50% to 90% of adults with thymoma-associated MG and may cross-react with anti-AChR antibodies. They are not specific for thymoma-associated MG because they can be present with or without anti-AChR antibodies in recipients of allogenic bone marrow transplants, patients receiving D-penicillamine treatment, and patients with primary lung carcinomas. The antibody titer decreases with thymectomy and may be a helpful marker for recurrence of thymoma after surgical removal.[21,22]

Anti–ryanodine receptor antibodies (detected by Western blot assay using rabbit muscle homogenate as the test antigen) are found in 50% of patients with thymoma-associated MG. Ryanodine receptors are calcium channel proteins in skeletal and cardiac muscle sarcoplasmic membranes that are involved in the excitation-contraction coupling of myofibers. These receptors share certain antigenic epitopes with AChR. They are specific but not very sensitive markers for thymoma-associated MG.[23,24]

Muscle Biopsy Findings

The skeletal muscle of patients with MG does not show exudative inflammatory or obvious myocytic necrosis. The neuromuscular junctions are relatively intact, the sarcoplasm is infiltrated by a few mononuclear inflammatory cells, and there are occasional necrotic myofibers surrounded by interstitial lymphocyte clusters (lymphorrhages). By electron microscopy, the infoldings at the neuromuscular junction are decreased, consistent with AChR loss and postsynaptic membrane destruction. Although these findings are consistent with neuromuscular junction disease, they are not MG specific. Thus, muscle biopsy is considered helpful but not essential for a diagnosis of myasthenia gravis.[1,6–8,25] Muscle biopsies are performed as outlined in **Table 20-2**.

Other Neuromuscular Diseases Mimicking Myasthenia Gravis

At least three types of neuromuscular diseases can have symptoms resembling MG: Lambert-Eaton myasthenia syndrome (LEMS), neurotoxic venomation from certain insect or snake bites, and botulism.

Lambert-Eaton myasthenia syndrome is an auto-immune paraneoplastic neuromuscular disorder characterized by proximal leg weakness, hyporeflexia, bulbar palsy, dry mouth, and bowel dysfunction. Up to 60% of LEMS patients harbor small cell lung carcinoma and LEMS may precede clinical tumor detection by 5 years. Testing for autoantibodies directed against presynaptic membrane voltage-gated calcium channel (VGCC) particles would help to diagnose LEMS, because fewer than 5% of MG patients have anti-VGCC autoantibodies. The cause of LEMS is thought to be decreased neurotransmission due to autoantibody-mediated depletion of the VGCC particles located in the presynaptic membrane "active zone" (**Figure 20-1A** to **20-1C**). From 5% to 15% of LEMS patients with lung carcinoma have anti-AChR antibodies.[26,30]

Table 20-2. Guidelines for Handling of Muscle Biopsy[26-29]

1. Needle or fine forcep tips are recommended to avoid excessive handling of biopsied tissue.
2. For both light and electron microscope studies, 2.5% glutaraldehyde (pH 7.35) is used as a tissue fixative. The tissue samples are fixed as soon as possible (preferably immediately after biopsy) and kept at room temperature to minimize contraction artifacts.
3. For immunofluorescence and histochemistry, the biopsy samples may be placed in Hanks' solution during transport from surgery to the laboratory. On arrival, the tissue is snap frozen in isopentane and liquid nitrogen or dry ice and stored at –70°C until cryostat frozen sections can be cut for immunostaining or incubation with various enzyme substrates.

Neurotoxic venoms from viper, cobra, and krait snakes and black widow spiders can cause neuromuscular junction dysfunction by fusing the synaptic vesicles to the terminal axon membranes, resulting in decreased transmitter release and unexcitability. Symptoms resembling those for MG—muscle weakness, proceeding in the order of ocular, masticular, palatal, neck, and proximal to distal limb usually develop within 4 hours after venomation.[7]

Botulism toxins cause presynaptic neuromuscular junction blockade by binding to receptors on the terminal axon membrane. Within 12 to 48 hours after ingestion of a toxin, affected individuals exhibit diplopia, ptosis, swallowing and speech difficulties, and quadriplegia; if untreated, they progress to cardiopulmonary arrest.[1,6]

Generalized and/or bulbar ocular muscle weakness can occur in other types of neuromuscular

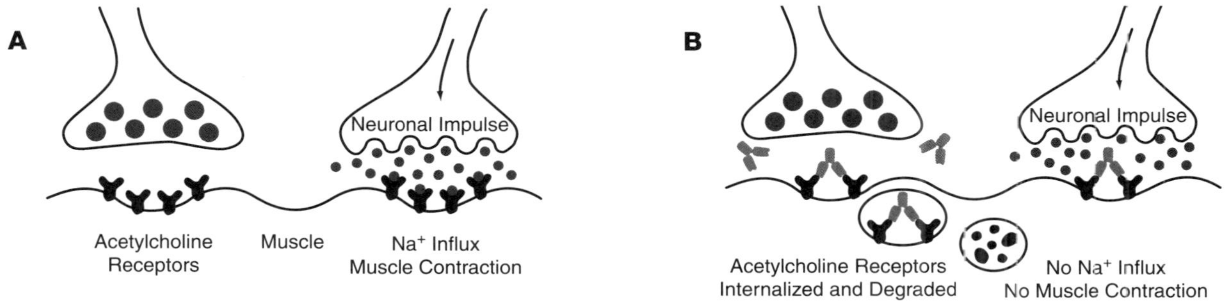

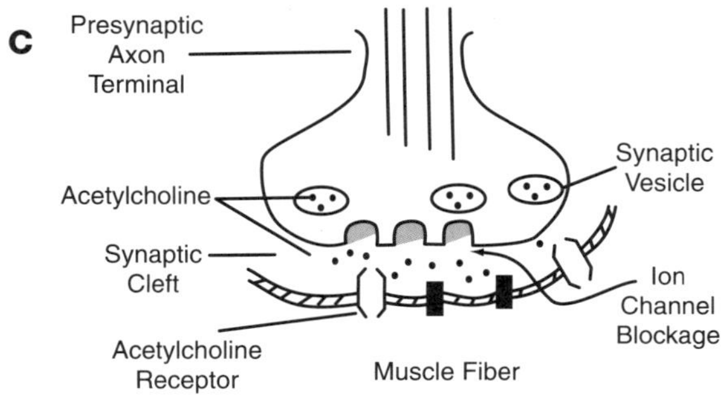

Figure 20-1. (**A**) Normally, muscle contracts when acetylchlorine (ACh) released from stimulated neurons at the neuromuscular junction (NMJ) binds to ACh receptors (AChRs) of postsynaptic muscle cell membrane clefts. (**B**) In myasthenia gravis, anti-AChR antibodies directed against alpha subunit epitopes of the AChR at the NMJ prevent response to motor neuron impulses. (**C**) In the Lambert-Easton myasthenia syndrome, anti–voltage-gated calcium channel antibodies directed against antigenic epitopes of "active zone" particles along presynaptic membrane vesicles from which neurotransmitters are released apparently block ion channels and prevent receipt of motor neuron impulses.

disorders such as Guillain-Barré syndrome, organophosphate poisoning, multiple sclerosis, brain stem lesions, and amyotrophic lateral sclerosis. Anti-AChR autoantibodies usually are not found in these disorders.[6,7]

Pathogenesis of Myasthenia Gravis

Role of the Thymus

There is consensus that the thymus is the site of initial T- and B-cell autosensitization against the AChR alpha subunit polypeptides in thymic myoid cells of patients with MG. Thymic hyperplasia occurs in 65% of these patients, and thymomas are found in 15% of patients with MG symptoms. As previously stated, thymoma-associated MG is most likely and should probably be regarded as an autoimmune paraneoplastic myasthenia syndrome type of neuromuscular disorder with paraneoplastic antistriational and anti-AChR antibodies. Thymectomy can ameliorate MG symptoms in over 80% of patients.[1,8,31–34]

Role of Genetic and Environmental Risk Factors

There is a definite association between MG and certain human leukocyte antigen (HLA) haplotypes. The HLA association in thymoma-associated MG is different from that in thymic hyperplasia MG. Early-onset MG in whites is associated with HLA-B8 and HLA-DR3 antigens: 72% and 60% of the patient group test positive for B8 and DR3, respectively, versus 28% and 23% of controls. Direct binding of AChR molecules to antigen-presenting cells that express HLA-DR3 have been demonstrated. Weaker associations with HLA-BW21, BW35, BW44, and BW51 (16% to 37% in the patient group versus 4% to 13% in controls) are noted in Asian, Indian, and Japanese patients. Association with immunoglobulin heavy chain (Gm) genes also have been reported in some studies. Such variability in HLA association reflects the polygenic, multifactorial nature of autoimmune diseases.[1,8,32,33]

Autoimmune Myositis

Disease Classification and Clinicopathologic Features

Autoimmune myositis is currently classified into five major and four minor groups by its distinctive clinicopathologic and laboratory characteristics (**Table 20-3**).[4,5,35] The five major groups are polymyositis, dermatomyositis, overlap myositis associated with systemic autoimmune diseases, juvenile myositis, and "inclusion body" myositis (IBM). The four minor groups are granulomatous

Table 20-3. Classification of Autoimmune Myositis and Clinicopathologic Features[4,5,35]

Types of Myositis	Distinguishing Clinicopathologic Features
Five major groups	
Polymyositis	Diagnosis by exclusion of the following features (other exclusions required): • Paraneoplastic myositis (cancer associated), most likely adenocarcinoma of the gastrointestinal tract or genitourinary tract or (less likely) of the lung • Infectious (viral, Lyme) or myotoxic myositis
Dermatomyositis	V and shawl or purplish eyelid rash; mechanic's hand (scaled cracked skin with cuticular overgrowth); vasculitis; good response to steroids
Overlap myositis	Associated with scleroderma, SLE, or Sjögren's syndrome
Juvenile myositis	Onset before age 18; subcutaneous calcified nodules; frequent skin and gastrointestinal tract ulcers due to vasculitis; responsive to steroids
Inclusion body myositis	Predominant in elderly men with symptoms of dysphagia, facial, and distal limb muscle weakness; possibly normal serum CK; does not respond to steroids or immunosuppression; muscle biopsy needed for definitive diagnosis
Four minor groups	
Granulomatous myositis	Exclusion of sarcoidosis, fungi, and mycobacteria required
Eosinophilic myositis	Exclusion of parasites, protozoa, and myotoxins required
Focal nodular myositis	Up to 5 cm in area; usually in lower extremities; may regress, but follow-up needed to exclude early form of polymyositis
Ocular myositis	Painful inflammation confined to extraocular muscles; exclusion of Graves' disease required

Abbreviations: SLE = systemic lupus erythematous; CK = creatine kinase.

myositis, eosinophilic myositis, focal nodular myositis, and ocular myositis.

Polymyositis, dermatomyositis, overlap myositis, and juvenile myositis are diverse groups of systemic inflammatory autoimmune diseases of connective tissue affecting not only the skeletal muscles but other organs such as skin, gastrointestinal tract, lung, and heart. Patients usually have fever, painful myalgia, and progressive muscle weakness with myopathic electromyographic findings. The muscle groups involved tend to be, but are not always, proximal and symmetric. Serum creatine kinase (CK) is increased in more than 95% of myositis patients. Most affected patients have either myositis-associated or myositis-specific autoantibodies.[4,5,33–36] The various clinical and immunopathologic disease characteristics, as well as laboratory tests useful for disease diagnosis and monitoring, are discussed in the next section.

Inclusion body myositis is a distinct, often painless, but therapy-resistant autoimmune myositis affecting elderly men during the sixth or seventh decade of life. Patients with IBM account for the majority of "polymyositis unresponsive to therapy" cases referred to the National Institutes of Health (NIH) for consultation. This disease was originally described in 1967 as chronic polymyositis with myxoviruslike particles in the nuclei and sarcoplasm of muscle fibers, but thus far no causal viral agents have been detected.[37–39] These "inclusion bodies" of IBM are described later in this chapter.

In contrast to the predominant symmetric pattern of proximal muscle involvement in polymyositis and dermatomyositis, IBM is characterized by asymmetric distal muscle weakness (foot extensor and finger flexor groups). Familial oculopharyngeal and fascioscapulohumeral myopathy or other systemic autoimmune diseases also may be present in 10% to 20% of IBM patients. Inclusion body myositis usually has an indolent disease course lasting from 10 to 20 years; rare associations with malignancies or sarcoidosis have been reported. Serum CK may be normal or elevated but not beyond 10 times the normal range. Patients with IBM may have myositis-specific and myositis-associated autoantibodies.[4,38,39]

The four minor groups of autoimmune myositis are more localized with granulomatous, eosinophilic, focal nodular, or ocular manifestations. These rare but distinct disease entities need to be included in the differential diagnosis of sarcoidosis, mycobacterial infection, parasitism, chemical- or toxin-induced myopathies, localized variants of polymyositis, and other types of bulbar neuromyopathies.[40–42]

Diagnostic Laboratory Testing

Most patients with autoimmune myositis show laboratory evidence of both humoral and cellular immunologic abnormalities, such as hypergammaglobulinemia, and circulating autoantibodies directed against cytoplasmic or intranuclear antigens. Activated lymphocytes are found in blood and inflammatory infiltrates in affected muscles.[5,27,28,35,43–45]

Human epithelial (HEp-2) cell immunofluorescence antinuclear antibody (IFM-ANA) is the most helpful myositis autoantibody screening test, because 60% to 90% of affected patients test positive.[46] Moreover, as shown in **Images 20-1A** to **20-1D**, the IFM-ANA staining patterns can be used to predict whether a patient has myositis-specific autoantibodies (MSAs)

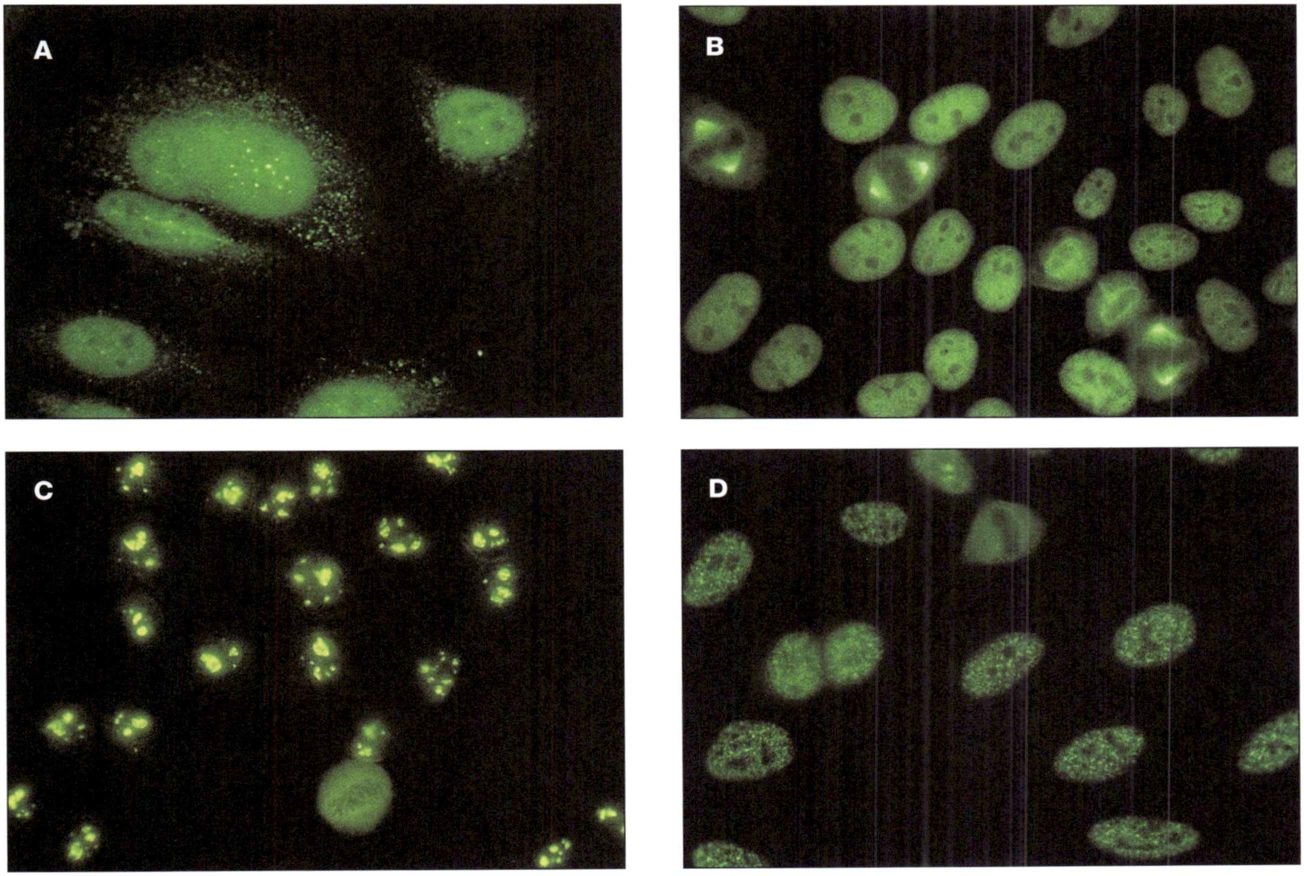

Image 20-1. (**A**) Anti-Jo-1 antibody staining on HEp-2 cells. There is a speckled cytoplasmic and nucleoplasmic staining. (**B**) Anti-PL-12 synthetase antibody staining on HEp-2 cells. PL-12 antibodies are directed against PL-12 (alanyl-tRNA synthetase) and demonstrate dense speckled cytoplasmic staining. (**C**) Anti-PM-Scl antigen is located in the granular component of the nucleolus. On HEp-2 cells, the anti-PM-Scl shows a homogeneous nucleolar staining and a negative staining of chromosomes in dividing cells. (**D**) Anti-Ku antibodies are directed against two proteins of 66 and 86 kd with different structure and function. The two proteins form a hetero-dimer that binds DNA with a possible role in transcriptional activation, DNA replication, and cell proliferation. On HEp-2 cells, the anti-Ku antibodies show a patchy homogeneous nucleoplasmic and nucleolar staining in interphase cells.

Table 20-4. Autoantibodies, Target Antigens, and HLA Associations in Autoimmune Myositis[5,36,47-53]

Antibody Type (Frequency %)	Target Antigen	Associated HLA Types and Disease Course
Myositis-specific autoantibodies		
	tRNA synthetases	DR3, DRw52, DQA1-0501
Anti-EJ (2%)	Glycyl	
Anti-Jo-1 (20%)	Histidyl	Most patients with anti-tRNA synthetase antibodies have either PM or DM with pulmonary interstitial fibrosis, fever, Raynaud's symptoms, and severe myalgia.
Anti-OJ (2%)	Isoleucyl	Disease response to steroids is variable.
Anti-PL-7 (3%)	Threonyl	Disease onset tends to cluster in spring.
Anti-PL-12 (3%)	Alanyl	Flare-ups occur when therapy is tapered. Five-year survival rate is 70%.
Anti-SRP (5%)	Signal recognition protein	DR5, DRw52, DQA1-0301 Most patients are black women with frequent cardiac conduction defects or arrhythmias and acute severe myalgia. Chemotherapy needed for disease control. Disease onset usually occurs in autumn. Five-year survival rate is around 25%.
Anti-Mi-2 (8%)	Unidentified nuclear protein	DR7, DRw53, DQA1-0201 Almost all patients have DM, mild disease, and good response to steroids. Five-year survival rate is near 100%.
Myositis-associated autoantibodies		
Anti-PM-Scl (8%)	Nucleolar protein complex	Most patients have polymyositis with overlap syndrome of scleroderma; also may have SLE symptoms.
Anti-U_1RNP (12%)	U_1 small nuclear protein	
Anti-U_2RNP (3%)	U_2 small nuclear protein	
Anti-Ku (1%)	DNA-binding protein	Most patients have dermatomyositis with overlap of Sjögren's syndrome or SLE and pulmonary hypertension.

Abbreviations: HLA = human leukocyte antigen; tRNA = transfer RNA; PM = polymyositis; DM = dermatomyositis

or myositis-associated autoantibodies (MAAs). Enzyme-linked immunosorbent assay (ELISA), double immunodiffusion, and immunoblot methods can be used to confirm and quantitate these myositis autoantibodies. **Table 20-4** lists the various types of myositis-specific and myositis-associated autoantibodies, their frequencies, HLA associations, and clinical disease characteristics.

Clinical and Prognostic Value of Myositis Autoantibodies

Myositis-specific autoantibodies occur in 25% to 40% of adult and pediatric patients. The targeted intracellular autoantigens involved in "translation-type" protein can inhibit, in vitro, the function of their respective target antigens. Tests for myositis-specific autoantibodies are useful because they help classify patients in groups sharing similar disease epidemiologic, immunogenetic, and prognostic features, and the antibody titers correlate with disease activities.[36,47–50,54–56] The three basic types of MSAs are

- Anti-tRNA synthetases
- Anti–signal recognition particle (anti-SRP)
- Anti–Mi-2, a cytoplasmic antigen

Anti-tRNA synthetase MSAs include histidine (anti–Jo-1), threonine (anti–PL-7), alanine (anti–PL-12), glycine (anti-EJ), and isoleucine (anti-OJ). Almost all patients with anti-tRNA synthetase autoantibodies share certain common clinical features designated as the "antisynthetase syndrome." This syndrome is characterized by interstitial lung fibrosis, erosive small joint arthritis, Raynaud's phenomenon, fever, and severe myalgia. Patients with these MSAs have a guarded prognosis, with a 5-year survival rate of around 70%; death is usually related to complications of pulmonary fibrosis.[4,36,49]

Anti-SRP MSAs are directed against the ribonucleoprotein complexes needed to escort and transport synthesized polypeptides to cytoplasmic endoplasmic reticulum. All patients (mostly black women) who test positive for these autoantibodies have acute disease onset, severe myositis, and frequent (at times fatal) cardiac arrhythmia or conduction defects. Such patients are resistant to steroid therapy, requiring cytotoxic agents for control of the clinical symptoms. Their 5-year survival rate is less than 25%.[5,36,54]

Anti–Mi-2 MSAs are directed against a complex of seven nuclear proteins. This type of MSA occurs exclusively in dermatomyositis patients with a "V and shawl" pattern skin rash and cuticle overgrowth. These patients respond to steroid therapy and usually have a good prognosis, with a 5-year survival rate of nearly 100%.[35,55,56]

There are four basic types of MAAs: anti–PM-Scl, anti-U_1RNP, anti-U_2RNP, and anti-Ku (see Table 22-4). Anti–SS-A/Ro, anti–SS-B/La, and anti-Sm antibodies also may be detected. This group of myositis patients usually have overlap myositis with concurrent scleroderma, systemic lupus erythematosus (SLE), or Sjögren's syndrome. Pulmonary fibrosis and hypertension can develop in MAA-positive patients, but the disease prognosis is usually better than that of MSA-positive patients.[51–53]

Although autoantibodies directed against endothelium, myosin, myoglobin, thyroglobulin, microsome, and rheumatoid factor can be detected in 5% to 10% of autoimmune myositis patients, their significance is unclear and may represent "epiphenomena" secondary to muscle damage.[4,46]

Muscle Biopsy Findings

The muscle biopsies from patients with autoimmune myositis show inflammatory mononuclear infiltrates accompanied by degenerative and regenerative changes. Immunostaining shows both CD4+ and CD8+ cells either surrounding or infiltrating endomysial and perivascular regions of necrotic and nonnecrotic muscle. Polymyositis muscle biopsies display prominent endomysial inflammatory patterns without perifascicular atrophy or vasculitis. In contrast, dermatomyositis muscle biopsies apparently show immune complex–type injury with perivascular and perifascicular inflammation, endothelial proliferation, intravascular deposits of membranolytic attack complex (MAC) components, and thrombus formation.[27–29,43,44,57]

The inclusion bodies that characterize the muscle biopsies from IBM patients are seen as vacuoles with small granules on cryostat sections stained with trichrome or hematoxylin-eosin and as whorls of membranous material or masses of tubulofilaments by electron microscopy. These inclusions have been interpreted as β-amyloid or prion-type filaments, but at present no viral nucleocapsid material has been identified.[59] Other studies have demonstrated ubiquitin immunoreactivity in these inclusion bodies. Up to 60% of IBM muscle biopsies do not have significant inflammatory or necrotic changes.[39,59,60]

Several studies[61–65] have shown that—except for IBM, which requires confirmation of inclusion bodies by electron microscopy—the information generated by laboratory tests and magnetic resonance imaging (MRI) is adequate to diagnose and classify autoimmune myositis without the need for muscle biopsy. In myositis, the creatine kinase–aminotransferase (CK:AST) ratio is always less than 40, in contrast to muscular dystrophy with a CK:AST ratio that is always greater than 40.[61,62] Magnetic resonance imaging can provide anatomic views of the involved muscle and delineate inflammatory patterns that correlate with clinical and laboratory parameters of disease activity. Moreover, magnetic resonance spectroscopy can estimate the levels of inorganic phosphate, phosphocreatine, and adenosine triphosphate (ATP), which are myositis markers.[63–65]

Additional Laboratory Tests for Monitoring Skeletal Muscle Diseases

Among the plethora of serum markers used to assess muscle damage, CK, aspartate transaminase (AST), myoglobin, and carbonic anhydrase III have been shown to be practical and useful biochemical markers for monitoring disease activities.[46,61]

Creatine kinase is increased 10 to 100 times in 75% to 95% of myositis patients. The MB isoenzymes of creatine kinase (CK-MB isozymes) from regenerating myoblasts usually comprise more than 2% of a patient's total CK. These enzyme increases usually precede disease flare-up by 1 to 2 months and decrease when therapy is effective. However, there may be 5% to 10% false-negative results due to a loss of muscle mass or circulating CK enzymatic inhibitors.[66,67]

Aspartate transaminase, although not specific for skeletal muscle, is a reliable indicator of muscle damage. In myositis, the CK:AST ratio is less than 40, whereas in muscular dystrophy, it is greater than 40, with a total CK almost always greater than 14,100 U/L.[61,62]

Myoglobins are oxygen-carrying proteins found only in heart and skeletal muscle. They are useful for assessment of disease activity and therapeutic effectiveness in myositis. However, patient blood samples need to be drawn at the same time of day to be useful for disease monitoring, because blood myoglobin level has a diurnal/circadian pattern.[68]

Carbonic anhydrase III (by radioimmunoassay) is a specific enzyme marker for skeletal muscle damage because it is not found in cardiac muscle. Myositis patients exhibit moderate increases in plasma, whereas muscular dystrophy patients have the highest.[69]

Creatine, produced in the liver, pancreas, and kidney for use as an energy source by muscle, is a helpful marker for differentiating steroid myopathy from myositis. Both serum and urine creatine levels are increased in patients with myositis, but only urine creatine levels are increased in those with steroid myopathy.[46,70]

Aldolase and lactate dehydrogenase (LDH) are not muscle-specific enzymes because they also increase with hemolysis and liver disease. Erythrocyte sedimentation rate (ESR) may be elevated in 50% of myositis patients but it does not correlate with disease activity.[35,46,61]

For juvenile myositis and dermatomyositis, which are usually associated with immune complex–mediated muscle damage, factor VIII–related antigen, antiendothelial antibody, thrombomodulin, and neopterin (indicators of vascular injury and activated mononuclear cells) may be helpful in assessing and monitoring disease activity.[71–74]

Other Diseases Mimicking Autoimmune Myositis

In evaluating patients for autoimmune myositis, several other types of myopathies need to be considered in the differential diagnosis.[60,75–80] The pertinent clinical and laboratory characteristics of these myopathies are described here.

Infectious Myositis

Bacterial myositis due to staphylococci, streptococci, *Yersinia*, or anaerobes is usually suppurative. Infected patients often are febrile and septic with neutrophilia and a very high ESR. The intramuscular abscesses often extend to and destroy the fascia. Lyme and legionnaires' diseases can trigger polymyositis-like symptoms, but affected patients usually do not have myositis autoantibodies.[75,76] Nevertheless, clinical and laboratory follow-ups are recommended.

Fungal myositis is often associated with prominent ischemic hemorrhagic muscle necrosis and vascular invasion by fungal hyphae or spores. This type of infection usually occurs in immunosuppressed patients.[60]

Parasitic myositis is usually associated with marked eosinophilia, fever, myalgia, and fatigue. Immunocompromised individuals are at risk for *Toxoplasma* myositis, whereas immunocompetent individuals may develop cysticercosis and trichinosis-associated myositis after ingestion of infected pork or beef products. Neurologic complications due to parasitic encystment in the brain can occur. These cysts eventually undergo calcific degeneration with seizure or "central nervous system mass effect" as consequences.[27,28,60]

Viral myositis due to coxsackievirus, echovirus, adenovirus, or influenza A or B virus can be complicated by severe muscle pain and swelling of the thigh and calf, or less often of the chest and abdomen. These symptoms may resolve in a few weeks without sequelae, but there may be rare fatal complications of rhabdomyolysis with myoglobulinuria or debilitating postviral chronic fatigue syndrome. Persistent enterovirus RNA has been demonstrated in affected muscle of some patients.[77–79]

Drug-, Toxin-, and Chemical-Induced Myositis

A distinct entity designated as eosinophilia-myalgia has been linked to the ingestion of contaminants in L-tryptophan, fatty acid anilides, and phenol-thiol compounds. The symptoms are diffuse muscle weakness, severe myalgia, edema to indurated skin, and blood eosinophilia. Muscle biopsies show prominent eosinophilic infiltration of endomysial, interstitial, and perivascular regions of muscle. Dermatomyositis-type fasciitis and skin rash also may occur.[80–82]

Leuprolide acetate used for prostate carcinoma treatment and D-penicillamine used to treat rheumatoid arthritis and Wilson's disease can induce polymyositis that regresses after drug withdrawal.[83–85] Ciguatera fish toxins cause polymyositis symptoms.[86] In certain genetically susceptible individuals, silicone and collagen implants may be associated with subacute myositis, but a direct causal relationship has not been established.[87,88]

Paraneoplastic (Cancer-Associated) Myopathies

Polymyositis, dermatomyositis, and other neuromyopathic paraneoplastic syndromes can occur in patients with carcinomas of the lung, gastrointestinal tract, prostate, breast, or ovary.[89–93] Autoantibodies to muscle antigens, including MSAs, may be present in a minority of cancer patients.[4,36,89] Some breast cancer patients may experience the diffuse, painful, tetanus-like, strychnine-type muscle spasm of stiff-man syndrome, associated with autoantibodies directed against amphiphysin, a postsynaptic vesicle membrane protein.[94] Close follow-up/monitoring of patients is recommended.

Systemic Autoimmune Diseases Associated With Myopathies

Patients with other systemic autoimmune diseases and vasculitides may have symptoms of myalgia and/or myositis. Muscle biopsies from patients with SLE or polyarteritis nodosa show fibrinoid necrosis of the vessel wall or transmural inflammatory disruption, usually with evidence of intravascular immunoglobulin and complement deposition.[95] Muscle biopsies from patients with polymyalgia rheumatica usually show type 2 fiber atrophy without significant inflammation. Muscle biopsies from patients with rheumatoid arthritis may have rheumatoid nodule–type inflammatory and fibrotic lesions in the perimysium.[28,96] Some patients with autoimmune myositis (most notably those older than 60 years) may have coexisting myasthenia gravis or other types of autoimmune diseases.[1,8,97]

Pathogenesis of Autoimmune Myositis

Role of Cytokines

Macrophages, effector T cells, and their associated cytokines such as interleukin (IL) 1, 2, and 8; tumor necrosis factor–alpha (TNF-α), and interferon gamma (IFN-γ) greatly affect and determine the severity of muscle damage in autoimmune myositis. These cytokines can induce the major histocompatibility complex (MHC) molecule and intercellular adhesion molecule (ICAM) expression on muscle and endothelial cells, so additional circulating immune cells can be recruited to sites of tissue inflammation and further expand muscle damage.[27,28,43–45]

Role of Genetic and Environmental Risk Factors

Genetic susceptibility plays a significant role in the development of autoimmune myositis. Numerous studies have reported increased familial incidence of these diseases, increased disease frequency in certain racial groups, and strong disease association with certain HLA antigens (eg, polymyositis with HLA-DR3, DRw5, and DQA1 0501; dermatomyositis with HLA-DR7, DRw53, and DQA1 0201; steroid-resistant polymyositis with HLA-DR5, DRw52, and DQA1 0301).[4,47]

Environmental events can affect the development of autoimmune myositis. This is evidenced by the clustering of anti–Jo-1–positive cases in spring and anti-SRP–positive cases in autumn; the acute onset of clinical disease during or following viral or bacterial illness; and the occurrence of subacute autoimmune myositis in genetically susceptible individuals after exposure to D-penicillamine, silicone, or collagen tissue implants.[36,54,80]

Summary

Myasthenia gravis, the prototype of autoimmune disease of neuromuscular junction, is associated with anti-AChR antibodies that may bind, block, and destroy postsynaptic AChRs and membranes. Assays to specify whether a given patient has binding-, blocking-, or modulating-type antibodies are useful because AChR-blocking and AChR-modulating antibodies correlate closely with disease activity. A positive anti-AChR antibody test confirms a diagnosis of MG, but a negative test does not exclude disease because 15% of MG patients (most notably neonatal and congenital MG) do not have detectable AChR antibodies. Five percent to 15% of patients with lung carcinoma and other autoimmune diseases have anti-AChR antibodies. Lambert-Eaton myasthenia syndrome needs to be considered in evaluating patients with symptoms of MG. Anti-VGCC autoantibody is a helpful marker for LEMS because it is present in more than 90% of lung cancer patients with LEMS but fewer than 5% of MG patients.[90]

Thymic hyperplasia is seen in 65% of MG patients; 15% of MG patients have thymoma. Antistriational or anti–ryanodine receptor antibodies are markers for thymoma-associated MG. The tests for these autoantibodies have low specificity because they are also found in lung cancer patients, patients treated with D-penicillamine, and bone marrow transplant recipients. They may be helpful markers for recurrence of thymoma after tumor resection. A negative result helps exclude the presence of thymoma.

Polymyositis and dermatomyositis are prototypes of autoimmune myositis, a necrotizing inflammatory myopathy. The most helpful laboratory tests for diagnosis are HEp-2 cell IFM-ANA and creatine kinase. Immunofluorescence tests are positive in 60% to 90% of affected patients who have myositis autoantibodies. Further testing by enzyme immunoassay, immunoprecipitation, or Western blot is needed to determine whether these autoantibodies are myositis specific or myositis associated. The test results can be useful, providing valuable guidelines for disease classification, choice of therapy, and prognosis (see Tables 20-3 and 20-4).

Elevated CK occurs in more than 90% of myositis patients, but 5% to 10% may have normal levels due to inhibitors in sera or chronic muscle atrophy. Other laboratory tests helpful for disease monitoring are creatine, myoglobin, white blood cell, and platelet counts. These parameters usually correlate with disease activity. Cytokine testing, when available for clinical use, is sensitive for active immune myocyte damage.

Several studies[61–65] have shown that—except in IBM, which requires electron microscopy to confirm inclusion bodies—the information generated by MRI and laboratory tests can adequately diagnose and classify autoimmune myositis without the need for muscle biopsy.

Current knowledge of skeletal muscle autoimmune diseases can be summarized as follows:

- Myasthenia gravis and autoimmune myositis occur in genetically susceptible individuals who are exposed to certain environmental risk factors such as drugs, toxins, or chemicals. Patients' HLA haplotypes apparently affect the clinical disease characteristics, types of autoantibodies produced, and disease prognosis (Table 20-4 and **Table 20-5**).
- D-Penicillamine can induce myasthenia gravis or autoimmune myositis in genetically susceptible patients, but the disease subsides on withdrawal of the drug.
- The neuromuscular junction damage in myasthenia gravis is autoantibody mediated. The myocytic damage in autoimmune polymyositis results from combined cytotoxic T cells and autoantibodies. The muscle injury in dermatomyositis is associated with ischemic-type necrosis caused by immune complex–mediated vasculitis.
- Myasthenia gravis and autoimmune myositis can coexist or overlap with other autoimmune diseases.

Table 20-5. HLA Associations in Myasthenia Gravis and Autoimmune Myositis[1,4,8,30,46,80]

HLA Antigens	MG	D-Pen MG	PM	D-Pen PM	RA	Healthy
A1	64	44	<1	38	38	42
B8*	54	22	43-61	23	36	28
B27	10	33	NA	0	8	4
DR1	20	73	NA	0	20	18
DR3	46	9	57-67	11	23	23
DR4	20	26	NA	78	67	32
A1, B8, DR3†	46	7	21	11	11	5-18
A2, B27, DR1‡	0	27	NA	0	<2	<1

Abbreviations: HLA = human leukocyte antigen; MG = myasthenia gravis; D-Pen MG = D-penicillamine-induced myasthenia gravis; PM = polymyositis; D-Pen PM = D-penicillamine-induced polymyositis; RA = rheumatoid arthritis.

**HLA-B8 has been associated with impaired nonspecific suppressor function and high-titer anti-AChR antibodies. HLA-B8 and DR3 antigens occur more often in patients with adult-onset polymyositis and dermatomyositis.*

†HLA-A1, B8, and DR3 supratypes are more closely associated with juvenile dermatomyositis.

‡HLA-A2, B27, and DR1 supratypes occur in the 1% of D-penicillamine-treated rheumatoid arthritis or Wilson's disease patients who develop MG with high-titer anti-AChR antibodies. MG symptoms and decreased anti-AChR titers after drug is withdrawn.

- Cancer-associated paraneoplastic neuromyopathies can mimic myasthenia gravis. Although LEMS is the most commonly cited example, thymoma-associated MG is also a paraneoplastic myasthenia syndrome with antistriational autoantibodies directed against thymic myoid cells but showing cross-reactivity with AChR epitopes.[90]
- Paraneoplastic autoimmune myositis symptoms can occur in up to 20% of patients with lung, gastrointestinal tract, prostate, breast, or ovary carcinoma as well as lymphoid malignancies. Awareness of these paraneoplastic myopathies is important because early detection may lead to effective treatment of the occult neoplasms and improved patient survival.

References

1. Dawkins RL, Garlepp MJ. Autoimmune diseases of muscle: Myasthenia gravis and myositis. In: Rose NR, Mackay IR, eds. *The Autoimmune Diseases*. New York, NY: Academic Press; 1985:591–615.
2. Medsger TA Jr, Dawson WN Jr, Masi AT. The epidemiology of polymyositis. *Am J Med*. 1970;48:715–723.
3. Oddis CV, Conte CG, Steen VD, et al. Incidence of polymyositis-dermatomyositis: A 20 year study of hospital diagnosed cases in Allegheny County, PA, 1963–1982. *J Rheumatol*. 1990;17:1329–1334.
4. Plotz PH. NIH Conference. Myositis: Immunologic contributions to understanding cause, pathogenesis, and therapy. *Ann Intern Med*. 1995;122:715–724.
5. Joffe MM, Love LA, Leff RL, et al. Drug therapy of the idiopathic inflammatory myopathies: Predictors of responses to prednisone, azathioprine, and methotrexate and a comparison of their efficacy. *Am J Med*. 1993;94:379–387.
6. Lopate G, Pestronk A. Autoimmune myasthenia gravis. *Hosp Pract (Off Ed)*. 1993;28:109–132.
7. Younger DS, Gordon PH. Diagnosis of neuromuscular diseases. *Neurol Clin*. 1996;14:135–159.
8. Newsom-Davis J, Vincent AC, Wilcox HNA. Autoimmune disorders of the neuromuscular junction. In: Lachmann PJ, Peters K, Rosen FS, et al, eds. *Clinical Aspects of Immunology*. Boston, MA: Blackwell Scientific; 1993:2091–2112.
9. Somnier FE. Clinical implementation of anti-acetylcholine receptor antibodies. *J Neurol Neurosurg Psychiatry*. 1993;56:496–504.
10. Lindstrom JM, Seybold ME, Lennon VA, et al. Antibody to acetylcholine receptor in myasthenia gravis: Prevalence, clinical correlates, and diagnostic value. *Neurology*. 1978;26:1054–1059.
11. Jacobson DM. Acetylcholine receptor antibodies in patients with Graves' ophthalmopathy. *J Neuroophthalmology*. 1995;15:166–170.
12. Smith CIE, Hammarstrom L, Lefvert AK, et al. Bone marrow grafting induces acetylcholine receptor antibody formation. *Lancet*. 1985;1:978.
13. Drachman DG, Adams RN, Josifek LF, et al. Functional activities of autoantibodies to AChR and the clinical severity of myasthenia gravis. *N Engl J Med*. 1982;307:769–775.
14. Drachman DB, Silva SD, Ramsay D, et al. Humoral pathogenesis of myasthenia gravis. *Ann N Y Acad Sci*. 1987;505:90–105.
15. Howard FM Jr, Lennon VA, Finley J, et al. Clinical correlations of antibodies that bind, block, or modulate human acetylcholine receptors in myasthenia gravis. *Ann N Y Acad Sci*. 1987;505:526–538.
16. Martino G, Twaddle G, Brambilla E. Detection of anti-acetylcholine receptor antibody by ELISA using human receptor from a rhabdomyosarcoma cell line. *Acta Neurol Scand*. 1994;89:218–222.
17. Steenkamp KJ, Duim W, Myer MS, et al. Measurement of anti-acetylcholine receptor autoantibodies in myasthenia gravis. *S Afr Med J*. 1995;85:1293–1294.
18. Wu JT, Astill M, Lloyd C, et al. Rhabdomyosarcoma cell line can be used for the isolation of soluble acetylcholine receptors and for assaying, blocking and modulating autoantibodies. *J Clin Lab Anal*. 1993;7:11–18.
19. Li Z, Forester N, Vincent A. Modulation of acetylcholine receptor function in TE671 (rhabdomyosarcoma) cells by non-AChR ligands: Possible relevance to seronegative myasthenia gravis. *J Neuroimmunol*. 1996;64:179–183.
20. Lutz CZ, Lu L, Hao ZS, et al. Antibody-secreting cells to AChR and to presynaptic membrane receptor in seronegative myasthenia gravis. *J Neuroimmunol*. 1993;43:145–149.
21. Ckikes N, Momoi MY, Williams CL, et al. Striational autoantibodies: Quantitative detection by enzyme immunoassay in myasthenia gravis, thymoma, and recipients of D-Penicillamine or allogeneic bone marrow. *Mayo Clin Proc*. 1988;63:474–481.
22. Kuks JB, Limburg PC, Horst G, et al. Antibodies to skeletal muscle in myasthenia gravis, Part 3: Relation with clinical course and therapy. *J Neurol Sci*. 1993;120:168–173.
23. Mygland A, Tysnes OE, Matre R, et al. Anti-cardiac ryanodine receptor antibodies in thymoma-associated myasthenia gravis. *Autoimmunity*. 1994;17:327–331.

24. Mygland A, Aarli JA, Matre R, et al. Ryanodine receptor antibodies related to severity of thymoma associated myasthenia gravis. *J Neurol Neurosurg Psychiatry*. 1994;57:843–846.

25. Hohlfeld R, Engel AG. The immunobiology of muscle. *Immunol Today*. 1994;15:269–274.

26. Maselli RA. Pathophysiology of myasthenia gravis and Lambert-Eaton syndrome. *Neurol Clin*. 1994;12:285–292.

27. Dalakas MC. Immunopathogenesis of inflammatory myopathies. *Ann Neurol*. 1995;37:S74–S86.

28. Kalovidouris AE. Mechanisms of inflammation and histopathology in inflammatory myopathy. *Rheum Dis Clin North Am*. 1994;20:881–897.

29. Oxenhandler R, Adelstein EH, Hart MN. Immunopathology of skeletal muscle. The value of direct immunofluorescence in the diagnosis of connective tissue diseases. *Hum Pathol*. 1977;8:322–328.

30. Lennon VA, Lambert EH. Autoantibodies bind solubilized calcium channel ω-conotoxin complexes from small cell lung carcinoma: A diagnostic aid for Lambert-Eaton myasthenia syndrome. *Mayo Clinic Proc*. 1989;64:1498–1504.

31. Merrill JE, Graves MC, Mulder DG. Autoimmune disease and the nervous system: Biochemical, molecular, and clinical update. *West J Med*. 1992;156:639–646.

32. Spurkland A, Gilhus NE, Ronningen KS, et al. Myasthenia gravis patients with thymic hyperplasia and myasthenia gravis patients with thymoma display different HLA associations. *Tissue Antigens*. 1991;37:90–93.

33. DeBates M, Vincent A. Myasthenia gravis. In: Bona CS, Siminovitch KA, Zanetti M, et al, eds. *The Molecular Pathology of Autoimmune Diseases*. San Francisco, CA: Academic Press; 1993:541–553.

34. Hohlfeld R, Wekerle H. The thymus in myasthenia gravis. *Neurol Clin*. 1994;12:331–342.

35. Rider LG, Miller FW. New perspectives on the idiopathic inflammatory myopathies of childhood. *Curr Opin Rheumatol*. 1994;6:575–582.

36. Miller FW. Myositis-specific autoantibodies: Touchstones for understanding the inflammatory myopathies. *JAMA*. 1993;270:1846–1849.

37. Chou DM. Myxovirus-like structures in a case of human chronic polymyositis. *Science*. 1967;158:1453–1455.

38. Carpenter S, Karparti G, Heller I, et al. Inclusion body myositis: A distinct variety of idiopathic inflammatory myositis. *Neurology*. 1987;28:8–17.

39. Dalakas MC. Polymyositis, dermatomyositis, and inclusion body myositis. *N Engl J Med*. 1991;325:1487–1498.

40. Hewlett RH, Brownell B. Granulomatous myopathy: Its relationship to sarcoidosis and polymyositis. *J Neurol Neurosurg Psychiatry*. 1975;38:1090–1099.

41. Heffner RR, Barron SA. Polymyositis beginning as a focal process. *Arch Neurol*. 1981;38:439–442.

42. Noel E, Tebib J, Walch G, et al. Focal myositis: A pseudotumoral form of polymyositis. *Clin Rheumatol*. 1991;10:333–338.

43. Targoff IN. Immune manifestations of inflammatory muscle disease. *Rheum Dis Clin North Am*. 1994;20:857–880.

44. Karparti G, Pouliot Y, Carpenter S. Expression of immunoreactive MHC products in human skeletal muscle. *Ann Neurol*. 1988;23:64–72.

45. Miller FW, Love LA, Barbieri SA, et al. Lymphocyte activation markers in idiopathic myositis: Changes with disease activity and differences among clinical and autoantibody subgroups. *Clin Exp Immunol*. 1990;81:373–379.

46. Rider LG, Miller FW. Laboratory evaluation of the inflammatory myopathies. *Clin Diagn Lab Immunol*. 1995;2:1–9.

47. Miller FW. Humoral immunity and immunogenetics in the idiopathic inflammatory myopathies. *Curr Opin Rheumatol*. 1991;3:902–910.

48. Gurley RC, Love LA, Targoff IN, et al. Association among myositis specific autoantibodies (MSAs) and HLA-DQA1 alleles. *Arthritis Rheum*. 1991;34(suppl): S137.

49. Targoff IN, Trieu EP, Plotz PH, et al. Antibodies to glycyl-transfer RNA synthetase in patients with myositis and interstitial lung disease. *Arthritis Rheum*. 1992;35:821–830.

50. Miller FW, Twitty SA, Biswas T, et al. Origin and regulation of a disease-specific autoantibody response: Antigenic epitope, spectrotype stability, and isotype restriction of anti-Jo-1 autoantibodies. *J Clin Invest*. 1990;85:468–475.

51. Oddis CV, Okano Y, Rudert WA, et al. Serum autoantibody to the nucleolar antigen PM-Scl: Clinical and immunogenetic associations. *Arthritis Rheum*. 1992;35:1217.

52. Baszczyk M, Jabonska S, Szymanska-Jagieo W, et al. Childhood scleromyositis: An overlap syndrome associated with PM-Scl antibody. *Pediatr Dermatol*. 1991;8:1–8.

53. Isern RA, Yaneva M, Weiner E, et al. Autoantibodies in patients with primary pulmonary hypertension: Association with anti-Ku. *Am J Med*. 1992;93:307–312.

54. Leff RL, Burgess SH, Miller FW, et al. Distinct seasonal pattern in the onset of adult idiopathic inflammatory myopathy in patients with anti-Jo-1 and anti-SRP autoantibodies. *Arthritis Rheum*. 1991;34:1391–1396.

55. Pachman L. Inflammatory myopathy in children. *Rheum Dis Clin North Am*. 1994;20:919–943.

56. Love LA, Leff RL, Fraser DD, et al. A new approach to the classification of idiopathic inflammatory myopathy: Myositis-specific autoantibodies define useful homogeneous patient groups. *Medicine*. 1991;70:360–374.

57. Kissel JT, Mendell JR, Rammohan KW. Microvascular deposition of complement membrane attack complex (MAC) in dermatomyositis. *N Engl J Med.* 1986;314:329–334.

58. Emslie-Smith AM, Engel AG. Microvascular changes in early and advanced dermatomyositis: A quantitative study. *Ann Neurol.* 1990;27:343–356.

59. Askanas V, Engel WK, Alvarez RB. Light and EM localization of beta-amyloid protein in muscle biopsies of patients with inclusion body myositis. *Am J Pathol.* 1992;141:31–36.

60. Heffner RR. Inflammatory myopathies: A review. *J Neuropathol Exp Neurol.* 1993;52:339–350.

61. Bohlmeyer TJ, Wu AHB, Perryman MB. Evaluation of laboratory tests as a guide to diagnosis and therapy of myositis. *Rheum Dis Clin North Am.* 1994;20:845–856.

62. Hood D, Van Lente F, Estes M. Serum enzyme alterations in chronic muscle disease: A biopsy-based diagnostic assessment. *Am J Clin Pathol.* 1991;95:401–407.

63. Fraser DD, Frank JA, Dalakas M, et al. Magnetic resonance imaging in the idiopathic inflammatory myopathies. *J Rheumatol.* 1991;18:1693–1700.

64. Hernandez RJ, Sullivan DB, Chenevert TL, et al. Magnetic resonance imaging in children with dermatomyositis: Musculoskeletal findings and correlation with clinical laboratory findings. *Am J Roentgenol.* 1993;161:359–366.

65. Park JH, Vital TL, Ryder M, et al. Magnetic resonance imaging and P-31 magnetic resonance spectroscopy provide unique quantitative data useful in the longitudinal management of patients with dermatomyositis. *Arthritis Rheum.* 1994;37:736–746.

66. Gran J, Myklebust G, Johansen S. Adult idiopathic polymyositis without elevation of CK: Case report and review of literature. *Scand J Rheumatol.* 1993;22:94–96.

67. Kagen LJ, Aram S. Creatine kinase activity inhibitor in sera from patients with muscle disease. *Arthritis Rheum.* 1987;30:213–217.

68. Bombardieri SA, Clerico L, Riente MG, et al. Circadian variations of serum myoglobin levels in normal subjects and patients with polymyositis. *Arthritis Rheum.* 1982;25:1419–1424.

69. Oht M, Itagaki Y, Itoh N, et al. Carbonic anhydrase III in serum in muscular dystrophy and other related neurological disorders: Relationship with creatine kinase. *Clin Chem.* 1991;36:36–39.

70. Askari A, Vignos PJ Jr, Moskowitz RW. Steroid myopathy in connective tissue disease. *Am J Med.* 1976;61:485–492.

71. Guzman J, Petty RE, Malleson PN. Monitoring disease activity in juvenile dermatomyositis: The role of von Willebrand factor and muscle enzymes. *J Rheumatol.* 1994;21:739–743.

72. Ohdama S, Takano S, Miyake T, et al. Plasma thrombomodulin as a marker of vascular injuries in collagen vascular disease. *Am J Clin Pathol.* 1994;101:109–113.

73. DeBenedetti F, DeAmici L, Aramini N, et al. Correlation of serum neopterin concentration with disease activity in juvenile dermatomyositis. *Arch Dis Child.* 1993;69:232–235.

74. Stein DP, Jordan SC, Toyoda O, et al. Anti–endothelial cell antibodies in dermatomyositis. *Neurology.* 1993;43:A356.

75. Christin L, Saosi GA. Pyomyositis in North America: Case reports and review. *Clin Infect Dis.* 1992;15:668–677.

76. Muller-Felber W, Reimer CD, de Koning J, et al. Myositis in Lyme borreliosis: An immunochemical study of seven patients. *J Neurol Sci.* 1993;118:207–212.

77. Sowa JM. Human T lymphotropic virus, myelopathy, polymyositis, and synovitis: An expanding rheumatic spectrum. *J Rheumatol.* 1992;19:316–318.

78. Archard LC, Bowle NE, Behan PO, et al. Postviral fatigue syndrome: Persistent enterovirus RNA in muscle and elevated creatine kinase. *J R Soc Med.* 1988;81:326–329.

79. Gold D, Bowden R, Sixbey J, et al. Chronic fatigue: A prospective clinical and virologic study. *JAMA.* 1991;264:48–53.

80. Miller FW. Noninfectious environmental agents associated with myopathies. *Curr Opin Rheumatol.* 1993;5:712–718.

81. Kamb ML, Murphy JJ, Jones JL, et al. Eosinophilia-myalgia syndrome in L-tryptophan exposed patients. *JAMA.* 1992;267:77–82.

82. Lin JD, Phelps RG, Gordon ML, et al. Pathologic manifestations of the eosinophilia-myalgia syndrome: Analysis of 11 cases. *Hum Pathol.* 1992;23:429–437.

83. Crayton H, Bohlmann T, Sufit R, et al. Drug-induced polymyositis secondary to leuprolide acetate (Lupron) therapy for prostate carcinoma. *Clin Exp Rheumatol.* 1991;9:525–528.

84. Christensen PD, Sorensen KE. Penicillamine-induced polymyositis with complete heart block. *Eur Heart J.* 1989;10:1041–1044.

85. Taneja V, Mehra N, Singh TN, et al. HLA-D region gene and susceptibility to D-Penicillamine-induced myositis. *Arthritis Rheum.* 1990;33:1445–1447.

86. Stommel EW, Parsonnet J, Jenkyn LR. Polymyositis after ciguatera toxin exposure. *Arch Neurol.* 1991;48:874–877.

87. Cukier J, Beauchamp RA, Spindler JS, et al. Association between bovine collagen dermal implants and a dermatomyositis or a polymyositis-like syndrome. *Ann Intern Med.* 1993;118:920–928.

88. Love LA, Weiner SR, Vasey FB, et al. Clinical and immunogenetic features of women who develop myositis after silicone implants. *Arthritis Rheum.* 1992;35:S46. [Abstract]

89. Callan JP. Relationship of cancer to inflammatory muscle diseases: Dermatomyositis, polymyositis, and IBM myositis. *Rheum Dis Clin North Am*. 1994;20:93–153.

90. Sherry DD, Haas JE, Milstein JM. Childhood myositis as a paraneoplastic phenomenon. *Pediatr Neurol*. 1993;9:155–156.

91. Sakon M, Monden M, Fujimoto Y, et al. Gastric carcinoma associated with dermatomyositis. *Acta Chir Scand*. 1989;155:365–366.

92. Pelucchi A, Ciceri E, Clementi F, et al. Calcium channel autoantibodies in myasthenia syndrome and small cell lung cancer. *Am Rev Resp Dis*. 1993;147: 1229–1232.

93. Lennon VA. Serological diagnosis of myasthenia gravis and the Lambert-Eaton myasthenia syndrome. In: Lisak RP, ed. *Handbook of Myasthenia Gravis and Myasthenic Syndromes*. New York, NY: Marcel Dekker; 1994:149–164.

94. Camilli PD, Thomas A, Roxanne C, et al. The synaptic vesicle-associated protein amphiphysin is the 128-kD autoantigen of stiff-man syndrome with breast cancer. *J Exp Med*. 1992;178:2219–2223.

95. Foote RA, Kimbrough SM, Stevens JC. Lupus myositis. *Muscle Nerve*. 1982;5:65–68.

96. Brooke MH, Kaplan H. Muscle pathology in RA, polymyalgia rheumatica, and polymyositis. A histochemical study. *Arch Pathol*. 1972;94:101–118.

97. Plotz PH, Dalakas M, Leff RL, et al. Current concept in the idiopathic inflammatory myopathies: Polymyositis, dermatomyositis, and related disorder. *Ann Intern Med*. 1989;111:143–157.

CHAPTER 21

Autoimmune Paraneoplastic Syndromes of the Central Nervous System

Robert M. Nakamura, MD, and LeMing Hang, MD

Autoimmune paraneoplastic syndromes (APSs) are clinical manifestations of autoimmune tissue injuries caused by neoplasms in which the sites of autoimmune organ/tissue damage are separate from the primary malignant tumor. The clinical symptoms of these syndromes are diverse; they can present as central nervous system degeneration, sensorimotor dysfunction, and various types of systemic autoimmune diseases.[1–3] Several organ-specific autoantibodies against neuronal and muscle antigens have been identified as serologic markers of these disorders.[1–10] The tumor antigens that stimulate production of paraneoplastic autoimmune antibodies may act as a co-immunogenic macromolecular complex of nuclear, cytoplasmic, and plasma membranes.[11–17]

Central nervous system (CNS) autoimmune paraneoplastic syndromes are found most frequently in patients with carcinomas of the lung, reproductive organs, and breast. In 50% to 66% of patients, the neurologic symptoms precede clinical detection of malignancy by several months to years. Other neoplasms that may be associated with CNS autoimmune paraneoplastic syndromes are Hodgkin's disease; childhood neuroblastomas; and occasional carcinomas of the colon, prostate, thymus, or thyroid.[2–10] The consequences of CNS autoimmune paraneoplastic syndromes are devastating to the patient, because the brain tissue damage is often irreversible. Symptoms can range from memory loss, ataxia, cerebellar degeneration, and encephalomyelitis to opsoclonus, myoclonus, sensorimotor deficits, painful tetanus-type motor rigidity, or myasthenia gravis–like muscle weakness. Yet, despite the permanent CNS tissue damage, rare patients experience spontaneous tumor regression, indicating the presence of concurrent "pathologic autoimmunity" and antitumor immunity.

Autoantibodies associated with CNS autoimmune paraneoplastic syndromes were first noted in 1965 when antineuronal antibodies were detected by immunofluorescence testing of sera from lung carcinoma patients with sensory neuropathy.[2] Subsequent studies gave evidence of in situ intrathecal antineuronal antibody synthesis in cancer patients with CNS autoimmune paraneoplastic syndromes.[12–14]

This chapter reviews the classifications of CNS autoimmune paraneoplastic syndromes, the types of APS-associated antineuronal antibodies, and the sites of CNS tissue damage and underlying malignancies; laboratory testing for APS-associated antineuronal antibodies; guidelines for interpreting antibody test results; and clinical and laboratory guidelines for managing patients with either neurologic or laboratory findings of possible CNS autoimmune paraneoplastic syndrome. The interrelationship of tumor immunity, autoimmunity, and immunopathogenesis of CNS autoimmune paraneoplastic syndromes also is discussed.

Classification of Autoimmune Paraneoplastic Syndromes

Central nervous system APSs can be classified into 5 distinct groups, according to specific neurologic symptoms, associated malignancies, onconeuronal autoantigens, autoantibodies, and patterns of CNS tissue injury.[15] The characteristic features of each of these 5 groups are listed in **Table 21-1**.

Paraneoplastic Cerebellar Degeneration

Paraneoplastic cerebellar degeneration is characterized by cerebellar dysfunction with superimposed encephalomyelopathic signs of lethargy, memory loss, bulbar palsy, and limb weakness. This condition is most frequently associated with small cell lung carcinoma and gynecologic malignancies. In more than 50% of cancer patients, paraneoplastic cerebellar degeneration symptoms may precede clinical detection of a tumor by several months to 5 years. The 2 antineuronal antibodies implicated in paraneoplastic cerebellar degeneration are anti-Yo (Purkinje's cell cytoplasmic antibody [PCA-1]) and anti-Hu (antineuronal nuclear antibody type 1 [ANNA-1]), named after the 2 patients in whom these autoantibodies were first detected.[16,17] Although the clinical manifestations of patients who are positive for anti-Yo and anti-Hu are those of cerebellar degeneration, the histopathology of CNS tissue injury is different.[12,15,18]

Anti-Yo antibodies apparently occur only in women; affected patients usually have müllerian/ovarian (75%) or breast (21%) carcinomas. The Yo antigens are 34- and 62-kd Purkinje's cell cytoplasmic regulatory proteins encoded by genes located near the fragile site of the X chromosome[19] (**Image 21-1**). The CNS histopathologies seen in anti-Yo–positive paraneoplastic cerebellar degeneration patients are characterized by extensive Purkinje's cell destruction with 50% to 100% neuron cell loss but minimal to no inflammatory infiltrates.[20]

Anti-Hu antibodies occur in both men and women with small cell lung carcinoma (>80%). The

Table 21-1. Classification of Autoimmune Paraneoplastic Syndromes, Associated Onconeuronal Autoantibodies, and Malignancies

Type of Syndrome (Neurologic Signs)	Associated Autoantibody (% False Positive)	Associated Malignancies (Frequency)
PCD/PEM/SN (cerebellar degeneration, encephalomyelitis, sensory neuropathy)	Anti-Hu (none) Anti-Yo (7%)	Small cell lung cancer (>80%) Gynecologic/müllerian cancer (74%) Breast cancer (20%)
Adult POMA (opsoclonus, myoclonus, ataxia)	Anti-Ri (none)	Breast and gynecologic cancer (>75%) Other sites (13%)
Stiff man syndrome associated with PND (tetanuslike muscle spasm and rigidity)	Antiamphiphysin (none known)	Breast cancer (most often), lung and colon cancer, Hodgkin's disease, thymoma
Lambert-Eaton myasthenia syndrome	Anti-P/Q-type VGCC (<10%)	Lung cancer, all types (65%)
Carcinoma-related retinopathy (blindness)	Antienolase and antirecoverin (none known)	Cancer of the lung, breast, gastrointestinal tract, or genitourinary tract (no predominant tumor type)

Abbreviations: PCD = paraneoplastic cerebellar degeneration; PEM = paraneoplastic encephalomyelitis; PND = paraneoplastic neurologic disorders; SN = sensory neuropathy; POMA = paraneoplastic opsoclonus-myoclonus ataxia; VGCC = voltage-gated calcium channel; CNS = central nervous system.

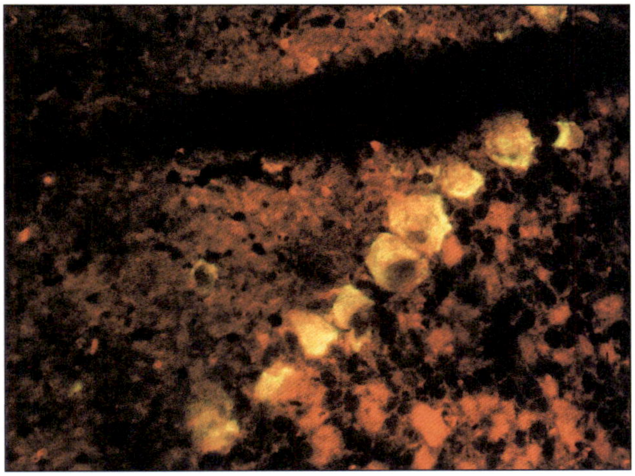

Image 21-1. Purkinje cell antibodies (Yo). Coarse granular cytoplasmic fluorescence in the Purkinje cells using tissue from human cerebellum. Yo antibodies occur in paraneoplastic cerebellar degeneration, which most often accompanies gynecological cancers, and is also seen in breast cancer and lung cancers. (Reproduced with permission from Krapf AR, von Mühlen CA, Krapf FE, Nakamura RM, Tan EM. *Atlas of Immunofluorescent Autoantibodies*. Baltimore, MD: Urban & Schwarzenberg; 1996:119.)

Hu antigens are 34- to 40-kd neuronal nuclear RNA–binding proteins that regulate the posttranscriptional processing of genes necessary for neuron maturation and maintenance.[21] Moreover, approximately 15% of anti-Hu–positive cancer patients have not only cerebellar dysfunction but also signs of multisystem neuronal degeneration such as polyneuritis, sensorimotor dysfunction, and enteric pseudoobstruction.[22,23] In contrast to anti-Yo–positive paraneoplastic degeneration women in whom CNS tissue destruction is limited to cerebellar Purkinje's cells with minimal lymphocytic infiltrates, the CNS tissue destruction in anti-Hu–positive patients is diffuse and multifocal with neuronal loss in the cerebrum, cerebellum, brain stem, spinal cord, dorsal roots, and autonomic ganglia and is accompanied by prominent perivascular and leptomeningeal lymphocytic infiltrates.[24]

Paraneoplastic Opsoclonus-Myoclonus Ataxia

Paraneoplastic opsoclonus-myoclonus ataxia (POMA) is characterized by brain stem, spinal cord, and cerebellar dysfunction with neurologic symptoms of opsoclonus ("dancing eye movements"), myoclonus, and ataxia. Adult patients with POMA usually have carcinoma of the breast (75%) as well as other sites (13%). The implicated autoantibody is anti-Ri (antineuronal nuclear antibody type 2 [ANNA-2]),[16,17] again named after the patient in whom it was first detected.[25,26] The Ri onconeuronal antigens are 55- to 61-kd and 79- to 84-kd neuronal RNA-binding proteins expressed by tumor and CNS neuronal cells.[25,26]

Paraneoplastic opsoclonus-myoclonus ataxia can be found in 2% to 3% of children with neuroblastomas. These patients have predominantly paraneoplastic opsoclonus symptoms and a good prognosis.[27] In contrast to adults with POMA, childhood neuroblastoma patients do not have detectable anti-Ri antibodies. Nevertheless, the opsoclonus and related neurologic symptoms respond dramatically to adrenocorticotropic hormone and immunosuppressive agents such as corticosteroids and cyclophosphamide. Moreover, the neuroblastomas in these patients show a higher incidence of spontaneous tumor regression or maturation to ganglioneuromas.[11,15]

Paraneoplastic Stiff-Man Syndrome

Paraneoplastic stiff-man syndrome is characterized by sustained muscle spasm at rest (resembling tetanus or strychnine poisoning), accompanied by fever and respiratory difficulties. This syndrome occurs most often in patients with breast carcinoma; other associated malignancies are lung and gastrointestinal tract adenocarcinomas, Hodgkin's disease, and (rarely) thymoma. The implicated autoantibody is antiamphiphysin. Amphiphysins are 128-kd synaptic membrane proteins, and the respective autoantibodies are thought to cause the painful tetanuslike muscle spasms by preventing the inhibitory synaptic functions of motor neurons.[28] Plasmapheresis, corticosteroids, and diazepam are used to relieve the muscle spasms and painful rigidity.[12,15]

Stiff-man syndrome also occurs in patients without cancer who have diabetes mellitus, hyperthyroidism, hypopituitarism, or epilepsy. Autoantibodies reactive with glutamic acid decarboxylase, not amphiphysin, are found in patients of this group.[29]

Lambert-Eaton Myasthenia Syndrome

Lambert-Eaton myasthenia syndrome (LEMS) is characterized by proximal muscle weakness, ptosis, dry mouth, anhidrosis, hyporeflexia, and constipation. Approximately 60% of LEMS patients harbor small cell lung carcinoma, while the remaining 40% have "hereditary LEMS" without carcinoma. In patients with malignancy-associated LEMS, the neurologic symptoms can precede clinical diagnosis of tumor by up to 5 years. The implicated antineuronal autoantibody is anti–voltage-gated calcium channel (VGCC). This is a presynaptic neuromuscular junction membrane particle antigen expressed by the patient's neuron and tumor cells. Voltage-gated calcium channel particles are needed for coupling of the depolarization to release acetylcholine. These VGCC autoantibodies apparently bind and deplete VGCC particles at the presynaptic membrane active zone, causing impaired calcium transport and decreased acetylcholine release to muscle end plates.[15,30]

Carcinoma-Associated Retinopathy

Carcinoma-associated retinopathy is an autoimmune retinopathy characterized by vision loss, abnormal electroretinography, and histologic evidence of photoreceptor cell depletion. Carcinoma-related retinopathy is associated with lung, breast, bladder, prostate, gastrointestinal tract, or salivary gland malignancies. The implicated autoantibodies are antienolase and antirecoverin, which are glycolic enzymes and proteins found in both patient tumor and retinal photoreceptor cells. These enzymatic proteins participate in the cyclic guanosine monophosphate signal transduction cascade of photoreceptors, and the respective autoantibodies apparently disrupt the phototransduction signaling pathway, causing photoreceptor cell degeneration. Other types of unidentified antiretinal antibodies also may be present and contribute to the retinopathy.[31,32]

Laboratory Testing for Autoimmune Paraneoplastic Syndrome Antineuronal Antibodies

The antineuronal nuclear and cytoplasmic autoimmune antibodies of defined specificities are readily identifiable by indirect immunofluorescence microscopy (IIFM). The interference by non–organ-specific autoimmune antibodies is eliminated by preliminary absorption of diluted sera with a homogenate of nonneural tissue and use of a composite block of neural and nonneural tissue sections as substrates.[16,17]

Serologic assessment by Western blot using native or recombinant neuronal proteins can be used as a primary or secondary confirmatory assay. However, IIFM results are sufficient for diagnosis, and the Western blot tests may be required only in unusual circumstances when IIFM results are uninterpretable due to interference by high-titer non–organ-specific autoimmune antibodies.[30]

The neuronal calcium channel binding antibodies are usually detected by radioimmunoprecipitation of detergent-solubilized synaptic membrane proteins complexed with the appropriate iodine 125–labeled ligand.[30]

Most APS-associated antineuronal antibodies, such as anti-Hu, anti-Ri, anti-Yo, and antiamphiphysin can be detected by evaluation of IIFM staining patterns (**Images 21-2** to **21-5**). The absorption of patient sera with nonneural tissue homogenate and the use of a composite block of neural-nonneural tissue as substrate are necessary to produce reliable IIFM results.[18] Western blot assays also are available and may be preferred as more specific and sensitive methods for the detection of APS-associated autoantibodies. These assays tend to avoid the false-positive results that occur with IIFM due to interferences by other types of autoantibodies in patients with concurrent systemic autoimmune diseases.[16,17,33,34]

Anti-VGCC antibodies are detected by immunoprecipitation of detergent-solubilized synaptic membrane proteins complexed with appropriate radioactive ligand.[30] The 3 different VGCC antigens—designated P/Q, N, and L subtypes—are based on DNA sequences of alpha-1 subunits. Each VGCC subtype has its distinct electrophysiologic neurotoxic peptide-binding properties and various roles in neurotransmitter release, membrane voltage sensing, and regulating apoptosis. Thus, the respective autoantibodies—designated anti-P/Q–type, anti-N–type, and anti-L–type VGCC—have different effects on cell survival. Enzyme-linked immunosorbent assay (ELISA) and immunoblot for these anti-VGCC antibody subtypes are commercially available.[16,17,35]

Antienolase and antirecoverin antibodies associated with carcinoma-related retinopathy can be detected by either ELISA or immunoblot.

Because a "positive" result for autoimmune paraneoplastic syndrome autoantibody implies the presence of malignancy, testing should be done by reliable reference laboratories with expertise, such as Mayo Clinic or Sloan-Kettering Cancer Center. Moreover, there should be timely, direct, and concise communication among the pathologist, the clinician, and the patient.

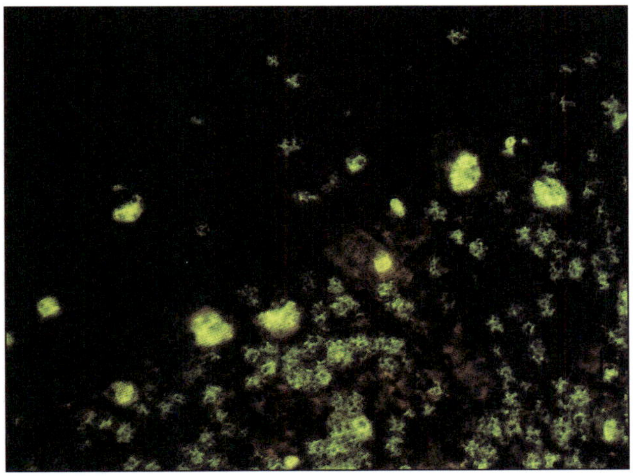

Image 21-2. Neuronal nuclear antibodies. This antibody is specific for neuronal nuclei, type II (Ri). There is irregular homogeneous nucleoplasmic staining of neuronal cells, with increased IgG staining at the peripheral portions of the neuronal nuclei. Human brain tissue. (Reproduced with permission from Krapf AR, von Mühlen CA, Krapf FE, Nakamura RM, Tan EM. *Atlas of Immunofluorescent Autoantibodies*. Baltimore, MD: Urban & Schwarzenberg; 1996:109.)

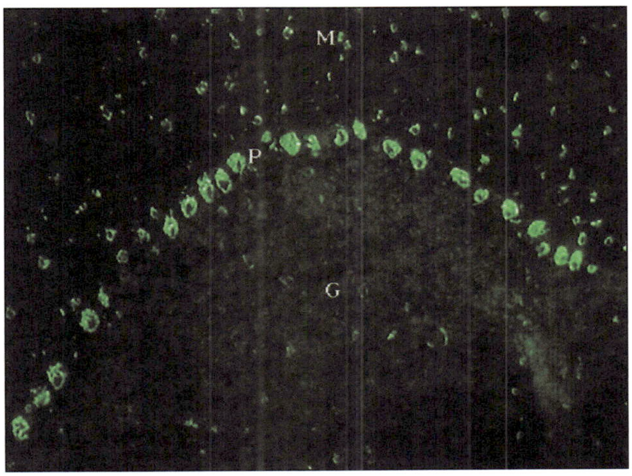

Image 21-3. Immunofluorescent staining pattern of anti-Yo (PCA-1) antibody. Note granular staining of cytoplasm of Purkinje's cells. Tissue is mouse cerebellar cortex. M = molecular layer, P = Purkinje's cell layer, G = granular layer. (Provided by Dr Vanda A. Lennon, Neuroimmunology Laboratory, Mayo Clinic, Rochester, MN; staining and photography performed by Ms Ann Schmeichel.)

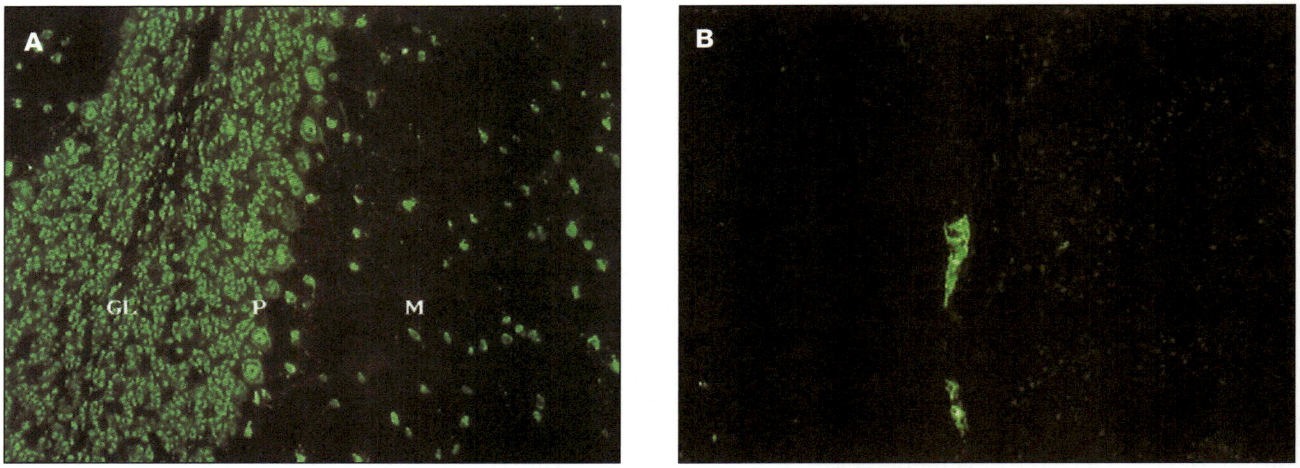

Image 21-4. Immunofluorescent staining pattern of anti-Hu (anti-neuronal nuclear antibody-1 [ANNA-1]) on mouse tissue. (**A**) Staining of ANNA-1 on section of mouse cerebellar cortex. Note irregular fine speckled staining of outer portions of neuronal cells in granular layer (GL). P = Purkinje's cell layer, M = molecular layer. (**B**) Staining of ANNA-1 mesenteric plexus of mouse. (Provided by Dr Vanda A. Lennon, Neuroimmunology Laboratory, Mayo Clinic, Rochester, MN; staining and photography performed by Ms Ann Schmeichel.)

Laboratory Interpretation of Autoimmune Paraneoplastic Syndrome Autoantibody Test Results

Clinical and Prognostic Significance of "Positive" versus "Negative" Results

Anti-Yo (high titer >1:1,000) is a useful and highly sensitive test for APSs in women because more than 90% of seropositive patients have müllerian-related or breast carcinomas. Rare association with salivary gland carcinoma has been reported. The genes coding for the Yo antigens are located in the X chromosome; thus, anti-Yo is rarely found in male cancer patients. The 7% false-positive rate (seropositive patients without tumor) may reflect microscopic tumor size or tumor regression because anti-Yo is apparently associated with effective antitumor immunity. More than 85% of anti-Yo–positive patients with gynecologic cancer have early stage tumors or limited metastasis[36–39] (Image 21-1, 21-3).

Anti-Hu (high titer >1:1,000) is a useful, highly specific marker for the presence of small cell lung carcinoma, because more than 80% of anti-Hu–positive patients with clinical signs of cerebellar degeneration have this malignancy.[15,18] Patients with gastrointestinal carcinoma, large cell lung carcinoma, and Hodgkin's disease may develop cerebellar and/or sensorimotor deficit symptoms without detectable anti-Hu antibodies.[40–44] These patients apparently have tumor cells that do not express major histocompatibility complex (MHC) class I or II molecules, but their clinical course is similar to that of seropositive patients.[15,31,45] Anti-Hu has occasionally been noted in children with neuroblastoma.[21] False-positive low-titer anti-Hu may occur when IIFM and ELISA are used. Immunoblot is the recommended confirmatory test.[37,40]

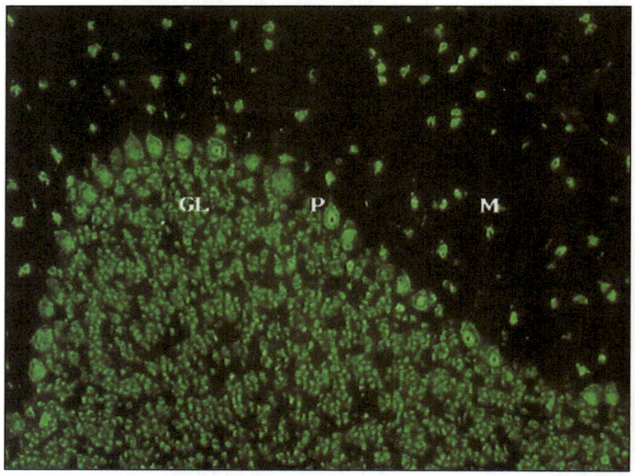

Image 21-5. Immunofluorescent staining pattern of anti-Ri (anti-neuronal nuclear antibody-2 [ANNA-2]). Staining of ANNA-2 autoantibody on mouse cerebellum In GL (granular layer) reveals a fine speckled staining of neuronal muclei. P = Purkinje's cell layer, M = molecular layer. (Provided by Dr Vanda A. Lennon, Neuroimmunology Laboratory, Mayo Clinic, Rochester, MN; staining and photography performed by Ms Ann Schmeichel.)

Anti-Ri (high titer >1:1,000) is useful for the evaluation of patients with POMA. This antibody test has high specificity (>90%) but only moderate sensitivity (40% to 60%). False negatives can occur. Thus, for individuals with risk factors (eg, family history) for breast or müllerian malignancies who present with POMA but no clinical tumor, meticulous gynecologic evaluation and close follow-up are recommended.[15,27]

High-titer anti-P/Q–type VGCC (>100 pmol/L) helps confirm the presence of LEMS-associated lung carcinoma, but low titers can be detected in 54% of patients with gynecologic malignancies, 24% of cancer patients without paraneoplastic syndromes, and up to 3% of noncancer patients with myasthenia gravis, scleroderma, or epilepsy.[30] When concurrent anti-P/Q–type VGCC antibodies are found in patients with other APS-associated antineuronal antibodies (anti-Hu, anti-Yo, or anti-Ri), the patients have neurologic symptoms of both LEMS and cerebellar degeneration. The LEMS symptoms can be ameliorated by plasmapheresis.[46–48]

Identification of high-titer anti-N–type VGCC supports a diagnosis of malignancy-related LEMS (test sensitivity, 73%) and helps rule out hereditary LEMS as well as neuropathies caused by chemotherapy. Thirty-six percent of anti-N–type VGCC–positive patients do not harbor malignancies. Anti-L–type VGCC antibodies are found in 75% of patients with sporadic amyotrophic lateral sclerosis; this antibody is not associated with malignancy.[16,17,30,35]

Antiamphiphysin, antienolase, and antirecoverin antibodies have high specificity but low sensitivity for their respective APSs. These are investigational tests.[29,31,32]

Currently, there are 2 major problems hindering accurate and meaningful interpretation of APS autoantibody test results:

- Laboratories do not use the same tissue test substrate antigens and procedures for IIFM. The criteria for interpretation of immunofluorescence staining patterns as positive or negative are not standardized.[16,17,49–51]
- Laboratories do not use the same terminology in naming the APS autoantibody.[17,49] For example, depending on the investigator's preference, anti-Yo may be referred to as APCA-1, anti-Hu as ANNA-1, and anti-Ri as anti-NOVA and/or ANNA-2.

A 1994 workshop conducted by the International Society of Neuroimmunology on paraneoplastic neurologic diseases held in the Netherlands proposed the following measures for resolution of these problems[51]:

- Use only human neuronal tissue for the preparation of test substrate.
- Adopt standardized procedures for end-point immunofluorescence staining and antigen purification.
- Perform both immunofluorescence screening and Western blot assay for all positive test results.
- Test samples within 2 days or keep the sample frozen until use.

The panel also explained that the terminology with numeric designations, such as ANNA-1, ANNA-2, and PCA-1, were originally based on the staining patterns seen with immunofluorescence/immunohistochemical assays. The terms "anti-Hu," "anti-Ri," and "anti-Yo" were based on determination by both immunohistochemistry and Western blot. These are only recommended guidelines; the ultimate decision as to the choice of assay methods for a specific test should be left to the experts in charge of the reference laboratory.

Clinical and Laboratory Guidelines for Evaluating Patients With Suspected Autoimmune Paraneoplastic Syndrome

Although most patients with APS already have irreversible CNS damage by the time of diagnosis, certain groups, such as adult patients with paraneoplastic stiff-man syndrome or POMA and children with paraneoplastic opsoclonus, benefit from plasmapheresis, corticosteroids, and cyclophosphamide with dramatic improvement of their neurologic symptoms.[15,52]

The following are recommended guidelines for evaluating patients who are positive for APS autoantibodies without clinically detectable malignancy.

Anti-Yo–Positive Patients

Concurrent high-titer anti-Yo antibodies and paraneoplastic cerebellar degeneration symptoms are diagnostic markers for gynecologic malignancies. Moreover, if only unrelated Yo-negative tumors are found in patients with anti-Yo, a search for Yo-positive tumors should continue with serum calcium 125 testing, computed tomography, or magnetic resonance imaging (MRI); endometrial sampling curettage; and repeat pelvic examination.[18,37,45] Female patients with cerebellar dysfunction and risk factors such as family history of breast or müllerian tumors may benefit from testing for anti-Yo antibodies.[40]

Anti-Hu–Positive Patients

Concurrent high-titer anti-Hu antibodies and paraneoplastic cerebellar degeneration are highly specific and sensitive markers for small cell lung carcinoma (>80%). Therefore, anti-Hu–positive adults with no obvious tumor need computed tomography and/or MRI of lung and mediastinal lymph nodes to search for such malignancy. Low-titer anti-Hu may be detected in patients with other carcinomas such as those of the colon or prostate, Hodgkin's disease, myxoid chondrosarcoma, and neuroblastoma; such patients usually do not have paraneoplastic cerebellar degeneration.[35,53]

Anti-Ri–Positive Patients

High-titer anti-Ri antibodies with POMA are useful markers for breast and müllerian carcinomas (>75%). Close follow-up of anti-Ri–positive patients without clinical evidence of tumor is indicated, because thus far no false-positive cases have been documented. Anti-Ri also may precede clinical tumor by months to years. In some patients, the tumor may be microscopic in size.[25]

Anti-P/Q–Type VGCC–Positive Patients

Because anti-P/Q–type VGCC (>100 pmol/L) is present in 60% of malignancy-related LEMS patients, detection of this autoantibody in asymptomatic individuals should lead to a search for lung, breast, or ovarian carcinoma, especially if the patient has risk factors, such as tobacco use or family members with these malignancies. It is important to note that false-negative cases may occur in immunosuppressed patients with occult tumor.[18,30,31]

Immunopathogenesis of Central Nervous System Autoimmune Paraneoplastic Syndromes

In most cases of CNS autoimmune paraneoplastic syndromes, the autoimmune responses appear to be directed against a single type of onconeuronal antigen and associated with a set of distinct neurologic symptoms. Thus, accurate classification of CNS signs and identification of APS-associated neuronal autoantibody types can often help predict the sites as well as the types of primary malignancy and the anatomic locations of CNS tissue damage.[32,37,54–56]

The APS-associated autoantibodies are believed to be genetically predetermined immunologic responses[15–17,30,32] because some patients whose tumors express similar onconeuronal antigens do not have detectable autoantibodies or clinical evidence of APS.[15,32]

Some APS-associated autoantibodies can suppress tumor growth; anti-Yo– and/or anti-Ri–positive patients may have localized tumors with limited staging and/or metastasis. Rare cases of tumors vanishing after the onset of neurologic diseases have been reported.

Based on these observations, it has been proposed that autoimmune paraneoplastic syndromes are initiated as appropriate antitumor immune responses; but in genetically susceptible patients with defects in cytokine regulation, aberrant MHC expression, or effector cell hyperactivity, these immune responses somehow progress to pathologic autoimmunity with clinical manifestations of neurologic diseases.[15,41]

Summary

Central nervous system APSs are autoimmune responses directed against onconeuronal antigens expressed by both normal neuronal and malignant tumor cells. Anti-Yo, anti-Hu, and anti-Ri are the most frequently encountered APS-associated autoantibodies.

The diagnostic value of a positive antineuronal antibody test in patients with APS is high, because the presence of underlying malignancy can be demonstrated in more than 90% of seropositive patients.[57] However, it is important to note that a negative test result does not exclude the presence of tumor. The incidence of false-negative results varies from 5% to 62%, depending on the clinical accuracy of APS classification as well as the patient's own environmental and genetic risk factors for the development of malignancy.

False-positive APS autoantibody immunofluorescence results are most likely due to inexperienced interpretation of staining patterns.[16,17,58] Investigators who have expertise in immunostaining and in-depth knowledge of the various types of APS-associated antineuronal antibodies feel that fewer than 15% of positive immunofluorescence results need Western blot confirmation. However, the consensus among participants in the 1994 workshop conducted by the International Society of Neuroimmunology on paraneoplastic neurologic diseases recommended both immunofluorescence/immunohistochemical and Western blot/immunoblot analysis for all patients who tested positive for APS autoantibody but in whom a clinical tumor could be demonstrated.[16,17,51]

Immunosuppressed patients may have false-negative antibody test results. Autoimmune paraneoplastic syndrome patients with Hodgkin's disease, non–small cell lung carcinomas, and gastrointestinal adenocarcinomas may have atypical antineuronal autoantibodies with different immunofluorescence and immunoblot patterns. It may be of interest that a 1991 survey of 150 patients with lung carcinoma found the APS prevalence rate to be approximately 4%, while 44% of these patients had neurologic symptoms related to neurotoxic chemotherapy agents, ischemic cerebrovascular disorders, or tumor metastasis.[59,60]

In conclusion, the development of CNS autoimmune paraneoplastic syndromes is a multistep autoimmune process that occurs in cancer patients who have a genetic susceptibility to immunologic defects of aberrant MHC expression as well as autoregulation of their immune effector cells and cytokines. These cellular and humoral immunoregulatory defects transform the initial appropriate physiologic immune responses against tumor cell antigens into pathologic autoimmune responses with the production of neuronal autoantibodies that apparently cause functional disruptions and permanent tissue damage of the central nervous system.

Autoimmune paraneoplastic syndrome neuronal autoantibodies can be of value in establishing the diagnosis of occult malignancies. The insights and knowledge gained from continued studies of APS will allow the design of tumor-specific immunotherapy that can intercept the irreversible autoimmune-mediated CNS tissue injury.

References

1. Zenone T. Autoimmunity and cancer: Paraneoplastic syndromes associated with small cell lung cancer. *Bull Cancer (Paris)*. 1992;79:837–853.
2. Wilkinson PC, Zeomski J. Immunofluorescent detection of antibodies against neurons in sensory carcinomatous neuropathy. *Brain*. 1965;88:529–538.
3. Graus F, Cordon-Cardo C, Posner JB. Demonstration of serum anti-Purkinje antibody in paraneoplastic cerebellar degeneration and preliminary antigen characterization. *Ann Neurol*. 1983;14:111. [Abstract]
4. Graus F, Elkon KB, Cordon-Cardo C, et al. Sensory neuronopathy and small cell lung carcinoma: Antineuronal antibody that also reacts with the tumor. *Am J Med*. 1986;80:45–52.
5. Steven MM, Mackay MR, Carnegie PR, et al. Cerebellar cortical degeneration with ovarian carcinoma. *Postgrad Med*. 1982;58:47–51.
6. Greenlee JE, Brashear HR. Antibodies to cerebellar Purkinje cells in patients with paraneoplastic cerebellar degeneration and ovarian carcinoma. *Ann Neurol*. 1983;14:609–613.
7. Dropcho EJ, Payne R. Paraneoplastic opsoclonus-myoclonus: Association with medullary thyroid carcinoma and review of the literature. *Arch Neurol*. 1986;43:410–415.
8. Baloh R, DeRossett S, Cloughesy T, et al. Novel brain stem syndrome associated with prostate carcinoma. *Neurology*. 1993;43:2591–2596.
9. Hammack JE, Kotanides H, Rosenblum MK, et al. Paraneoplastic cerebellar degeneration: Clinical and immunological findings in 21 patients with Hodgkin's disease. *Neurology*. 1992;42:1938–1943.
10. Kiessling LS, Marcotte AC, Culpepper L. Antineuronal antibodies in movement disorders. *Pediatrics*. 1993;92:39–43.
11. Fisher PG, Singer HS. Paraneoplastic opsoclonus with and without tumor. *Neurology*. 1995;45:1421–1426.
12. Merrill JE, Graves MC, Mulder DG. Autoimmune disease and the nervous system—Biochemical, molecular, and clinical update. *West J Med*. 1992;156:639–646.
13. Darnell RB, DeAngelis LM. Regression of small-cell lung carcinoma in patients with paraneoplastic neuronal antibodies. *Lancet*. 1993;341:21–22.
14. Furneaux HF, Reich L, Posner JB. Autoantibody synthesis in the CNS of patients with paraneoplastic syndromes. *Neurology*. 1990;40:1085–1091.
15. Dropcho EJ. Autoimmune central nervous system paraneoplastic disorders: Mechanisms, diagnosis, and therapeutic options. *Ann Neurol*. 1995;37(suppl 1):S102–S113.
16. Lennon VA. Views and reviews: Paraneoplastic autoantibodies: The case for a descriptive generic nomenclature. *Neurology*. 1994;44:2236–2240.
17. Lennon VA. Special correspondence: The case for a descriptive generic nomenclature: Clarification of immunostaining criteria for PCA-1, ANNA-1 and ANNA-2 autoantibodies. *Neurology*. 1994;44:2412–2415.

18. Lennon VA. Anti-Purkinje cell cytoplasmic and neuronal autoantibodies aid in diagnosis of paraneoplastic autoimmune neurologic disorders. *J Neurol Neurosurg Psychiatry*. 1989;42:1438–1439.

19. Siniscalo M, Oberle I, Melis P, et al. Physical and genetic mapping of the CDR gene with particular reference to its position with respect to the FRAXA site. *Am J Med Genet*. 1991;38:357–362.

20. Sindic CJ, Anderson M, Boucquey D, et al. Anti-Purkinje cells antibodies in two cases of paraneoplastic cerebellar degeneration. *Acta Neurol Belg*. 1993;93:65–77.

21. Fisher P, Wechsler D, Singer H. Anti-Hu antibody in a neuroblastoma-associated paraneoplastic syndrome. *Pediatr Neurol*. 1994;10:309–312.

22. Lennon VA, Sas DF, Busk MF, et al. Enteric neuronal autoantibodies in pseudo-obstruction with small cell lung carcinoma. *Gastroenterology*. 1991;100:137–142.

23. Chu G, Wilson, PG, Carter C, et al. Intestinal pseudo-obstruction: Type 1 anti-neuronal nuclear antibodies and small cell lung carcinoma. *J Gastroenterol Hepatol*. 1993;8:604–606.

24. Kiers L, Altermatt HJ, Lennon VA. Paraneoplastic anti-neuronal nuclear IgG autoantibodies (type 1) localize antigen in SCLC. *Mayo Clin Proc*. 1991;55: 1209–1216.

25. Luque FA, Furneaux HM, Ferziger R, et al. Anti-Ri: An antibody associated with paraneoplastic opsoclonus and breast carcinoma. *Ann Neurol*. 1991;29:241–251.

26. Graus F, Rowe G, Fueyo J, et al. The neuronal nuclear antigen recognized by the human anti-Ri autoantibody is expressed in central but not peripheral nervous system neurons. *Neurosci Lett*. 1993;150:212–214.

27. Budde-Steffen C, Anderson NE, Rosenblum MK, et al. An anti-neuronal autoantibody in paraneoplastic opsoclonus. *Ann Neurol*. 1988;23:528–531.

28. Camilli PD, Thomas A, Roxanne C, et al. The synaptic vesicle-associated protein amphiphysin is the 128-kD autoantigen of stiff-man syndrome with breast cancer. *J Exp Med*. 1992;178:2219–2223.

29. David C, Solimena S, Camilli PD. Autoimmunity in stiff-man syndrome with breast cancer is targeted to the C-terminal region of human amphiphysin. *FEBS Lett*. 1994;351:73–79.

30. Lennon VA. Calcium channel and related paraneoplastic disease autoantibodies. In: Peter JB, Shoenfeld Y, eds. *Autoantibodies*. Amsterdam, the Netherlands: Elsevier Science; 1996:139–147.

31. Adamus G, Aptsiauri G, Guy J, et al. The occurrence of serum autoantibodies against enolase in cancer-associated retinopathy. *Clin Immunol Immunopathol*. 1996;78:120–129.

32. Darnell RB. Onconeural antigens and the paraneoplastic disorders: At the intersection of cancer, immunity, and the brain. *Proc Natl Acad Sci U S A*. 1996;93:4529–4536.

33. Dalmau JO, Furneaux HM, Gralla RJ, et al. Detection of the anti-Hu antibody in serum of patients with small cell lung cancer: A quantitative Western blot analysis. *Ann Neurol*. 1990;27:544–552.

34. Dalmau JO, Rosenfeld MR. Characterization of neuronal antigens and anti-neuronal antibodies. *Methods Neurosci*. 1995;24:261–271.

35. Smith RG, Appel SH. Calcium channel autoantibodies and amyotrophic lateral sclerosis. In: Peter JB, Shoenfeld Y, eds. *Autoantibodies*. Amsterdam, the Netherlands: Elsevier Science; 1996:148–152.

36. Peterson K, Rosenblum MK, Kotanides H, et al. Paraneoplastic cerebellar degeneration. A clinical analysis of 55 anti-Yo antibody-positive patients. *Neurology*. 1992;42:1931–1937.

37. Dalmau JO, Posner JD. Purkinje cell autoantibodies, type 1 (Yo). In: Peter JB, Shoenfeld Y, eds. *Autoantibodies*. Amsterdam, the Netherlands: Elsevier Science; 1996:655–659.

38. Hammack JE, Kimmel DW, O'Neill BP. Paraneoplastic cerebellar degeneration: A clinical comparison of patients with and without Purkinje cell cytoplasmic antibodies. *Mayo Clin Proc*. 1990;65:1423–1431.

39. Brashear HR, Greenlee JE, Jaeckle KA, et al. Anti-cerebellar antibodies in neurologically normal patients with ovarian carcinoma. *Neurology*. 1989;39: 1605–1609.

40. Furneaux HM. Neuronal nuclear autoantibodies, type 1 (Hu). In: Peter JB, Shoenfeld Y, eds. *Autoantibodies*. Amsterdam, the Netherlands: Elsevier Science; 1996:551–554.

41. Graus F, Elkon KB, Lloberes P, et al. Neuronal antinuclear antibody (anti-Hu) in paraneoplastic encephalomyelitis simulating acute polyneuritis. *Acta Neurol Scand*. 1987;75:249–252.

42. Dalmau J, Graus F, Rosenblum MK, et al. Anti-Hu-associated paraneoplastic encephalomyelitis/ sensory neuropathy: A study of 71 patients. *Medicine*. 1992;71:59–72.

43. Luchinetti CF, Kimmell DW, Lennon VA. Clinical, oncological and serological profiles of patients seropositive for type 1 antineuronal nuclear antibody (ANNA-1, a.k.a. "anti-Hu"). *Neurology*. 1994;44:A156.

44. Greenlee JE, Jaeckle KA, Brashear HR. Anti-Hu antibody in suspected paraneoplastic syndromes other than small cell lung cancer and initial detection of antibody at very low titer. *Ann Neurol*. 1991;30:308. [Abstract]

45. Dalmau JO, Graus F, Cheung N-KU, et al. Major histocompatibility proteins, anti-Hu antibodies, and paraneoplastic encephalomyelitis in neuroblastoma and small cell lung carcinoma. *Cancer*. 1995;75:99–109.

46. Clouston PD, Saper CB, Arbizu T, et al. Cerebellar degeneration, cancer, and the LEMS. *Neurology*. 1992;42:1944–1950.

47. O'Suilleabhain PE, Lambert EH, Lennon VA. Anti-VGCC antibodies in women with paraneoplastic cerebellar degeneration (PCD) and seropositivity for type 1 anti-Purkinje cell antibody (PCAb). *Neurology*. 1994;44(suppl 2):A157.

48. Blumfeld AM, Recht LD, Chad DA, et al. Coexistence of LEMS and subacute cerebellar degeneration: Differential effect of treatment. *Neurology*. 1991;41:1682–1685.

49. Dalmau JO, Posner JB. Neurologic paraneoplastic antibodies (anti-Yo; anti-Hu; anti-Ri): The case for a nomenclature based on antibody and antigen specificity. *Neurology*. 1994;44:2241–2246.

50. Sillevis-Smitt P, Manley G, Moll JW, et al. Pitfalls in the diagnosis of autoantibodies associated with paraneoplastic neurologic diseases. *Neurology*. 1996;46: 1739–1741.

51. Moll JWB, Antoine JC, Brashear HR, et al. Guidelines on the detection of paraneoplastic anti-neuronal-specific antibodies. *Neurology*. 1995;45:1937–1941.

52. Dropcho EJ, Kline LB, Riser J. Antineuronal (anti-Ri) antibodies with steroid-responsive opsoclonus-myoclonus. *Neurology*. 1993;43:207–211.

53. Verschuuren J, Twijnstra A, De Baets M, et al. Hu antigens and anti-Hu antibodies in a patient with myxoid chondrosarcoma. *Neurology*. 1994;44:1551–1552.

54. Furneaux HM, Rosenblum MK, Dalmau J, et al. Selective expression of Purkinje cell antigen in tumor tissue from patients with paraneoplastic cerebellar degeneration. *N Engl J Med*. 1990;322:1844–1851.

55. Hartzel DJ, Stanhope CR, O'Neill BO, et al. Gynecological cancer in patients with subacute degeneration predicted by anti-Purkinje cell antibodies and limited in metastatic volume. *Mayo Clin Proc*. 1990;65:1558–1563.

56. Tanaka K, Igarashi S, Yamazaki M, et al. Paraneoplastic cerebellar degeneration: Successful early detection and treatment of cancer through characterization of the anti-Purkinje cell antibody. *Intern Med*. 1992;31: 1339–1342.

57. Moll JWB, Henzen-Logmans SC, Splinter TAW, et al. Diagnostic value of anti-neuronal antibodies for paraneoplastic disorders of the nervous system. *J Neurol Neurosurg Psychiatry*. 1990;53:940–943.

58. Nemni R, Camerlingo M, Fazio R, et al. Serum antibodies to Purkinje cells and dorsal root ganglia neurons in sensory neuropathy without malignancy. *Ann Neurol*. 1993;34:848–854.

59. Elrington GM, Murray NM, Spiro SG, et al. Neurological paraneoplastic syndromes in patients with small cell lung carcinoma. A prospective survey of 150 patients. *J Neurol Neurosurg Psychiatry*. 1991;54:764–767.

60. Cascino TL. Neurologic complications of systemic cancer. *Med Clin North Am*. 1993;77:265–278.

CHAPTER 22

Autoimmune Neuropathies

David F. Carney, PhD

Of the large number of patients with immune-mediated neurologic disorders, many have demonstrated high titers of circulating autoantibodies to a variety of antigens found in neural tissues.[1–4] This chapter focuses primarily on 2 of the groups of autoantibodies most commonly found in these patients, namely those directed against gangliosides and those directed against sulfated carbohydrates. Autoantibodies associated with neurologic diseases that are directed against phospholipid antigens and autoantibodies found in paraneoplastic syndromes and systemic lupus erythematosus neuropathies are covered in separate chapters.

It is estimated that up to 25% of idiopathic neuropathies are autoimmune in nature.[5] Categorization of a neuropathy as an autoimmune disorder is important for ruling out other causes, including inherited disorders, systemic diseases such as diabetes, deficiency states, toxins, and ischemia.[6] The demonstration of high-titer autoantibodies to a specific neural antigen is highly suggestive of an autoimmune neuropathy but is rarely diagnostic for a specific neuropathy. However, many studies have shown that specific autoantibodies are commonly associated with specific patterns of neuropathy.[7] Thus, screening neuropathy patients for the presence of specific autoantibodies should be guided by the classification of the neuropathy. Neuropathies are classified using several criteria, including the following[7]:

- Patterns of nerves affected
- Proximal to distal level of neuron involvement
- Cell type involved
- Time course (acute, chronic, subacute, and so forth)
- Pathologic reaction (parenchymatous versus interstitial)
- Evidence of demyelination or axonal degeneration
- Pathologic classification (ie, inflammatory, granulomatous, infiltrative)
- Inherited or acquired

Some patients with autoimmune-mediated neuropathy have shown clinical improvement when treated with immunosuppressive therapy.[8–10] Neuropathy patients with high titers of antimonosialoganglioside-SMI (anti-GM1), anti–myelin-associated glycoprotein (anti-MAG), or anti-GQ1b have exhibited reductions in titer and clinical improvement when treated with cyclophosphamide, plasmapheresis, or both.[8–10] The role of these antibodies in neurologic disease is not yet clear. However, the results of experimental passive transfer models have suggested that antibodies against some neural antigens can induce the clinical and pathologic features of neuropathy, suggesting that these antibodies may play a pathogenic role in these diseases.[11] Repeat assays for autoantibodies to neural antigens in patients undergoing such treatments may be useful for monitoring the immunosuppressive effectiveness of therapy.[8,10]

Ganglioside Antigens

Gangliosides belong to a family of acidic glycolipids composed of a ceramide and a carbohydrate moiety that may contain up to 4 sialic acids (**Table 22-1**).[2] Gangliosides are located in the plasma membrane of neuronal cells and processes, where they are believed to participate in a variety of cellular and membrane functions.[2] Antiganglioside antibodies associated with autoimmune neuropathies include those directed against GM1 and asialo GM1, GD1b, GD1a, GT1b, and GQ1b.[1,9,12,13] Gangliosides differ in the number and location of sialic acid residues, with the letters M, D, T, and Q constituting 1 to 4 sialic acids per molecule, respectively (see Table 22-1). The antigenic epitope in gangliosides has been localized to the Gal β1-3 GalNAc portion of the carbohydrate moiety[12,14]; therefore, it is known that significant antibody cross-reactivity exists within this group of antigens. It is believed that differences in antibody specificities to the different gangliosides are due to steric effects contributed by the sialic acid groups; although in some cases, antibodies specifically directed against the sialic acids also occur.[15] Two other clinically important ganglioside antigens are sialosyl paragloboside, also referred to as LM1, which is the major ganglioside in human peripheral nerve myelin, and sialosyl lactosaminyl paragloboside. Antibodies to these two paraglobosides are found in patients with inflammatory demyelinating polyneuropathies.[16,17]

Sulfated Carbohydrate Antigens

A number of autoantibodies against sulfated carbohydrate–containing neural antigens are associated with autoimmune neuropathies. Sulfatides, which are sulfated galactose–containing glycolipids, constitute one of the major glycolipids of this class of antigens.[18] Sulfatides contain the antigenic

Table 22-1. Structures of Antigens Involved in Autoimmune Neuropathies

Neural Antigen	Structure
GM1	Galβ1-3GalNAcβ1-4(NeuAcα2-3)Galβ1-4Glcβ1-1'Cer
Asialo GM1	Galβ1-3GalNAcβ1-4Galβ1-4Glcβ1-1'Cer
GD1a	NeuAcα2-3Galβ1-3GalNAcβ1-4(NeuAcα2-3)Galβ1-4Glcβ1-1'Cer
GD1b	Galβ1-3GalNAcβ1-4(NeuAcα2-8NeuAcα2-3)Galβ1-4Glc1-1'Cer
GT1b	NeuAcα2-3Galβ1-3GalNAcβ1-4(NeuAcα2-3NeuAcα2-8)Galβ1-4Glcβ1-1'Cer
GQ1b	Galβ1-3GalNAcβ1- (NeuAcα2-8NeuAcα2NeuAcα2-8NeuAcα2) 4Galβ1-4Glc1-1'Cer
SPG	(NeuAcα2-3)Galβ1-4GlcNAcβ1-3Galβ1-4Glcβ1-1'Cer
SLPG	(NeuAcα2-3)Galβ1-4GlcNAcβ1-3Galβ1-4GlcNAcβ1-3Galβ1-4Glcβ1-1'Cer
Sulfatide	SO_4-3Galβ1-1'Cer
SGPG	SO_4-3GlcAβ1-4GlcNAcβ1-3Galβ1-4Glcβ1-1'Cer

Abbreviations: Gal = galactose; GalNAc = N-acetylgalactosamine; NeuAc = N-acetylneuraminic acid; Glc = glucose; Cer = ceramide; SPG = sialosyl paragloboside; GlcNAc = N-acetylglucosamine; SLPG = sialosyl lactosaminyl paragloboside; SGPG = sulfoglucuronyl paragloboside; GlcA = glucuronic acid.

epitope SO_4-3-galactose, which is attached to a ceramide (see Table 22-1). Heterogeneity among the sulfatides is due to differences in the composition of the fatty acid portion of the cerebroside. Another important group of glycolipids in this class are the sulfated glucuronic–containing glycolipids, particularly sulfoglucuronyl paragloboside (SGPG) and sulfoglucuronyl lactosaminyl paragloboside (see Table 22-1).[19–21] The glycoproteins MAG and P_0 also belong to this antigen class, based on the fact that antibodies that bind to the glucuronyl sulfate epitope of SGPG also cross-react with MAG and P_0.[22,23] These results suggest that SGPG, MAG, and P_0 contain an epitope with common structural features.

Assay Methods

The immunoassay method of choice for autoantibodies associated with neuropathy syndromes is dependent on the antigen used. For most glycolipids, including the gangliosides and sulfated galactose– and glucuronic–containing glycolipids, the 2 preferred immunoassays are enzyme-linked immunosorbent assay (ELISA) and thin-layer chromatography (TLC) immuno-overlay.[24,25] The ELISA is usually preferred over TLC because of the former's high sensitivity and specificity, simplicity, and low cost. Thin-layer chromatography, however, is advantageous in that highly purified antigen preparations are not required and only a single lane is used to screen each patient serum for antibodies to multiple neural antigens that become separated during the chromatographic process. The TLC method suffers from being relatively labor-intensive and requires the use of large quantities of highly volatile organic solvents.

Although a number of ELISAs using glycolipid antigens with a variety of modifications have been reported, most methods share many common features.[26–28] Sulfatides and many of the gangliosides are commercially available in purified forms, and thus can be coated directly onto ELISA plates. Sulfated glucuronic–containing glycolipids are not available commercially in purified form and must be purified from neural tissues such as cauda equina or sciatic nerve using organic solvents.[29] For the glycolipid antigens, hydrophobic plates are preferred because they give low nonspecific binding as well as higher specificity among closely related epitopes compared with hydrophilic plates.[28] Glycolipid antigens are dissolved and coated in ELISA wells in an organic solvent such as methanol, ethanol, chloroform, or various mixtures of these solvents. After solvent evaporation, a blocking step is performed, which usually consists of incubating antigen-coated wells with 1% to 3% bovine serum albumin.[26,28]

Different laboratories are inconsistent in the use of detergents in wash buffers for ELISAs using glycolipid antigens.[26,28] Tween-20 (polyoxyethylene sorbitan monolaurate) (0.05%) is reported to significantly reduce nonspecific binding of serum antibodies to glycolipid antigens.[26,27,30] Because low nonspecific reactivity is observed when detergent washes are used, some laboratories that use detergent do not include wells for nonspecific binding.[24] However, detergents also dramatically reduce specific antibody binding.[26,27] For example, anti-GM1 titers are up to 3 to 10 times higher when detergent is avoided.[2] In one survey of the literature on ELISAs of antiganglioside antibodies, about 50% (10 of 21) of the laboratories surveyed did not use detergent in the assay.[28]

Several strategies have been reported for evaluating the significance of elevated serum antibody levels against neuronal glycolipid antigens. Results are most often expressed as a titer and less often as an arbitrary unit value.[12,31–33] Many laboratories define the absolute titer for antiglycolipid antibodies as the highest serial dilution of patient serum at which the optical density is 0.05 to 0.1 unit above the nonspecific binding control.[32] Although the use of this method is acceptable for initially defining titer units, its routine use for patient samples may be unreliable due to variabilities inherent in the ELISA related to antigen coating, reagents used, washing steps, and reaction times and temperatures. Incorporation of a standard curve or calibrator using a patient serum with an assigned titer (or arbitrary unit value) may be preferable to correct for plate-to-plate and day-to-day variations in the assay.

Interpretation of neuropathy autoantibody titers is typically accomplished by comparing patient titers with titers obtained from a panel of disease-free donors.[9,13,34,35] Some laboratories consider a titer positive when the value is above the highest normal value obtained.[31] Statistical methods are more reliable for obtaining the cutoff value to distinguish negative (normal) titers from those that are significantly elevated. According to the National Committee for Clinical Laboratory Standards, patient values above the 97.5th percentile of the distribution of healthy normal individuals are considered statistically elevated.[36,37] Alternatively, investigators have set the cutoff for antibody titers at 2 to 3 or more standard deviations above the mean values obtained from a panel of normal healthy individuals to improve the clinical specificity of the assay.[9,13,34,35]

Several groups of researchers have observed that differences exist in the cutoff titer among different antiglycolipid antibodies, ranging from as low as 1:100 or less to as high as 1:1,600 or more.[1,32,37] Therefore, cutoff titers should be established independently for each antigen. In addition, cutoff titers for antibodies to a single antigen can differ for different isotypes by as much as a factor of 6.[38] Most laboratories perform immunoglobulin (Ig) M and G (and, less frequently, A) isotyping for most of the neuropathy autoantibodies, establishing independent cutoffs for each antibody isotype.

Assays for MAG are typically done by Western blot, although improved methods of MAG purification have justified the use of an ELISA for this purpose.[39] For the Western blot method, proteins in purified human myelin are separated by polyacrylamide electrophoresis and blotted onto nitrocellulose. The blotted nitrocellulose membranes are then incubated with diluted patient sera and immunostained by standard techniques. Anti-MAG detection by ELISA offers many obvious advantages over Western blot. Unfortunately, minor contaminants that can cause false-positive reactions in the ELISA may be present in purified MAG preparations. If contaminants present in MAG preparations cannot be removed before use in an ELISA, detection of anti-MAG activity should be confirmed by Western blot.[39]

Autoantibodies in Peripheral Neuropathies

Motor and Sensory Neuropathies

Autoantibodies to neural antigens have been demonstrated in a variety of patients with predominantly motor, predominantly sensory, and sensorimotor neuropathies with or without evidence of conduction block and/or axonal loss. Patients with predominantly motor neuropathies frequently demonstrate high IgM anti-GM1 titers.[1,30] For example, more than 80% of patients with high-titer anti-GM1 have either multifocal motor neuropathy or lower motor neuron syndromes.[1,2,27] Although high titers of anti-GM1 are very specific for these neuropathies, such results are present in only 20% to 50% of affected patients, with the remainder having low-to-intermediate anti-GM1 titers.[1,27,40] High titers of GM1 have also been observed in some patients with sensorimotor neuropathy.[12] Anti-GM1 titers are low or inconsistent in patients with amyotrophic lateral sclerosis.[34] Approximately 10% of patients with high IgM anti-GM1 titers have monoclonal gammopathies[4] and should be evaluated accordingly. Autoantibodies to asialo GM1 and GD1b are found in many of the same neuropathies that demonstrate anti-GM1, but with lower frequency.[12,37] Asialo GM1 has shown similar antigenic specificity to GM1, with high-titer antibodies to asialo GM1 occurring in up to 36% of patients with lower motor neuron syndromes.[1]

Patient screening for antiganglioside antibodies other than anti-GM1 may be useful, because high titers of these antibodies are sometimes present when the anti-GM1 titer is low.[15] For example, high titers of antibodies to GD1b and GT1b are sometimes observed in patients with predominantly sensory neuropathy.[41,42] High titers of antisulfatide antibodies are also present with varying frequency in motor and sensory neuropathies, but are more frequently associated with demyelinating neuropathies.[35,43] Patients with autoimmune neuropathy[12,30,37] syndromes can demonstrate high or low titers of one or multiple antiganglioside antibodies. However, high titers of antiganglioside antibodies are usually seen only in autoimmune neuropathy syndromes, whereas low titers of antiganglioside antibodies may be seen in many diseases other than autoimmune neuropathy syndromes.[2,12,30,37] For example, low anti-GM1 titers are found in 20% to 30% of patients with nonimmune neurologic diseases and nonneurologic autoimmune diseases (**Figure 22-1**).[12,37] Therefore, high titers, but not low titers, of antiganglioside antibodies are specific for autoimmune neuropathy syndromes.

Demyelinating Peripheral Neuropathies

Neuropathy patients with evidence of demyelination with or without axonal degeneration frequently demonstrate high-titer antibodies to MAG, SGPG, and P_0.[21] High-titer IgM anti-MAG is observed in 25% to 35% of patients with predominantly sensory or sensorimotor demyelinating neuropathy, which is usually slowly progressive, symmetric, and distal.[21] Although anti-MAG titers have not been shown to correlate with disease activity, therapeutic reduction of anti-MAG titers often shows clinical improvement.[10] Up to 50% of patients with monoclonal gammopathy and peripheral neuropathy with evidence of demyelination have high anti-MAG titers.[32] Some of these patients also demonstrate high titers of antisulfatide.[18,44]

Patients with acquired inflammatory demyelinating polyneuropathies, which include Guillain-Barré syndrome (GBS) and chronic inflammatory demyelinating polyradiculoneuropathy (CIDP), often demonstrate serum autoantibodies.[45] Up to 50% of GBS patients demonstrate elevated anti-GM1 titers that are

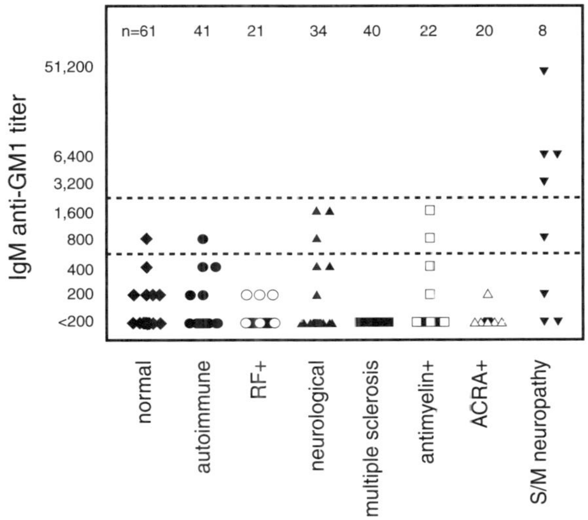

Figure 22-1. Immunoglobulin M anti-GM1 titers obtained for patients from various disease groups. Abbreviations: normal (◆) = healthy, disease-free volunteers; autoimmune (●) = patients with systemic lupus erythematosus, Sjögren's syndrome, or rheumatoid arthritis; RF+ (○) = rheumatoid factor positive; neurological (▲) = neurologic disorders other than sensorimotor or motor neuropathies; multiple sclerosis (■) = patients diagnosed with chronic progressive or relapsing remitting multiple sclerosis; antimyelin+ (positive) (□) = determined by indirect imunofluorescence microscopy; ACRA+ (△) = acetylcholine receptor antibody–positive; S/M neuropathy (▼) = patients with sensorimotor or motor neuropathy. Patients with titers below the 97.5th percentile of the titer distribution of normal individuals (less than 1:800) were considered negative for IgM anti-GM1. Titers between 1:800 and 1:1,600 (demarcated with dashed lines) are intermediate-positive titers. Titers in this category did not correlate with specific neuropathy syndromes. High titers greater than or equal to 1:3,200 showed a positive correlation with sensorimotor or motor neuropathies. The enzyme-linked immunosorbent assay method used at the Scripps Reference Laboratory is the same as described in Table 22-2.

most frequently IgG, as well as elevated titers of other glycolipid antibodies.[16,17] Although the correlation between GBS and antiganglioside antibodies remains controversial, the clearest association is between anti-GM1 and the predominantly axonal forms of GBS, such as acute motor axonal neuropathy (AMAN).[46] High-titer IgG anti-GM1 have been found in up to 50% of patients with AMAN, frequently following infection with *Campylobacter jejuni*.[7,47] Interestingly, antigens from *C jejuni* cross-react with anti-GM1, suggesting a possible link between the 2 antibodies.[48,49]

Patients with Miller-Fisher syndrome—a variant of GBS characterized by ophthalmoplegia, gait ataxia, and areflexia—frequently have high titers of GQ1b.[50] Among the gangliosides, GQ1b has demonstrated the best correlation with a specific clinical syndrome, appearing in more than 90% of patients with Miller-Fisher syndrome.[9,50]

Patients with CIDP, some of whom present with a monoclonal gammopathy, typically do not have elevated ganglioside titers.[45] However, anti-SGP has been found in up to 67% of CIDP patients.[16] More than 80% of CIDP patients have elevated titers of anti-sulfatides and 50% to 60% have high titers of anti–β-tubulin.[16,51] The presence of anti–β-tubulin may be a specific marker for CIDP because these antibodies are rare in other demyelinating polyneuropathies.[45]

Multiple Sclerosis

Of the demyelinating autoimmune neuropathies of the central nervous system, multiple sclerosis (MS) is the principal disease in humans. Laboratory diagnostic testing for MS typically involves evaluation of immunoglobulins in the cerebrospinal fluid. In patients with MS, cerebrospinal fluid total protein is commonly normal while IgG is elevated.[52] In addition, the demonstration of an oligoclonal banding pattern for cerebrospinal fluid immunoglobulins by electrophoresis is characteristic of but not specific for MS.[52] Anti–myelin basic protein (anti-MBP) has been found in the cerebrospinal fluid or serum of more than 90% of patients having either the acute relapsing or the progressive form of MS.[53] However, anti-MBP is not specific for MS and is also found with high frequency in many other neurologic diseases, including acute idiopathic neuritis, Alzheimer's disease, and acquired immunodeficiency syndrome dementia complex.[53]

Quality Assurance

Two independent studies performed interlaboratory comparisons for the determination of anti-GM1, which may serve as a model for most of the lipid-based neural antigens that include gangliosides and sulfatides.[26,27] Both studies found good correlation for sera with high and low titers; however, significant variation was observed for titers between these 2 ranges. The authors found similar results when comparing the results of a GM1 assay performed in their laboratory with those of several other laboratories (**Table 22-2**). Controlled proficiency surveys would

Table 22-2. Immunoglobulin M Anti-GM1 Titer Correlation Among Clinical Laboratories

Sample #	SRL*	Lab 1	Lab 2	Lab 3	Lab 4
1	51,200	3,200		68,000	
2	6,400	3,200	25,600	39,000	
3	6,400		1,600		
4	3,200				HI POS
5	1,600	800		3,700	
6	1,600	<800			
7	800	800	1,600		
8	800	1600	400		
9	800	800			
10	800	800	200		
11	800	<800			
12	400	<800			
13	400	<800	800		
14	400	<800	100		
15	<400	<800			
16	<400	<800	400		
17	<400	<800	200		
18	<400		200		
19	<400		100		
20	<400		NEG		
21	<400		NEG		
22	<400		NEG		
23	<400		100		
24	<400		NEG		
25	<400	<800	NEG		
26	<400	<800			
27	<400				NEG
28	<400				NEG
29	<400				NEG
30	<400				NEG
31	<400				NEG

Abbreviations: SRL = Scripps Reference Laboratory; HI POS = highly positive; NEG = negative.

**The anti-GM1 assay at Scripps Reference Laboratory was performed as follows. ELISA wells were coated with 500 ng of GM1 in methanol and then blocked with 1% bovine serum albumin. Diluted patient sera were added to wells with and without GM1 and incubated at room temperature for 90 minutes. All washes were performed without detergent. Antibody binding was detected with peroxidase-conjugated goat-antihuman IgM and 2,2'-Azino-di-[3-ethyl-benzthiazoline sulfonate]. Specific GM1 binding for each patient was calculated by subtracting the OD490 values of wells without GM1 from wells coated with GM1. These values were compared to a standard curve consisting of a patient serum with a known GM1 titer to assign titer values for each patient.*

Table 22-3. Neuropathies Associated With High-Titer Autoantibodies to Neural Antigens

Antibody	Neuropathy	References
GM1	MMN, SMN, LMND, GBS	1, 30, 31
Asialo GM1	MMN, SMN, LMND, GBS	1, 2, 38
GD1b	PSN, MMN, SMN, LMND, GBS	1, 4, 12
GD1a	GBS	13
GQ1b	MFS, GBS, PSN	9, 49
SPG	GBS, CIDP	16, 17
SLPG	GBS, CIDP	16, 17
Sulfatide	PSN, SMN, GBS, CIDP, SMDN, PSDN	16, 18
MAG	PSDN, SMDN	18
P_0	PSDN, SMDN	23
SGPG	PSDN, SMDN, CIDP	20, 54
β-Tubulin	CIDP	51
MBP	MS, AIN, AD, ADC	53

Abbreviations: MMN = multifocal motor neuropathy; SMN = sensorimotor neuropathy; LMND = lower motor neuron disease; GBS = Guillain-Barré syndrome; PSN = predominantly sensory neuropathy; MFS = Miller-Fisher syndrome; SPG = sialosyl paragloboside; CIDP = chronic inflammatory demyelinating polyneuropathy; SLPG = sialosyl lactosaminyl paragloboside; SMDN = sensorimotor demyelinating neuropathy; PSDN = predominantly sensory demyelinating neuropathy; MAG = myelin-associated glycoprotein; SGPG = sulfoglucuronyl paragloboside; MBP = myelin basic protein; MS = multiple sclerosis; AIN = acute idiopathic neuritis; AD = Alzheimer's disease; ADC = AIDS dementia complex.

be helpful as an initial step toward standardization of these assays. However, none are as yet available for autoantibodies associated with neuropathies.

Summary

The detection and monitoring of high-titer autoantibodies associated with autoimmune neuropathies is useful diagnostically for some autoimmune neuropathies such as multifocal motor neuropathy and Miller-Fisher syndrome. The demonstration of autoantibodies to neural antigens is also useful for subclassifying patients with monoclonal gammopathies and to exclude diagnoses of non–immune-mediated neuropathies (**Table 22-3**). Many of these diseases are treatable with conventional immunosuppressive therapy, which can sometimes be monitored by serial measurement of serum titers of certain autoantibodies.[8–10] It is apparent that individual laboratories are using several significant modifications when performing immunoassays that detect autoantibodies in neurologic disease.[26–28] Based on the variability in test results observed in interlaboratory comparative studies[26,27] (see Figure 22-1), standardization of these assays must be encouraged. Another area of concern is the variable assignment of titer values or arbitrary unit values, indicating the need for establishment of World Health Organization standards or their equivalent for these values. The use of an internal calibrator or standard curve for ELISAs is encouraged to adjust for plate-to-plate and day-to-day variations, as well as reagent lot-to-lot differences. Finally, the assignment of disease correlations for patients with low-to-intermediate titers should be considered carefully due to the lack of disease specificity.[12,31,37,40]

References

1. Pestronk A, Chaudhry V, Feldman EL, et al. Lower motor neuron syndromes defined by patterns of weakness, nerve conduction abnormalities, and high titers of antiglycolipid antibodies. *Ann Neurol.* 1990;27:316–326.
2. Pestronk A. Invited review: Motor neuropathies, motor neuron disorders, and antiglycolipid antibodies. *Muscle Nerve.* 1991;14:927–936.
3. Zeballos RS, McPherson RA. Update of autoantibodies in neurologic disease. *Clin Lab Med.* 1992;12:61–83.
4. Latov N. Pathogenesis and therapy of neuropathies associated with monoclonal gammopathies. *Ann Neurol.* 1995;37:S32–S42.
5. Dyck PJ, Oviatt KF, Lambert EH. Intensive evaluation of referred unclassified neuropathies yields improved diagnosis. *Ann Neurol.* 1981;10:222–226.
6. Bosch EP, Mitsumoto H. Disorders of peripheral nerves, plexuses in neurology in clinical practice: the neurological disorders. In: Bradley WB, Daroff RB, Fenichel GM, et al, eds. *Neurology in Clinical Practice.* Stone, MA: Butterworth-Heinemann; 1991:1719–1804.
7. Griffin JW, Hsieh S-T, McArthur JC, et al. Laboratory testing in peripheral nerve disease. *Neurol Clin.* 1996;14:119–133.
8. Pestronk A, Cornblath DR, Ilyas AA, et al. A treatable multifocal motor neuropathy with antibodies to GM1 ganglioside. *Ann Neurol.* 1988;24:73–78.
9. Yuki N, Sato S, Tsuji S, et al. Frequent presence of anti-GQ1b antibody in Fisher's syndrome. *Neurology.* 1993;43:414–416.

10. Blume G, Pestronk A, Goodnough LT. Anti-MAG antibody-associated polyneuropathies: Improvement following immunotherapy with monthly plasma exchange and IV cyclophosphamide. *Neurology*. 1995;45:1577–1580.

11. Steck AJ. Antibodies in the neurology clinic. *Neurology*. 1990;40:1489–1492.

12. Sadiq SA, Thomas FP, Kilidireas K, et al. The spectrum of neurologic disease associated with anti-GM1 antibodies. *Neurology*. 1990;40:1067–1072.

13. Yuki N, Yamada M, Sato S, et al. Association of IgG anti-GD1a antibody with severe Guillain-Barré syndrome. *Muscle Nerve*. 1993;16:642–647.

14. Shy ME, Heiman-Patterson T, et al. Lower motor neuron disease in a patient with autoantibodies against Gal(b1-3)GalNAc in gangliosides GM1 and GD1b: Improvement following immunotherapy. *Neurology*. 1990;40:842–844.

15. Ben Younes-Chennoufi A, Léger J-M, Hauw J-J, et al. Ganglioside GD1b is the target antigen for a biclonal IgM in a case of sensorimotor axonal polyneuropathy: Involvement of *N*-acetylneuraminic acid in the epitope. *Ann Neurol*. 1992;32:18–23.

16. Fredman P, Vedeler CA, Nyland H, et al. Antibodies in sera from patients with inflammatory demyelinating polyradiculoneuropathy react with ganglioside LM1 and sulphatide of peripheral nerve myelin. *J Neurol*. 1991;238:75–79.

17. Ilyas AA, Mithen FA, Dalakas MC, et al. Antibodies to acidic glycolipids in Guillain Barré syndrome and chronic inflammatory demyelinating polyneuropathy. *J Neurol Sci*. 1992;107:111–121.

18. Pestronk A, Li F, Griffin J, et al. Polyneuropathy syndromes associated with serum antibodies to sulfatide and myelin-associated glycoprotein. *Neurology*. 1991;41:357–362.

19. McGinnis S, Kohriyama T, Yu RK, et al. Antibodies to sulfated glucuronic acid containing glycosphingolipids in neuropathy associated with anti-MAG antibodies and in normal subjects. *J Neuroimmunol*. 1988;17:119–126.

20. Yuki N, Tagawa Y, Handa S. Autoantibodies to peripheral nerve glycosphingolipids SPG, SLPG, and SGPG in Guillain-Barré syndrome and chronic inflammatory demyelinating polyneuropathy. *J Neuroimmunol*. 1996;70:1–6.

21. Link H. Myelin-associated glycoprotein autoantibodies. In: Peter JB, Shoenfeld Y, eds. *Autoantibodies*. Amsterdam, the Netherlands: Elsevier Science; 1996:513–519.

22. Ariga T, Kohriyama T, Freddo L, et al. Characterization of sulfated glucuronic acid containing glycolipids reacting with IgM M-proteins in patients with neuropathy. *J Biol Chem*. 1987;262:848–853.

23. Bollensen E, Steck AJ, Schachner M. Reactivity with the peripheral myelin glycoprotein P0 in serum from patients with monoclonal IgM gammopathy and polyneuropathy. *Neurology*. 1988;38:1266–1270.

24. Freddo L, Yu RK, Latov N, et al. Gangliosides GM1 and GD1b are antigens for IgM M-protein in a patient with motor neuron disease. *Neurology*. 1986;36:454–458.

25. Gregson NA, Jones D, Thomas PK, et al. Acute motor neuropathy with antibodies to GM1 ganglioside. *J Neurol*. 1991;238:447–451.

26. Zuraw BL, Chambers SL. Prevalence of auto-anti-C1 inhibitor (C1INH) antibodies in acquired C1INH deficient patients. *J Allergy Clin Immunol*. 1990;85:208. [Abstract]

27. Kornberg AJ, Pestronk A. The clinical and diagnostic role of anti-GM1 antibody testing. *Muscle Nerve*. 1994;17:100–104.

28. Ravindranath MH, Ravindranath RMH, Morton DL, et al. Factors affecting the fine specificity and sensitivity of serum antiganglioside antibodies in ELISA. *J Immunol Methods*. 1994;169:257–272.

29. Chou DKH, Ilyas AA, Evans JE, et al. Structure of sulfated glucuronyl glycolipids in the nervous system reacting with HNK-1 antibody and some IgM paraproteins in neuropathy. *J Biol Chem*. 1986;261:11717–11725.

30. Adams D, Kuntzer T, Burger D, et al. Predictive value of anti-GM1 ganglioside antibodies in neuromuscular diseases: A study of 180 sera. *J Neuroimmunol*. 1991;32: 223–230.

31. van den Berg LH, Marrink J, deJager AEJ, et al. Anti-GM1 antibodies in patients with Guillain-Barré syndrome. *J Neurol Neurosurg Psychiatry*. 1992;55:8–11.

32. Nobile-Orazio E, Manfredini E, Carpo M, et al. Frequency and clinical correlates of anti-neural IgM antibodies in neuropathy associated with IgM monoclonal gammopathy. *Ann Neurol*. 1994;36:416–424.

33. von Wulffen H, Hartard C, Scharein E. Seroreactivity to *Campylobacter jejuni* and gangliosides in patients with Guillain-Barré syndrome. *J Infect Dis*. 1994;170: 828–833.

34. Pestronk A, Adams RN, Clawson L, et al. Serum antibodies to GM1 ganglioside in amyotrophic lateral sclerosis. *Neurology*. 1988;38:1457–1461.

35. van den Berg LH, Lankamp CLAM, deJager AEJ, et al. Anti-sulphatide antibodies in peripheral neuropathy. *J Neurol Neurosurg Psychiatry*. 1993;56:1164–1168.

36. Sasse EA, Aziz KJ, Harris EK, et al. Analysis of reference values. In: *How to Define and Determine Reference Intervals in the Clinical Laboratory; Approved Guideline*. Villanova, PA: National Committee for Clinical Laboratory Standards; 1995:15–25.

37. García Guijo C, García-Merino A, Rubio G. Presence and isotype of anti-ganglioside antibodies in healthy persons, motor neuron disease, peripheral neuropathy, and other diseases of the nervous system. *J Neuroimmunol*. 1995;56:27–33.

38. Kornberg AJ, Pestronk A. Chronic motor neuropathies: Diagnosis, therapy, and pathogenesis. *Ann Neurol*. 1995;37:S43–S50.

39. Pestronk A, Li F, Bieser K, et al. Anti-MAG antibodies: Major effects of antigen purity and antibody cross-reactivity on ELISA results and clinical correlation. *Neurology*. 1994;44:1131–1137.

40. Nobile-Orazio E, Carpo M, Legname G, et al. Anti-GM1 IgM antibodies in motor neuron disease and neuropathy. *Neurology*. 1990;40:1747–1750.

41. Yuki N, Miyatani N, Sato S, et al. Acute relapsing sensory neuropathy associated with IgM antibody against B-series gangliosides containing a GalNAcb1-4 (Gal3-2aNeuAc8-2aNeuAc)b1 configuration. *Neurology*. 1992;42:686–689.

42. Daune GC, Farrer RG, Dalakas MC, et al. Sensory neuropathy associated with monoclonal immunoglobulin M to GD1b ganglioside. *Ann Neurol*. 1992;31:683–685.

43. Nemni R, Fazio R, Quattrini A, et al. Antibodies to sulfatide and to chondroitin sulfate C in patients with chronic sensory neuropathy. *J Neuroimmunol*. 1993;43:79–86.

44. Ilyas AA, Cook SD, Dalakas MC, et al. Anti-MAG IgM paraproteins from some patients with polyneuropathy associated with IgM paraproteinemia also react with sulfatide. *J Neuroimmunol*. 1992;37:85–92.

45. van der Meché FGA, van Doorn PA. Guillain-Barré syndrome and chronic inflammatory demyelinating polyneuropathy: Immune mechanisms and update on current therapies. *Ann Neurol*. 1995;37:S14–S31.

46. Yuki N, Yoshino H, Sato S, et al. Acute axonal polyneuropathy associated with anti-GM1 antibodies following *Campylobacter enteritis*. *Neurology*. 1990;40:1900–1902.

47. Ogino M, Nobile-Orazio E, Latov N. IgG anti-GM1 antibodies from patients with acute motor neuropathy are predominantly of the IgG1 and IgG3 subclasses. *J Neuroimmunol*. 1995;58:77–80.

48. Yuki N, Taki T, Takahashi M, et al. Molecular mimicry between GQ1b ganglioside and lipopolysaccharides of *Campylobacter jejuni* isolated from patients with Fisher's syndrome. *Ann Neurol*. 1994;36:791–793.

49. Jacobs BC, Endtz HP, van der Meché FGA, et al. Serum anti-GQ1b IgG antibodies recognize surface epitopes on *Campylobacter jejuni* from patients with Miller Fisher syndrome. *Ann Neurol*. 1995;37:260–264.

50. Chiba A, Kusunoki S, Shimizu T, et al. Serum IgG antibody to ganglioside GQ1b is a possible marker of Miller Fisher syndrome. *Ann Neurol*. 1992;31:677–679.

51. Connolly AM, Pestronk A, Trotter JL, et al. High-titer selective serum anti-beta-tubulin antibodies in chronic inflammatory demyelinating polyneuropathy. *Neurology*. 1993;43:557–562.

52. Noronha A, Arnason B. Demyelinating diseases. In: Rich RR, Fleisher TA, Schwartz BD, et al, eds. *Clinical Immunology Principles and Practice*. St. Louis, MO: Mosby Year Book; 1996:1364–1376.

53. Li S. Myelin basic protein autoantibodies. In: Peter JB, Shoenfeld Y, eds. *Autoantibodies*. Amsterdam, the Netherlands: Elsevier Science; 1996:520–526.

54. van den Berg L, Hays AP, Nobile-Orazio E, et al. Anti-MAG and anti-SGPG antibodies in neuropathy. *Muscle Nerve*. 1996;19:637–643.

CHAPTER 23

Autoimmune Diseases of the Thyroid and Adrenal Glands

C. Lynne Burek, PhD, ABMLI

The term *autoimmune disease* is properly reserved for conditions in which structural or functional damage, or both, are produced by humoral and/or cell-mediated immune reactions to normal components of the body. Stringent criteria for this designation of an autoimmune disease were proposed by Witebsky et al[1] in 1957 based on Koch's postulates. The postulates include the following:

- The relevant antibodies or cell-mediated reactivities should be demonstrated.
- The responsible antigen should be defined, isolated, and used to induce an immunologic response in experimental animals.
- The pathologic changes similar to those seen in human disease should appear in the corresponding tissue of the immunized animal.

A modification of these criteria was proposed by Rose and Bona[2] in 1993 to include the definition of the pathogenic lymphocytes mediating the autoimmune diseases. However, in many cases, the actual antigens have not been identified. In these cases, strong indirect evidence should be sufficient to warrant a designation as an autoimmune disorder. Thus, the more conventional interpretation of autoimmune disease is one in which there is a strong autoimmune element associated with the particular disorder, even though no direct experimental evidence proves that the autoimmunity is causing the disease.

This chapter deals with laboratory methods for the evaluation of autoantibodies found in the organ-specific autoimmune diseases of the thyroid and adrenal glands (**Table 23-1**). Although the autoimmune responses to these organs frequently involve both humoral and cell-mediated immunity directed to tissue-specific antigens, at present, the detection of humoral responses (autoantibodies) has greater clinical utility. The empiric association between an autoantibody and a particular disease may provide a clinically useful diagnostic tool, even in the absence of a cause-and-effect relationship.

The recognition that there is an autoimmune basis for certain endocrinopathies was made in the mid-1950s by 2 different groups of investigators. First, in Buffalo, New York, Witebsky and Rose conducted an experimental study with thyroglobulin (Tg), a major protein of the thyroid gland. They chose Tg because previous reports indicated that this protein was specific for the thyroid gland and that Tg of different species were antigenically related. They made the surprising observation that Tg from rabbits injected into other rabbits elicited antibody that reacted with rabbit Tg.[3] Furthermore, the immunized rabbit's own thyroid gland was infiltrated by mononuclear cells, denoting the presence of autoimmune thyroiditis. Stimulated by the resemblance of this experimentally induced disease to human chronic thyroiditis, they collected sera from patients with Hashimoto's disease and related disorders. They found that many patients with chronic thyroiditis produced antibodies to human Tg and therefore proposed that human thyroiditis is an example of a human autoimmune disease.[1]

At approximately the same time in London, England, Roitt et al[4] followed up earlier clinical observations that many patients with Hashimoto's disease had elevated levels of circulating gamma globulins. They therefore examined serum samples from a number of patients with Hashimoto's disease and discovered that many contained precipitating antibodies to human Tg. Since these seminal discoveries, there has been ample confirmation that most patients with chronic thyroiditis develop autoantibodies to human Tg.

The Utility of Autoantibody Detection

In some cases, autoantibodies may actually cause disease, such as the thyroid-stimulating antibody found in Graves' disease. However, they are more frequently used as markers in a variety of ways:

Autoantibodies may be used as an aid in diagnosing disease, either by inclusion or exclusion, depending on the sensitivity and specificity of the association of antibody with the particular disorder. For example, virtually all patients with autoimmune thyroiditis have autoantibodies to one or both of the commonly detected antigens of the thyroid—Tg or thyroperoxidase (TPO), formerly known as the microsomal antigen. The sensitivity of the association between thyroiditis and these autoantibodies is high. Combined with other signs and symptoms of disease and biochemical markers (elevated thyroid-stimulating hormone [TSH]) and reduced thyroid hormones, diagnosis of autoimmune thyroiditis can be confirmed. However, the antibodies also may be found in other disorders, such as Graves' disease and thyroid carcinoma, or even in euthyroid individuals. Thus, the specificity of these autoantibodies does not relate to thyroiditis alone, because patients with other conditions also present with these antibodies. However, if a patient lacks these antibodies, autoimmune thyroiditis may virtually be excluded.

Table 23-1. Laboratory Tests for Autoantibodies Found in Autoimmune Thyroid and Adrenal Diseases

Organ	Autoantigen	Test	Utility	Comments
Thyroid	Thyroglobulin (Tg)	IIF—fixed primate thyroid	2nd colloid antigen, rarely used	Historical assay, not sensitive
		HA	Aid in diagnosis	Commercially available
		ELISA	Aid in diagnosis	Commercially available
		ELISA—quantitative	Research availability	Objective measure of total Tg antibody or of specific isotypes; performed in specialized laboratories only
		ELISA—epitope analysis	Research availability	May be a more specific test than total antibody levels; performed in specialized laboratories only
	Thyroperoxidase/ microsomal (TPO/M)	IIF	Aid in diagnosis	Superseded by more objective tests such as HA or ELISA
		HA	Aid in diagnosis	Commercially available
		ELISA	Aid in diagnosis	Commercially available
		ELISA—epitope analysis	Research	Performed in specialized laboratories only
	Thyrotropin receptor (TSHR)	Bioassay	Aid in diagnosis	Specific for functional antibodies, stimulating or blocking Performed in specialized laboratories only
		Binding assay	Aid in diagnosis	Not specific for stimulating antibodies Commercially available
Adrenal	Adrenal cortex cytoplasmic antigens	IIF on primate adrenal	Aid in diagnosis	Only clinically available test
		ELISA—specific antigens of the adrenal	Research	
		Western blot	Research	

Abbreviations: IIF = indirect immunofluorescence; HA = hemagglutination; ELISA = enzyme-linked immunosorbent assay.

Autoantibodies may help distinguish between different forms of a condition, which in turn may result in the use of different therapeutic strategies. For example, it is important to differentiate a case of adrenal insufficiency due to an infectious cause from a case associated with autoimmunity. The presence of adrenal autoantibodies tends to be a specific but not a sensitive marker of autoimmune adrenalitis. Thus, antibodies can confirm a diagnosis but not rule one out.

A change in antibody quantity may be a monitor of successful therapy or a predictor of disease exacerbation. For diseases of endocrine origin, however, changes in titer have less relevance in the management of the disorder. In these diseases, a change in titer is frequently unrelated to clinical status. Often the symptoms are treated without "curing" the disease. Replacement therapy for hyporesponsiveness is initiated to normalize the signs and symptoms of disease without treating the underlying immunologic cause. In many cases, the immunologic mechanism of the disease has not yet been clarified and is the topic of considerable research. Until the etiology and immunopathogenesis have been determined, immunologic interventions are unlikely to succeed.

Autoantibodies may be used as indicators of individuals who are at risk of future disease, as in the case of endocrinopathies that have genetic predisposition. Thyroiditis and Graves' disease can be familial disorders. Children are at much higher risk of either thyroiditis or Graves' disease if both parents have thyroid autoantibodies.[5] Autoantibodies also may be predictive of postpartum thyroiditis, because the presence of thyroid autoantibodies before pregnancy or the development of such autoantibodies during pregnancy imparts a much higher risk of postpartum thyroiditis.[6] Subclinical autoimmune thyroiditis also may be identified by the presence of autoantibodies in conjunction with elevated TSH but normal levels of thyroid hormones. Affected patients should be monitored closely, because their risk of developing clinical thyroiditis is very high.

Autoantibodies are found secondary to an initial infection or other tissue injury, as in postinfarction syndrome or postinfectious encephalomyelitis. In these situations, the demonstration of autoantibodies may be valuable in recognizing an autoimmune state and distinguishing it from the initial injury.

In certain patients, autoantibodies may cause the disease; however, this has proved true in only a few systems. Such instances include autoantibodies that are directed to the erythrocyte surface (autoimmune hemolytic anemia), to TSH receptors in Graves' disease, to acetylcholine receptors of the neuromuscular junctions in myasthenia gravis, and to antigens of the epidermis as found in bullous skin diseases such as pemphigus vulgaris. Even in these cases, the pathogeneses are largely unknown and are topics of continuing investigation. An interesting note about autoimmune thyroiditis: even after 40 years of research, the relative contribution of infiltrating cells as the cause of disease and the role of autoantibodies in initiating disease have not yet been clarified.

In general, autoantibody tests should not be used as the sole criterion for diagnosis of disease. The whole patient must be taken into account. Autoantibodies are found in normal individuals who have no clinical illness, ranging in frequency according to age and sex. Generally, the lowest frequency is in young men and the highest in elderly women. Consequently, the demonstration of autoantibodies is not necessarily synonymous with autoimmune disease. However, as a marker of disease, the presence of autoantibodies is the clinical laboratory assay used most frequently as an aid to identify autoimmune conditions.

Rationale of Test Selection for Autoimmune Thyroid and Adrenal Diseases

Techniques for demonstrating autoantibodies are prescribed by the location and properties of the antigen and the required level of sensitivity. Early assays, some of which are still used today, included agglutination and precipitation techniques. Precipitation in fluid or agar media (eg, immunodiffusion) is less sensitive than most assays and is not used as a routine clinical test for endocrine autoantibodies. However, it is still appropriate for the demonstration of antibodies to complex mixture-soluble antigens, such as certain nuclear antigens that have not yet been purified.

Indirect immunofluorescence microscopy (IIFM) is the most commonly used test for the detection of tissue-specific autoantibodies because of its versatility. Indirect immunofluorescence can detect multiple antibodies on a single tissue or on a multiple tissue block; thus, it has considerable value as a screening test. Autoantibody isotype can be determined by using heavy chain–specific anti-immunoglobulin conjugates. Indirect immunofluorescence is particularly valuable in testing for autoantibodies for which the antigen has not yet been characterized and for unexpected antibodies. Autoantibodies may be missed by an assay using a single purified antigen. With IIFM, the reaction site can be seen. Thus, the location of the cellular antigen can be determined, and other antibodies to the tissue can be detected. Indirect immunofluorescence can be considered semiquantitative, because a serum titer can be established for a particular sample. A titer is the reciprocal of the last serum dilution to give a positive reaction. Before the identification of the thyroid microsomal antigen, IIFM was the primary technique to identify these antibodies. The test is still used and is still valid. However, other tests, such as those described in this chapter, have for the most part superseded this technique. Indirect immunofluorescence is still the major assay used to identify adrenal autoantibodies.

The major autoantigen associated with a particular autoimmune disorder is eventually isolated, as in the case of the major thyroid antigens Tg and TPO. Subsequently, more sensitive semiquantitative tests, such as hemagglutination (HA), enzyme-linked immunosorbent assay (ELISA), or radioimmunoassay (RIA), have been developed using the isolated antigen fraction and have replaced or supplemented IIFM. Autoantibody isotype detected in these indirect tests can be evaluated by using heavy chain–specific or subclass-specific anti-immunoglobulin conjugated to a detection marker (fluorochrome or enzyme). The results of these tests can be expressed as a titer if serial dilutions are performed. An alternative is to develop ranges of reactivity (eg, nonreactive, low, medium, high) that can be compared with previously determined control values. Many of the commercial ELISA or RIA kits evaluate sera in this fashion. Another way to express the results is based on international units. Few autoantibody tests use this method, because it requires an international standard of antibody preparation that is widely available (and that does not yet exist). Expression of results as international units has the advantage of comparing one laboratory result with another. This should be considered as a goal for the future. A further method of expressing results that is truly quantitative is expressing specific immunoglobulins in actual amounts of µg/mL. For this method of expression, an affinity-purified antibody that has been assayed for total immunoglobulin (Ig) G and IgG subclasses is necessary.

Autoimmune Thyroiditis

Autoimmune thyroiditis is known by many names. It has been referred to as lymphocytic thyroiditis, chronic lymphocytic thyroiditis, Hashimoto's disease, and simply thyroiditis. The term *Hashimoto's disease* has become synonymous with the goitrous form of chronic autoimmune thyroiditis. End-stage disease results in signs and symptoms of hypothyroidism, including fatigue, mental impairment, cold intolerance, and weight gain. Biochemical signs of disease are low levels of the thyroid hormones, such as thyroxine (T_4) or triiodothyronine (T_3), and high levels of TSH. However, not all hypothyroidism has an autoimmune etiology. The immunologic hallmarks for autoimmune thyroiditis are autoantibodies to 2 of the major autoantigens of the thyroid gland, Tg and TPO. These autoantibodies are accompanied by lymphocytic infiltration of the thyroid gland with inflammation and destruction of the thyroid follicles. The mechanism by which the immunologic response contributes to the thyroid cell destruction has still not been explained. Autoimmune thyroiditis is considered a multifactorial disease with both genetic and environmental components contributing to it.

Other thyroid conditions associated with the Tg and TPO antibodies include myxedema, certain types of goiter, thyroid cancer, and Graves' disease. Myxedema is thought to be the result of long-standing autoimmune thyroiditis with the accumulation of glycosaminoglycans in subcutaneous and other interstitial tissue. Graves' disease is the hyperthyroid condition caused by autoantibodies binding to and stimulating the TSH receptor, which is discussed later. Some individuals with normal thyroids also possess autoantibodies to Tg. Interestingly, thyroiditis patients frequently develop autoantibodies to other thyroid-specific antigens, especially TPO. Unlike Tg, however, TPO does not appear capable of initiating the autoimmune process in most animals. There is evidence, in fact, that it may be the consequence of initial autoimmune damage.[7] Some observers therefore have concluded that antibodies to TPO make better indicators of active thyroid inflammation than do antibodies to Tg.

Interestingly, there is a tendency for more than one autoimmune disorder to occur in the same individual. The overlaps are generally within the same category of disease, as seen in a patient with multiple endocrine disorders (such as thyroiditis and adrenalitis) or multiple connective tissue diseases (such as patients with Sjögren's keratoconjunctivitis sicca and lupus). In addition, there is a significantly higher incidence of autoantibodies to unrelated organ-specific antigens in patients with an autoimmune disease. For example, 25% of patients with thyroiditis have antibodies to gastric parietal cells, while almost 50% of patients with pernicious anemia have antibodies to a thyroid antigen. Antibodies to thyroid antigen occur in 25% of patients with Addison's disease (adrenal insufficiency) and in 20% of patients with diabetes mellitus, suggesting that a shared autoimmune factor is involved in those diseases. The aggregation of autoimmune responses to immunologically distinct organ-specific antigens cannot be explained except as a genetic predisposition to the development of autoimmune responses.

Laboratory Evaluation of Thyroid Autoantibodies

When autoimmune thyroiditis is suspected as the underlying cause of hypothyroidism, the laboratory detection of thyroid autoantibodies helps confirm a diagnosis.[8] As previously discussed, the most commonly detected thyroid autoantibodies are to the antigens Tg and TPO. Autoantibodies to the TSH receptor are not part of routine testing. This is a very specialized test and is available only in special centers. It is complex, requires a high level of technical skill, and uses very specialized reagents.[9,10]

The College of American Pathologists conducts a proficiency survey for the detection of autoantibodies to Tg and TPO antigens. It is part of the Diagnostic Immunology Series 2 Survey. More information can be obtained from the College of American Pathologists, 325 Waukegan Road, Northfield, IL 60093-2750; 800-323-4040.

International biologic standards for Tg and microsomal antigen antibodies are available through the National Institute for Biological Standards and Control. Information about obtaining a sample can be obtained by contacting the organization at PO Box 1193, Potters Bar, Hertfordshire EN6 3QH, United Kingdom; e-mail: standards@nibsc.ac.uk.

Autoantigens

Thyroglobulin

Thyroglobulin is one of the main autoantigens of the thyroid; it constitutes the main component of the colloid within the thyroid follicle. It plays an essential role in the storage of iodine and synthesis of the iodinated thyroid proteins T_4 and T_3. It is a 660-kd glycoprotein consisting of 2 apparently identical 330-kd polypeptide chains.

Thyroglobulin biochemistry has been reviewed in depth elsewhere,[11] so this chapter only summarizes some of the major findings. The gene for human Tg has been discovered on chromosome 8. Molecular cloning from complementary DNA (cDNA) prepared from thyroid glands indicates that the messenger RNA (mRNA) is composed of 8,448 base pairs.[12] Subsequent protein expression and sequencing of overlapping peptides has shown that the monomer of the molecule consists of 2,767 amino acids.[12] Of these amino acids, 67 are tyrosines, for a total of 134 per molecule. The iodinated tyrosines are the amino acids that make up the thyroid hormones. Thyroglobulin is highly glycosylated, with 10% carbohydrate by weight. It also undergoes other posttranslational modifications of phosphorylation, sulfations, and iodinations.

The amino acid structure shows 3 types of internal homologies. The N-terminal portion of the molecules has a sequence of approximately 60 amino acids, each of which is repeated 10 times. Cysteine, proline, and glycine are highly represented in this domain, possibly for maintaining a rigid conformation to promote hormonogenesis. A second domain found in the central part of the molecule consists of 3 segments of 14 to 17 amino acids. The final domain appears 5 times between residues 1603 and 2186. The C-terminal part of Tg shares no homology with the N-terminal part of the molecule. Strikingly, however, the C-terminus is about 90% homologous with the sequence of acetylcholinesterase.[13] The functional importance of this homology is unknown, but there is speculation about the evolutionary aspects of the respective genes. Another interesting homology is a portion of the N-terminal part of the molecule that has similarities to the invariant chain of the Ia protein of the murine major histocompatibility complex antigen.[14]

There also is considerable homology among species. For example, human and bovine Tg share approximately 70% of the same protein sequence.[15] It is surprising, therefore, that the serologic response to Tg in patients does not show more species cross-reactivity. Studies on the fine specificities of Tg autoantibodies from the author's laboratory (Johns Hopkins University) confirm that patients develop autoantibodies that react with those parts of the molecule that are human-specific rather than cross-reactive.[16]

Thyroglobulin autoantibodies can be demonstrated by several procedures, such as precipitation in agar, IIF, indirect HA of cells coated with Tg, RIA, and ELISA. At present, HA is the most commonly employed technique for the detection of antibodies against Tg. The ELISA is increasingly used for the measurement of antibodies to Tg. It also detects antibodies that are nonagglutinating. Indirect immunofluorescence is rarely used. At least one laboratory has reported a quantitative ELISA assay for Tg antibodies.[17] This assay uses an affinity-purified anti-Tg antibody that was well characterized for immunoglobulin quantity. Radioimmunoassay using iodine 125 (^{125}I)–labeled antigens also has proven useful but has limited availability.[18]

Assay Methods

The methods described here for detecting Tg autoantibodies include only the most frequently used assays: HA, IIF, and ELISA. Most of these methodologies are similar for the individual autoantibodies with differences in tissue substrates or antigens.

Hemagglutination employs stable suspensions of erythrocytes coated with the appropriate soluble antigen. Autoantibodies cross-link the coated particles that form the complex lattice structure of agglutination. Group O red blood cells are used routinely in this procedure to prevent agglutination due to blood group antibodies. Passive HA tests with the use of tanned erythrocytes (tanned-cell hemagglutination [TCH]) or chromic chloride–treated erythrocytes (chromic chloride hemagglutination [CCH]) are very sensitive. Experimental details are described elsewhere.[10] Thus, these techniques detect antibodies to

Tg in a variety of conditions other than thyroiditis, a possible disadvantage for diagnosis.

Erythrocytes treated with tannic acid are capable of adsorbing protein antigens on their surface. When added to serial dilutions of patient serum, these erythrocytes react with the appropriate antibody, if present, giving a visible agglutination reaction. Tanned erythrocytes coated with thyroid extract or purified Tg are employed to detect antibodies to Tg. The method is highly sensitive but requires fresh erythrocytes and reagents for best results. It may be replaced by the CCH method for adsorption of antigen to the red blood cells.

Chromic chloride can be used to couple Tg to erythrocytes, providing a simpler alternative to the tannic acid method.[10] However, this test is not commercially available. Setting up and creating a "homemade" assay makes the chromic chloride assay less attractive to most clinical laboratories, even though the assay may have certain advantages. The chromic chloride assay has been shown to be equally sensitive to ELISA in research.[19]

Several commercially available kits are widely used. They vary in sensitivity, and no standardized assessment of the different kits has been performed. However, their availability has allowed many laboratories to perform evaluation of Tg antibodies without the onus of reagent preparation of Tg or preparation of antigen-coated red blood cells. Information about these Tg assays has been reviewed in the literature.[20]

Enzyme-linked immunosorbent assay is an indirect method of antibody assessment. It uses specialized microtiter plates and individual antigens for coating the plates. Antibody dilutions are incubated in the wells, and any antibody binds to the antigen. Excess proteins are washed away. The second antibody, anti-human immunoglobulin, is conjugated to an enzyme. This reagent is incubated in the wells and, again, excess proteins are washed away. An enzyme substrate is added to the wells and hydrolyzed, causing a color change in the substrate. The change in color is dose dependent on the initial antibody bound. This can be read in a spectrophotometer and expressed as a particular optical density. The results are compared with known positives and negatives. It is essential to have a conjugate-only control to determine nonspecific reactivity of the conjugate itself. Details of the ELISA procedure have been described previously.[10,21] Factors to consider when preparing an ELISA are

- Antigen coating of the plate (concentration, volume, and so forth)
- The necessity of a blocking step
- Incubation times for the individual steps
- Anti-human immunoglobulin concentration
- Time of substrate incubation
- Expression of results
- Interpretation of findings

Requirements for an ELISA for Tg autoantibodies also have been described.[19,22] Commercially available ELISAs are available, and it is essential to follow the manufacturer's instructions rigorously. The method is especially useful for large-scale studies. An advantage of the ELISA is that it can detect thyroid autoantibodies that are not hemagglutinating antibodies. Another advantage is that specific isotypes of the Tg antibody can be determined.[23,24] Although at present this may be a controversial issue and the test should be regarded as a research tool, additional investigation of isotypes may provide insight into the subsets of the disease. A quantitative ELISA has been developed that expresses the amount of individual Tg-specific IgG subclasses in μg/mL.[17]

Although ELISA readily detects antibody to Tg in those sera that have medium to high titers of autoantibodies determined by HA, it may not readily discriminate between negatives and those samples with low titers.[19] The reason for this is unclear, especially because ELISA has proved to be as sensitive as the isotopic assay in other antibody detection systems. Possibly, the ELISA is less sensitive to particular subclasses of antibody to Tg.

Recent evidence shows that there is a difference in the antigenic specificity of autoantibodies to Tg in patients with thyroiditis compared with people with antibody but no disease. The naturally occurring antibodies from normal individuals are directed primarily to sites on the molecule that are shared among species (ie, conserved), whereas those found primarily in patients with thyroiditis are directed to human-specific regions.[25]

Indirect immunofluorescence is rarely used for the detection of Tg autoantibodies. If IIF is used, special handling of the thyroid tissue is necessary because Tg is water-soluble and leaches off the slide. Therefore, the tissue is fixed in methanol at 56°C for 3 minutes. The staining pattern obtained when methanol-fixed sections are used is characteristic and has a floccular, "puffy" appearance. Details of the IIF procedure are described fully in the section on TPO antibodies.

Radioimmunoassay also is rarely used. Many of the RIA procedures are being superseded by ELISA techniques. One RIA uses ^{125}I-labeled Tg to identify Tg autoantibodies.[26] However, this sensitive assay has limited availability.

The prevalence of Tg autoantibodies varies with the sensitivity of the assay from 25% using IIF to 100% in very sensitive HA, ELISA, or RIA tests.[20] These antibodies are found in individuals with chronic thyroiditis, myxedema, Graves' disease, goiter, thyroid tumors, and other polyendocrine disorders. The highest titers are found in patients with autoimmune thyroid disorders. Low titers of Tg antibodies may be found in normal individuals. Low but significant titers also may be found in children.[5,27] The prevalence of such antibodies in patients without overt thyroid disease is higher in women. The incidence also increases with age, so that 18% of women older than 40 years may have antibodies to Tg. Total Tg antibody is not a specific marker of autoimmune thyroiditis, because so many other conditions also show the presence of this antibody. Recent evidence suggests, however, that there may be disease-related epitope specificity of the autoantibody.[25] The disease-related antibodies were detected by competitive inhibition ELISA experiments of murine monoclonal antibodies.

Thyroid Peroxidase

The microsomal antigen was discovered by Holborow et al[28] and found to be an integral part of the smooth endoplasmic reticulum.[29] Later, Mariotti et al[30] showed an intimate association between microsomal antigen and the lipid bilayer of the membrane. Microsomal antigen is available on the membrane in thyroid cell cultures, where it is located on the apical surface of acinar cells,[31] but it also can appear on the basal side under certain experimental conditions.[32] The microsomal antigen also is found on the surface of cultured rat thyroid cells,[33] although its expression is dependent on the presence of TSH in the medium.

Thyroid peroxidase has been identified as an antigen that reacts with human antimicrosomal antibodies.[34,35] Antibody to the microsomal antigen binds complement and may participate in complement-mediated cytotoxicity,[36] as well as in antibody-dependent cell-mediated cytotoxicity.[37]

Recent studies have provided some information on the biochemical and immunochemical character of the antigen. There are difficulties in purifying TPO, because after isolation and solubilization of the microsomes, contaminating substances (especially Tg) have been found.[30,38–40] Despite this problem, 2 independent groups of investigators used immunoprecipitation[39,40] and Western immunoblot[40] techniques to identify a protein with a molecular weight of about 105 kd. This protein binds to antimicrosomal antibody from patients with autoimmune disease.[34,35,39] Intrachain disulfide bonds may be present; Banga et al[39] found a difference in the mobility of the antigen in polyacrylamide gel electrophoresis when comparing reducing versus nonreducing conditions. At least 2 epitopes bind antibodies from patient sera. One of the antigenic sites is a sequential epitope, while the other may be a conformational epitope dependent on the integrity of the intrachain disulfide bonds. Some reviews have explored the immunologic and molecular characteristics of the TPO autoantigen.[41,42]

Although TPO has been identified as an antigen that reacts with human antimicrosomal antibodies,[34,35] purified TPO is not readily available for use in diagnostic tests. The most commonly used tests for the microsomal autoantibodies are IIF using primate thyroid tissue, a commercially available HA assay, ELISA, and at least one radioimmunoassay. One commercial test now uses chemiluminescence.

Assay Methods

For many years, the test of choice for the detection of microsomal antigens was complement fixation using an optimal dilution of thyrotoxic thyroid extract.[28] The immunofluorescence method that replaced this test was found to be more sensitive, and IIF remains one of the most commonly used tests for microsomal autoantibody. The substrate consists of frozen human or monkey thyroid tissue that is air dried and unfixed. A positive test of patient sera on unfixed slides appears as bright fluorescence of the cytoplasm of the follicular epithelial cells. Commercially available HA tests are now replacing IIF because of the speed of the former and its increased sensitivity. This increased sensitivity, however, may lead to reduced specificity, because normal individuals may also exhibit these autoantibodies.

While titers of TPO by IIF may reach 1,200 or higher, those obtained by HA may reach well over 25,000. The antibodies to TPO belong predominantly to the IgG class and, when detected by IIF, stain the cytoplasm of thyroid cells. Indirect immunofluorescence for antibodies to TPO is positive in approximately 70% to 90% of patients with chronic thyroiditis. It is also positive in 64% of patients with primary hypothyroidism, 50% of patients with thyrotoxicosis, 10% of patients with simple goiters, and 17% of patients with thyroid tumor. It can be found in normal individuals at a low frequency and titer.

In performing IIF, serum is placed on a frozen tissue section (4 µm thick). If autoantibodies are present, they bind to the appropriate antigen. Excess serum is washed away. A second reagent, antihuman immunoglobulin conjugated to a fluorescent dye (usually fluorescein isothiocyanate [FITC]) is then incubated with the tissue section. Unbound reagent is again washed away. Autoantibodies are detected by microscopes with an appropriate light source (usually mercury vapor or halogen quartz) and filter system that enables the fluorescent markers to be seen.

The most important variables involved in producing a standardized technique are (1) the type of substrate, including source, storage, and preparation; (2) the duration of staining and washing; and (3) the specificity and sensitivity of the conjugate. An essential part of each test is the incorporation of known positive and negative reactive sera as controls. The most readily available substrate tissue for IIF is primate thyroid. Rabbit or goat antisera, prepared by immunization with human globulin or with individual isotypes of immunoglobulins (eg, heavy chain or subclass specific) and conjugated to FITC, are used to detect the site of the reaction between tissue substrate and antibody from the patient's serum. Plasma is less useful in IIF, because the fibrinogen causes considerable nonspecific fluorescence of tissue substrate; therefore, serum is the sample of choice. Because concentrated serum also causes nonspecific staining and results in unclear results, an initial serum dilution using phosphate buffered saline (PBS) of 1:10 or greater is recommended, depending on the sensitivity of the assay. Screening of patient sera may be performed initially using 2 or more dilutions. Positive sera should be retested using serial dilutions until the reaction is negative so that an end point titer can be determined. The titer is considered to be the reciprocal of the last dilution that gives a positive (+1) response. Until standard sera are generally available, each laboratory must establish its own set of standards regarding quantitation. Each assay that is run should include controls for tissue autofluorescence and conjugate specificity, and known positive and negative sera. Fluorescein isothiocyanate conjugate combined with an optional counterstain of rhodamine B-BSA (Rh B-BSA) or Evans blue provides good contrast to the FITC conjugate. Indirect immunofluorescence is less sensitive but reportedly can detect nonagglutinating antibodies that are missed by other procedures. It can also detect antibodies to CA2 (the second colloid antigen), which are undetectable by HA.

Several HA and ELISA kits for TPO/microsomal autoantibodies are available. However, some tests may be labeled TPO but actually use a microsomal preparation for coating. These preparations of "TPO" from human tissue invariably contain Tg contaminants. Manufacturers mitigate these contaminants by adding absorbents to the diluent. However, a false-positive result may occur if the sample contains a high titer of Tg autoantibodies. Tests using recombinant antigen are not subject to this potential failing.

With any kit, it is essential to follow the manufacturer's instructions exactly. When changing lots or techniques for the evaluation of autoantibodies, parallel testing of the old and new is also necessary. Documentation of parallel testing should be maintained.

The sensitivity of HA or ELISA for TPO/antimicrosomal antibodies is greater than with IIF. However, the antigens are not readily available for development of these assays in individual laboratories. Most laboratories depend on the commercially available tests.

Graves' Disease

Graves' disease is an exception to the concept that disease causes organ hyporesponsiveness. Graves' disease results in hyperthyroidism due to autoantibody binding to the thyrotropin receptor, mimicking the action of TSH. No feedback loop is in operation; therefore, signs and symptoms of hyperthyroidism, such as hyperactivity, fatigue, heat intolerance, change in weight (usually loss), palpitations, and ophthalmopathy, result. The biochemical signs of Graves' disease are elevated T_4 and reduced TSH levels. The immunologic marker and cause of the condition are autoantibodies to the thyrotropin receptor called thyroid-stimulating antibody (TSAb). Additional details about these clinical conditions are covered elsewhere in the literature.[43] The detection of TSAb is not yet a routine part of the laboratory detection of Graves' disease, although certain clinical situations indicate that such detection could be useful.[3]

Autoantigen: Thyrotropin Receptor

The thyroid-stimulating hormone (thyrotropin receptor [TSHR]) is present on the thyrocyte cell surface, primarily on the basilar or basolateral pole of the cell.[44] The frequency of these molecules on the surface is very low, with only 10^3 to 10^4 sites per cell.[9] The receptor has been cloned from dogs, humans, and rats[45–47] and is described here briefly.[48] The protein from cDNA has 764 amino acids, with approximately 21 serving as a signal peptide. The protein is composed of approximately 743 amino acids, with an estimated molecular weight of 84.5 kd. There also are about 15-kd carbohydrate moieties, so the entire molecule is approximately 100 kd. The extracellular amino terminal part of the molecule consists of 397 amino acids and is heavily glycosylated. The carboxyl terminal part of the receptor spans the plasma membrane 7 times and ends with a cytoplasmic tail of 82 amino acids. Additional details can be found elsewhere in the literature.[48]

Autoantibodies binding to the TSHR on the surface of thyroid epithelial cells are the primary cause of the hyperthyroidism in Graves' disease. Initially called long-acting thyroid stimulator (LATS), the antibody was first identified as a stimulatory serum factor present in a few patients with Graves' disease when measured by bioassay in mice.[49,50] However, not all antibodies bind to mouse thyroid, the basis of the LATS bioassay. Another subset of these receptor antibodies, called long-acting thyroid stimulator-protector (LATS-P), was found to bind only to human thyroid and not to mouse thyroid. This subset was named for its function, because it prevented or "protected" neutralization of LATS when human thyroid tissue was added to serum before the LATS bioassay.[51]

As a whole, these antibodies are conventionally called thyrotropin receptor antibodies (TRAbs). The TSAbs bind near to or with the TSHR and mimic TSH activity, resulting in uncontrolled stimulation because there is no negative feedback control.

Clinical Utility

Diagnosis of hyperthyroidism depends on the demonstration of elevated thyroid hormones, which may not always be due to autoimmune disease. The prevalence of TSAbs, by definition, should be 100%. However, many assays lack the needed sensitivity or use systems that do not express the particular epitopes that will bind to these antibodies. For example, the use of rat cell lines or xenogeneic antigens (bovine or porcine TSHRs) reduces the utility of these tests because not all antibodies cross-react to foreign antigens.

Thus, the detection of these antibodies in patients with Graves' disease ranges from 55% to 95%, depending on the assay. The TSAb assay is of greatest utility in conditions where conventional test results are equivocal or where clinical signs and symptoms are minimal. An example of this is where patients exhibit thyroid-associated ophthalmopathy in the absence of other symptoms.[52] Moreover, the TSAb assay is usually negative for patients with thyrotoxicosis in association with thyroid nodules, cancer, or subacute thyroiditis.[53] Therefore, a positive test establishes a diagnosis of Graves' disease with a high degree of confidence. The assay can be used to monitor patient therapy; successful treatment of Graves' disease with propylthiouracil or methimazole may result in lower levels of TSAbs. Therefore, monitoring these antibodies may help to predict the clinical course of disease.[54] The assay also has proven useful in the diagnosis of neonatal thyrotoxicosis (in which the maternal antibodies cross the placenta and cause thyrotoxicosis in the infant). There is at least one reported case of a hypothyroid mother whose newborn child suffered severely from this disorder.[55] On testing the mother, a high level of TSAb was found, which was a completely unexpected finding based on her medical history.

Assay Methods

Tests for TSAbs are primarily of 2 types: bioassays or binding assays. Autoantibodies that are detected by bioassay and demonstrate the ability to stimulate the thyroid are properly called stimulating antibodies. All antibodies detected by binding assays may not be biologically functional. If not, the antibodies are referred to as thyrotropin-binding antibodies or thyrotropin-binding inhibitory immunoglobulin (TBII), depending on the relevant assay. Each of these tests is highly complex and requires specialized reagents.

Most bioassays have limited utility because they are cumbersome and require scarce materials, such as viable slices of fresh human thyroid tissue or cultured cell lines. Bioassays evaluate functional aspects of the antibodies, such as adenylate cyclase activation or cyclic adenosine monophosphate (cAMP) increase, as their end point.[56]

Binding assays are based on competition between ^{125}I-labeled TSH and patient immunoglobulin for binding to thyroid preparations. However, these assays do not discriminate among the heterogeneous types of autoantibodies that may be bound (ie, stimulating versus blocking). Therefore, a true value of TSAb cannot be evaluated. The TSAb and TBII may represent different specificities of autoantibodies to the thyroid epithelial cell surface on or near the TSHR. The heterogeneity of the autoantibodies and the diversity of the assays for their demonstration has created some confusion. The antibodies and their tests have been reviewed in the literature.[9,10]

An assay using a cloned line of rat thyroid cells (FRTL-5) is very promising, because these cells can be maintained in tissue culture. This assay is based on the stimulation of adenylate cyclase in the cell membranes of FRTL-5 by patient sera. The amount of cAMP is measured and compared with the effect of normal sera, and a "thyroid-stimulating immunoglobulin index" is calculated. At least 2 groups of investigators have found good correlation between an elevated index and Graves' disease.[53,57] Kits for cAMP measurement are commercially available.

Chinese hamster ovary cells have been adapted for this assay. The human recombinant TSHR has been introduced to this cell line.[58,59] Theoretically, this combines the advantages of having (1) human antigens instead of a foreign species and (2) a convenient source of a "standard" cell line instead of relying on the availability of fresh thyroid tissue. Indeed, several reports have shown the utility of this approach as cells for a bioassay, in the purification of the soluble receptors for binding assays, or for flow cytometry.[60–62] One investigation extended this approach by expressing a biotinylated human TSHR in HeLa cells and using this reagent to develop an assay for Graves' disease autoantibodies.[63]

In the next few years, with improvements in the techniques to measure TSAbs, the assays will be more widespread and more information will become available. This will ultimately lead to a better understanding of the etiology and pathogenesis of autoimmune thyroid disease.

Idiopathic Autoimmune Addison's Disease

The idiopathic form of primary adrenocortical insufficiency (Addison's disease) is frequently associated with autoimmune phenomena. Antibodies bind to (usually unidentified) antigens associated with the cytoplasm of cells. However, some progress has been made in identifying major antigens of the adrenal gland that are rarely found in healthy individuals. Indirect immunofluorescence is the predominant method of autoantibody detection and the only one clinically available at this time.

The presence of these antibodies suggests that the disease is idiopathic, potentially of immune origin, and not of malignant, infectious, or other nature. However, it is not uncommon for patients with autoantibodies to one endocrine organ to have multiple endocrine reactivities. Based on prospective studies,[64] the presence of adrenal autoantibodies in healthy individuals may serve as a predictive sign of incipient adrenal failure. Furthermore, not all patients with a particular disorder have the autoantibodies, so a negative test result does not exclude a particular diagnosis. On the other hand, a positive test is not necessarily diagnostic, because the patient may have other autoantibodies to endocrine organs without clinical disease.

Idiopathic Addison's disease is frequently associated with other autoimmune conditions and their respective autoantibodies. In certain patients, the autoantibodies cross-react with steroid-secreting cells of the theca interna of the ovary or with the interstitial cells of the testis. In female patients with Addison's disease and in those with primary ovarian failure, clinical evidence of ovarian failure is correlated with the presence of these autoantibodies. Adrenal antibodies are found with differing frequency, ranging from 20% of certain groups of Addison's disease patients to 100% of patients with ovarian failure.[65]

Autoantigens

In recent years, a major antigen of the adrenal gland has been identified. The cytochrome P450 enzyme 21 hydroxylase (21-OH) was recognized by the presence of antibodies to it in patients with idiopathic Addison's disease or other autoimmune endocrinopathies.[66] One longitudinal study[67] indicates that disappearance of adrenal-specific autoantibodies can occur in individuals without clinical symptoms of disease. Furthermore, the disappearance of antibodies, even if induced by corticosteroid therapy, correlated with a return of adrenal function in patients with Addison's disease.[67] As is the case in thyroiditis, the autoimmune response to individual epitopes may predict benign autoimmunity compared with a malignant progression of autoimmunity. Epitope analysis using recombinant antigens has been initiated and has revealed that over 80% of antibody-positive patients react to a conserved part of the molecule.[68] Further test development with individual autoantigenic epitopes may provide more useful information in the future.

Clinical Laboratory Assays

Currently, autoantibodies to the adrenal cortex are demonstrated by IIF on primate adrenal tissue substrate. The same reagents and procedures previously described for the thyroid TPO IIF test are used. Frozen (unfixed and air dried) sections of monkey or human adrenal glands are used as tissue substrate. Because titers of antibody are low and are rarely found in the normal population, starting dilutions can be as low as 1:2. However, it is important to include a negative control serum at the same dilution, because nonspecific binding is high at these concentrations of sera.

The autoantibodies may react with individual zones or with all 3 zones of the adrenal cortex. Most sera stain the whole cortex, with a brighter fluorescence in the glomerular zone. A few sera stain only the fascicular and reticular zones, and not the glomerular zone. The latter pattern has been reported with sera that also stain the interstitial cells of the testis and the theca interna cells of the ovary. The antibodies belong predominantly to the IgG class and, in general, have low titers (not higher than 100). The specific antigens in more quantitative tests, such as ELISA, have been used in clinical research projects as mentioned previously. However, until the antigens are widely available, usage will remain limited.

Summary

Several concepts are clear:

- Autoimmunity and autoimmune disease are not synonymous.
- Autoimmunity or autoimmune disease may involve humoral and cell-mediated reactivities.
- Autoantibodies are often associated with autoimmune disorders and are easier to evaluate than cell-mediated reactions.
- Measurement of these autoantibodies help in disease definition, are useful markers for diagnostic purposes, or in some cases, are part of the pathogenesis and can correlate with disease severity.

However, as useful as these autoantibodies are in the above processes, we must not forget that autoantibodies must not be used as the sole criteria for the diagnosis of a disorder. Many healthy people also develop autoantibodies unrelated to any biological disorder. Therefore, the total clinical picture of an individual must be considered. Future directions for diagnostic capabilities include the further discrimination between benign autoimmune reactivities and those associated with disease.

References

1. Witebsky E, Rose NR, Terplan K, et al. Chronic thyroiditis and autoimmunization. *JAMA*. 1957;164: 1439–1447.
2. Rose NR, Bona C. Defining criteria for autoimmune diseases (Witebsky's postulates revisited). *Immunol Today*. 1993;14:426–430. [Review]
3. Rose NR, Witebsky E. Studies on organ specificity, V: Changes in the thyroid glands of rabbit following active immunization with rabbit thyroid extracts. *J Immunol*. 1956;76:417–427.
4. Roitt IM, Doniach D, Campbell PN, et al. V: Autoantibodies in Hashimoto's disease. *Lancet*. 1956;2:820–821.
5. Burek CL, Hoffman WH, Rose NR. The presence of thyroid autoantibodies in children and adolescents with autoimmune thyroid disease and in their siblings and parents. *Clin Immunol Immunopathol*. 1982;25:395–404.
6. Stagnaro-Green A. Postpartum thyroiditis: Prevalence, etiology, and clinical implications. *Thyroid*. 1993;16:1–12.
7. Rose NR, Skelton FR, Kite JHJ, et al. Experimental thyroiditis in the rhesus monkey, 3: Course of the disease. *Clin Exp Immunol*. 1966;1:171–188.
8. Singer PA, Cooper DS, Levy EG, et al. Treatment guidelines for patients with hyperthyroidism and hypothyroidism. Standards of Care Committee, American Thyroid Association. *JAMA*. 1995;273:808–812.
9. Volpe R. Thyrotropin receptor autoantibodies. In: Peter JB, Shoenfeld Y, eds. *Autoantibodies*. Amsterdam, the Netherlands: Elsevier Biomedical; 1996:822–829.
10. Bigazzi PE, Burek CL, Rose NR, et al. Endocrinopathies. In: Rose NR, Conway de Macario E, Folds JD, et al, eds. *Manual of Clinical Laboratory Immunology*. 5th ed. Washington, DC: American Society for Microbiology; 1997:972–988.
11. Dunn JT. Thyroglobulin: Chemistry and biosynthesis. In: Braverman LE, Utiger RD, eds. *The Thyroid*. 6th ed. New York, NY: JB Lippincott Co; 1991:98–110.
12. Malthiery Y, Lissitzky S. Primary structure of human thyroglobulin deduced from the sequence of its 8448-base complementary DNA. *Eur J Biochem*. 1987;165: 491–498.

13. Swillens S, Ludgate M, Mercken L, et al. Analysis of sequence and structure homologies between thyroglobulin and acetylcholinesterase: Possible functional and clinical significance. *Biochem Biophys Res Commun*. 1986;137:142–148.

14. Koch N, Lauer W, Habicht J, et al. Primary structure of the gene for the murine Ia antigen-associated invariant chains (Ii): An alternatively spliced exon encodes a cysteine-rich domain highly homologous to a repetitive sequence of thyroglobulin. *EMBO J*. 1987;6:1677–1683.

15. Mercken L, Simons MJ, Swillens S, et al. Primary structure of bovine thyroglobulin deduced from the sequence of its 8,431-base complementary DNA. *Nature*. 1985;316:647–651.

16. Wildberger E, Von Gruenigen C, Kohler J, et al. Regulation of enzymatic iodothyronine synthesis in thyroglobulin by low concentrations of iodide. *Eur J Biochem*. 1983;130:485–490.

17. Kuppers RC, Outschoorn IM, Hamilton RG, et al. Quantitative measurement of human thyroglobulin-specific antibodies by use of a sensitive enzyme-linked immunoassay. *Clin Immunol Immunopathol*. 1993;67:68–77.

18. Prentice LM, Phillips DI, Sarsero D, et al. Geographical distribution of subclinical autoimmune thyroid disease in Britain: A study using highly sensitive direct assays for autoantibodies to thyroglobulin and thyroid peroxidase. *Acta Endocrinol (Copenh)*. 1990;123:493–498.

19. Voller A, Bidwell DE, Burek CL. An enzyme-linked immunosorbent assay (ELISA) for antibodies to thyroglobulin. *Proc Soc Exp Biol Med*. 1980;163:402–405.

20. Burek CL, Rose NR. Thyroglobulin autoantibodies. In: Peter JB, Shoenfeld Y, eds. *Autoantibodies*. Amsterdam, the Netherlands: Elsevier Biomedical; 1996:810–815.

21. Voller A, Bidwell D, Bartlett A. Enzyme-linked immunosorbent assay. In: Rose NR, Friedman H, eds. *Manual of Clinical Immunology*. 2nd ed. Washington, DC: American Society for Microbiology; 1980:359–371.

22. Bigazzi PE, Burek CL, Rose NR. Antibodies to tissue-specific endocrine, gastrointestinal, and surface-receptor antigens. In: Rose NR, Conway de Macario E, Fahey JL, et al, eds. *Manual of Clinical Laboratory Immunology*. 4th ed. Washington, DC: American Society for Microbiology; 1992:765–774.

23. Parkes AB, McLachlan SM, Bird P, et al. The distribution of microsomal and thyroglobulin antibody activity among the IgG subclasses. *Clin Exp Immunol*. 1984;57:239–243.

24. Rose NR, Outschoorn IM, Burek CL, et al. IgG subclass distribution of anti-Tg antibodies among thyroid disease patients and their relatives and in high and low responder mouse strains. In: Pinchera A, Ingbar SH, McKenzie JM, et al., eds. *Thyroid Autoimmunity—Thirtieth Anniversary: Memories and Perspectives*. New York, NY: Plenum Publishing Corp; 1987:189–198.

25. Bresler HS, Burek CL, Hoffman WH, et al. Autoantigenic determinants on human thyroglobulin, II: Determinants recognized by autoantibodies from patients with chronic autoimmune thyroiditis compared to autoantibodies from healthy subjects. *Clin Immunol Immunopathol*. 1990;54:76–86.

26. Beever K, Bradbury J, Phillips D, et al. Highly sensitive assays of autoantibodies to thyroglobulin and to thyroid peroxidase. *Clin Chem*. 1989;35:1949–1954.

27. Loeb PB, Drash AL, Kenny FM. Prevalence of low-titer and "negative" antithyroglobulin antibodies in biopsy-proved juvenile Hashimoto's thyroiditis. *J Pediatr*. 1973;82:17–21.

28. Holborow EJ, Brown PC, Roitt IM, et al. Cytoplasmic localization of "complement-fixing" auto-antigen in human thyroid epithelium. *Br J Exp Pathol*. 1959;40: 583–588.

29. Roitt IM, Ling NR, Doniach D, et al. The cytoplasmic auto-antigen of the human thyroid, I: Immunological and biochemical characteristics. *Immunology*. 1964;7:375–393.

30. Mariotti S, Pinchera A, Marcocci C, et al. Solubilization of human thyroid microsomal antigen. *J Clin Endocrinol Metab*. 1979;48:207–212.

31. Khoury EL, Bottazzo GF, Roitt IM. The thyroid "microsomal" antibody revisited. Its paradoxical binding in vivo to the apical surface of the follicular epithelium. *J Exp Med*. 1984;159:577–591.

32. Hanafusa T, Pujol-Borrell R, Chiovato L, et al. In vitro and in vivo reversal of thyroid epithelial polarity: Its relevance for autoimmune thyroid disease. *Clin Exp Immunol*. 1984;57:639–646.

33. Chiovato L, Vitti P, Lombardi A, Kohn LD, et al. Expression of the microsomal antigen on the surface of continuously cultured rat thyroid cells is modulated by thyrotropin. *J Clin Endocrinol Metab*. 1985;61:12–16.

34. Portmann L, Hamada N, Heinrich G, et al. Anti-thyroid peroxidase antibody in patients with autoimmune thyroid disease: Possible identity with anti-microsomal antibody. *J Clin Endocrinol Metab*. 1985;61:1001–1003.

35. Czarnocka B, Ruf J, Ferrand M, et al. Purification of the human thyroid peroxidase and its identification as the microsomal antigen involved in autoimmune thyroid diseases. *FEBS Lett*. 1985;190:147–152.

36. Khoury EL, Hammond L, Bottazzo GF, et al. Presence of the organ-specific "microsomal" autoantigen on the surface of human thyroid cells in culture: Its involvement in complement-mediated cytotoxicity. *Clin Exp Immunol*. 1981;45:316–328.

37. Bonger U, Schleusener H, Wall JR. Antibody-dependent cell mediated cytotoxicity against human thyroid cells in Hashimoto's thyroiditis but not Graves' disease. *J Clin Endocrinol Metab*. 1984;59: 734–738.

38. Goodburn R, Williams DL, Marks V. The preparation of thyroid microsomal antigen for use in the indirect micro-ELISA method for the detection of anti-thyroid microsomal autoantibody. *Clin Chim Acta.* 1982;119:291–297.

39. Banga AP, Pryce G, Hammond L, et al. Structural features of the autoantigens involved in thyroid autoimmune disease. *Mol Immunol.* 1985;22:629–642.

40. Hamada N, Grimm C, Mori H, et al. Identification of a thyroid microsomal antigen by Western blot and immunoprecipitation. *J Clin Endocrinol Metab.* 1985;61:120–128.

41. Banga JP, Barnett PS, McGregor AM. Immunological and molecular characteristics of the thyroid peroxidase autoantigen. *Autoimmunity.* 1991;8:335–343.

42. McLachlan SM, Rapoport B. The molecular biology of thyroid peroxidase: Cloning, expression, and role as autoantigen in autoimmune thyroid disease. *Endocr Rev.* 1992;13:192–206.

43. Braverman LE, Utiger RD. *Werner and Ingbar's The Thyroid.* 7th ed. New York: Lippincott-Raven; 1996.

44. Nicholson LB, Vlase H, Graves P, et al. Monoclonal antibodies to the human TSH receptor: Epitope mapping and binding to the native receptor on the basolateral plasma membrane of thyroid follicular cells. *J Mol Endocrinol.* 1996;16:159–170.

45. Parmentier M, Libert F, Lefort A, et al. Molecular cloning of the thyrotropin receptor. *Science.* 1989;246:1620–1622.

46. Nagayama Y, Kaufman KD, Seto P, et al. Molecular cloning, sequence and functional expression of the cDNA for the human thyrotropin receptor. *Biochem Biophys Res Commun.* 1989;165:1184–1190.

47. Akamizu T, Ikuyama S, Saji M, et al. Cloning, chromosomal assignment, and regulation of the rat thyrotropin receptor: Expression of the gene is regulated by thyrotropin, agents that increase cAMP levels, and thyroid autoantibodies. *Proc Natl Acad Sci U S A.* 1990;87:5677–5681.

48. Rapoport B, Spaulding SW. Mechanisms of action of thyrotropin and other thyroid growth factors. In: Braverman LE, Utiger RD, eds. *Werner and Ingbar's The Thyroid.* 7th ed. New York, NY: Lippincott-Raven; 1996:207–219.

49. Mathiesen T, Chiodi F, Broliden P-A, et al. Analysis of a subclass-restricted HIV-1 gp41 epitope by omission peptides. *Immunology.* 1989;67:1–9.

50. McKenzie JM, Zakarija M. LATS in Graves' disease. *Recent Prog Horm Res.* 1976;33:29–57.

51. Adams DD, Kennedy TH. Evidence to suggest that LATS protector stimulates the human thyroid gland. *J Clin Endocrinol Metab.* 1971;33:47–51.

52. Turner M, Feldmann M. Comparison of patterns of expression of tumour necrosis factor, lymphotoxin and interleukin-6 mRNA. *Biochem Biophys Res Commun.* 1988;153:1144–1151.

53. Jiang NS, Fairbanks VF, Hay ID. Assay for thyroid stimulating immunoglobulin. *Mayo Clin Proc.* 1986;61:753–755.

54. Takasu N, Oshiro C, Akamine H, et al. Thyroid-stimulating antibody and TSH-binding inhibitor immunoglobulin in 277 Graves' patients and in 686 normal subjects. *J Endocrinol Invest.* 1997;20:452–461.

55. Hoffman WH, Sahasrananan P, Ferandos SS, et al. Transient thyrotoxicosis in an infant delivered to a long-acting thyroid stimulator (LATS) and LATS protector-negative, thyroid-stimulating antibody-positive woman with Hashimoto's thyroiditis. *J Clin Endocrinol Metab.* 1982;54:354–356.

56. Zakarija M, McKenzie JM. Assays for thyroid-stimulating antibody and their clinical application. In: Soto RJ, De Nicola A, Blaqier J, eds. *Physiopathology of Endocrine Diseases: Mechanisms of Hormone Action.* New York, NY: Alan R. Liss; 1981:147–152.

57. Vitti P, Rotella CM, Valente WA, et al. Characterization of the optimal stimulatory effects of Graves' monoclonal and serum immunoglobulin G on adenosine 3′,5′-monophosphate production in fRTL-5 thyroid cells: A potential clinical assay. *J Clin Endocrinol Metab.* 1983;57:782–791.

58. Murakami M, Miyashita K, Kakizaki S, et al. Clinical usefulness of thyroid-stimulating antibody measurement using Chinese hamster ovary cells expressing human thyrotropin receptors. *Eur J Endocrinol.* 1995;133:80–86.

59. Vitti P, Chiovato L, Fiore E, et al. Use of cells expressing the human thyrotropin (TSH) receptor for the measurement of thyroid stimulating and TSH-blocking antibodies. *Acta Med Austriaca.* 1996;23:52–56.

60. Metcalfe RA, Oh YS, Stroud C, et al. Analysis of antibody-dependent cell-mediated cytotoxicity in autoimmune thyroid disease. *Autoimmunity.* 1997;25:65–72.

61. Takano T, Sumizaki H, Amino N. Detection of thyroid-stimulating antibody using frozen stocks of Chinese hamster ovary cells transfected with cloned human thyrotropin receptor. *Endocr J.* 1997;44:431–435.

62. Jaume JC, Kakinuma A, Chazenbalk GD, et al. Thyrotropin receptor autoantibodies in serum are present at much lower levels than thyroid peroxidase autoantibodies: Analysis by flow cytometry. *J Clin Endocrinol Metab.* 1997;82:500–507.

63. Minich WB, Weymayer JD, Loos U. Expression of a biotinylated human thyrotropin receptor in HeLa cells using recombinant vaccinia virus and its application for the detection of Graves' autoantibodies. *Thyroid.* 1998;8:3–7.

64. Betterle C, Zannette F, Zanchetta R, et al. Complement-fixing adrenal autoantibodies as a marker for predicting onset of idiopathic Addison's disease. *Lancet.* 1983;1:1238–1241.

65. Hoek A, Wulffraat NM, Drexhage HA. Steroid cell autoantibodies. In: Peter JB, Shoenfeld Y, eds. *Autoantibodies*. New York, NY: Elsevier Biomedical; 1996:798–804.

66. Winqvist O, Karlsson FA, Kampe O. 21-hydroxylase, a major autoantigen in idiopathic Addison's disease. *Lancet*. 1992;339:1559–1562.

67. De Bellis A, Bizzarro A, Rossi R, et al. Remission of subclinical adrenocortical failure in subjects with adrenal autoantibodies. *J Clin Endocrinol Metab*. 1993;76:1002–1007.

68. Song YH, Connor EL, Muir A, et al. Autoantibody epitope mapping of the 21-hydroxylase antigen in autoimmune Addison's disease. *J Clin Endocrinol Metab*. 1994;78:1108–1112.

CHAPTER 24

Autoimmune Disorders That Influence Carbohydrate Metabolism

William Ernest Winter, MD

There are several distinct disorders in which autoimmunity to islet cells, insulin, or the insulin receptor leads to a disruption of normal carbohydrate metabolism.[1,2] Depending on the specific disorder, either hyperglycemia or hypoglycemia may result. This chapter discusses the following disorders: autoimmune diabetes mellitus (type 1 diabetes mellitus), alpha-cell autoimmunity, type B insulin-resistant diabetes mellitus, insulinomimetic hypoglycemia, and autoimmune hypoglycemia. Several autoantibodies are associated with these disorders. Islet cell cytoplasmic autoantibodies (ICAs),[3,4] insulin autoantibodies (IAAs),[5] glutamic acid decarboxylase autoantibodies (GADAs),[6] and IA-2/ICA512 autoantibodies (IA-2As)[7] are collectively referred to as "islet autoantibodies" throughout this chapter. Previews of the metabolic and immunologic findings are found in **Tables 24-1** and **24-2**, which can be referred to throughout.

In one 1988 report, researchers described "Graves' disease of the beta cell." They identified a patient's serum that appeared to stimulate beta-cell release of insulin and hypoglycemia. There have been no further reports of beta-cell stimulatory autoantibodies; the existence of this condition must be considered controversial and is not included here.[8]

Clinical Description

Autoimmune (Type 1) Diabetes

Cell-mediated autoimmune destruction of pancreatic beta cells is responsible for the development of autoimmune diabetes[9–14] (**Figure 24-1**). The clinical phenotype of autoimmune diabetes is most commonly recognized as immune-mediated type 1 diabetes (formerly insulin-dependent diabetes mellitus), which presents clinically with acute onset polyuria, polydipsia, weight loss, and ketonuria or ketoacidosis. Before the development of ketosis (which can cause nausea), many affected patients report polyphagia. Classically, 2 or more years after onset, there is no detectable endogenous insulin production. Approximately 75% of patients with type 1 diabetes develop the disease before age 18. Although disease onset occurs primarily in youth, type 1 diabetes can strike at any age, and there is a slight predominance of men to women. This is unusual because most autoimmune diseases affect women more often than men. The only other autoimmune diseases that display a male predominance are polyarteritis nodosa and ankylosing spondylitis. Ankylosing spondylitis displays a strong association with the HLA-B27 allele of the HLA-B locus.

Table 24-1. Metabolic Overview of Autoimmune Disorders That Directly Perturb Carbohydrate Metabolism

	Analyte Concentrations	
	Insulin	C Peptide
Autoimmune diabetes	–	–
Alpha-cell autoimmunity	N	N
Type B insulin-resistant diabetes mellitus	+	+
Insulinomimetic hypoglycemia	–, N, +	–
Autoimmune hypoglycemia	+	–

Abbreviations: N = normal; + = increased; – = decreased.

Table 24-2. Autoantibody Overview of Autoimmune Disorders That Directly Perturb Carbohydrate Metabolism

	ICA, GADA, and/or IA-2A	IAA	Insulin Receptor Autoantibody
Autoimmune diabetes	+	±	–
Alpha-cell autoimmunity	–	–	–
Type B insulin-resistant diabetes mellitus	–	–	+
Autoimmune hypoglycemia	–	–	+
Insulinomimetic hypoglycemia	–	+	–

Abbreviations: ICA = islet cell cytoplasmic autoantibodies; GADA = glutamic acid decarboxylase autoantibodies; IA-2A = IA-2/ICA512 autoantibodies; IAA = insulin autoantibodies; + = present; – = absent; ± = sometimes present.

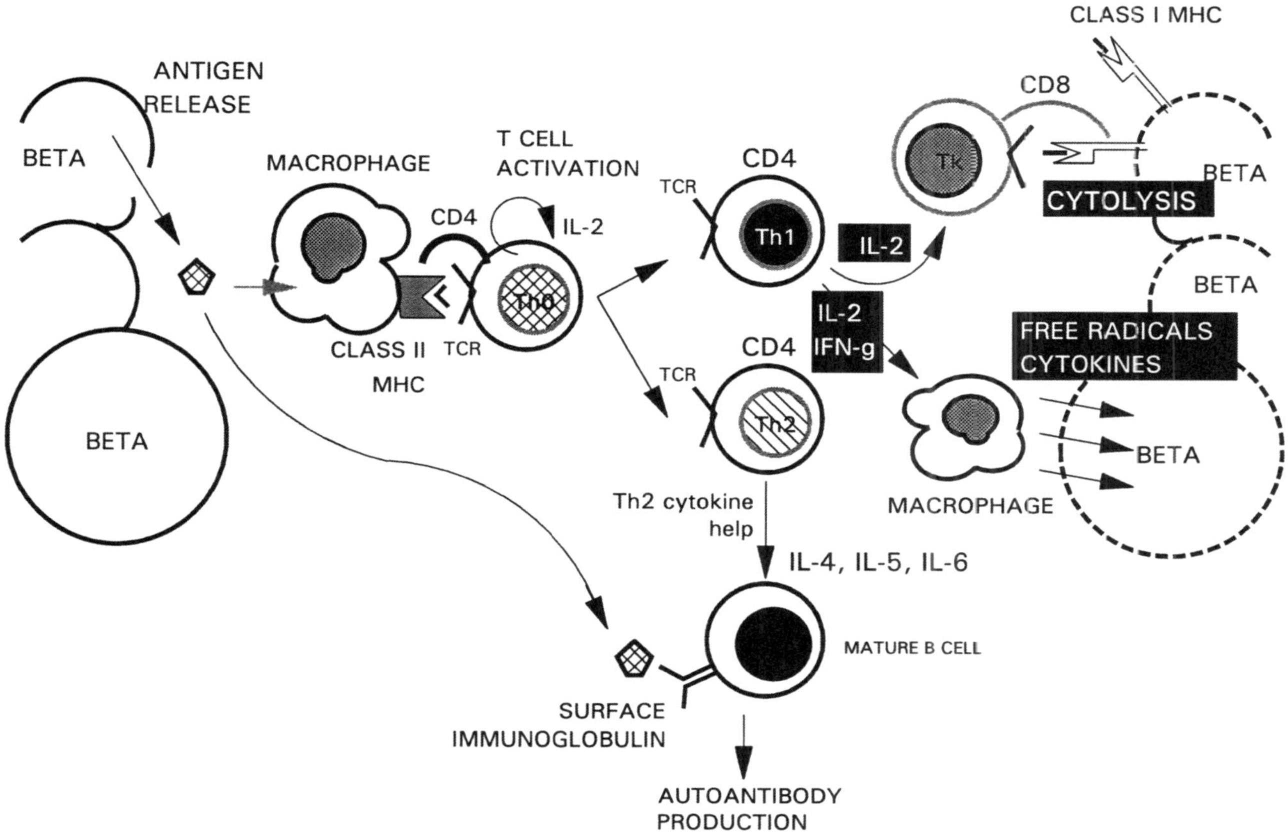

Figure 24-1. Hypothetical model of autoimmune beta-cell destruction. Beta-cell autoantigens are released (for unclear reasons) and peptides from these proteins are presented to CD4 T cells by class II major histocompatibility complex (MHC) molecules that are present on macrophages. The CD4 molecules of the T cells interact with the class II MHC molecules and function as coreceptors. The initial type of CD4 T cell that is activated (the Th0 cell) is not yet committed to the Th1 or Th2 line. Interleukin-2 (IL-2) is secreted by the activated T cell to cause proliferation. The Th0 cell pool provides some Th1 cells and others that may develop as Th2 cells. Th1 cells drive the cell-mediated immune response (activation of CD8 killer T cells, natural killer cells, and macrophages). Th2 cells drive the humoral immune response that results in antibody (or autoantibody) production. Th1 cells activate CD8 T cells by secreting IL-2 and activate macrophages by secreting interferon gamma (IFN-γ). Via recognition of the peptides presented by class I MHC molecules, CD8 T cells target beta cells for cytolysis, which mainly results in target cell apoptosis (programmed cell death). Activated macrophages damage beta cells through secretion of toxic cytokines (eg, tumor necrosis factor-α, tumor necrosis factor-β, and IFN-γ) and free radicals. Th2 cells activate B cells by secreting IL-4, IL-5, and/or IL-6.

In contrast to individuals with type 2 diabetes (formerly known as non–insulin-dependent diabetes mellitus [NIDDM]), type 1 patients are generally lean (especially at the time of diagnosis). Type 1 diabetes represents approximately 10% of all cases of diabetes in the United States. Whites, especially Northern Europeans, are at relatively high risk for type 1 diabetes (from about 1 in 250 to 1 in 500 individuals[15,16]) compared with Asians or African Americans. Although the frequency of type 1 diabetes in Finland is nearly 1 in 100 individuals, in Japan the figure is closer to 1 in 10,000. African Americans develop the disease at half the rate observed in white Americans.

Potentially as common as classic type 1 diabetes is latent autoimmune diabetes of adulthood (LADA). This disease results from slowly progressive beta-cell destruction. Affected patients present with a type 2 phenotype of mild, nonketotic hyperglycemia that may be controlled initially with diet, exercise, or oral hypoglycemic agents without the immediate need for exogenous insulin replacement. However, after months to years of the traditional type 2 phenotype,

LADA patients become insulin-dependent, similar to patients with classic type 1 diabetes. Latent autoimmune diabetes of adulthood can be referred to as "autoimmune NIDDM." Beta-cell autoimmunity should be suspected in patients who present with classic type 1 diabetes or LADA.

Alpha-Cell Autoimmunity

The first humoral markers of islet cell autoimmunity, ICAs, were described in 1974.[3,17–19] Islet cell autoantibodies are detected in about 3 of 4 patients presenting with new-onset type 1 diabetes. Indirect immunofluorescence for ICAs can detect autoantibodies directed solely against the glucagon-secreting alpha cells.[20] This species of islet cell autoantibody is termed alpha cell autoantibodies (ACAs). Such autoantibodies are directed against a cytoplasmic component of the alpha cell, but not against glucagon. Rare autoantibodies to delta cells have been detected.[21]

In a general population study of healthy school children in Pasco County, Florida,[20] ACAs were found as commonly as ICAs (eg, approximately 1 in 250 children tested positive for either ICAs or ACAs). Studies of individuals with ACAs have failed to detect glucagon deficiency or an increased risk for later-onset type 1 diabetes or hypoglycemia.[20,22,23] Therefore, alpha-cell autoimmunity is a benign phenomenon that is often detected during ICA screening of nondiabetic populations. Autoantibodies to glucagon have also been described in a subject with diabetes.[23,24] If ACAs are detected on the basis of a positive ACA test, there is no indication for further clinical or laboratory evaluations.

Type B Insulin-Resistant Diabetes Mellitus

When autoantibodies that function as insulin antagonists are directed against the insulin receptor, insulin action is blocked, producing a type 2 phenotype and type B insulin-resistant diabetes (**Figure 24-2**).[25,26]

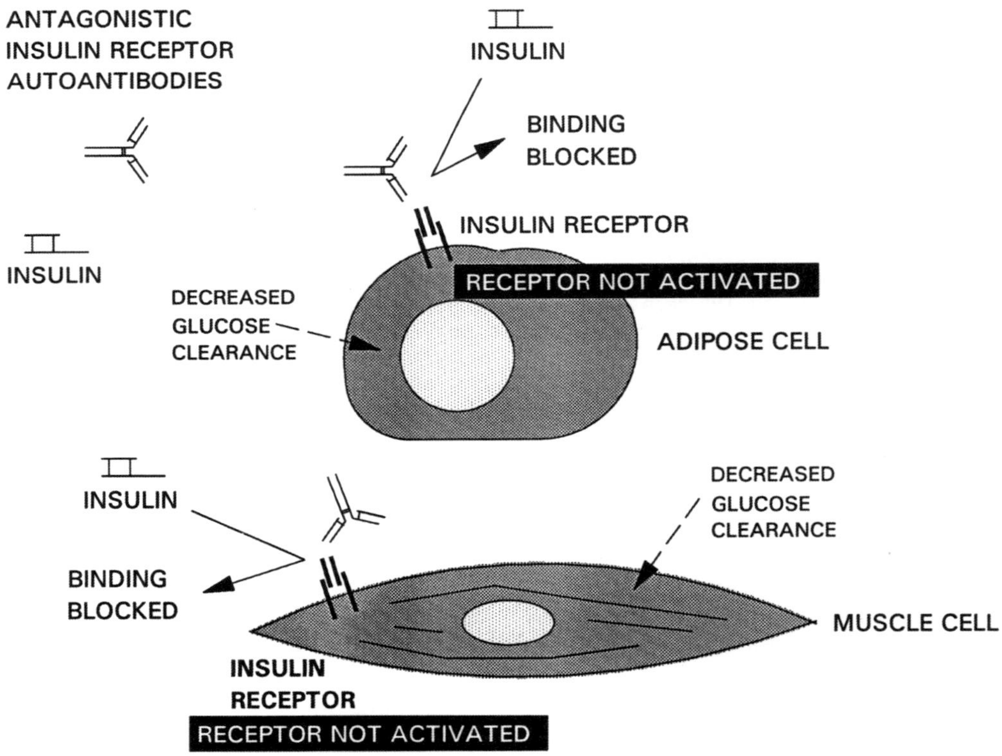

Figure 24-2. Type B insulin-resistant diabetes mellitus. Antagonistic autoantibodies directed against the insulin receptor block insulin binding, yet there is no receptor activation. Glucose is not taken up at normal rates by adipose or muscle tissue, and hyperglycemia results.

Type A insulin resistance is a genetic deficiency of insulin receptors. Most patients are women and exhibit polycystic ovary disease (ie, hirsutism and amenorrhea) and accelerated growth.

Acanthosis nigricans is a frequent clinical finding in insulin-resistant forms of diabetes. It appears as waxy, raised plaques that occur in skin folds, especially around the neck and upper trunk. Type B patients may have other findings that suggest immunodysregulation, including antinuclear antibodies (ANAs), anti-DNA antibodies, episodic hypocomplementemia, hypergammaglobulinemia, and leukopenia. A number of type B patients have been reported with systemic lupus erythematosus, scleroderma, Sjögren's syndrome, and ataxia-telangiectasia.[27]

Massive doses of insulin may be required to treat type B insulin-resistant diabetes patients. Insulin doses of greater than 20,000 IU per day may not be effective in controlling hyperglycemia. Insulin resistance produces endogenous hyperinsulinism with insulin levels as high as 40,000 μIU/mL. Because insulin resistance can resolve spontaneously, accounts of improvement in insulin sensitivity with immunosuppressive therapy are difficult to evaluate.[28] Upregulation of insulin receptor number may occur as a compensatory event.

Type B insulin-resistant diabetes should be suspected in patients with type 2 diabetes and acanthosis nigricans who require large doses of insulin (>100 to 1,000 IU/day) for treatment of hyperglycemia. The coexistence of non–organ-specific autoantibodies (eg, ANAs) or non–organ-specific autoimmune diseases increases the likelihood of type B disease in type 2 patients who are resistant to standard doses of insulin.

Insulinomimetic Hypoglycemia

When insulin receptor autoantibodies function as insulin mimics (eg, insulin receptor agonists), life-threatening hypoglycemia can develop (**Figure 24-3**). This is the opposite of type B insulin-resistant diabetes.

The clinical phenotype is that of hyperinsulinism in the absence of detectable insulin concentrations, because endogenous insulin secretion is suppressed by hypoglycemia. **Table 24-3** provides a differential diagnosis for syndromes of hypoglycemia in which hyperinsulinism is present. The hyperinsulinism phenotype consists of severe and/or recurrent hypoglycemia in the absence of plasma or urine ketones, and normal or suppressed levels of glucagon, free fatty acids, and branched chain amino acids.

Insulinomimetic insulin receptor autoantibodies have been described in adults with Hodgkin's disease[29] and lupus erythematosus[30,31] as well as in otherwise healthy children.[32] As is the case with type B insulin resistance, associated autoimmune disorders or autoantibodies are common in insulinomimetic hypoglycemia.

The biologic effect of insulin receptor autoantibodies appears to be concentration-dependent. At low concentrations, their agonist effects are dominant. At high concentrations—possibly through increased insulin receptor turnover—they are antagonistic to insulin action. (Hence, patients with a type B syndrome may have a history of hypoglycemia.) Insulinomimetic hypoglycemia should be suspected in patients with the clinical phenotype of hyperinsulinism who display insulin receptor autoantibodies. Glucocorticoids, plasmapheresis, and alkylating agents have been used to treat patients with this disease.

Autoimmune Hypoglycemia

Insulin autoantibodies as markers of beta-cell autoimmunity are discussed in the next section. In rare instances, IAAs interfere with normal carbohydrate metabolism by sequestering insulin and, it is theorized, lowering free insulin concentrations, producing hyperglycemia, glucose intolerance on oral glucose tolerance testing, or reactive hypoglycemia (**Figure 24-4**).[33] At other times, IAAs may spontaneously release excess insulin, leading to elevated free insulin concentrations that are inappropriate for metabolic needs. This produces hypoglycemia and the syndrome of autoimmune hypoglycemia, also known as the insulin autoimmune syndrome. An alternative explanation for the hypoglycemia is that IAAs increase insulin bioactivity. If one IAA molecule has bound 2 insulin molecules and each insulin molecule can interact with a separate insulin receptor, IAAs lead to insulin receptor cross-linking and activation.

Another theory to explain how IAAs cause autoimmune hypoglycemia proposes that some IAAs may bind to the insulin receptor binding domain of insulin. Therefore, if an anti-idiotypic antibody to IAAs arose, this anti-idiotype antibody would possess a structure similar to that of native insulin. The anti-idiotype antibody could then interact with the insulin receptor to activate the receptor.

The presence of IAAs in a patient with hypoglycemia who has not been treated with exogenous insulin is consistent with the autoimmune hypoglycemia

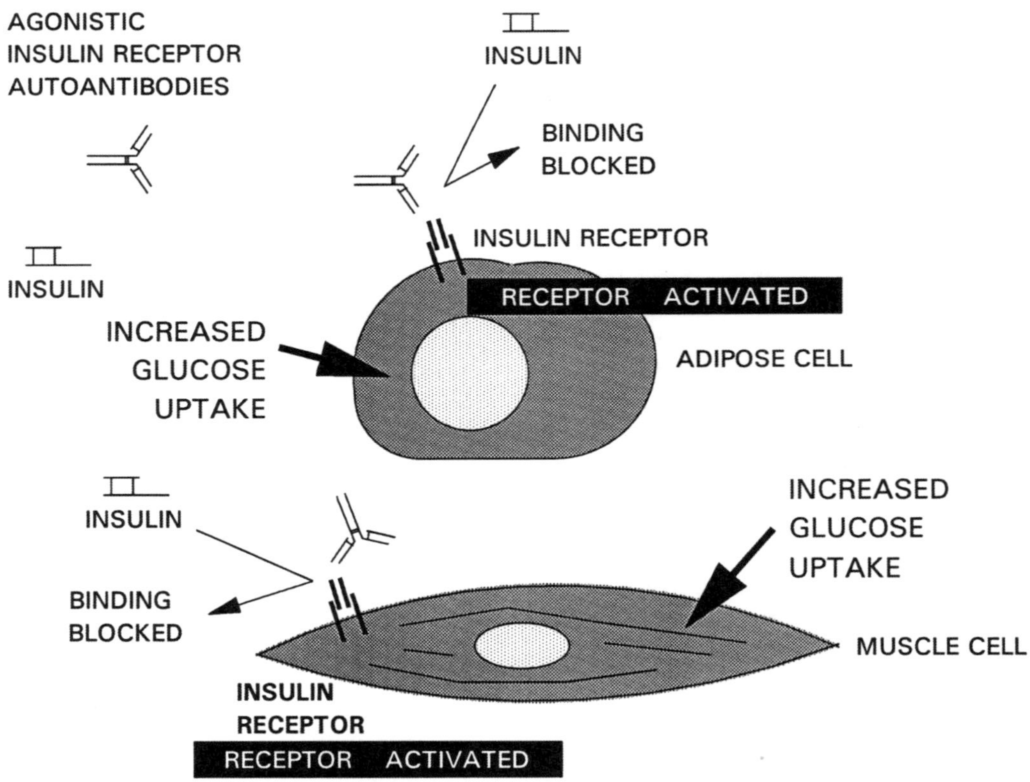

Figure 24-3. Insulinomimetic hypoglycemia. Agonistic autoantibodies directed against the insulin receptor block insulin binding and activate the receptor. Glucose is taken up at excessive rates by adipose and muscle tissue, producing hypoglycemia.

syndrome. Insulin autoantibodies in autoimmune hypoglycemia are polyclonal[34] and bind to human insulin but not porcine or bovine insulins. Outside of Japan, reports of autoimmune hypoglycemia are infrequent.[35,36] In Japan, autoimmune hypoglycemia is reported to cause about 33% of hypoglycemia cases, representing approximately 15% of patients with spontaneous hypoglycemia.[37,38] We have observed autoimmune hypoglycemia in a patient in our hospital.

Autoimmune hypoglycemia should be suspected in patients with the clinical syndrome of hyperinsulinism who lack radiologic evidence of an insulinoma and display IAAs. Many patients who develop autoimmune hypoglycemia have been treated with methimazole for Graves' disease.[39] In the natural

Table 24-3. Hypoglycemic Syndromes in Which Hyperinsulinism Is Present

	Insulin	C Peptide	IAA	Note
Insulinoma	+	+	−	Beta-cell tumor
Sulfonylurea poisoning	+	+	−	Beta-cell stimulation
Exogenous insulin administration	+	−	+	Development of IAA after several injections
Autoimmune hypoglycemia	+	−	+	Other possible autoimmune disorders
Insulinomimetic autoantibodies	+*	−	−	Insulin receptor autoantibody positive

Abbreviations: IAA = insulin autoantibodies; + = increased; − = decreased.
**Insulin levels may be increased from decreased clearance.*

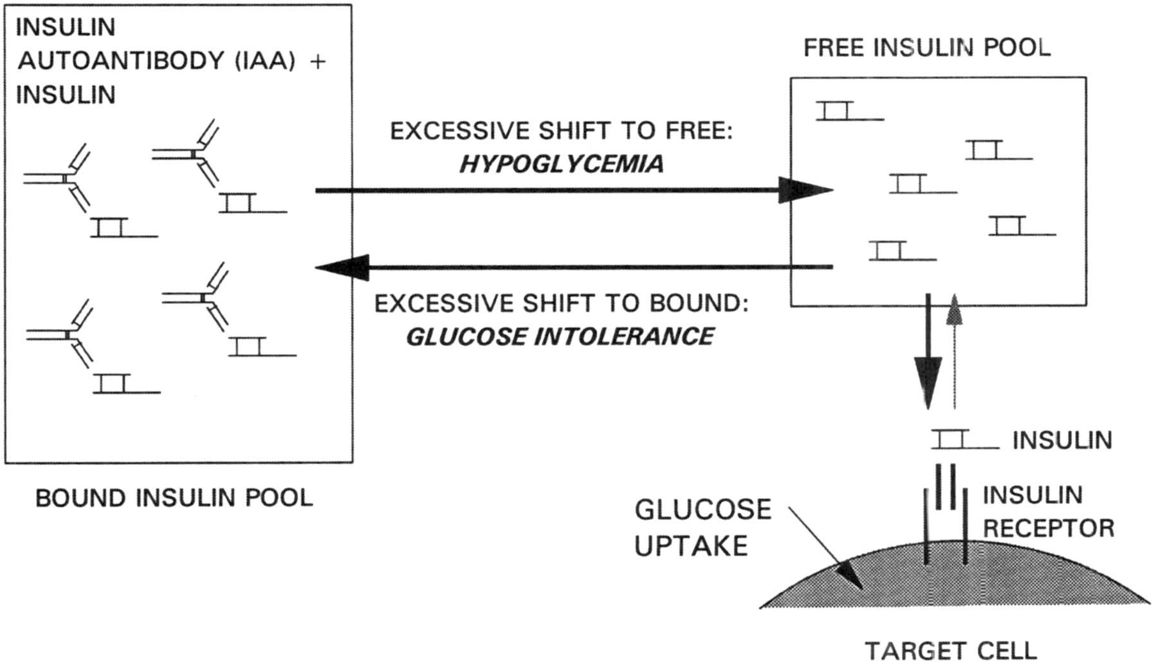

Figure 24-4. Autoimmune hypoglycemia. Insulin autoantibodies may hoard insulin, producing glucose intolerance, or release insulin out of proportion to metabolic needs, producing hypoglycemia.

history of autoimmune hypoglycemia, the disorder is said to be transient and conservative therapy (eg, frequent small meals) is recommended. Prednisone is typically ineffective.[40]

Laboratory Evaluation of Autoimmune Disorders That Affect Carbohydrate Metabolism

Autoimmune (Type 1) Diabetes

Diagnosis

The standard 1997 American Diabetes Association criteria are used to diagnose diabetes. These criteria are the same for type 1 and type 2 diabetes, and there are no longer different criteria for children and adults. Type 1 and type 2 diabetes are clinically differentiated based on the severity of clinical presentation and the need for insulin. Type 1 diabetes is of acute onset, whereas the onset of type 2 diabetes is usually subtle. Although either type can develop in individuals older than 40 years, type 2 diabetes is more common after that age. The patient's weight and body mass index may also be helpful in diagnosis; 80% or more of type 2 diabetes patients are obese, whereas obesity at the time of onset of type 1 diabetes is uncommon. Latent autoimmune diabetes of adulthood is diagnosed in patients with type 2 diabetes who develop clinical insulin dependence and express islet autoimmunity.[41–46]

When autoimmunity to islet cells or beta-cell products is detected in a patient who carries the biochemical diagnosis of diabetes, the etiology of the diabetes can be ascribed to autoimmune beta-cell destruction. The most useful autoantibody markers for the diagnosis of autoimmune diabetes are ICAs,[3,4] IAAs,[5] GADAs,[6] and IA-2As. Numerous other autoantibodies occur in new-onset type 1 patients, including autoantibodies to the insulin receptor,[47] GLUT2 (the beta-cell glucose transporter[48]), carboxypeptidase H,[49] 51-kd aromatic-L-amino-acid decarboxylase,[50] proinsulin,[51] glima 38,[52] 38-kd reactive autoantbodies,[53] peripherin, DNA topoisomerase II,[54] 30-kd pancreatic chymotrypsinogen-related autoantigen,[55] 52-kd protein of rat insulinoma cell line,[56] and GM2-1.[57] However, these autoantibodies have not proven as clinically valuable as the 4 mentioned above in the detection of autoimmunity in type 1 diabetes. The relevance of other autoantibodies in type 1 diabetes, such as heat shock protein 59 and

ICA69 autoantibodies,[58,59] is controversial. Cellular reactivity of lymphocytes from patients with type 1 diabetes to various islet autoantigens (eg, GAD,[60,61] imogen 38,[62] insulin secretory granule proteins,[63] and others[64–66]) has been demonstrated.

Islet Cell Cytoplasmic Autoantibodies

As noted previously, ICAs were the first type 1 diabetes–associated autoantibodies to be described. Islet cell cytoplasmic autoantibodies are detected by indirect immunofluorescence using cryocut tissue sections; therefore, ICA tests detect autoantibodies to intracellular, cytoplasmic antigens. Although only the beta cells are destroyed in type 1 diabetes and LADA, ICAs react with all cells of the islet: alpha cells that produce glucagon, beta cells that produce insulin, delta cells that produce somatostatin, and PP cells that produce pancreatic polypeptide. Because antibodies normally do not penetrate intact cells and ICAs react with cytoplasmic antigens, ICAs do not appear to be pathogenic. Furthermore, in murine models of autoimmune diabetes (eg, BioBreeding [BB] rats and nonobese diabetic [NOD] mice), serum is unable to transfer acute diabetes. Only when lymphocytes are transferred from an acutely diabetic animal to a syngeneic nondiabetic animal is diabetes transferred. Finally, ICAs that cross the placenta from a woman with type 1 diabetes to her fetus cause no apparent disease.

Islet cell cytoplasmic autoantibodies are detected at the time of onset of type 1 diabetes in 60% to 85% of whites.[67,68] In African Americans, only about 40% of individuals with youth-onset diabetes of less than 2 years' duration are ICA-positive. This suggests that conditions other than autoimmune diabetes are responsible for a large percentage of cases of youth-onset diabetes in African Americans. One example of such a heterogeneous etiology is atypical diabetes mellitus in African Americans.[69,70] This is a nonautoimmune familial disorder that causes at least 10% of cases of diabetes in young black individuals. In the general population, ICA frequency is 0.1% to 0.3% in whites.

The frequency of ICAs falls after the time of diagnosis of type 1 diabetes. Five to 10 years after onset, less than 5% to 10% of whites remain positive for ICAs. This probably reflects the fact that as beta-cell mass approaches zero, the autoantigens that elicit and maintain ICA titers are completely lost. Thus, without continued autoantigen stimulation, the immune system's production of ICAs wanes.

Sera that are ICA-positive react to a sialoglycoconjugate and/or glycolipid[71,72] in the islet cell cytoplasm and also frequently react with GAD[73] and IA-2A,[74] which are both found in the cytoplasm of the islet cells.[75] During indirect immunofluorescence using tissue sections mounted on glass slides, ICAs do not detect autoantibodies to the surface of islet cells. However, islet cell surface autoantibodies (ICSAs) have been described using suspensions of viable islets.[76–82] Some of these species have been shown to be cytotoxic in vitro. [83] Because of the need for living islet cells that can be placed in suspension, ICSA testing will likely always be limited to the research laboratory. Even in the research studies that screen for prediabetes (discussed later in this chapter), ICSAs are not employed because much better markers (eg, GADA and IA-2A as well as traditional ICA testing) have been developed.

Insulin Autoantibodies

In 40% to 50% of children with new-onset type 1 diabetes, autoantibodies to insulin can be detected before the institution of exogenous insulin replacement.[5,84] After exposure to injected insulin, regardless of the source (eg, porcine, bovine, or human), insulin antibodies frequently develop. The IAA assay does not discriminate between insulin antibodies and autoantibodies. The presence of IAAs in adults is far less common than in children who develop type 1 diabetes. Insulin autoantibodies are seen in patients with other autoimmune diseases such as thyroiditis. In autoimmune diabetes, insulin is the only autoantigen that appears to be absolutely beta-cell specific. Insulin autoantibodies can improve the predictive value of ICA for the later development of type 1 diabetes. [85]

Glutamic Acid Decarboxylase Autoantibodies

In the early 1980s, Baekkeskov and colleagues[86] demonstrated that sera from patients with type 1 diabetes were able to immunoprecipitate a unique islet cell protein with a molecular weight of 64 kd. The autoantibodies immunoprecipitating the 64-kd autoantigen were termed 64 KA. In this procedure, human or murine islets were labeled in vivo with (^{35}S)-methionine. The islets were disrupted and the membrane portion of the islet was extracted with triton X-114. This material was initially cleared by immunoprecipitation with control sera to remove proteins recognized by normal sera. Similar to control sera, sera from type 1 patients were employed next to immunoprecipitate the radiolabeled islet cell extract. After incubating the sera with the islet extract, antigen-antibody complexes were precipitated by binding to staphylococcal protein A, which was in turn bound to sepharose beads. After incubation, the sepharose beads were washed and the antigen-antibody complexes were released by boiling. The material was then size-fractionated using polyacrylamide gel electrophoresis. Bands were visualized by autoradiography. This procedure is very complex and expensive, requires living islets, and is not suited for routine clinical use.

The 64 KAs are predictive of type 1 diabetes in nondiabetic individuals[13,86] and are detected in 78% to 90% of new-onset patients. These autoantibodies are also found in NOD mice[87] and BB rats.[88,89] To develop an assay that was inexpensive, rapid, and automated, the autoantigen responsible for 64 KA reactivity had to be identified.

The breakthrough identification of the predominant 64-kd autoantigen came in 1990 when Baekkeskov and colleagues[6] demonstrated that the 64-kd autoantigen was glutamic acid decarboxylase (GAD).[92] The researchers recognized that one third of patients with stiff-man syndrome, a rare neurologic disease, developed type 1 diabetes and that GAD was a recognized autoantigen in this syndrome.[90] Furthermore, GAD had a "convenient" molecular weight of near 64,000 d. Baekkeskov et al showed that sera from type 1 diabetes patients without stiff-man disease could immunoprecipitate GAD. Preclearing islet extracts using GAD-6 (a sheep anti-GAD monoclonal antibody) eliminated the apparent 64 KA reactivity of patient sera because the autoantigen had been removed.

Glutamic acid decarboxylase activity is represented by 2 enzymes encoded by 2 separate genes: GAD_{65} (65,000-d molecular weight; chromosome 2q31) and GAD_{67} (67,000-d molecular weight; chromosome 10p11.2-p12).[91] Glutamic acid decarboxylase is responsible for the conversion of glutamic acid to gamma-aminobutyric acid (GABA), an inhibitory neurotransmitter. GAD_{65} and GAD_{67} display 70% amino acid homology. Glutamic acid decarboxylase is expressed predominantly in the central and peripheral nervous systems but also is found in the testis, ovary, adrenal gland, pituitary gland, thyroid, islets, and kidney. Glutamic acid decarboxylase autoantibodies react preferentially with GAD_{65}.[93-95]

Like ICAs, GADAs are detected in approximately 70% to 80% of white patients with new-onset type 1 diabetes. Whereas ICA frequency declines remarkably in the years following diagnosis, GADA presence appears to be more persistent. Therefore, GADA is a better marker to address the question of an autoimmune etiology for diabetes 2 or more years after diagnosis.

IA-2/ICA512 Autoantibodies (IA-2A)

IA-2/ICA512 is a 979–amino acid, 106-kd islet cell autoantigen and a member of the protein tyrosine phosphatase (PTP) family of proteins, which includes CD45, LAR, DLAR, DPTP, HPTPα, HPTPβ, and HPTPε.[95,96] Protein tyrosine phosphatases appear to function as cytoplasmic signal-transducing enzymes. IA-2 is composed of a 26–amino acid signal peptide (residues 1 through 26), a 551–amino acid extracellular domain (residues 27 through 577), a 23–amino acid transmembrane domain (residues 578 through 600), and a 379–amino acid intracellular domain (residues 601 through 979). In Northern blot analysis, IA-2 is expressed in brain, pituitary gland, adrenal gland, pancreas, and certain brain tumor cells.

IA-2 maps to chromosome 2q35-q36.198.[97] It is a full-length protein; ICA512 is a fragment of IA-2. ICA512 autoantigens were initially discovered by screening a cDNA expression library for clones that reacted with sera from patients with type 1 diabetes.

The biologic role of IA-2 is unclear. ICA512 is identified in beta-cell secretory granules, as well as in other neurosecretory granule peptide-secreting endocrine cells and neurons.[98] Following exposure at the cell surface, ICA512 is cleaved at its luminal domain, transported to the Golgi complex, and re-sorted into new secretory granules.

Because IA-2 has been cloned, immunoassays have been developed that should be adaptable to automation and eventual population screening.

Human Leukocyte Antigen Typing

Although certain HLA types (eg, DR3, DR4, DQB1*0302, DQB1*0201) occur more frequently in patients with autoimmune diabetes than in the general population,[99–108] the diagnosis of autoimmune diabetes cannot be inferred from HLA typing data alone. Therefore, even if a patient is HLA typed, supportive serologic evidence of islet autoimmunity is necessary to make a diagnosis of autoimmune diabetes. The question then arises as to why HLA typing should be performed if autoantibodies must still be measured. Such typing might be of value diagnostically only when patients have had long-standing diabetes and all serologic markers are negative. If a diabetic patient is typed DR3/DR4, or DQB1*0302/DQB1*0201, the likelihood that his or her diabetes is of autoimmune origin is greatly increased. DR3/DR4 is seen in approximately 40% of white type 1 diabetic patients versus only approximately 3% of the healthy general population. Finding DQB1*0602 may be of value in difficult diagnostic cases because this allele is very rare in type 1 diabetes patients. However, DQB1*0602 does not prevent the development of islet autoantibodies.[109] In fact, DQB1*0602 is considered protective against autoimmune diabetes, for example, type 1 diabetes is less likely to occur in subjects positive for DQB1*0602. The finding of DQB1*0602 is used as an exclusion criteria in nondiabetic subjects with islet autoantibodies who are considered for inclusion in trials designed to prevent type 1 diabetes (eg, the Diabetes Prevention Trial 1 discussed later in this chapter).

Identification of Prediabetes

Advances have been made in the treatment of type 1 diabetes by providing intensive insulin therapy guided by frequent home blood glucose monitoring. Insulin can be injected several times per day or infused continuously into the subcutaneous space using an insulin pump supplemented by premeal insulin boluses. In patients without end-stage complications, tight diabetic control can decrease the frequency of microvascular complications (eg, retinopathy, nephropathy, neuropathy) by at least 50%.[109] Nevertheless, insulin does not cure type 1 diabetes.[110]

Current efforts are directed at developing techniques to prevent autoimmune beta-cell destruction. Pancreas and islet cell transplants offer hope for individuals with established diabetes; but the cost and complexity, as well as the limited availability of organs for transplant, preclude application of transplant therapies to all but a small percentage of patients. Even with a syngeneic human donor (eg, identical twin), immunosuppression of the recipient appears necessary to prevent a reoccurrence of beta-cell destruction.[111–115]

Immunosuppressive treatment of type 1 diabetes at onset was explored in the 1980s as a potential method for preserving or even restoring beta-cell function.[116] Although drugs like cyclosporin A[116–122] and azathioprine (with or without prednisone)[122–125] induced a modest remission in approximately 50% of new-onset patients treated,[126] few patients became insulin independent and none experienced permanent remission once the immunosuppressive agents were discontinued.[127] Other agents attempted include anti-CD3 antibodies,[128] anti-CD4 antibodies,[129] anti-CD5 antibody conjugated to the ricin A chain,[130] anti–IL-2 receptor monoclonal antibody,[131] antiblast monoclonal antibody CBL1,[132] IL-2 conjugated with diphtheria toxin,[133] buffy coat transfusions,[134] lymphocyte transfusion,[135] pancreas irradiation,[136] ciamexone,[137] interferon,[138,139] intravenous immunoglobulin (Ig) G,[140] antithymocyte globulin,[141] levamisole,[142] BCG,[143] prednisone,[144,145] thymopentin,[146] thymostimulin,[147] FK506,[148] photophoresis,[149] and plasmapheresis.[150–152]

Although these preliminary results seemed to indicate that the natural history of type 1 diabetes could be altered through immunointervention, it appeared that by the time the disease was diagnosed, irreparable beta-cell damage and beta-cell loss had occurred, which was only temporized by such agents. Researchers realized that to effectively, and perhaps permanently, modify the natural history of beta-cell destruction in "prediabetes," intervention must begin long before the clinical diagnosis of diabetes was evident. This implies treating individuals who have autoantibody markers of beta-cell autoimmunity that display beta-cell dysfunction yet who are normoglycemic. Treating asymptomatic nondiabetic individuals with immunosuppression does not appear justified because the immunosuppression itself has considerable complications, such as nephropathy from cyclosporin A,[153] predisposition to lymphoma from azathioprine, and increased susceptibility to infection from either agent.

Instead of suppressing the immune system, as in the management of an organ transplant recipient, researchers asked if tolerance to the beta cell and its autoantigens could be induced through a more benign and less risky approach.[154–158] In an animal model of multiple sclerosis studied in the late 1980s, experimental allergic encephalomyelitis (EAE) could be prevented by feeding genetically susceptible animals myelin basic protein before the intracerebral injection of myelin basic protein that usually precipitates EAE. This tolerogenic approach of providing autoantigen exposure to prevent disease was also efficacious in an animal model of rheumatoid arthritis induced by collagen immunization. Oral antigen feeding also produced tolerance in animal models of autoimmune diabetes.[159–161] Shortly thereafter, clinical trials involving feeding myelin basic protein to human patients with multiple sclerosis demonstrated improvement in their clinical course.[162] However, it is necessary to determine which autoantigen might be used to produce beta-cell tolerance in type 1 diabetes.

Studies in the 1980s in both BB rats and NOD mice showed that insulin injections given before the expected time of onset of type 1 diabetes prevented onset of the disease.[163] In at least one study, insulitis in NOD mice was also retarded by insulin injection. In autoimmune diabetes, insulitis is the pathognomonic histologic lesion that consists of a mononuclear and lymphocytic infiltrate of the pancreatic islets.[164–169] More recently, oral insulin has been shown to prevent type 1 diabetes in NOD mice. Feeding the A chain of insulin to mice is ineffective in preventing disease, but feeding the B chain is effective. Because oral insulin has no insulin-like biologic effect, alimentary insulin exposure must alter the immune system in some way. One theory proposes that oral insulin induces CD8+ suppressor T cells that travel to the islet to induce tolerance. It is not known how either oral or subcutaneous insulin functions in generating tolerance. Intensive insulin treatment at the onset of disease in humans can improve beta-cell function.[170]

It has been theorized that insulin injection can "rest" the beta cell by exogenously lowering blood glucose, subjecting the beta cell to less "stress." Furthermore, suppression of endogenous insulin production could downregulate autoantigen production and expression, leading to less beta-cell targeting by the immune system.

There is limited human data to support the concept that insulin pretreatment of prediabetic individuals prevents type 1 diabetes.[121] In a very small study from the Joslin Diabetes Clinic in Boston,[171] insulin treatment of islet autoantibody marker–positive nondiabetic individuals was efficacious in the short term in preventing disease.

Combining the existing animal data and the human data, in the mid 1990s, the National Institutes of Health funded the Diabetes Prevent Trial-1 (DPT-1), which was designed to determine whether the onset of type 1 diabetes can be delayed or prevented using subcutaneous insulin injections or oral insulin ingestion. Optimistically, insulin injections could prevent type 1 diabetes onset altogether.[172] Individuals can enter the DPT-1 study if they have a first-degree relative with type 1 diabetes and have repeatedly tested positive for ICAs. Such marker-positive individuals then undergo biochemical examination via intravenous glucose tolerance testing. If the 1-minute plus 3-minute insulin value (eg, the first-phase insulin response) is repeatedly less than the first percentile, the individual can be randomized to placebo or subcutaneous insulin treatment. Such individuals have a greater than 50% chance of otherwise developing type 1 diabetes during 5 years of follow-up. Insulin therapy in the study consists of 0.25 U/kg per day injected subcutaneously in 2 doses. In comparison, most type 1 patients require about 1 U/kg per day. For individuals with a 5-year risk of 25% to 50% for type 1 diabetes, oral insulin therapy is being studied as a preventive measure.

In the Finnish Diabetes Prediction and Prevention (DIPP) trial, nasal insulin is being investigated as a form of diabetes prevention. Other autoantigens, such as GAD or IA-2/ICA512, may be used in the future in tolerance programs.[116,161]

In New Zealand, Europe, Texas, and Canada (the European Nicotinamide Intervention Trial [ENDIT] includes Texas and Canada), nicotinamide is being used experimentally to prevent type 1 diabetes based on its antioxidant properties.[173–176] Nicotinamide may function as a free radical scavenger and an inhibitor of a DNA repair enzyme.[174] It is controversial whether nicotinamide will be effective.[177–179]

Multiple studies from the United States and Europe clearly demonstrate that islet autoantibodies in nondiabetic individuals predict a later development of type 1 diabetes.[180–186] Such markers predict type 1 regardless of whether the subject has a first-degree relative with the disease.[20] Higher titers of ICA are associated with increased risk for type 1 diabetes.[187–189] Higher titers of ICA are also able to fix complement.[190,191] In children who have a first-degree relative with type 1 diabetes, are ICA positive, and display a depressed first-phase insulin response to intravenous glucose infusion,[192–199] the risk of developing type 1 diabetes during 5 years is greater than 50%.[20,200] During 10 years, this risk may approach 100%. In ICA-positive individuals who eventually develop the disease, first-phase insulin release diminishes at a rate of approximately 20 to 40 µIU/mL per year.[195] Acute insulin response to intravenous glucagon, arginine, and tolbutamide may be maintained temporarily in response to intravenous glucose despite insulinopenia.[201] Eventually, insulin response to all secretagogues is lost.

Just as ICA in nondiabetic individuals is a strong predictor of the later development of type 1 diabetes, GADA,[202] IAA,[203] and IA-2A also predict the disease. In a variety of retrospective and prospective studies, having more than one islet autoantibody further increases an individual's risk of developing type 1 diabetes.[204–208] For example, positivity for ICA and IAA is a more powerful risk factor than positivity for ICA alone. Although the DPT-1 study is based primarily on the finding of ICA, future prevention trials will doubtless use other markers to screen for prediabetes.

The optimal choice of markers for prediabetes screening has not been established.[197–206,209,210] However, if multiple autoantibodies could be tested for simultaneously, a single assay for IAA, GADA, and IA-2A might be optimal. Testing for ICA cannot be automated because this is an indirect immunofluorescence procedure. Some researchers report that by screening for IAA, GADA, and ICA512 autoantibodies, 100% of prediabetic individuals can be recognized.[211] In a study from England of relatives of patients with type 1 diabetes, individuals with 3 or more islet autoantibodies had an 88% chance of developing the disease during 19 years of follow-up.[207,212]

Until effective and safe therapy to prevent or delay the onset of type 1 diabetes is available, autoantibody screening for prediabetes in nondiabetic individuals should be restricted to those participating in research studies. None of the autoantibody tests described here have been approved by the US Food and Drug Administration (FDA), nor are they reimbursable under Medicare. However, once diabetes can be prevented, it is reasonable to argue that federal or state screening programs for prediabetes should be put into place. Several approaches might be employed.

One proposal for detection of prediabetes would be to screen all children in kindergarten or early elementary school for islet autoantibodies. Systems would need to be developed to detect GADA, IA-2A, and IAA in a spot of blood placed on filter paper, similar to blood collection procedures for newborn screening (eg, screening for phenylketonuria and congenital hypothyroidism). These technical problems have been resolved for the anonymous detection of human immunodeficiency virus (HIV) antibodies in filter paper blood spots mailed to a central laboratory with a product that is FDA approved and sold as the Confide HIV test (Johnson & Johnson, New Brunswick, NJ). The technology is so sophisticated that blood spots initially positive for HIV antibody by enzyme immunoassay (EIA) can be repeated and confirmed by Western blot if the sample is indeed repeatedly EIA positive.

Other approaches to detecting islet autoantibodies might involve the measurement of IgA islet autoantibodies in saliva or of islet autoantibodies in urine. Manufacturers are working on both IgA and urine techniques for HIV antibody screening. OraSure (OraSure Technologies, Bethlehem, PA) is FDA approved for detection of HIV IgA antibody; Seradyn Clinical Diagnostics (Indianapolis, IN) and Calypte Biomedical Corporation (Alameda, CA) have developed the urine HIV antibody screening test.

Because of the vast number of children who would require islet autoantibody testing, phlebotomy is probably too expensive and too invasive to be accepted as part of a public screening program involving young children. It is unreasonable to restrict islet autoantibody screening to children who have a first-degree relative with type 1 diabetes, because only 15% of type 1 patients have a first-degree relative with the disease. Assuming that nearly 100% of prediabetic individuals could be detected using a combination of islet autoantibodies (eg, GADA plus IA-2A plus IAA), if only children who have a relative with type 1 diabetes are screened, 85% of children destined to develop the disease will be missed.

Every year, screening programs would need to test 3 to 4 million children (the number of children born yearly in the United States). If children were screened for islet autoantibodies twice (eg, at an early age before or just after entry into school and at a later age such as 8 or 10 years), 6 to 8 million islet antibody tests would need to be performed each year as part of the prediabetes screening program. However, it is possible that islet autoantibodies may appear much earlier than currently anticipated and that screening in early infancy could be accomplished on a single occasion. The German Multicenter BABY-DIAB study has shown that islet autoantibodies can arise in infancy.[213]

To limit the number of children tested serologically, genetic prescreening could involve identification of children who are genetically susceptible to autoimmune diabetes through newborn HLA typing and typing for alleles associated with type 1 diabetes at other genetic loci.[214] This would identify children at highest risk for the disease (eg, children who carry DQB1*0302 and DQB1*0201) and target such children for later islet autoantibody screening. Although this would reduce the total number of islet autoantibody tests performed each year, there would be a substantial initial expense for HLA typing 3 to 4 million newborns per year. In the more than 9,000 cord blood specimens tested in the Diabetes Autoimmunity Study in Youth (DAISY) project, about 2% of infants were identified as high risk for type 1 diabetes (DR3/DR4, DQB1*0302). It could be argued that much valuable DNA data might also be acquired about risks of other diseases by performing newborn genetic testing,[215–218] because the HLA typing would likely involve molecular methods that require DNA extraction from a newborn screening blood spot.

Genetic prescreening for type 1 diabetes would not be foolproof. It is highly likely that a few children who lack all of the recognized markers of genetic predisposition for type 1 diabetes would still develop the disease. These children would be recognized as screening system failures, because, given the results of genetic prescreening, they would never undergo islet autoantibody testing. However, it is naive to think that screening all children for islet autoantibodies would be error-free and would detect 100% of children destined to develop type 1 diabetes. The islet autoantibody tests are unlikely to be perfect (despite optimism to the contrary); samples may not be obtained; samples may be lost or mislabeled; and, even after the detection of islet autoantibodies, there may be a failure of clinical follow-up and/or tolerance-induction therapy. Furthermore, in the real world it is unlikely that any therapy in the near future will be 100% effective in preventing type 1 diabetes. If a parallel can be drawn to the treatment of childhood leukemia, efforts at preventing autoimmune diabetes are similar to those of researchers in the early 1950s when chemotherapy was first applied to treat acute lymphocytic leukemia.

When a sibling of a patient with type 1 diabetes is considering donating a kidney for transplantation to the diabetic sibling, the donor's risk for the disease should be assessed by ICA testing. Type 1 diabetes can develop after donation in the previously unaffected sibling.[218]

Monitoring

The serologic markers discussed here (including ICA, IAA, GADA, and IA-2A) have a diagnostic value in providing evidence of an autoimmune etiology for diabetes. However, once autoimmune diabetes has been diagnosed, the serologic markers of islet autoimmunity provide little or no useful information about the prognosis of the disease.[219,220] By the time type 1 diabetes is clinically manifested, it is estimated that more than 90% of the beta cells have already been destroyed. Japanese researchers have suggested that GADA at diagnosis predicts higher C peptide levels after 5 years of follow-up[221]; however, this has been disputed by another group.[222]

Because several autoimmune diseases occur at increased frequencies in patients with autoimmune diabetes, once autoimmune diabetes is confirmed or suspected based on the clinical diagnosis of type 1 diabetes, patients should be screened for both autoimmune thyroid disease and chronic lymphocytic gastritis.[223–226] Thyroid microsomal or thyroperoxidase autoantibodies are most useful for the diagnosis of autoimmune thyroid disease. Such screening needs to be performed only once. About 1 in 4 girls diagnosed with type 1 diabetes display serologic evidence of thyroid autoimmunity; 1 in 8 are positive for gastric parietal cell autoantibodies, whose presence is consistent with chronic lymphocytic gastritis. Autoimmune thyroid disease and chronic lymphocytic gastritis are half as common in boys with type 1 diabetes as in girls with the disease. Fifty percent of children who test positive for thyroid autoantibodies display thyroid dysfunction. Of these children, 80% will be hypothyroid and 20% will be hyperthyroid. Hyperthyroidism may precede the clinical presentation of type 1 diabetes. The clinical course of chronic lymphocytic gastritis in these patients is protracted because, even with complete destruction of the parietal cells and loss of intrinsic factor secretion, the liver still maintains an approximate 10-year store of vitamin B_{12}.[227]

If thyroid or gastric autoimmunity is present, adrenal autoimmunity should be determined by testing for adrenal cortical cytoplasmic autoantibodies.[228] Approximately 6% of children with type 1 diabetes and thyroiditis have adrenalitis as determined by adrenal autoantibody testing. Half of these children have elevated adrenocorticotropic hormone levels and/or elevated renin levels consistent with frank or compensated adrenal insufficiency.[229] Therefore, recognizing that a case of diabetes is autoimmune in etiology can provide important information about the subsequent need to test for associated organ-specific autoimmune diseases.[230–232] These disorders are potentially serious or even life-threatening if Addisonian crisis should develop as a consequence of adrenalitis.

Alpha-Cell Autoimmunity

Clinical Diagnosis

Because alpha-cell autoimmunity is a laboratory phenomenon and an artifact of ICA testing, the laboratory that reports the presence of alpha-cell autoantibodies should communicate to the researcher and clinician that these autoantibodies, as currently understood, are not associated with any recognized pathologic processes or clinical conditions. The physician should decide whether it is appropriate to report to the patient that alpha-cell autoantibodies are present. Because ACAs have no clinical significance, informing patients in the clinical setting that they are positive for ACAs may only engender anxiety. On the other hand, most study patients would probably accept this information without developing any traumatic psychological stress.

Disease Prediction and Monitoring

Because ACAs are not associated with any recognized pathologic processes involving the islets, other endocrine glands, or other tissues or organ systems, there is no indication to screen for ACAs. However, ACAs are detected during ICA screening, and this information may be communicated to the patient.

Type B Insulin-Resistant Diabetes

Diagnosis

The metabolic diagnosis of diabetes is based on the American Diabetes Association criteria already described. The clinical indications that antagonistic insulin receptor autoantibodies may be present include hyperglycemia that is resistant to large doses of exogenous insulin, a history of other autoimmune diseases in the patient, and the presence of acanthosis nigricans.

Tests for ICA, GADA, IAA, and IA-2A are expected to be negative in this situation. If islet autoantibodies are detected, beta-cell destruction should be suspected. However, such destruction does not produce the insulin resistance seen in type B syndrome. The clinical phenotype of the type B syndrome is of extreme insulin resistance as opposed to type 1 diabetes, where patients are clearly sensitive to exogenous insulin replacement and demonstrate a decline in blood glucose on daily doses of insulin not much greater than 1 to 1.2 U/kg per day.

Insulin receptor autoantibodies that bind to the insulin receptor but do not stimulate the receptor are diagnostic of the type B syndrome. Assays for insulin receptor autoantibodies are available only through research laboratories. These assays usually do not differentiate agonistic from antagonistic activities.

Prediction of Type B Insulin Resistance

There is no clinical indication to screen for insulin receptor autoantibodies as a predictive measure of susceptibility. Although type B disease is autoimmune, there does not appear to be a familial predisposition to the disorder. Furthermore, type B disease is a rare condition in the general population.

Monitoring

There is no information to suggest that measuring the titer of insulin receptor autoantibodies provides useful information in the management of this condition. However, the detection of insulin receptor autoantibodies in a patient with extreme insulin resistance differentiates this condition from type A insulin resistance, which is caused by a deficiency in insulin receptor number. This clinical differentiation is of therapeutic importance because there are case reports of patients with type B disease who have been successfully treated with immunosuppressive drugs (eg, prednisone) that apparently ameliorated the autoimmune condition and improved insulin sensitivity.

Insulinomimetic Hypoglycemia

Diagnosis

The diagnosis of hypoglycemia is established when 3 criteria are documented:

- Symptoms compatible with hypoglycemia are identified. Common adrenergic symptoms of hypoglycemia include tachycardia, palpitations, pounding heart, sweating, tremulousness, anxiety, nervousness, feeling cold and sweating. Neuroglycopenia (low blood glucose in the brain) can be manifested as decreased consciousness, tiredness or drowsiness, faintness, confusion, blurred or double vision, hemiparesis, behavioral changes, dizziness, paresthesias (pins and needles feelings), incoordination, slurred speech, hunger and headache.
- There is laboratory verification of a depressed blood glucose concentration (serum or plasma glucose <45 mg/dL) at the time the patient has symptoms.
- The symptoms are alleviated promptly with the rapid administration of glucose.

The absence of urine ketones, a normal serum or plasma level of β-hydroxybutyrate, and normal or suppressed levels of glucagon, free fatty acids, and branched chain amino acids are consistent with hyperinsulinism. C-peptide and insulin levels are usually depressed (insulin/glucose ratio <0.25 [μIU/mg] • 10). However, in some cases, insulin concentrations may be highly elevated in the face of depressed C peptide. Insulin may still be detectable in patients with insulinomimetic hypoglycemia because although insulin is normally degraded through the insulin receptor, the insulin receptor is anatomically blocked in the presence of insulin receptor autoantibodies, thus slowing insulin degradation.

The identification of insulin receptor autoantibodies in a patient with a "hyperinsulinemic" hypoglycemia that is otherwise unexplained (eg, the insulin level is not elevated) confirms the diagnosis of insulinomimetic hypoglycemia.[233–235] Fatalities due to uncontrolled insulinomimetic hypoglycemia have been reported. Tests for islet autoantibodies are expected to be negative in these cases.

Prediction of Insulinomimetic Hypoglycemia

Because this syndrome is extremely rare, there is no indication to measure insulin receptor autoantibodies unless a patient has unexplained hypoglycemia or insulin-resistant diabetes.

Monitoring

There are no data to suggest that measuring the titer of insulin receptor autoantibodies provides useful information in the management of insulinomimetic hypoglycemia.

Autoimmune Hypoglycemia

Diagnosis

The clinical diagnosis of hypoglycemia is always based on the same criteria, regardless of the etiology of the fasting hypoglycemia (see the above discussion of insulinomimetic hypoglycemia). In patients with hypoglycemia, free insulin levels are elevated (eg, free insulin/glucose ratio ≥0.25 [μIU/mg] • 10) and various biochemical parameters are consistent with hyperinsulinism (eg, suppressed ketones). Free insulin levels can be determined analytically after antigen-antibody complexes are removed from the serum by treatment with polyethylene glycol. Insulin concentrations greater than 200,000 pmol/L have been reported in patients with autoimmune hypoglycemia, while insulin values are usually 10 to 100 times higher than normal when tested using double-antibody radioimmunoassays for insulin. If charcoal or polyethylene glycol (PEG) is used, IAAs artifactually lower the insulin measurement. Because the IAAs in this disorder may "hoard" insulin, glucose intolerance or reactive hypoglycemia may be observed during oral glucose tolerance testing.

This clinical picture combined with the detection of insulin antibodies suggests autoimmune hypoglycemia in a patient who is not under insulin treatment.[236] The clinician must be careful in interpreting insulin autoantibody results; once exogenous insulin has been injected on several occasions, insulin antibodies will develop. With both exogenous insulin administration and autoimmune hypoglycemia, insulin is elevated, C peptide is suppressed, and insulin antibodies are detected. Thus, the clinical history of whether or not exogenous insulin has been injected is important. Serum iodine 125 (^{125}I)–insulin binding in autoimmune hypoglycemia usually exceeds 30% (reference range, approximately <5% ^{125}I-insulin binding by serum).

In a sample that demonstrates hyperinsulinism, the origin of the insulin (eg, human versus animal) can be determined by high-performance liquid chromatography (HPLC). However, if exogenous human insulin is injected, HPLC identification of the insulin origin is uninformative. As is the case in type B insulin resistance, tests for islet autoantibodies are expected to be negative.

Although not diagnostic, the presence of HLA-DR4 is very common in autoimmune hypoglycemia syndrome.[237,238]

Prediction of Autoimmune Hypoglycemia

This is a rare condition outside of Japan. Screening for IAAs other than as part of a research prediabetes screening program is not indicated.

Monitoring

At this time, there is no clinical reason to measure the titer of insulin antibodies in a patient with autoimmune hypoglycemia.

Assay Methods

Islet Cell Cytoplasmic Autoantibodies

These autoantibodies are polyclonal,[239] and indirect immunofluorescence is used to detect them.[3,67] To avoid the potential confusion of isohemagglutinins reacting with tissue ABO antigens, blood group O pancreata are used. Similarly, unfixed tissue is used to avoid the potential problem of detecting insulin antibodies or autoantibodies, because tissue insulin is retained when the pancreas or pancreatic tissue is fixed. With unfixed tissue, insulin is eluted from the tissue during the many wash steps.

Pancreata from cadaveric organ donors are collected by the transplantation service and delivered on ice to the ICA laboratory. After sectioning into approximately 1-cm^3 portions, the "cubes" are snap-frozen in isopentane and cooled in a dry ice acetone bath. The tissue blocks can then be mounted on a chuck for cryostatic sectioning or saved at –70°C to –80°C in a 50-mL screw-top tube.

When cleaved into 4-µm slices, the sections are transferred from the microtome blade by placing room temperature glass slides against the tissue; the tissue immediately attaches to the slide. Undiluted patient serum is then applied to the tissue. After 30 minutes of incubation, the slide is washed 3 times with phosphate buffered saline (PBS). Then a PBS solution containing fluorescein isothiocyanate–labeled goat antihuman IgG conjugate is layered over the tissue. After another series of PBS washes and removal of the excess liquid, glycerol is layered over the tissue, followed by the addition of a coverslip. As observed through the fluorescent microscope, green immunofluorescence of the islet cytoplasm indicates that ICAs are present.

Methodology variations[71] have included increasing the incubation time[239] (eg, overnight incubation); using nonhuman tissue[240,241] (eg, rat, mouse, or monkey); counterstaining alpha cells or proinsulin[242] for the identification of islets; and use of horseradish peroxidase (HRP)–labeled secondary antibodies.[243] Although each of these permutations may offer a specific benefit, most research laboratories continue to employ the basic ICA technique as outlined by Bottazzo et al in 1974.[3] Most technologists can perform 2 ICA runs per day, totaling about 80 specimens per run, including negative and positive controls. Although the materials for the ICA assay are relatively inexpensive, the microtome is costly (more than $10,000), and labor costs are relatively high.

An ICA titering system has been developed under the auspices of the Juvenile Diabetes Foundation International; the unit used is the "JDF" unit.[244] Sera with values less than 10 JDF units are considered to represent low-titer sera and predict no increased risk for type 1 diabetes compared with sera with JDF titers of at least 10 JDF units. The lowest positive value reported is usually 5 JDF units. Sera with titers of at least 20 JDF units are considered strongly positive. In nondiabetic individuals, sera with low JDF titers may occasionally revert to negative. With JDF titers of 20 units or more, reversion to negative is unusual.

Despite its methodologic simplicity, ICA testing requires a rigorous quality assurance and control program to provide accurate and reproducible results.[245] To date, an automated ICA assay system has not been developed. Because the ICA assay is labor-intensive, nonautomated, and difficult to quality control, ICA testing should be restricted to research laboratories that have a long-term commitment to the assay.

Insulin Autoantibodies

Insulin autoantibodies are detected using a liquid-phase assay. When measured by enzyme-linked immunosorbent assay (ELISA), the presence of insulin autoantibodies does not predict type 1 diabetes in nondiabetic individuals.[246,247] Therefore, ELISAs should not be used to measure IAAs.

Measurement is performed by determining to what extent patient serum is able to immunoprecipitate radiolabeled insulin.[5] Two tubes are set up for IAA measurement. Both tubes contain patient serum and ^{125}I-labeled A14 insulin, but one also contains excess cold insulin. This second tube is to determine nonspecific binding (NSB). Following 7 days, incubation, PEG is added to precipitate insulin-IAA immune complexes. Bound and free ^{125}I-insulin are then separated by centrifugation. The supernatant is discarded, the pellet is washed, and the radioactivity in the pellet is counted. The number of counts in the pellet (minus NSB) is divided by the total counts (minus NSB) to calculate the percentage of insulin that was immunoprecipitated. This figure is proportional to the IAA concentration.

The upper limit of normal is described as the control mean plus 3 standard deviations. Given the quantitative amount of radiolabeled insulin in the assay, IAA concentrations can be expressed as the nanograms of insulin that are precipitated. Insulin autoantibodies are considered to be present when more than 102 ng of insulin is precipitated according to the University of Florida Diabetes Research Laboratory assay protocol.

Glutamic Acid Decarboxylase Autoantibodies

The 64 KA assay is inappropriate for screening large numbers of specimens. It is expensive and complex and requires viable islet cells. However, GADA testing has few of these intrinsic limitations because GADAs can be detected by several different assays.

Glutamic acid decarboxylase autoantibodies can be measured by the ability of patient serum to immunoprecipitate radioactively labeled GAD (eg, in radiobinding assays [RBAs]).[248–252] Glutamic acid decarboxylase can isolated from pig brain and iodinated with ^{125}I or produced by recombinant DNA technology using in vitro translation with a solution containing ^{35}S-methionine. It also can be tritiated (eg, ^{3}H-GAD). Patient serum is added to and incubated with the radiolabeled GAD. Antigen-antibody complexes are separated using staphylococcal protein A sepharose or antihuman Ig antibody bound to sepharose. After filtering and centrifugation, the beads are washed and counted. The GADA concentration is proportional to the percentage of the total radioactivity found in the pellet. The Kronus GADA assay (Boise, ID) uses ^{125}I-labeled GAD_{65}.

Another GADA screening technique, the enzyme immunoprecipitation assay, involves measuring the enzymatic activity of GAD in the immunoprecipitate. The GAD in the precipitate is used to convert carbon 14 (^{14}C)–glutamic acid to GABA, liberating carbon dioxide 14 ($^{14}CO_2$). The $^{14}CO_2$ is collected and counted, and the amount released is proportional to the GADA titer. In these assays, GAD has been isolated from rat, human, or pig brains. Furthermore, the GAD may be affinity-purified using a GAD monoclonal antibody that has been bound to a column.

The immunotrapping enzyme activity assay is a variation of the enzyme immunoprecipitation assay in which human serum (potentially containing GADAs) is absorbed onto protein A sepharose beads.[253] Purified GAD is then added. If GADAs are present in the serum, GAD is linked to the bead via the GADA. The ^{14}C-glutamic acid is added, and liberated $^{14}CO_2$ is then measured. Liberated $^{14}CO_2$ is proportional to the GADA concentration.

In the capture ELISA technique, all wells of a 96-well tray are coated with GAD-6, a GAD monoclonal antibody. Glutamic acid decarboxylase is then added and bound by the GAD monoclonal antibody. This spaces GAD out from the wall of the well and preserves the native conformation of GAD. If GAD is denatured, it will not be recognized by serum from type 1 diabetes patients. Glutamic acid decarboxylase autoantibodies from type 1 diabetic serum cannot be detected by Western blot because in Western blot assays, the GAD antigen is denatured. However, GADAs in sera from patients with stiff-man syndrome can be detected by Western blot because GADAs in such sera recognize linear epitopes and GADAs in stiff-man syndrome are present in very high titers.

The term "capture" ELISA is used for this assay because GAD is secured or arrested (ie, "captured") by the GAD-6 monoclonal antibody. Patient serum is added and if GADAs are present in the serum, they bind to GAD. Following washing, human Ig antibody labeled with HRP is added. Following another washing, substrate is added, producing a color change catalyzed by HRP that can be read with a spectrophotometer.

A "noncapture" (ie, traditional) ELISA has been developed in which 3 overlapping recombinant fusion proteins derived from a mouse brain GAD cDNA are expressed and coated onto wells. However, the sensitivity of this "noncapture" test in new-onset type 1 diabetes patients is low (only 46% positive).[254]

Another variation of the GADA assay is the depletion ELISA. In this assay, GAD in solution is labeled with biotin. Avidin is bound to the wall of the ELISA plate. Unless patient serum contains GADAs, GAD-biotin is bound to the plate via the avidin-biotin interaction. Bound GAD-biotin is detected by addition of a GAD antibody labeled with HRP. Addition of a substrate produces a color change. When patient serum contains GADAs, the GADAs bind to the soluble GAD-biotin and interfere with GAD-biotin binding to the avidin that has been used to coat the tube. Therefore, the assay is depleted of GAD and the signal declines (thus the name "depletion ELISA").

Theoretically, any of these techniques can be automated and used to measure GADA. Undoubtedly, new techniques will continue to be described. Two international workshops have been conducted comparing GADA assays.[255,256] Among these assays, the RBAs demonstrate the highest sensitivity (about 76%) versus the ELISAs (about 36%) and enzyme immunoprecipitation assays (about 50%) in new-onset type 1 diabetes patients.

IA-2/ICA512 Autoantibodies

These assays involve radioactively labeled IA-2 or fragments of IA-2 (eg, ICA512) that are immunoprecipitated by patient serum.[95,212] Such an approach is not fundamentally different from the immunoprecipitation GADA assays. IA-2/ICA512 can be labeled in vitro with ^{35}S-methionine.[257] There is a variation in which fragments of IA-2 are expressed and used as target autoantigen in the assays.[212] When autoantibodies to fragments of IA-2 are sought, the intracellular domain, especially the C-terminal region, displays immunoreactivity with human serum containing IA-2A.[258] The ICA512bdc assay measures autoantibodies to amino acid residues 256 to 979 of IA-2.[207]

When type 1 diabetic serum is trypsinized, 50-, 40-, and 37-kd fragments are derived.[259,260] The 50-kd protein is derived from GAD; the 40-kd fragment originates from IA-2; and the 37-kd autoantigen is released from IA-2β, a recently described 1,004–amino acid 112-kd member of the PTP family,[257,261] also known as phogrin.[262] Postranslationally, IA-2β is processed by proteolytic sectioning into 60-kd and 64-kd proteins. In the PTP domain, phogrin exhibits 80% amino acid sequence homology with IA-2 and, overall, about 43% homology with IA-2. IA-2β and IA-2 share several epitopes, whereas other epitopes are unique to each protein.

Antibodies to the 37-kd protein (eg, phogrin) have been detected in 56% of new-onset type 1 diabetes patients and in 59% of first-degree relatives of patients who later developed the disease.[257] Autoantibodies to IA-2β appear to be most predictive of rapid progression to type 1 diabetes in nondiabetic, marker-positive individuals.[263,264] At the time of diagnosis, more than 90% of patients are positive for autoantibodies to 50- 40-, and/or 37-kd fragments, and 70% have autoantibodies to all 3.[265] A third PTP autoantigen target has been described: islet cell antigen-related PTP, a 990–amino acid protein.[266]

IA-2As display a specificity of greater than 99% and a sensitivity of 62% for autoimmune diabetes. This suggests that IA-2A may be the single best autoantibody for prediabetes screening.[267] However, as discussed previously, the presence of more than one islet autoantibody appears to be the best predictor of type 1 diabetes. In a study by Verge and colleagues,[207] 100% of individuals who were positive for IAA, GADA, and ICA512 autoantibodies and were first-degree relatives of patients with type 1 diabetes developed the disease during 4.5 years of follow-up.

Insulin Receptor Autoantibodies

There are several different approaches to the detection of insulin receptor autoantibodies. Most commonly, the ability of patient serum to inhibit the binding of ^{125}I-labeled insulin to insulin receptors is determined.[236] This procedure is similar to a thyrotropin-binding inhibitory immunoglobulin assay. Lymphocytes are used as target cells because they naturally express insulin receptors.

An alternative method is to evaluate the immunoprecipitation of radioactively labeled, solubilized insulin receptors by patient serum. The molecular weight of the receptor can be identified by SDS-polyacrylamide electrophoresis of the proteins in the pellet. This is followed by autoradiography. Finally, the biologic insulin-like effect of insulin receptor autoantibodies can be measured.

Because type B insulin resistance and insulinomimetic hypoglycemia are rare conditions and are rarely considered in the diagnosis of carbohydrate disorders, there should be little clinical demand for this assay. Unless they are distinguished by bioassay, finding insulin receptor autoantibodies does not define whether these autoantibodies are agonistic or antagonistic. This differentiation is best made through review of the clinical case; type B insulin resistance would imply the presence of antagonistic insulin receptor autoantibodies, whereas insulinomimetic hypoglycemia would imply the presence of agonistic insulin receptor autoantibodies.

Combined Assays

Researchers are developing methods to screen for several islet autoantibodies simultaneously; for example, immunoprecipitation assays that contain radiolabeled insulin, GAD, and IA-2/ICA512 in the same test tube. If such a screen is positive, individual assays for IAA, GADA, and IA-2A can then be carried out. Scandinavian researchers are experimenting with labeling insulin, GAD, and IA-2 each with a different rare earth element that would allow simultaneous, one-tube detection of IAA, GADA, and IA-2A. A combined IA-2A–GADA immunoprecipitation assay has been described in which IA-2/ICA512 is labeled with ^{35}S-methionine and GAD is labeled with ^{3}H-leucine.[268] In such screening scenarios, ICA testing could be reserved for individuals who screen positive with the multi-islet autoantibody test.

Comments and Recommendations

Testing for islet autoantibodies should be ordered only in special circumstances. One circumstance is to confirm the autoimmune etiology of diabetes in patients presenting with an acute onset. In this instance, results are clinically interesting and may be diagnostically helpful. Patients with autoimmune diabetes should be screened for associated autoimmune disorders involving the thyroid gland and gastric parietal cells.[230] If autoantibodies indicative of either of these disorders are detected, clinical evaluation is indicated, along with testing for adrenal autoantibodies. The argument also can be made that if a patient presents with acute-onset type 1 diabetes, because autoimmunity is the overwhelming statistical cause of this disease, islet autoantibody testing can be bypassed and that all type 1 patients should be screened for thyroid and gastric parietal cell autoantibodies as described.[269]

A waterfall approach to testing should be considered in type 1 patients. A combined assay for GADA/IA-2A or GADA/IA-2A/IAA could be the initial screen. If positive, ICA testing could be performed as a confirmation.

The second situation in which a screen should be performed for islet autoantibodies is when a patient with type 2 diabetes becomes insulin-dependent. Finding islet autoantibodies[43–46] would confirm an autoimmune etiology, suggesting that exogenous insulin treatment should replace attempts at diabetic control with oral hypoglycemic agents. Four percent to 17% of patients with type 2 diabetes are positive for ICA.[44-47] Type 2 patients who are ICA-positive proceed to insulin dependence at a higher rate than those who are ICA-negative, exhibit lower C-peptide levels[92] than ICA-negative patients, and display higher frequencies of HLA-DR3 and HLA-DR4 than ICA-negative patients. Glutamic acid decarboxylase autoantibodies have been reported to be persistent in patients with LADA and following the diagnosis of type 1 diabetes.[249,250,270] Relatives of patients with LADA are expected to be at increased risk for autoimmune diabetes. There are no data about the frequency of associated autoimmunities in LADA.

In prediabetes screening, testing for islet autoantibodies should only be undertaken as part of a research protocol. When type 1 diabetes can finally be prevented, childhood screening for islet autoantibodies could become as common as immunizations. This would represent a huge market for islet autoantibody testing.

In addition to the preceding circumstances, IAA should be ordered for evaluation of possible autoimmune hypoglycemia. Insulin receptor autoantibody tests should be ordered when type B insulin resistance or insulinomimetic hypoglycemia are clinical considerations.

References

1. Winter WE. Autoimmune endocrinopathies. In: Kappy MS, Blizzard RM, Migeon CJ, eds. *Wilkin's Diagnosis and Treatment of Endocrine Disorders in Childhood and Adolescence*. 4th ed. Springfield, IL: Charles C Thomas; 1994:317–382.
2. Winter WE, Maclaren NK. Autoimmune endocrinopathies. In: Stiehm ER, ed. *Immunologic Disorders in Infants and Children*. 4th ed. Philadelphia, PA: WB Saunders; 1996:824–854.
3. Bottazzo GF, Florin-Christensen A, Doniach D. Islet-cell autoantibodies in diabetes mellitus with autoimmune polyendocrine deficiencies. *Lancet*. 1974;2:1279–1283.
4. Gianani R, Pugliese A, Bonner-Weir S, et al. Prognostically significant heterogeneity of cytoplasmic islet cell antibodies in relatives of patients with type I diabetes. *Diabetes*. 1992;41:347–353.
5. Palmer JP, Asplin CM, Raghu PK, et al. Anti-insulin antibodies in insulin dependent diabetes before insulin treatment: A new marker for autoimmune B cell damage. *Diabetes*. 1983;32:76A.
6. Baekkeskov S, Aanstoot HJ, Christgau S, et al. Identification of the 64K autoantigen in insulin-dependent diabetes as the GABA-synthesizing enzyme glutamic acid decarboxylase. *Nature*. 1990;347:151–156.
7. Verge CF, Gianani R, Yu L, et al. Late progression to diabetes and evidence for chronic beta-cell autoimmunity in identical twins of patients with type I diabetes. *Diabetes*. 1995;44:1176–1179.
8. Wilkin TJ, Hammonds P, Mirza I, et al. Graves' disease of the beta cell: glucose dysregulation due to islet-cell stimulating antibodies. *Lancet*. 1988;2: 1155–1158.
9. Cahill GF, McDevitt HO. Insulin-dependent diabetes mellitus: The initial lesion. *N Engl J Med*. 1981;304: 1454–1465.
10. Doniach D, Bottazzo GF, Cudworth AG. Etiology of type I diabetes mellitus: Heterogeneity and immunological events leading to clinical onset. *Ann Rev Med*. 1983;34:13–20.
11. Nerup J, Lernmark A. Autoimmunity in insulin-dependent diabetes mellitus. *Am J Med*. 1983;70:135–141.
12. Marx JZ. Diabetes: A possible autoimmune disease. *Science*. 1984;225:1381–1383.
13. Atkinson MA, Maclaren NK. What causes diabetes? *Sci Am*. 1990;262:62–71.
14. Thai A-C, Eisenbarth GS. Natural history of IDDM. *Diabetes Rev*. 1993;1:1–14.
15. Sperling MA. Diabetes mellitus. *Pediatr Clin North Am*. 1979;26:149–170.
16. Winter WE. Diabetes mellitus: Pathophysiology, etiologies, complications, management, and laboratory evaluation. *Am Assoc Clin Chem*. 1994;12:1–84. [Monograph]
17. Lendrum R, Walker G, Gamble DR. Islet-cell antibodies in juvenile diabetes mellitus of recent onset. *Lancet*. 1975;1:880–883.
18. Lendrum R, Walker G, Cudworth AG, et al. Islet-cell antibodies in diabetes mellitus. *Lancet*. 1976;2: 1273–1276.

19. Lernmark A, Baekkeskov S. Islet cell antibodies: Theoretical and practical implications. *Diabetologia.* 1981;21:431–435.

20. Winter WE, Maclaren NK, Riley WJ, et al. Pancreatic alpha cell autoantibodies and glucagon response to arginine. *Diabetes.* 1984;33:435–437.

21. Bottazzo GF, Lendrum R. Separate autoantibodies to human pancreatic glucagon and somatostatin cells. *Lancet.* 1976;2:873–876.

22. Schatz D, Krischer J, Horne G, et al. Islet cell antibodies predict insulin-dependent diabetes in United States school age children as powerfully as in unaffected relatives. *J Clin Invest.* 1994;93:2403–2407.

23. Del Prete GF, Tiengo A, Nosadini R, et al. Glucagon secretion in two patients with autoantibodies to glucagon-producing cells. *Horm Metab Res.* 1978;10:260–261.

24. Baba S, Morita S, Mizuno N, et al. Autoimmunity to glucagon in a diabetic not on insulin. *Lancet.* 1976;2:585.

25. Sanke T, Kondo M, Moriyama Y, et al. Glucagon binding autoantibodies in a patient with hyperthyroidism treated with methimazole. *J Clin Endocrinol Metab.* 1983;57:1140–1144.

26. Kahn CR, Flier JS, Bar RS, et al. The syndromes of insulin resistance and acanthosis nigricans: Insulin-receptor disorders in man. *N Engl J Med.* 1976;294: 739–745.

27. Wilkin TJ. Receptor autoimmunity in endocrine disorders. *N Engl J Med.* 1990;323:1318–1324.

28. Bloise W, Wajchenberg BL, Moncada VY, et al. Atypical antiinsulin receptor antibodies in a patient with type B insulin resistance and scleroderma. *J Clin Endocrinol Metab.* 1989;68:227–231.

29. Duncan JA, Shah SC, Shulman DI, et al. Type B insulin resistance in a 15-year-old white youth. *J Pediatr.* 1983;103:421–424.

30. Braund WJ, Naylor BA, Williamson DH, et al. Autoimmunity to insulin receptor and hypoglycaemia in patient with Hodgkin's disease. *Lancet.* 1987;1:237–240.

31. Moller DE, Ratner RE, Borenstein DG, et al. Autoantibodies to the insulin receptor as a cause of autoimmune hypoglycemia in systemic lupus erythematosus. *Am J Med.* 1988;84:334–338.

32. Varga J, Lopatin M, Boden G. Hypoglycemia due to antiinsulin receptor antibodies in systemic lupus erythematosus. *J Rheumatol.* 1990;17:1226–1229.

33. Elias D, Cohen IR, Schechter Y, et al. Antibodies to insulin receptor followed by anti-idiotype: Antibodies to insulin in child with hypoglycemia. *Diabetes.* 1987;36:348–354.

34. Goldman J, Baldwin D, Rubenstein AH, et al. Characterization of circulating insulin and proinsulin-binding antibodies in autoimmune hypoglycemia. *J Clin Invest.* 1979;63:1050–1059.

35. Dozio N, Sodoyez Goffaux F, Koch M, et al. Polymorphism of insulin antibodies in six patients with insulin-immune hypoglycaemic syndrome. *Clin Exp Immunol.* 1991;85:282–287.

36. Burch HB, Clement S, Sokol MS, et al. Reactive hypoglycemic coma due to insulin autoimmune syndrome: Case report and literature review. *Am J Med.* 1992;92:681–685.

37. Meschi F, Dozio N, Bognetti E, et al. An unusual case of recurrent hypoglycaemia: 10-year follow up of a child with insulin autoimmunity. *Eur J Pediatr.* 1992;151:32–34.

38. Takayama S, Hirata Y. Incidence of insulin autoimmune hypoglycemia in Japan during the three-year period from 1979 to 1981. *Diabetes.* 1983;32:150A.

39. Takayama S, Eguchi Y, Sato A, et al. Insulin autoimmune syndrome is the third leading cause of spontaneous hypoglycemic attacks in Japan. *Diabetes Res Clin Pract.* 1990;10:211–214.

40. Hirata Y. Methamizole and insulin autoimmune syndrome with hypoglycemia. *Lancet.* 1983;2:1037–1038.

41. Schlemper RJ, Uchigata Y, Frolich M, et al. Recurrent hypoglycaemia caused by the insulin autoimmune syndrome: The first Dutch case. *Neth J Med.* 1996;48:188–192.

42. Irvine WJ, McCallum CJ, Gray RS, et al. Clinical and pathogenic significance of pancreatic islet-cell antibodies in diabetics treated with oral hypoglycemic agents. *Lancet.* 1977;1:1025–1027.

43. Gray RS, Irvine WJ, Cameron EH, et al. Glucose and insulin responses to oral glucose in overt non-insulin-dependent diabetics with and without the islet cell antibody. *Diabetes.* 1980;29:312–316.

44. Di Mario U, Irvine WJ, Borsey DQ, et al. Immune abnormalities in diabetic patients not requiring insulin at diagnosis. *Diabetologia.* 1983;25:392–395.

45. Ohgawara H, Hirata Y. Islet cell surface antibodies in diabetes and their possible influence on glucose tolerance. *Tohoku J Exp Med.* 1984;142:211–216.

46. Niskanen L, Karjalaienen J, Sarlund H, et al. Five year follow-up of islet-cell antibodies in type 2 (non-insulin dependent) diabetes mellitus. *Diabetologia.* 1991;34:402–408.

47. Maron R, Elias D, DeJongh BM, et al. Autoantibodies to the insulin receptor in juvenile onset insulin-dependent diabetes. *Nature.* 1983;303:817–818.

48. Johnson JH, Crider BP, McCorkle K, et al. Inhibition of glucose transport into rat islet cells by immunoglobulins from patients with new-onset insulin-dependent diabetes mellitus. *N Engl J Med.* 1990;332:653–659.

49. Castano L, Russo E, Zhou L, et al. Identification and cloning of a granule autoantigen (carboxypeptidase-H) associated with type I diabetes. *J Clin Endocrinol Metab.* 1991;73:1197–1201.

50. Rorsman F, Husebye ES, Winqvist O, et al. Aromatic-L-amino-acid decarboxylase, a pyridoxal phosphate-dependent enzyme, is a beta-cell autoantigen. *Proc Natl Acad Sci U S A*. 1995;92:8626–8629.

51. Bohmer K, Keilacker H, Kuglin B, et al. Proinsulin autoantibodies are more closely associated with type 1 (insulin-dependent) diabetes mellitus than insulin autoantibodies. *Diabetologia*. 1991;34:830–834.

52. Aanstoot HJ, Kang SM, Kim J, et al. Identification and characterization of glima 38, a glycosylated islet cell membrane antigen, which together with GAD_{65} and IA2 marks the early phases of autoimmune response in type 1 diabetes. *J Clin Invest*. 1996;97:2772–2783.

53. Pak CY, Cha CY, Rajotte RV, et al. Human pancreatic islet cell specific 38 kilodalton autoantigen identified by cytomegalovirus-induced monoclonal islet cell autoantibody. *Diabetologia*. 1990;33:569–572.

54. Chang YH, Hwang J, Shang HF, et al. Characterization of human DNA topoisomerase II as an autoantigen recognized by patients with IDDM. *Diabetes*. 1996;45:408–414.

55. Kim YJ, Zhou Z, Hurtado J, et al. IDDM patients' sera recognize a novel 30-kD pancreatic autoantigen related to chymotrypsinogen. *Immunol Invest*. 1993;220:219–227.

56. Karounos DG, Thomas JW. Recognition of common islet antigen by autoantibodies from NOD mice and humans with IDDM. *Diabetes*. 1990;39:1085–1090.

57. Dotta F, Gianani R, Previti M, et al. Autoimmunity to the GM2-1 islet ganglioside before and at the onset of type I diabetes. *Diabetes*. 1996;45:193–196.

58. Atkinson MA, Holmes LA, Scharp DW, et al. No evidence for serological autoimmunity to islet cell heat shock proteins in insulin dependent diabetes. *J Clin Invest*. 1991;87:721–724.

59. Pietropaolo M, Castaño L, Babu S, et al. Islet cell autoantigen 69 kD (ICA69): Molecular cloning and characterization of a novel diabetes-associated autoantigen. *J Clin Invest*. 1993;92:359–371.

60. Lampasona V, Ferrari M, Bosi E, et al. Sera from patients with IDDM and healthy individuals have antibodies to ICA69 on Western blots but do not immunoprecipitate liquid phase antigen. *J Autoimmun*. 1994;7:665–674.

61. Atkinson MA, Kaufman DL, Campbell L, et al. Response of peripheral blood mononuclear cells to glutamate decarboxylase in insulin-dependent diabetes. *Lancet*. 1992;339:458–459.

62. Harrison LC, Honyman MC, DeAizpurua HJ, et al. Inverse relation between humoral and cellular immunity to glutamic acid decarboxylase in subjects at risk of insulin-dependent diabetes. *Lancet*. 1993;431:1365–1369.

63. Arden SD, Roep BO, Neophytou PI, et al. Imogen 38: A novel 38-kD islet mitochondrial autoantigen recognized by T cells from a newly diagnosed type 1 diabetic patient. *J Clin Invest*. 1996;97:551–561.

64. Roep BO, Arden SD, de Vries RRP, et al. T-cell clones from a type-1 diabetes patient respond to insulin secretory granule proteins. *Nature*. 1990;345:632–634.

65. Roep BO, Kallan AA, Hazenbos WL, et al. T-cell reactivity to 38 kD insulin-secretory-granule protein in patients with recent-onset type 1 diabetes. *Lancet*. 1991;337:1439–1441.

66. Roep BO, Kallan AA, Duinkerken G, et al. T-cell reactivity to beta-cell membrane antigens associated with beta-cell destruction in IDDM. *Diabetes*. 1995;44:278–283.

67. Hummel M, Durinovic-Bello I, Ziegler A-G. Relation between cellular and humoral immunity to islet cell antigens in type I diabetes. *J Autoimmun*. 1996;9:427–430.

68. Neufeld M, Maclaren NK, Riley WJ, et al. Islet cell and other organ-specific autoantibodies in U.S. Caucasians and African Americans with insulin-dependent diabetes mellitus. *Diabetes*. 1980;29:589–592.

69. Riley WJ, Maclaren NK. Islet cell autoantibodies. In: Samios E, ed. *The Endocrine Pancreas*. New York, NY: Raven Press; 1991:409–422.

70. Winter WE, Maclaren NK, Riley WJ, et al. Maturity-onset diabetes of youth in black Americans. *N Engl J Med*. 1987;316:285–291.

71. Winter WE. Atypical diabetes in African Americans. *Clin Diabetes*. 1991;9:49–56.

72. Nayak RC, Omar MAK, Rabizadeh A, et al. Cytoplasmic islet cell antibodies. *Diabetes*. 1985;34:617–619.

73. Cabrera-Rode E, Diaz-Horta O, Fernandez LE, et al. Glycolipids as the major autoantigens of cytoplasmatic islet cell antibodies. *Autoimmunity*. 1995;20:145–151.

74. Atkinson MA, Kaufman DL, Newman D, et al. Islet cell cytoplasmic autoantibody reactivity to glutamate decarboxylase in insulin-dependent diabetes. *J Clin Invest*. 1993;91:350–356.

75. Lan MS, Wasserfall C, Maclaren NK, et al. IA-2, a transmembrane protein of the protein tyrosine phosphatase family, is a major autoantigen in insulin-dependent diabetes mellitus. *Proc Natl Acad Sci U S A*. 1996;93:6367–6370.

76. Myers MA, Rabin DU, Rowley MJ. Pancreatic islet cell cytoplasmic antibody in diabetes is represented by antibodies to islet cell antigen 512 and glutamic acid decarboxylase. *Diabetes*. 1995;44:1290–1295.

77. Maclaren NK, Huang S-W. Antibody to cultured human insulinoma cells in insulin-dependent diabetes. *Lancet*. 1975;1:997–999.

78. Lernmark A, Freedman ZR, Hofmann C, et al. Islet-cell-surface antibodies in juvenile diabetes mellitus. *N Engl J Med*. 1978;299:375–380.

79. Maclaren NK, Huang S-W. Cell-mediated immunity in insulin dependent diabetes. In: Irvine WF, ed. *The Immunology of Diabetes*. Edinburgh, Scotland: Tevoit Scientific Publications; 1980:185–193.

80. Eisenbarth GS, Morris MA, Sceararce RM. Cytotoxic antibodies to cloned islet cells in serum of patients with diabetes mellitus. *J Clin Invest*. 1981;67:403–408.

81. Sai P, Boitard C, Debray-Sachs M, et al. Complement-fixing islet cell antibodies from some diabetic patients alter insulin release in vitro. *Diabetes*. 1981;30:1051–1057.

82. Van Der Winkel M, Smets G, Gepts W. Islet cell surface antibodies from insulin-dependent diabetics bind specifically to pancreatic cells. *J Clin Invest*. 1982;70:41–49.

83. Maruyama T, Takei I, Matsuba I, et al. Cell-mediated cytotoxic islet cell surface antibodies to human pancreatic beta cells. *Diabetologia*. 1984;26:30–33.

84. Atkinson MA, Maclaren NK, Riley WJ, et al. Are insulin autoantibodies markers for insulin-dependent diabetes mellitus? *Diabetes*. 1986;35:894–898.

85. Landin-Olsson M, Palmer JP, Lernmark A, et al. Predictive value of islet cell and insulin autoantibodies for type 1 (insulin-dependent) diabetes mellitus in a population-based study of newly-diagnosed diabetic and matched control children. *Diabetologia*. 1992;35: 1068–1073.

86. Baekkeskov S, Nielson JH, Marner B, et al. Autoantibodies in newly diagnosed diabetic children immunoprecipitate human pancreatic islet cell proteins. *Nature*. 1982;298:167–169.

87. Atkinson MA, Maclaren NK, Scharp DW, et al. 64,000 Mr autoantibodies as predictors of insulin-dependent diabetes. *Lancet*. 1990;335:1357–1360.

88. Atkinson MA, Maclaren NK. Autoantibodies in nonobese diabetic mice immunoprecipitate 64,000-Mr islet antigen. *Diabetes*. 1988;37:1587–1590.

89. Baekkeskov S, Dryberg T, Lernmark A. Autoantibodies to a 64-kilodalton islet cell protein precede the onset of spontaneous diabetes in the BB rat. *Science*. 1984;224:1348–1350.

90. Solimena M, Folli F, Aparisi R, et al. Autoantibodies to GABA-ergic neurons and pancreatic beta cells in stiff-man syndrome. *N Engl J Med*. 1990;322:1555–1560.

91. Kaufman DL, Erlander MG, Clare-Salzler M, et al. Autoimmunity to two forms of glutamate decarboxylase in insulin-dependent diabetes mellitus. *J Clin Invest*. 1992;89:283–292.

92. Christie MR, Hollands JA, Brown TJ, et al. Detection of pancreatic islet 64,000 M(r) autoantigens in insulin-dependent diabetes distinct from glutamate decarboxylase. *J Clin Invest*. 1993;92:240–248.

93. Hagopian WA, Michelsen B, Karlsen AE, et al. Autoantibodies in IDDM primarily recognize the 65,000-M(r) rather than the 67,000-M(r) isoform of glutamic acid decarboxylase. *Diabetes*. 1993;42:631–636.

94. Luhder F, Schlosser M, Mauch L, et al. Autoantibodies against GAD_{65} rather than GAD_{67} precede the onset of type 1 diabetes. *Autoimmunity*. 1994;19:1–80.

95. Lan MS, Lu J, Goto Y, et al. Molecular cloning and identification of a receptor-type protein tyrosine phosphatase, IA-2, from human insulinoma. *DNA Cell Biol*. 1994;13:505–514.

96. Rabin DU, Pleasic SM, Shapiro JA, et al. Islet cell antigen 512 is a diabetes-specific islet autoantigen related to protein tyrosine phosphatases. *J Immunol*. 1994;152:3183–3188.

97. van den Maagdenbert AMJM, Weghuis DO, Rijss J, et al. Assignment of the human gene for receptor-type protein tyrosine phosphatase IA-2 (PTPRN) to chromosome region 2q35 q36.1 and identification of an intragenic genetic marker. *Cytogenet Cell Genet*. 1996;73:145–148.

98. Solimena M, Dirkx R Jr, Hermel JM, et al. ICA 512, an autoantigen of type I diabetes, is an intrinsic membrane protein of neurosecretory granules. *EMBO J*. 1996;15:2102–2114.

99. Nerup J, Platz P, Andersen OO. HL-A antigens and diabetes mellitus. *Lancet*. 1974;2:864–866.

100. Cudworth AG, Wolf E. The genetic susceptibility to type I (insulin-dependent) diabetes mellitus. *Clin Endocrinol Metab*. 1982;11:389–407.

101. Owerbach D, Lernmark A, Platz P, et al. HLA-D region beta-chain DNA endonuclease fragments differ between HLA-DR identical healthy and insulin-dependent diabetic individuals. *Nature*. 1983;303: 815–817.

102. Owerbach D, Hagglof B, Lernmark A, et al. Susceptibility to insulin-dependent diabetes defined by restriction enzyme polymorphism of HLA-D region genomic DNA. *Diabetes*. 1984;33:958–965.

103. Bottazzo GF, Todd I, Pujol-Borrell R. Hypotheses on genetic contributions to the aetiology of diabetes mellitus. *Immunol Today*. 1984;5:230–231.

104. Michelsen B, Lernmark A. Molecular cloning of a polymorphic DNA endonuclease fragment associates insulin-dependent diabetes mellitus with HLA-DQ. *J Clin Invest*. 1987;79:1144.

105. Todd JA, Bell JI, McDevitt HO. HLA-DQ? gene contributes to susceptibility and resistance to insulin-dependent diabetes mellitus. *Nature*. 1987;329:599–604.

106. Morel PA, Dorman JS, Todd JA, et al. Aspartic acid at position 57 of the HLA-DQ? chain protects against type I diabetes: A family study. *Proc Nat Acad Sci U S A*. 1988;85:8111–8115.

107. Maclaren N, Riley W, Skordis N, et al. Inherited susceptibility to insulin-dependent diabetes is associated with HLA-DR1, while DR5 is protective. *Autoimmunity*. 1988;1:197–205.

108. Baisch JM, Weeks T, Giles R, et al. Analysis of HLA-DQ genotypes and susceptibility in insulin-dependent diabetes mellitus. *N Engl J Med*. 1990;322:1836–1841.

109. Pugliese A, Gianani R, Moromisato R, et al. HLA-DQB1*0602 is associated with dominant protection from diabetes even among islet cell antibody-positive first-degree relatives of patients with IDDM. *Diabetes*. 1995;44:608–613.

110. The Diabetes Control and Complications Trial Research Group. The effect of intensive treatment of diabetes on the development and progression of long-term complications in insulin-dependent diabetes mellitus. *N Engl J Med*. 1993;329:977–986.

111. Rosenbloom AL. Long term complications of type 1 (insulin-dependent) diabetes mellitus. *Pediatr Ann*. 1983;12:655–683.

112. Sutherland DE, Goetz FC, Najarian JS. Pancreas transplants from related donors. *Transplantation*. 1984;38:625–633.

113. Sutherland DER, Goetz FC, Najarian JS. Recent experience with 89 pancreas transplants at a single institution. *Diabetologia*. 1984;27:149–153.

114. Sutherland DE, Sibley R, Xu XZ, et al. Twin-to-twin pancreas transplantation: Reversal and reenactment of the pathogenesis of type I diabetes. *Trans Assoc Am Physicians*. 1984;97:80–87.

115. Sutherland DE, Gores PF, Farney AC, et al. Evolution of kidney, pancreas, and islet transplantation for patients with diabetes at the University of Minnesota. *Am J Surg*. 1993;166:456–491.

116. Tyden G, Reinholt FP, Sundkvist G, et al. Recurrence of autoimmune diabetes mellitus in recipients of cadaveric pancreatic grafts. *N Engl J Med*. 1996;335: 860–863.

117. Marx J. Testing of autoimmune therapy begins. *Science*. 1991;252:272–278.

118. Stiller CR, Dupre J, Gent M, et al. Effects of cyclosporin immunosuppression in insulin-dependent diabetes mellitus of recent onset. *Science*. 1984;223:1362–1367.

119. Assan R, Feutren G, Debray-Sachs M, et al. Metabolic and immunological effects of cyclosporin in recently diagnosed type I diabetes mellitus. *Lancet*. 1985;1: 67–71.

120. Feutren G, Papoz L, Assan R, et al. Cyclosporin increases the rate and length of remissions in insulin-dependent diabetes of recent onset: Results of a multicentre double-blind trial. *Lancet*. 1986;2:119–124.

121. Dupre J, Stiller CR, Gent M, et al. Clinical trials of cyclosporin in IDDM. *Diabetes Care*. 1988;11(suppl 1): 37–44.

122. Chase HP, Butler-Simon N, Garg SK, et al. Cyclosporine A for the treatment of new-onset insulin-dependent diabetes mellitus. *Pediatrics*. 1990;85:241–245.

123. Bougneres PF, Carel JC, Castano L, et al. Factors associated with early remission of type I diabetes in children treated with cyclosporine. *N Engl J Med*. 1990;318:663–670.

124. Harrison LC, Colman PG, Dean B, et al. Increase in remission rate in newly diagnosed type I diabetic subjects treated with azathioprine. *Diabetes*. 1985;34:1306–1308.

125. Riley WJ, Maclaren NK, Spillar RP. Reversal of deteriorating glucose tolerance with azathioprine in prediabetes. *Transplant Proc*. 1986;18:819–822.

126. Silverstein J, Maclaren N, Riley W, et al. Immunosuppression with azathioprine and prednisone in recent-onset insulin-dependent diabetes mellitus. *N Engl J Med*. 1988;319:599–604.

127. Martin S, Schernthaner G, Nerup J, et al. Follow-up of cyclosporin A treatment in type 1 (insulin-dependent) diabetes mellitus: Lack of long-term effects. *Diabetologia*. 1991;34:429–434.

128. Marks JB, Skyler JS. Clinical review 17: Immunotherapy of type I diabetes mellitus. *J Clin Endocrinol Metab*. 1991;72:3–9.

129. Bach JF, Feutren G, Boitard C. Immunoprevention of insulin-dependent diabetes by cyclosporin. In: Andreani D, Kolb H, Pozzilli P, eds. *Immunotherapy of Type I Diabetes*. Chichester, England: John Wiley & Sons; 1989:125–136.

130. Sanders ME. Clinical trial of chimeric anti-CD4-monoclonal antibody for insulin dependent diabetes mellitus. *Diabetes Prev Ther*. 1991;5:28.

131. Skyler JS, Lorenz TJ, Schwartz S, et al. Effects of an anti-CD5 immunoconjugate (CD5-plus) in recent onset type I diabetes mellitus: A preliminary investigation. The CD5 Diabetes Project Team. *J Diabetes Complications*. 1993;7:224–232.

132. Vialettes B, Vague P. Treatment of diabetes by monoclonal antibodies: Lessons from a pilot study using anti-IL-2 receptor MoAb in recently diagnosed diabetic patients. *Diabetes Prev Ther*. 1991;5:21–22.

133. Culler FL, O'Connor R, Kaufmann S, et al. Immunospecific therapy for type I diabetes mellitus. *N Engl J Med*. 1985;313:695–696.

134. Boitard C, Timsit J, Assan R, et al. Treatment of type I diabetes mellitus with DAB486-IL-2, a toxin conjugate which targets activated T-lymphocytes. *Diabetologia*. 1992;35(suppl 1):A218. [Abstract]

135. Cavanaugh J, Chopek M, Binimelis J, et al Buffy coat transfusions in early type I diabetes. *Diabetes*. 1987;36:1089–1093.

136. Krug J, Verlohren HJ, Bierwolf B, et al. Lymphocyte transfusion in recent onset type I diabetes mellitus: A one-year follow-up of cell-mediated anti-islet cytotoxicity and C-peptide secretion. *J Autoimmun*. 1990;3: 601–609.

137. Dempe A, Baaske W, von-Baehr R, et al. Remission of the newly diagnosed type 1 diabetes by radiation of the pancreas. *Exp Clin Endocrinol*. 1988;92:123–125.

138. Usadel KH, Teuber J, Schmeidl R, et al. Management of type I diabetes with ciamexone. *Lancet*. 1986;2:567. [Letter]

139. Koivisto VA, Aro A, Cantell K, et al. Remissions in newly diagnosed type I (insulin-dependent) diabetes: Influence of interferon as an adjunct to insulin therapy. *Diabetologia*. 1984;27:193–197.

140. Rand KH, Rosenbloom AL, Maclaren NK, et al. Human leukocyte interferon treatment of two children with insulin-dependent diabetes. *Diabetologia.* 1981;21:116–119.

141. Pococco M, De-Campo C, Cantoni L, et al. Effect of high doses intravenous IgG in newly diagnosed diabetic children. *Helv Paediatr Acta.* 1987;42:289–295.

142. Silverstein J, Riley W, Barrett D, et al. Immunosuppressive therapy (IT) for newly diagnosed insulin dependent diabetes mellitus (IDD) with antithymocyte globulin (ATG) and prednisone (pred). *Pediatr Res.* 1984;71:295A.

143. Cobb WE, Molitch M, Reichlin S. Levamisole in insulin-dependent diabetes mellitus. *N Engl J Med.* 1980;303:1065–1066.

144. Shehadeh N, Calcinaro F, Bradley BJ, et al. Effect of adjuvant therapy on development of diabetes in mouse and man. *Lancet.* 1994;343:706–707.

145. Elliott RB, Crossley JR, Berryman CC, et al. Partial preservation of pancreatic β-cell function in children with diabetes. *Lancet.* 1981;2:1–4.

146. Jackson R, Dolinar R, Srikanta S, et al. Prednisone therapy in early type I diabetes: Immunological effects. *Diabetes.* 1982;31:48A.

147. Giordano C, Panto F, Amato MP, et al. Early administration of an immunomodulator and induction of remission in insulin-dependent diabetes mellitus. *J Autoimmun.* 1990;3:611–617.

148. Moncada E, Subira ML, Oleaga A, et al. Insulin requirements and residual beta-cell function 12 months after concluding immunotherapy in type I diabetic patients treated with combined azathioprine and thymostimulin administration for one year. *J Autoimmun.* 1990;3:625–638.

149. Carroll PB, Tzakis AG, Ricordi C, et al. The use of FK 506 in new-onset type I diabetes in man. *Transplant Proc.* 1991;23:3351–3353.

150. Harrison LC, Honeyman M, Steele C, et al. Photophoresis trial in IDDM: An interim report. *Proc Aust Diabetes Society.* 1992;91. [Abstract]

151. Leslie RDG, Pyke DA. Immunosuppression of acute insulin-dependent diabetes. In: Irvine WJ, ed. *The Immunology of Diabetes.* Edinburgh, Scotland: Tevoit Scientific Publications; 1980:345–347.

152. Ludvigsson J, Heding L, Lernmark A, et al. An attempt to break the autoimmune process at the onset of IDDM by the use of plasmapheresis and high doses of prednisolone. *Bull Int Study Group Diabetes Young.* 1982;6:11–12.

153. Ludvigsson J, Heding L, Gudrun L, et al. Plasmapheresis in the initial treatment of insulin-dependent diabetes mellitus in children. *Br Med J.* 1983;286:176–178.

154. Myers BD, Ross J, Newton L, et al. Cyclosporin associated chronic nephropathy. *N Engl J Med.* 1984;311:699–705.

155. Atkinson MA, Maclaren NK, Luchetta R. Insulitis and diabetes in NOD mice reduced by prophylactic insulin therapy. *Diabetes.* 1990;39:933–937.

156. Thivolet CH, Goillot E, Bedossa P, et al. Insulin prevents adoptive cell transfer of diabetes in the autoimmune non-obese diabetic mouse. *Diabetologia.* 1991;34:314–319.

157. Muir A, Peck A, Clare-Salzler M, et al. Insulin immunization of nonobese diabetic mice induces a protective insulitis characterized by diminished intraislet interferon-gamma transcription. *J Clin Invest.* 1995;95:628–634.

158. Daniel D, Wegmann DR. Protection of nonobese diabetic mice from diabetes by intranasal or subcutaneous administration of insulin peptide B-(9-23). *Proc Natl Acad Sci U S A.* 1996;93:956–960.

159. Muir A, Ramiya V. New strategies in oral immunotherapy for diabetes prevention. *Diabetes Metab Rev.* 1996;12:1–14.

160. Zhang ZJ, Davidson L, Eisenbarth G, et al. Suppression of diabetes in nonobese diabetic mice by oral administration of porcine insulin. *Proc Natl Acad Sci U S A.* 1991;88:1025–1026.

161. Tisch R, Yang XD, Liblau RS, et al. Administering glutamic acid decarboxylase to NOD mice prevents diabetes. *J Autoimmun.* 1994;7:845–850.

162. Weiner HL, Friedman A, Miller A, et al. Oral tolerance: Immunologic mechanisms and treatment of animal and human organ-specific autoimmune diseases by oral administration of autoantigens. *Annu Rev Immunol.* 1994;12:809–837.

163. Sosroseno W. A review of the mechanisms of oral tolerance and immunotherapy. *J R Soc Med.* 1995;88:14–17.

164. Hancock WW, Polanski M, Zhang J, et al. Suppression of insulitis in non-obese diabetic (NOD) mice by oral insulin administration is associated with selective expression of interleukin-4 and -10, transforming growth factor-beta, and prostaglandin-E. *Am J Pathol.* 1995;147:1193–1199.

165. Gepts W. Pathologic anatomy of the pancreas in juvenile diabetes mellitus. *Diabetes.* 1965;14:619–633.

166. Gepts W, Lecompte PM. The pancreatic islets in diabetes. *Am J Med.* 1981;70:105–115.

167. Bottazzo GF, Dean BM, McNally JM, et al. In situ characterization of autoimmune phenomena and expression of HLA molecules in the pancreas in diabetic insulitis. *N Engl J Med.* 1985;313:353–360.

168. Foulis AK, Stewart JA. The pancreas in recent-onset type 1 (insulin-dependent) diabetes mellitus: Insulin content of islets, insulitis and associated changes in the exocrine acinar tissue. *Diabetologia.* 1984;26:456–461.

169. Foulis AK, Liddle CN, Farquharson MA, et al. The histopathology of the pancreas in type 1 (insulin-dependent) diabetes mellitus: A 25-year review of deaths in patients under 20 years of age in the United Kingdom. *Diabetologia*. 1986;29:267–274.

170. Shah SC, Malone JI, Simpson NE. A randomized trial of intensive insulin therapy in newly diagnosed insulin-dependent diabetes mellitus. *N Engl J Med*. 1989;320:550–554.

171. Keller RJ, Eisenbarth GS, Jackson RA. Insulin prophylaxis in individuals at high risk of type I diabetes. *Lancet*. 1993;341:927–928.

172. Winter WE, Maclaren NK. Type I insulin dependent diabetes: An autoimmune disease that can be arrested or prevented with immunotherapy? In: Barness L, ed. *Advances in Pediatrics*. Chicago, IL: Year Book Medical Publishers; 1985:159–175.

173. Drash AL. Is it time to draw the curtain on immune intervention trials in newly diagnosed patients with IDDM? *Diabetes Care*. 1995;18:1499–1501.

174. Vague P, Picq R, Bernal M, et al. Effect of nicotinamide treatment on the residual insulin secretion in type 1 (insulin-dependent) diabetic patients. *Diabetologia*. 1989;32:316–321.

175. Elliott RB, Chase HP. Prevention or delay of type 1 (insulin-dependent) diabetes mellitus in children using nicotinamide. *Diabetologia*. 1991;34:362–365.

176. Lewis CM, Canafax DM, Sprafka JM, et al. Double-blind randomized trial of nicotinamide on early-onset diabetes. *Diabetes Care*. 1992;15:121–123.

177. Pozzilli P, Visalli N, Boccuni ML, et al. Randomized trial comparing nicotinamide and nicotinamide plus cyclosporin in recent onset insulin-dependent diabetes (IMDIAB 1). The IMDIAB Study Group. *Diabet Med*. 1994;11:98–104.

178. Herskowitz RD, Jackson RA, Soeldner JS, et al. Pilot trial to prevent type I diabetes: Progression to overt IDDM despite oral nicotinamide. *J Autoimmun*. 1989;2:733–737.

179. Manna R, Migliore A, Martin LS, et al. Nicotinamide treatment in subjects at high risk of developing IDDM improves insulin secretion. *Br J Clin Pract*. 1992;46: 177–179.

180. Pozzilli P, Kolb H, Browne PD. Meta-analysis of nicotinamide treatment in patients with recent-onset IDDM. *Diabetes Care*. 1996;19:1357–1363.

181. Irvine WJ, Gray RS, McCallum CJ. Pancreatic islet-cell antibody as a marker for asymptomatic and latent diabetes and prediabetes. *Lancet*. 1976;2:1097–1102.

182. Wolf BM, Bottazzo GF, Cudworth AG. Evidence of a long prediabetic period in type I (insulin-dependent) diabetes mellitus. *Lancet*. 1981;2:1363–1365.

183. Betterle C, Zanette F, Tiengo A, et al. Five-year follow-up on non-diabetes with islet-cell antibodies. *Lancet*. 1982;1:284–285.

184. Riley WJ, Spillar RP, Waltz J, et al. Predictive value of islet cell autoantibodies (ICA): 6 years experience. *Diabetes*. 1984;33:44A.

185. Deschamps I, Boitard C, Hors J, et al. Life table analysis of the risk of type 1 (insulin-dependent) diabetes mellitus in siblings according to islet cell antibodies and HLA markers: An 8-year prospective study. *Diabetologia*. 1992;35:951–957.

186. Landin-Olsson M, Palmer JP, Lernmark A, et al. Predictive value of islet cell and insulin autoantibodies for type 1 (insulin-dependent) diabetes mellitus in a population-based study of newly-diagnosed diabetic and matched control children. *Diabetologia*. 1992;35:1068–1073.

187. Schatz D, Krischer J, Wasserfall C, et al. ICA, GAD_{65}A, IAA and IA-2 to screen for IDD in school children and unaffected relatives. *Diabetes*. 1996;45(suppl 2):80A.

188. Bonifacio E, Bingley PJ, Shattock M, et al. Quantification of islet-cell antibodies and prediction of insulin-dependent diabetes. *Lancet*. 1990;335:147–149.

189. Ziegler AG, Herskowitz RD, Jackson RA, et al. Predicting type I diabetes. *Diabetes Care*. 1990;13:762–765.

190. Bingley PJ, Christie MR, Bonifacio E, et al. Combined analysis of autoantibodies improves prediction of IDDM in islet cell antibody-positive relatives. *Diabetes*. 1994;43:1304–1310.

191. Bottazzo GF, Dean BM, Gorsuch AN, et al. Complement-fixing islet-cell antibodies in type-I diabetes: Possible monitors of active beta-cell damage. *Lancet*. 1980;1:668–672.

192. Riley WJ, Neufeld M, Maclaren NK. Complement-fixing islet-cell antibodies: A separate species? *Lancet*. 1980;1:1133.

193. Srikanta S, Ganda OP. Chronic progressive beta cell dysfunction in relatives of patients with type 1 diabetes. *Diabetes*. 1983;32:51A.

194. Srikanta S, Ganda OP, Eisenbarth GS, et al. Islet-cell antibodies and beta-cell function in monozygotic triplets and twins initially discordant for type I diabetes mellitus. *N Engl J Med*. 1983;308:322–325.

195. Srikanta S, Ganda OP, Gleason RE, et al. Pre-type 1 diabetes, linear loss of beta cell response to intravenous glucose. *Diabetes*. 1984;33:717–720.

196. Srikanta S, Ganda OP, Jackson RA, et al. Type 1 diabetes mellitus in monozygotic twins: chronic progressive beta cell dysfunction. *Ann Intern Med*. 1983;99:320–326.

197. Srikanta S, Ganda OP, Jackson RA, et al. Pre-type 1 (insulin-dependent) diabetes: common endocrinological course despite immunological and immunogenetic heterogeneity. *Diabetologia*. 1984;27:146–148.

198. Bleich D, Jackson RA, Soeldner JS, et al. Analysis of metabolic progression to type I diabetes in ICA+ relatives of patients with type I diabetes. *Diabetes Care*. 1990;13:111–118.

199. Chase HP, Garg SK, Butler-Simon N, et al. Prediction of the course of pre-type I diabetes. *J Pediatr.* 1991;118:838–841.

200. Vardi P, Crisa L, Jackson RA. Predictive value of intravenous glucose tolerance test insulin secretion less than or greater than the first percentile in islet cell antibody positive relatives of type 1 (insulin-dependent) diabetic patients. *Diabetologia.* 1991;34:93–102.

201. Riley WJ, Maclaren NK, Krischer J, et al. A prospective study of the development of diabetes in relatives of patients with insulin-dependent diabetes. *N Engl J Med.* 1990;323:1167–1172.

202. Ganda OP, Srikanta S, Brink SJ, et al. Differential sensitivity to beta-cell secretagogues in early, type 1 diabetes mellitus. *Diabetes.* 1984;33:516–521.

203. Tuomilehto J, Zimmet P, Mackay IR, et al. Antibodies to glutamic acid decarboxylase as predictors of insulin-dependent diabetes mellitus before clinical onset of disease. *Lancet.* 1994;343:1383–1385.

204. Yassin N, Seissler J, Gluck M, et al. Insulin autoantibodies as determined by competitive radiobinding assay are positively correlated with impaired beta-cell function: The Ulm-Frankfurt Population Study. *Klin Wochenschr.* 1991;69:736–741.

205. Krischer JP, Schatz D, Riley WJ, et al. Insulin and islet cell autoantibodies as time-dependent covariates in the development of insulin-dependent diabetes: A prospective study in relatives. *J Clin Endocrinol Metab.* 1993;77:743–749.

206. Bonifacio E, Genovese S, Braghi S, et al. Islet autoantibody markers in IDDM: Risk assessment strategies yielding high sensitivity. *Diabetologia.* 1995;38:816–822.

207. Verge CF, Gianani R, Kawasaki E, et al. Prediction of type I diabetes in first-degree relatives using a combination of insulin, GAD, and ICA512bdc/IA-2 autoantibodies. *Diabetes.* 1996;45:926–933.

208. Bingley PJ. Interactions of age, islet cell antibodies, insulin autoantibodies, and first-phase insulin response in predicting risk of progression to IDDM in ICA+ relatives, the ICARUS data set. *Diabetes.* 1996;45:1720–1728.

209. Verge CF, Gianani R, Kawasaki E, et al. Number of autoantibodies (against insulin, GAD or ICA512/IA2) rather than particular autoantibody specificities determines risk of type I diabetes. *J Autoimmun.* 1996;9: 379–383.

210. Gorsuch AN, Spencer KM, Lister J, et al. Evidence for a long prediabetic period in type I (insulin-dependent) diabetes mellitus. *Lancet.* 1981;2:1363–1365.

211. Schott M, Schatz D, Atkinson M, et al. GAD_{65} autoantibodies increase the predictability but not the sensitivity of islet cell and insulin autoantibodies for developing insulin dependent diabetes mellitus. *J Autoimmun.* 1994;7:865–872.

212. Gianani R, Rabin DU, Verge CF, et al. ICA512 autoantibody radioassay. *Diabetes.* 1995;44:1340–1344.

213. Roll U, Christie MR, Fuchtenbusch M, et al. Perinatal autoimmunity in offspring of diabetic parents: The German Multicenter BABY-DIAB study: Detection of humoral immune responses to islet antigens in early childhood. *Diabetes.* 1996;45:967–973.

214. Tarn AC, Thomas JM, Dean BM, et al. Predicting insulin-dependent diabetes. *Lancet.* 1988;1:845–850.

215. Bell GI, Horita S, Karam JH. A polymorphic locus near the human insulin gene is associated with insulin-dependent diabetes. *Diabetes.* 1984;33:176–183.

216. Bain SC, Prins JB, Hearne CM, et al. Insulin gene region-encoded susceptibility to type 1 diabetes is not restricted to HLA-DR4-positive individuals. *Nat Genet.* 1992;2:212–215.

217. Julier C, Hyer RN, Davies J, et al. Insulin-IGF2 region on chromosome 11p encodes a gene implicated in HLA-DR4-dependent diabetes susceptibility. *Nature.* 1991;354:155–159.

218. Owerbach D, Gabbay KH. The search for IDDM susceptibility genes: The next generation. *Diabetes.* 1996;45:544–551.

219. Riley WJ, Maclaren NK, Spillar RP. Development of IDDM after donating kidney to diabetic sibling. *Diabetes Care.* 1990;13:883–885.

220. Christie MR, Daneman D, Champagne P, et al. Persistence of serum antibodies to 64,000-Mr islet cell protein after onset of type I diabetes. *Diabetes.* 1990;39: 653–656.

221. Karjalainen J, Knip M, Mustonen A, et al. Insulin autoantibodies at the clinical manifestation of type I (insulin-dependent) diabetes—a poor predictor of clinical course and antibody response to exogenous insulin. *Diabetologia.* 1988;31:129–133.

222. Yokota I, Shirakawa N, Shima K, et al. Relationship between GAD antibody and residual β-cell function in children after overt onset of IDDM. *Diabetes Care.* 1996;19:74–75.

223. Kordonouri O, Danne T, Weber B. Do GAD antibodies at IDDM onset predict the clinical course of diabetes in children? *Diabetes Care.* 1996;19:901–902.

224. Riley WJ, Maclaren NK, Lezotte D, et al. Thyroid autoimmunity in insulin-dependent diabetes mellitus: The case for routine screening. *J Pediatr.* 1981;98: 350–354.

225. Riley W, Maclaren N, Rosenbloom A. Thyroid disease in young diabetics. *Lancet.* 1982;2:489–490.

226. Riley WJ, Winer A, Goldstein D. Coincident presence of thyrogastric autoimmunity at onset of type I diabetes. *Diabetologia.* 1983;24:418–421.

227. Maclaren NK, Riley WJ. Thyroid, gastric, and adrenal autoimmunities associated with insulin-dependent diabetes mellitus. *Diabetes Care.* 1985;8(suppl 1):34–38.

228. Riley WJ, Toskes PP, Maclaren NK, et al. Predictive value of gastric parietal cell autoantibodies as a marker for gastric and hematological abnormalities associated with insulin-dependent diabetes. *Diabetes.* 1982;32:1051–1055.

229. Riley W, Maclaren N, Neufeld M. Adrenal autoantibodies and Addison's disease in insulin dependent diabetes mellitus. *J Pediatr*. 1980;97:191–195.

230. Ketchum C, Riley WJ, Maclaren NK. Adrenal dysfunction in asymptomatic patients with adrenocortical autoantibodies. *J Clin Endocrinol Metab*. 1984;58: 1166–1170.

231. Neufeld M, Maclaren N, Blizzard R. Autoimmune polyglandular syndromes. *Pediatr Ann*. 1980;9:43–53.

232. Neufeld M, Maclaren N, Blizzard R. Two types of autoimmune Addison's disease associated with polyglandular syndromes. *Medicine*. 1981;60:355–362.

233. Winter WE, Maclaren NK. To what extent is "polyendocrine" serology related to the clinical expression of disease. In: Doniach D, Bottazzo GF, eds. *Clinical Immunology and Allergy*. Vol. 1. Kent, UK: Bailliere Tindall; 1987:109–123.

234. Flier JS, Kahn DR, Roth J. Receptors, antireceptor antibodies and mechanisms of insulin resistance. *N Engl J Med*. 1979;330:413–419.

235. Taylor SI, Grunberger G, Marcus-Samuels B, et al. Hypoglycemia associated with antibodies to the insulin receptor. *N Engl J Med*. 1982;307:1422–1425.

236. Taylor SI, Barbetti F, Accili D, et al. Syndromes of autoimmunity and hypoglycemia. Autoantibodies directed against insulin and its receptor. *Endocrinol Metabol Clin North Am*. 1989;18:123–143.

237. Uchigata Y, Kuwata S, Tokunaga K, et al. Strong association of insulin autoimmune syndrome with HLA-DR4. *Lancet*. 1992;339:393–394.

238. Uchigata Y, Kuwata S, Tsushima T, et al. Patients with Graves' disease who developed insulin auto-immune syndrome (Hirata disease) possess HLA-Bw62/Cw4/DR4 carrying DRB1*0406. *J Clin Endocrinol Metab*. 1993;77:249–254.

239. Schatz DA, Barrett DJ, Maclaren NK, et al. Polyclonal nature of islet cell antibodies in insulin-dependent diabetes. *Autoimmunity*. 1988;1:45–50.

240. Pilcher C, Elliott RB. Improved sensitivity of islet cell cytoplasmic antibody assay in diabetics. *Lancet*. 1984;1:1352.

241. Dib SA, Colman PG, Dotta F, et al. Expression of cytoplasmic islet cell antigens by rat pancreas. *Diabetes*. 1987;36:982–985.

242. Dib SA, Colman PG, Dotta F, et al. Assay for cytoplasmic islet cell antibodies using two-color immunofluorescence and rat pancreas. *Adv Exp Med Biol*. 1988;246:63–67.

243. Madsen OD, Olsson ML, Bille G, et al. A two-colour immunofluorescence test with a monoclonal human proinsulin antibody improves the assay for islet cell antibodies. *Diabetologia*. 1986;29:115–118.

244. Colman PG, Tautkus M, Rabizadeh A, et al. Assay for islet cell antibodies with rat pancreas and peroxidase protein A. *Diabetes Care*. 1988;11:367–368.

245. Gleichmann H, Bottazzo GF. Progress toward standardization of cytoplasmic islet cell-antibody assay. *Diabetes*. 1987;36:578–584.

246. Greenbaum CJ, Palmer JP, Kuglin B, et al. Insulin autoantibodies measured by radioimmunoassay methodology are more related to insulin-dependent diabetes mellitus than those measured by enzyme-linked immunosorbent assay: Results of the Fourth International Workshop on the Standardization of Insulin Autoantibody Measurement. *J Clin Endocrinol Metab*. 1992;74:1040–1044.

247. Levy-Marchal C, Bridel MP, Sodoyez-Goffaux F, et al. Superiority of radiobinding assay over ELISA for detection of IAAs in newly diagnosed type I diabetic children. *Diabetes Care*. 1991;14:61–63.

248. Clare-Salzler M, Kaufman D, Tobin A. Glutamate decarboxylase on IDDM autoantigen. *Diabetes Care*. 1992;15:132–135.

249. DeAizpurua HJ, Wilson YM, Harrison LC. Glutamic acid decarboxylase autoantibodies in preclinical insulin-dependent diabetes. *Proc Natl Acad Sci U S A*. 1992;89:9841–9845.

250. Rowley MJ, Mackay IR, Chen Y, et al. Antibodies to glutamic acid decarboxylase discriminate major types of diabetes mellitus. *Diabetes*. 1992;41:548–551.

251. Kawasaki E, Takino H, Yano M, et al. Evaluation of islet-specific autoantibodies in Japanese patients with insulin-dependent diabetes mellitus: A comparison between autoantibodies to glutamic acid decarboxylase, autoantibodies to 64 kDa islet cell protein and islet cell antibodies. *J Autoimmun*. 1994;7:791–802.

252. Petersen JS, Hejnaes KR, Moody A, et al. Detection of GAD65 antibodies in diabetes and other autoimmune diseases using a simple radioligand assay. *Diabetes*. 1994;43:459–467.

253. Martino GV, Tapopaz ML, Graghi S, et al. Autoantibodies to glutamic acid decarboxylase (GAD) detected by an immuno-trapping enzyme activity assay: Relation to insulin-dependent diabetes mellitus and islet cell antibodies. *J Autoimmun*. 1991;4:915–923.

254. DeAizpurua HJ, Harrison LC, Cram DS. An ELISA for antibodies to recombinant glutamic acid decarboxylase in IDDM. *Diabetes*. 1992;41:1182–1187.

255. Schmidli RS, Colman PG, Bonifacio E. Disease sensitivity and specificity of 52 assays for glutamic acid decarboxylase antibodies. The Second International GADAB Workshop. *Diabetes*. 1995;44:636–640.

256. Schmidli RS, Colman PG, Bonifacio E, et al. High level of concordance between assays for glutamic acid decarboxylase antibodies. The First International Glutamic Acid Decarboxylase Antibody Workshop. *Diabetes*. 1994;43:1005–1009.

257. Kawasaki E, Eisenbarth GS, Wasmeier C, et al. Autoantibodies to protein tyrosine phosphatase-like proteins in type I diabetes, overlapping specificities to phogrin and ICA512/IA-2. *Diabetes*. 1996;45:1344–1349.

258. Zhang B, Lan MS, Notkins AL. Autoantibodies to IA-2 in IDDM, location of major antigenic determinants. *Diabetes*. 1997;46:40–43.

259. Bonifacio E, Lampasona V, Genovese S, et al. Identification of protein tyrosine phosphatase-like IA2 (islet cell antigen 512) as the insulin-dependent diabetes-related 37/40K autoantigen and a target of islet-cell antibodies. *J Immunol*. 1995;155:5419–5426.

260. Payton MA, Hawkes CJ, Christie MR. Relationship of the 37,000- and 40,000-M(r) tryptic fragments of islet antigens in insulin-dependent diabetes to the protein tyrosine phosphatase-like molecule IA-2 (ICA512). *J Clin Invest*. 1995;96:1506–1511.

261. Lu J, Li Q, Xie H, et al. Identification of a second transmembrane protein tyrosine phosphatase, IA-2beta, as an autoantigen in insulin-dependent diabetes mellitus: Precursor of the 37-kDa tryptic fragment. *Proc Natl Acad Sci U S A*. 1996;93:2307–2311.

262. Hawkes CJ, Wasmeier C, Christie MR, et al. Identification of the 37-kDa antigen in IDDM as a tyrosine phosphatase-like protein (phogrin) related to IA-2. *Diabetes*. 1996;45:1187–1192.

263. Christie MR, Tun RY, Lo SS, et al. Antibodies to GAD and tryptic fragments of islet 64K antigen as distinct markers for development of IDDM. Studies with identical twins. *Diabetes*. 1992;41:782–787.

264. Christie MR, Genovese S, Cassidy D, et al. Antibodies to islet 37k antigen, but not to glutamate decarboxylase, discriminate rapid progression to IDDM in endocrine autoimmunity. *Diabetes*. 1994;43:1254–1259.

265. Christie MR, Vohra G, Champagne P, et al. Distinct antibody specificities to a 64-kD islet cell antigen in type 1 diabetes as revealed by trypsin treatment. *J Exp Med*. 1990;172:789–794.

266. Cui L, Yu W-P, DeAizpurua HJ, et al. Cloning and characterization of islet cell antigen-related protein-tyrosine phosphatase (PTP), a novel receptor-like PTP and autoantigen in insulin-dependent diabetes. *J Biol Chem*. 1996;271:24817–24823.

267. Pietropaolo M, Hutton JC, Eisenbarth GS. Protein tyrosine phosphatase-like proteins: Link with IDDM. *Diabetes Care*. 1997;20:208–214.

268. Kawasaki E, Yu L, Gianani R, et al. Evaluation of islet cell antigen (ICA) 512/IA-2 autoantibody radioassays using overlapping ICA512/IA-2 constructs. *J Clin Endocrinol Metab*. 1997;82:375–380.

269. Irvine WJ. The association of atrophic gastritis with autoimmune thyroid disease. *Clin Endocrinol Metab*. 1975;4:351–377.

270. Kobayashi T, Nakanishi K, Okubo M, et al. GAD antibodies seldom disappear in slowly progressive IDDM. *Diabetes Care*. 1996;19:1031.

CHAPTER 25

Autoimmune Response and Autoimmune Lesions in Cardiovascular Diseases

LeMing Hang, MD, and Robert M. Nakamura, MD

The cardiovascular lesions in patients with systemic autoimmune disease seem to be related to the various types of autoantibodies generated by the underlying "pathogenic autoimmune responses." However, autoimmune responses to various myocardial tissue antigens occur in 5% to 35% of healthy individuals as well as 40% to 90% of patients with rheumatic heart disease, viral myocarditis, idiopathic dilated cardiomyopathy, ischemic infarcts, post–cardiac surgery, and cardiac trauma. Similarly, autoantibodies to oxidized low-density lipoprotein (oxLDL) are found in individuals with and without clinical symptoms of atherosclerosis.[1–3] Earlier studies[2,3] attempted to but could not unequivocally establish pathogenic relationships between myocardial autoantibodies and the development of cardiovascular disease. More recent studies[4–6] using advanced research tools in subcellular and molecular immunobiology provided evidence that under certain conditions, some of these myocardial autoantibodies can be pathogenic. Similarly, better standardized and defined assays for cholesterol metabolites and autoantibodies to oxLDL showed that anti-oxLDL antibodies contribute not only to atherogenesis but also to acceleration of coronary and systemic atherosclerosis.[7]

This chapter reviews the various types of autoantibodies found in cardiovascular disease patients, the laboratory methods used to identify these autoantibodies, the specific autoantibodies implicated in rheumatic heart disease and related cardiac conduction disorders, the specific autoantibodies implicated in idiopathic dilated cardiomyopathy, the various types of cardiovascular lesions and autoantibodies associated with systemic autoimmune diseases, and the role of anti-oxLDL antibodies in atherogenesis and atherosclerotic cardiovascular diseases. Issues regarding the diagnostic sensitivity and specificity of endomyocardial biopsy and immunospecific therapy for disease prevention are also discussed.

Types of Autoantibodies Detected in Various Cardiovascular Diseases

Table 25-1 lists the types and frequencies of autoantibodies detected in sera from healthy controls as well as from patients with rheumatic carditis, pericarditis, viral myocarditis, dilated cardiomyopathy, postpericardiotomy, coronary arteriosclerosis, post–myocardial infarct, and heart transplant rejections. **Table 25-2** lists the autoantibodies found in sera from patients with various types of cardiac conduction disorders.[4,8–11] As indicated in the tables, the more common myocardial autoantibodies are those showing reactivity with sarcolemma and myosin, but they do not appear to be disease specific. The less common myocardial autoantibodies are directed against myocyte mitochondrial membrane protein–adenine nucleotide translocator (ANT) and cardiac conduction tissue. The anti-ANT antibody appears to be a specific and sensitive marker for viral myocarditis–related dilated cardiomyopathy, whereas antisinus and anti-atrioventricular (anti-AV) node antibodies are specific but not sensitive indicators of rheumatic carditis–related conduction disorders.

Because antisarcolemma and antimyosin antibodies are also found in 5% to 35% of healthy controls, the induction and production of these myocardial autoantibodies most likely represent a physiologic autoimmune response for defense against infectious agents and elimination of damaged myocardial tissue.[2,4,8] However, studies have shown that antisarcolemma and antimyosin antibodies in sera from patients with rheumatic heart disease and viral myocarditis–related dilated cardiomyopathy cause in vitro complement-dependent cytolytic and cytotoxic damage of cardiac muscle cells. In addition, sera from patients with coxsackievirus B myocarditis and dilated cardiomyopathy contain anti-ANT antibodies that can inhibit in vitro myocyte energy metabolism and contractility.[4,5,10] The pathogenic potentials of these myocardial autoantibodies are discussed later in this chapter.

Laboratory Tests for Autoantibodies in Cardiovascular Diseases

Myocardial Autoantibodies

Indirect immunofluorescence microscopy (IIFM) tests are commercially available and useful to screen for the presence of myocardial autoantibodies (**Table 25-3**). Antisarcolemma and antimyosin antibodies show membrane and/or intermyofibrillar immunofluorescence staining patterns. However, sera from patients with other diseases, such as Epstein-Barr virus, rheumatoid arthritis, chronic liver diseases, and thymoma-related myasthenia gravis, also may show positive staining.[19] Anti-ANT autoantibodies usually display cytoplasmic immunofluorescence staining patterns. Autoantibodies to cardiac sinus and AV nodal tissue also are detected by IIFM, using human

Table 25-1. Types and Frequencies of Autoantibodies in Cardiovascular Diseases*

Types of Disease	No. of Patients	Autoantibody Type and Frequency (% Positive)		
		Antisarcolemma	Antimyosin	Anti-ANT
Healthy controls	>200	5–35	3–5	0
Rheumatic carditis	>100	90–100	23–67	0
Viral myocarditis	>300	40–90	23–50	79†
Dilated cardiomyopathy	120	10–42	20–33	90†
Pericarditis	20	60–100	10–67	0
Postpericardiotomy	67	90–100	12–92	0
Coronary arteriosclerosis	>170	4–36	4–8	0
Post–myocardial infarct	12	50–100	0–20	0
Heart transplant rejection	>300	42–100	3–6	0

Abbreviations: ANT = adenine nucleotide translocator (mitochondrial adenosine diphosphate/adenosine triphosphate carrier protein).

**Data shown are compiled from several independent surveys by investigators in the United States and Europe.*[4,8,10,11]

†Enzyme-linked immunosorbent assay was used to identify anti-ANT autoantibodies. Increased titers were noted in 79% of patients with acute coxsackievirus B myocarditis and 90% of patients who developed dilated cardiomyopathy. No increased anti-ANT titers were detected in patients with alcoholic cardiomyopathy, coronary heart disease, lupus, or other rheumatic diseases.

Table 25-2. Autoantibodies Detected in Various Cardiac Conduction Disorders[9,12,13]

Types of Conduction Disorders	No. of Patients	Types of Autoantibody (% Positive)		
		Antisinus Node	Anti-AV Node	Anti–SS-A/Ro*
Sick sinus syndrome	45	29	18	0
Atrioventricular block	55	24	22	0
Congenital heart block	48	0	0	92
Ischemic heart block (bundle branch)	102	0	0	0
Bundle branch block in polymyositis†	14	0	0	50–80
Bundle branch block in pulmonary fibrosis not related to autoimmune polymyositis	56	0	0	0

Abbreviation: Anti-AV, antiatrioventricular.

**Anti–SS-A/Ro is the autoantibody associated with neonatal lupus, Sjögren's syndrome, and adult lupus.*

†This subset of patients with autoimmune polymyositis also have anti–signal recognition particle, a myositis-specific autoantibody directed against a cytoplasmic transport protein. Enzyme-linked immunosorbent assay is used to identify this antibody because it cannot be detected by an immunofluorescent antinuclear antibody screen. This test is useful but not essential for diagnosis of autoimmune myositis–associated cardiac conduction disorders.

cardiac conduction tissue as substrate. Sera positive for these antibodies would, after absorption with myocardial ventricle tissue, show staining within the cardiac sinus and AV nodal regions.[9,11]

When indicated, enzyme-linked immunosorbent assay (ELISA) and/or Western blot can confirm and specify the antigenic epitopes of these myocardial autoantibodies. These assay methods offer better sensitivity and specificity; they also can characterize the various myocardial antigens by their individual molecular mass. For example, ELISA is more sensitive and specific for the detection of anti-ANT antibodies. Several studies have reported elevated anti-ANT titers in 75% to 90% of patients with dilated cardiomyopathy (versus 15% by IIFM), but no increased titers in patients with alcoholic cardiomyopathy, ischemic heart disease, and lupus or in healthy controls.[4,10,11]

Table 25-3. Methods for Detection of Autoantibodies in Cardiovascular Diseases[4,9,14–18]

Methods	Antigen Source	Sensitivity and Use
Indirect immunofluorescent microscopy	Tissue sections; cell lines	Sensitive assay for screening for myocardial autoantibodies
Western blot	Tissue/cell line extracts	Very sensitive for detection of antibodies to specific antigenic epitopes of myocytes
Enzyme-linked immunosorbent assay (ELISA)*	Purified native or recombinant antigens	Very sensitive and quantitative; also used to determine antibody class
Complement-mediated microcytotoxic assay†	Human fetal cardiac cell lines	Sensitive and specific for assessing antibody function; very labor intensive

**The ELISA methods used to detect anti-oxLDL (oxidized low-density lipoprotein) autoantibodies may differ among individual reference laboratories. A commercially developed kit (oLAB ELISA by Biomedica) is available. Anti-oxLDL antibody assay is not on the routine test menu of most hospitals.*

†Complement-mediated microcytotoxic assays for antisarcolemma and antimyosin autoantibodies are usually performed by reference or research laboratories.

Autoantibodies in Various Systemic Autoimmune Diseases

Human epithelial (HEp-2) cell immunofluorescence antinuclear antibody and rheumatoid factor testing are helpful for screening patients suspected of developing systemic autoimmune disease–related cardiac and vascular lesions. Western blot and/or ELISA can be used to confirm the antigenic specificity (ie, anti-dsDNA, anti-SS-A/Ro, or anti-Scl-70) of these autoantibodies.

Autoantibodies in Atherosclerotic Cardiovascular Diseases

Anti-oxLDL antibodies are quantitated by ELISA. Testing for anti-oxLDL is considered helpful but not essential for diagnosis of atherosclerotic cardiovascular diseases. Due to the various types of procedure modifications adopted by individual reference centers, the anti-oxLDL test results for a given patient generated by different laboratories may not be comparable.[7] Interlaboratory correlation of anti-oxLDL antibody test results have been made difficult by the lack of standardized assay methods. Significant differences in test results can be caused by the choice of blocking agents, test substrates, incubation temperatures, serum dilution factors, and formulas used to calculate immunoglobulin (Ig) G binding to oxLDL. Quantitation of anti-oxLDL antibodies also can be affected by cross-reactive cardiolipin autoantibodies and naturally occurring anti-oxLDL antibodies.[20–22] Future standardization of anti-oxLDL assay procedures should help clarify some of the current conflicting data regarding the role of these autoantibodies in the pathogenesis of atherosclerotic cardiovascular diseases.

Myocardial Autoantibodies Implicated in Rheumatic Heart Disease

Rheumatic fever is an acute inflammatory disease primarily involving the heart, joints, subcutaneous tissues, and central nervous system. It occurs in 3% of individuals with streptococcal pharyngitis. Rheumatic carditis, which develops in at least 50% of patients with rheumatic fever, is triggered by cross-reactive autoimmune events in response to infection by rheumatogenic strains of streptococci (M serotypes 1, 3, 5, 6, and 18). The M proteins and group A carbohydrate of these strains share antigenic epitopes with human cardiac sarcolemma-myosin proteins and *N*-acetylglucosamine of valvular tissue as well as with various types of cellular antigens, such as laminin, vimentin, DNA, and collagen.[23]

Pathogenic Antibodies Implicated in Rheumatic Carditis

The pathogenic antibodies in rheumatic carditis are those that cross-react with antistreptococcal antibodies directed against the group A carbohydrate and M proteins but with concurrent antisarcolemma, antimyosin, anti–heart valve, and anti–conduction tissue activities. They are found in patients with rheumatic fever–related carditis, valvulitis, and AV nodal conduction disorders.[5,8,9,11] Some studies have shown that streptococcal toxins can activate cytotoxic T cells.[6,23] Patients with clinical signs of streptococcal pharyngitis and suspected cardiovascular symptoms should be tested for these autoantibodies, because their presence would help support the diagnosis of rheumatic fever–related carditis and conduction disorders.

However, although these pathogenic cross-reactive myocardial autoantibodies may initiate the various types of rheumatic heart disease symptoms and tissue injury, autoreactive T cells and their cytokines, such as interleukins (ILs) and interferon gamma, ultimately determine the extent of irreversible myocardial damage. These cytokines can apparently induce expression of major histocompatibility complex molecules and intercellular adhesion molecules on cardiac muscle and valvular endothelium to recruit additional immune cells to sites of myocardial inflammation. These concerted humoral and cellular activities perpetuate and expand the antibody-initiated immune tissue damage.[5,23]

Endomyocardial biopsies are helpful but not essential for the diagnosis of rheumatic carditis because the histologic findings do not always reflect a patient's clinical symptoms, probably due to the focal nature of the inflammatory process and tissue damage. The biopsied tissues usually show lymphocytic infiltrate with myofiber necrosis most obvious near Aschoff bodies and around blood vessels. Biopsies from rheumatic fever patients with heart block symptoms show disruption of sinus and AV nodal regions by inflammatory infiltrates and fibrosis. Deposits of immunoglobulins and complement may be seen in areas of tissue damage.[1,5,6]

Role of Laboratory Tests in Predicting Disease Course or Prognosis

The natural course of rheumatic fever is hard to predict during the early stages of disease. The development of rheumatic carditis and the severity of clinical disease do not directly correlate with antibody types, titers, biopsy findings, or antibiotic therapy. However, genetic susceptibility (HLA-DR2, HLA-DR4, or HLA-DR7 haplotypes) appears to be a determining factor in disease course and prognosis.[2,5,6,11,24,25]

The current therapeutic regimens for rheumatic fever and heart disease are

- Prompt institution of antibiotic treatment for streptococcal pharyngitis and prophylaxis for higher-risk patients who have had carditis during initial attacks of rheumatic fever
- Suppression of the tissue inflammation with salicylates or corticosteroids
- Supportive care for symptoms of congestive heart failure and conduction disorders
- Efforts to develop multivalent vaccines against rheumatogenic strains of group A streptococcus are ongoing.[5,23]

Myocardial Autoantibodies Implicated in Idiopathic Dilated Cardiomyopathy

Patients with idiopathic dilated cardiomyopathy have congestive heart failure and cardiomegaly but no history or clinical findings of hypertension, rheumatic valvulitis, coronary arteriosclerosis, or exposure to myocardial toxins. Unlike rheumatic heart disease, the cause of idiopathic dilated cardiomyopathy is unknown. However, there is consensus that the majority of cases are sequelae of chronic myocarditis.[4,5,10,26–28] Genetic susceptibility also may be a risk factor because 27% to 46% of patients who develop idiopathic dilated cardiomyopathy are HLA-DR4 and/or HLA-B17 positive.[10,14,28]

In North America, 50% of patients with myocarditis and idiopathic dilated cardiomyopathy show immunologic evidence of enterovirus (most notably coxsackievirus B) infection. Circulating antibodies to coxsackievirus B are found in up to 50% of these patients, and viral RNA is identified in 17% to 25% of the endomyocardial biopsies.[26–28] Individuals infected with the human immunodeficiency virus and occasional peripartum patients develop similar dilated cardiomyopathy.[15,16]

In South America, most patients who develop idiopathic dilated cardiomyopathy have chronic myocarditis associated with *Trypanosoma cruzi* infection.[17]

Pathogenic Antibodies Implicated in Dilated Cardiomyopathy

Autoantibodies to adenine nucleotide translocator, the adenosine diphosphate/adenosine triphosphate (ADP/ATP) carrier protein of the inner mitochondrial membrane, are found in more than

75% of patients with viral myocarditis and cardiomyopathy. Antisarcolemma and/or antimyosin antibodies with cytolytic and cytotoxic properties also may be detected.[10,27–30] Anti-ANT autoantibodies are capable of inhibiting ADP/ATP energy transport activities of cardiac muscle cell cultures.[12,13,31] Endomyocardial biopsies from affected patients show immunoglobulin deposits and lymphocytic infiltrates in both the necrotic and fibrotic myocardium.[4,10,11]

Diagnostic Laboratory Tests for Dilated Cardiomyopathy

It is apparent that in genetically susceptible individuals, persistent coxsackievirus B infection can lead to the production of pathogenic myocardial autoantibodies. Some studies have noted that viral myocarditis patients with detectable anti-ANT antibodies in the early phase of disease are more likely to develop dilated cardiomyopathy. At present, anti-ANT antibody is regarded as an investigational and helpful test to support diagnosis of viral myocarditis–related dilated cardiomyopathy; it is not a diagnostic test. As in cases of rheumatic carditis, the early events of immunologic injury in dilated cardiomyopathy can be initiated and mediated by myocardial autoantibodies, but the types and severity of tissue damage are greatly affected by autoreactive effector T cells and their cytokines.[32–34]

Cardiovascular Lesions and Autoantibodies in Systemic Autoimmune Diseases

Several different types of myocardial and vascular lesions are seen in patients with systemic autoimmune diseases. Examples include

- Congenital heart block in neonatal lupus
- Cardiac conduction defects in autoimmune myositis
- Coronary arteritis in rheumatoid arthritis
- Endomyocarditis and valvulitis in systemic lupus erythematosus (SLE)
- Coronary and myocardial lesions in scleroderma
- Coronary aneurysms and necrotizing arteritis in Kawasaki syndrome
- Aortitis and coronary arteritis in Takayasu's disease
- Endomyocardial fibroelastosis (EMF) with hypereosinophilia
- Granulomatous eosinophilic angiitis in Churg-Straus's syndrome

The autoantibodies and other causal factors implicated in the pathogenesis of these lesions are discussed in this section.

Congenital Heart Block in Neonatal Lupus

The congenital heart block in infants with neonatal lupus is caused by transplacental maternal IgG anti–SS-A/Ro antibodies.[35,36] These autoantibodies apparently react with SS-A/Ro antigens expressed by fetal cardiac conduction tissue, triggering complement activation and immune tissue destruction. Anti–SS-A/Ro antibodies are found in fetal heart tissue eluates, and the fetal AV node shows healed inflammatory changes of fibrous disruption with variable dystrophic calcification. Vasculitis similar to that in SLE also may be seen in fetal myocardium. Infants who survive may develop subacute cutaneous lupus, interstitial pneumonitis, glomerulonephritis, leukopenia, or thrombocytopenia during the first 3 months of life. These symptoms resolve as the titer of the passively transferred maternal anti–SS-A/Ro decreases.[36]

Cardiac Conduction Defects in Autoimmune Myositis

Bundle branch heart block occurs in a subset of patients with autoimmune myositis. These patients experience severe myalgia, frequent cardiac arrhythmias, heart block, and congestive heart failure,[37] symptoms which often require cytotoxic immunosuppressive agents for relief. Anti–SS-A/Ro antibodies, found in 50% to 80% of affected patients, have been implicated as the cause of cardiac bundle branch block and tissue damage.[9,38] Some patients also may have anti–signal recognition particle (anti-SRP) antibodies that are specific for autoimmune myositis, but the pathogenic potentials of anti-SRP are unclear.[37]

Coronary Arteritis in Rheumatoid Arthritis

Rheumatoid arthritis patients with symptoms of heart block are noted to have necrotizing and/or granulomatous arteritis involving small to medium-sized coronaries. Rheumatoid factor immune complexes have been implicated as the cause of inflammatory damage to the endothelium and surrounding myocardium.[1,39]

Endomyocarditis and Valvulitis in Systemic Lupus Erythematosus

Up to 50% of patients with SLE develop endomyocarditis with aseptic valvular vegetations, predominantly on the mitral valve surface. The early lesions are necrotic with lymphoplasmacytic infiltrates, whereas later lesions are fibrotic and calcified. Anti-dsDNA and anti–SS-A/Ro antibodies have been implicated in their pathogenesis.[1,40]

Coronary and Myocardial Lesions in Scleroderma

Scleroderma patients develop stenotic intimal sclerosis of coronaries with ischemic myocardial damage. Fibrin deposition, concentric intimal thickening, and medial fibrosis are noted in both arterioles and capillaries. The intimal injury is thought to be mediated by cytotoxic antiendothelial antibodies, enhanced by inflammatory cytokines IL-1 and tumor necrosis factor–alpha.[41,42] Renovascular hypertension can be a fatal complication of scleroderma.[1]

Coronary Aneurysms and Necrotizing Arteritis in Kawasaki Syndrome

Kawasaki syndrome is an autoimmune disease occurring mostly in children younger than 5 years and triggered by staphylococcal toxins and/or *Yersinia* mitogens.[43–45] The disease symptoms are skin rash, conjunctivitis, facial edema, enlarged cervical lymph nodes, and necrotizing polyarteritis nodosa–type arteritis. The coronaries are frequently affected with thrombotic occlusion and myocardial infarct in the acute stage. Coronary aneurysms and myocardial fibrosis are the late-stage lesions. Activated T cells producing excessive immunostimulatory and cytotoxic cytokines have been implicated as the cause of the coronary arteritis. Circulating cryoglobulins and cytotoxic antiendothelial antibodies are detected in some patients during the acute disease stage.[46,47] Intravenous immunoglobulin and anti-inflammatory agents can ameliorate disease symptoms.[1,43]

Aortitis and Coronary Arteritis of Takayasu's Disease

Takayasu's disease is a chronic vasculitis with tissue destruction centered around the endothelium and adventitia of the aorta and coronary vessels. The presenting symptoms are hypertension, upper limb claudication, and muscle pain. Histologically, it is a granulomatous arteritis with variable intimal fibrosis, medial scarring, patchy inflammatory transmural infiltrates, and luminal obstruction. Direct cytotoxic endothelial damage due to excessive cytokine production and release by activated cytotoxic and helper T cells has been implicated as the cause of disease. Various microbial pathogens may play a role in the induction of this "autoimmune" arteritis. Although steroid treatment can improve the clinical symptoms, renovascular hypertension may be a late-stage disease complication. No disease-specific or diagnostic tests for this condition have been developed.[1,48–50]

Endomyocardial Fibroelastosis with Hypereosinophilia

Endomyocardial fibroelastosis is a necrotizing and eventually fibrotic cardiomyopathy associated with hypereosinophilia (>1,500/mm^3) that endures at least 6 months. In Western countries, EMF can be associated with underlying myeloproliferative disorders, carcinoma, T-cell lymphoma, or severe systemic allergies. In the tropics, it is usually associated with filaria or other helminthic infections. More than 80% of EMF patients develop cardiac dysfunction by 5 years after the onset of hypereosinophilia, and endomyocardial biopsies show either necrotic and thrombotic lesions permeated with eosinophilic granules or fibrosis with elastic degeneration and valvular scarring.[51,52] Endomyocardial fibroelastosis may be slowed by long-term corticosteroid treatment. Prophylactic thrombolysis and/or thrombectomy may avert systemic emboli. Prosthetic valvular replacement can help ameliorate late-stage congestive heart failure.

Granulomatosis Eosinophilic Angiitis in Churg-Strauss Syndrome

This is a systemic necrotizing and granulomatous angiitis associated with eosinophilia and elevated IgE affecting patients with chronic asthma, severe systemic allergies, or proliferative disorders of eosinophils. The blood vessels of the lungs, skin, heart, peripheral nerves, brain, gastrointestinal tract, and kidneys are permeated by eosinophils, histiocytes, lymphocytes, and neutrophils. Up to 50% of affected patients develop pericarditis, myocardial infarcts, and hypertension. Renal and/or cardiopulmonary failure with gastrointestinal and cerebral hemorrhage are fatal complications.[53,54]

The pathologic lesions in EMF and Churg-Strauss syndrome are associated with cytokine dysregulation. Excessive release of IL-3, IL-5, and toxic granules from activated T lymphocytes and eosinophils apparently cause necrotizing, granulomatous, and fibrotic tissue damage.[5,51,53] Corticosteroid and immunosuppressive agents are currently used to treat both diseases. Specific immunotherapy with cytokine inhibitors, such as IL-10 and/or anti–IL-3 and anti–IL-5 monoclonal antibodies, have been considered, and clinical trials are being implemented.[51]

The development of irreversible cardiovascular injury and tissue lesions in patients with systemic autoimmune diseases involve autoantibodies, immune complexes, cytokines, and effector T cells.

Role of Myocardial Biopsy for Diagnosis of Autoimmune Cardiac Lesions

Cardiologists traditionally have used endomyocardial biopsies to facilitate the clinical diagnosis of myocarditis and cardiomyopathies with histopathologic confirmation. However, clinical studies have not shown adequate correlation among biopsy histopathology, severity of clinical symptoms, disease prognosis, and response to therapy. The diagnostic sensitivity of endomyocardial biopsy is less than 30%.[1,4–6]

At present, most endomyocardial biopsies are done to evaluate patients with cardiac transplants or unexplained cardiomyopathies or those receiving cardiotoxic chemotherapy drugs. A minimum of 4 samples from different sites are required. Glutaraldehyde (2.5%; pH 7.35) is used as a tissue fixative for both light and electron microscopy. Snap-frozen biopsy samples in isopentane/liquid nitrogen are stored at –70°C for immunohistochemical studies. Viral RNA identification by polymerase chain reaction, if indicated, can be performed on thawed tissue or paraffin block sections of the biopsy.[1,27]

Role of Oxidized Low-Density Lipoprotein Autoantibodies in Atherogenesis

Low-density lipoprotein oxidation occurs in macrophages, endothelial cells, and smooth muscle cells of blood vessels. Oxidized low-density lipoproteins are immunogenic. Immunoglobulin M–type anti-oxLDL antibodies are found in healthy individuals as well as those with atherosclerosis. The autoantibody titers are affected by an individual's dietary habits, lifestyle, physical activities, and genetic makeup.[7,55] Immune complexes containing oxLDL and anti-oxLDL antibodies can be detected in atheromatous plaques and sera from patients with coronary heart diseases, carotid stenosis, and systemic hypertension.[56–61] Anti-oxLDL antibodies can activate and induce various immune cells to release inflammatory, immunostimulatory, chemotactic, and cytotoxic cytokines to cause vascular injury and promote atherogenesis. Anti-oxLDL immune complexes are found in atherosclerotic plaques of stenotic coronary, carotid, and other diseased blood vessels from patients with ischemic heart disease and/or systemic hypertension. Anti-oxLDL antibodies also have been implicated in the development of accelerated atheromatous vasculopathies of SLE, diabetes, preeclampsia, and uremia.[18,62–68]

Summary

Immune-mediated cardiac and vascular tissue damage is found in patients with various types of cardiovascular disease. Autoantibodies, autoreactive effector cells, and cytokines contribute to the development of these lesions. Although myocardial autoantibodies can initiate the disease-related immunologic events, the types and severity of irreversible injury and cardiovascular tissue lesions are determined by the activities of autoreactive T cells and cytokines. Certain HLA-DR haplotypes (genetic susceptibility) can be risk factors in the development of immune-mediated cardiovascular lesions.

Rheumatic heart disease is associated with cross-reacting antistreptococcal antibodies directed against group A carbohydrate and M protein with concurrent antisarcolemma, antimyosin, and anti–heart valve glycoprotein reactivities. These cross-reactive antibodies are found in 60% to 90% of patients with rheumatic carditis and valvulitis. Rheumatic cardiac conduction disorders are related to antibodies with antisinus and anti-AV node tissue cross-reactivities. Streptococcal toxin–activated cytotoxic T cells and cytokines most likely contribute to and cause the irreversible cardiac tissue damage. Identification of these cross-reacting antistreptococcal antibodies in symptomatic patients supports a diagnosis of rheumatic carditis. Antisinus and anti-AV node antibodies are specific but not sensitive indicators of rheumatic carditis–related conduction disorders. The severity of clinical disease cannot be predicted from the types and titers of these antibodies or endomyocardial biopsy findings, but genetic susceptibility (HLA-DR2, HLA-DR4, and HLA-DR7 haplotypes) is a risk factor in determining the disease course and prognosis.

Idiopathic dilated cardiomyopathy occurring in North American and European patients is associated with anti-ANT, antisarcolemma, and antimyosin antibodies. These myocardial autoantibodies apparently inhibit myocyte energy metabolism, impair contractility, and cause cytotoxic damage. Persistent or recurrent coxsackievirus B infections have been implicated in the production of these myocardial autoantibodies in genetically susceptible individuals. Anti-ANT antibodies appear to be specific markers for viral myocarditis–related dilated cardiomyopathy, but tests for these autoantibodies are currently regarded as investigational. Most South American patients with dilated cardiomyopathy have chronic chagasic myocarditis.

Identification of anti–SS-A/Ro antibodies establishes the diagnosis of congenital heart block in neonatal lupus and cardiac conduction defects in autoimmune polymyositis. Rheumatoid factor and anti-DNA immune complexes contribute to the coronary, myocardial, and valvular lesions found in patients with rheumatoid arthritis and SLE. Although cytotoxic antiendothelial antibodies can be detected in some patients with scleroderma, Takayasu's disease, and Kawasaki syndrome, autoreactive T cells and their cytokines also contribute to irreversible cardiovascular tissue damage.

The cardiovascular lesions seen in EMF and granulomatous eosinophilic angiitis are related to eosinophil dysregulation with excessive release of myotoxic eosinophil granules as well as IL-3 and IL-5. Persistent hypereosinophilia (>1,500/mm^3) that lasts longer than 6 months and increased serum IgE are helpful, useful tests for diagnosis of these disease entities, when other underlying causes, such as parasitism, myeloproliferative disorder, T-cell lymphoma, and occult carcinomas, have been excluded. In addition to the current use of immunosuppressive agents, specific immunotherapy with cytokine inhibitors and antagonists, such as IL-10 and anti–IL-3/anti–IL-5 monoclonal antibodies, have been considered and implemented.

Autoantibodies to oxLDL contribute to atherogenesis and atherosclerosis by forming immune complexes that induce the synthesis and release of cytokines, causing injury to endothelial and smooth muscle cells of the blood vessels. Identification of anti-oxLDL antibody help suggest an autoimmune etiology for a given patient's atherosclerotic disease, but this test is not essential for diagnosis. Its prognostic value has not been established.

It is important that researchers continue to investigate the various humoral, cellular, and cytokine activities that affect the cardiovascular system. Familiarity with the various types of immunopathogenic events that occur during the different phases of a given disease allow institution of appropriately timed and specific immunotherapy.[68–71] Therapy options may include suppression of autoantibody production, inactivation of T cells, interception of cytokine effects, or protection of genetically susceptible individuals against myocarditic agents with recombinant vaccines. These measures help avert the permanent immune cardiovascular tissue damages that can have debilitating and at times fatal consequences.

References

1. Fenoglio JJ, Marboe CC. Endomyocardial biopsy. In: Sternberg SS, ed. *Diagnostic Surgical Pathology*. New York, NY: Raven Press; 1989:877–895.
2. Maisch B. Retrospective and perspective in the immunology of cardiac diseases. *Springer Semin Immunopathol*. 1989;11:479–482.
3. Steinberg D. Modified forms of LDL and atherosclerosis. *J Intern Med*. 1993;233:227–232.
4. Rose NR, Neumann DA, Burek CL, et al. Autoimmune heart disease. In: Rose NR, Mackay IR, eds. *The Autoimmune Diseases*. Vol 2. New York, NY: Academic Press; 1992:303–315.
5. Kavinsky CJ, Parillo JE. Rheumatic fever and other cardiovascular diseases. In: Frank MM, Austen KF, Claman HN, et al, eds. *Samter's Immunologic Diseases*. 5th ed. Vol 2. Boston, MA: Little Brown; 1995:823–840.
6. Haffejee I. Rheumatic fever and rheumatic heart disease: The current status of its immunology, diagnostic criteria, and prophylaxis. *Q J Med*. 1992;84:641–658.
7. Lopes-Virella MF, Virella G. Atherosclerosis versus autoimmunity. *Clin Immunol Immunopathol*. 1994;73:155–167.
8. De Scheerder I, Vandekerckhove J, Robbrecht J, et al. Post-cardiac injury syndrome and an increased humoral immune response against the major contractile proteins (actin and myosin). *Am J Cardiol*. 1985;56:631-633.
9. Lotze U, Maisch B. Humoral immune response to cardiac conducting tissue. *Springer Semin Immunopathol*. 1989;11:409–422.
10. Neumann DA, Burek CL, Baughman KL, et al. Circulating heart-reactive antibodies in patients with myocarditis or cardiomyopathy. *J Am Coll Cardiol*. 1990;16:839–846.

11. Maisch B. Autoreactivity to the cardiac myocyte, connective tissue, and the extracellular matrix in heart disease and post-cardiac injury. *Springer Semin Immunopathol*. 1989;11:369–395.

12. Schulze K. Antibodies to ADP-ATP carrier—an autoantigen in myocarditis and dilated cardiomyopathy—impair cardiac function. *Circulation*. 1990;81:959–999.

13. Schultheiss HP, Bolte HD. Immunological analysis of autoantibodies against the adenine nucleotide translocator in dilated cardiomyopathy. *J Mol Cell Cardiol*. 1985;17:603–617.

14. Anderson JL, Calquist JF, Lutz JR, et al. HLA-A, B, and DR typing in idiopathic dilated cardiomyopathy: A search for immune response factors. *Am J Cardiol*. 1984;53:1326–1330.

15. Cohen IS, Anderson DW, Virmani R, et al. Congestive cardiomyopathy in association with the acquired immunodeficiency syndrome. *N Engl J Med*. 1986;315:628–631.

16. Homans DC. Peripartum cardiomyopathy. *N Engl J Med*. 1985;312:1432–1435.

17. Santos-Boch CA, Acosta AM. Immunology of chagasic heart disease. In: Zabriskie JB, Engle MA, Villareal H, eds. *Clinical Immunology of the Heart*. New York, NY: Wiley Press; 1981:1443–1490.

18. Lyons TJ. Oxidized LDL: A role in the pathogenesis of atherosclerosis in diabetes. *Diabet Med*. 1991;8:441–449.

19. Twomey SL, Bernett GE. Immunofluorescence method for detecting antimyocardial antibodies, and its use in diagnosing heart disease. *Clin Chem*. 1975;21:1903–1906.

20. Craig WY. Autoantibodies against oxidized LDL: A review of clinical findings and assay methods. *J Clin Lab Anal*. 1995;9:70–74.

21. Vaarala O, Alfthan ZG, Juahiaimen M, et al. Cross-reaction between antibodies to oxidized LDL and to cardiolipin in SLE. *Lancet*. 1994;341:923–925.

22. Craig WY, Poulin SE, Neveuz LM, et al. Anti-oxidized LDL antibodies and antiphospholipid antibodies in healthy subjects: Relationship with lipoprotein and oxidation-related analytes. *J Autoimmun*. 1995;8:713–726.

23. Cunningham MW. Streptococci and rheumatic fever. In: Friedman H, Rose NR, Bendinelli M, eds. *Microorganisms and Autoimmune Diseases*. New York, NY: Plenum Press; 1996:13–65.

24. Ayoub EM, Barrett J, Maclaren MK, et al. Association of class II HLA with rheumatic fever. *J Clin Invest*. 1986;77:2019–2026.

25. Carlquist JF, Ward RH, Meyer KJ, et al. Immune response factor in rheumatic heart disease: Meta-analysis of HLA-DR associations and evaluation of additional class II alleles. *J Am Coll Cardiol*. 1995;26:452–457.

26. Marboe CC, Knowles DM, Weiss MB, et al. Characterization of the inflammatory infiltrate in human myocarditis—An endomyocardial biopsy study. In: Bolte HD, ed. *Viral Heart Disease*. New York, NY: Springer-Verlag; 1984:74–82.

27. Beisel KW, Rose NR. The relationship of Coxsackie virus to cardiac autoimmunity. In: Bendinelli M, Friedman H, eds. *Coxsackie Virus: A General Update*. New York, NY: Plenum Press; 1988:271–292.

28. Muir P, Tilzey, AJ, English TAH, et al. Chronic relapsing pericarditis and dilated cardiomyopathy: Serological evidence of persistent enterovirus infection. *Lancet*. 1989;1:804–807.

29. Latif N, Smith J, Dunn MJ, et al. Complement-mediated cytotoxic activity of anti-heart antibodies present in sera of patients with dilated cardiomyopathy. *Autoimmunity*. 1994;198:99–104.

30. Maisch B, Deeg P, Liebau G, et al. Diagnostic relevance of humoral and cytotoxic immune reactions in primary and secondary dilated cardiomyopathy. *Am J Cardiol*. 1983;52:1072–1078.

31. Drude L, Weimer F, Maisch B. Impaired myocyte function in vitro incubated with sera from patients with myocarditis. *Eur Heart J*. 1991;12(suppl D):36–38.

32. Neumann DA, Lane JR, Allen GS, et al. Viral myocarditis leading to dilated cardiomyopathy: Do cytokines contribute to pathogenesis? *Clin Immunol Immunopathol*. 1993;68:181–190.

33. Ansari AA, Neckelmann N, Wang YC, et al. Immunologic dialogue between cardiac myocytes, endothelial cells, and monocytes. *Clin Immunol Immunopathol*. 1993;68:208–214.

34. Rose NL, Herskowitz A, Neumann DA. Autoimmunity in myocarditis: Models and mechanism. *Clin Immunol Immunopathol*. 1993;68:95–99.

35. Lee LA, Coulter S, Erner S, et al. Cardiac immunoglobulin deposition in congenital heart block associated with maternal anti-Ro autoantibodies. *Am J Med*. 1987;83:793–797.

36. Scott JS, Taylor PV. Anti-Ro and anti-La antibodies in congenital heart block. *Springer Semin Immunopathol*. 1989;11:401–410.

37. Love LA, Leff RL, Fraser DD, et al. A new approach to the classification of idiopathic inflammatory myopathy: Myositis-specific autoantibodies define useful homogeneous patients groups. *Medicine*. 1991;70:360–374.

38. Behan WMH, Behan PO, Gairus J. Cardiac damage in polymyositis associated with auto-antibodies to tissue ribonucleoproteins anti-SS-A/Ro. *Br Heart J*. 1987;57:176–180.

39. Ahern M, Lever JV, Cosh J. Complete heart block in rheumatoid arthritis. *Ann Rheum Dis*. 1983;42:389–394.

40. Petri M. Systemic lupus erythematosus and the cardiovascular system: The heart. In: Lahita RG, ed. *Systemic Lupus Erythematosus*. 3rd ed. New York, NY: Academic Press; 1999:687-706.

41. Sternberg EM. Pathogenesis of scleroderma: The interrelationship of the immune and vascular hypothesis. *Surv Immunol Res.* 1985;4:69–80.

42. Marks RM, Czerniecki M, Andrews BS, et al. The effects of scleroderma serum on human microvascular endothelial cells. *Arthritis Rheum.* 1988;31:1524–1534.

43. Weatherall DJ, Ledingham JG, Warrell DA. Kawasaki's disease. In: Kawasaki R, ed. *Oxford Textbook of Medicine.* New York, NY: Oxford University Press; 1987:241–324.

44. Leung DY, Meissner HC, Fulton DR, et al. Toxic shock syndrome: Toxin secreting *Staphylococcus aureus* in Kawasaki syndrome. *Lancet.* 1993;342:1385–1388.

45. Sato K, Ouchi K, Taki M. *Yersinia pseudotuberculosis* infection in children resembling Kawasaki syndrome. *Pediatr Infect Dis J.* 1993;2:123–126.

46. Leung DYM, Geha RS, Newberger JW, et al. Two cytokines, IL-1 and TNF-α render cultured vascular endothelial cells susceptible to lysis by antibodies circulating during Kawasaki syndrome. *J Exp Med.* 1986;164:1958–1994.

47. Herold BC, Davis AT, Arroyave CM, et al. Cryoprecipitates in Kawasaki syndrome: Association with coronary artery aneurysm. *Pediatr Infect Dis J.* 1988;7:255–257.

48. Wolff SM. The vasculitic syndromes. In: Cecil RL, ed. *Textbook of Medicine.* 19th ed. Philadelphia, PA: WB Saunders; 1992:1533–1537.

49. Hall S, Barr W, Lie JT, et al. Takayasu arteritis: A study of 32 North American patients. *Medicine.* 1985;64:89–99.

50. Behar SM, Procelli SA. Mechanism of autoimmune disease induction: The role of the immune response to microbial pathogens. *Arthritis Rheum.* 1995;38:458–476.

51. Spry CJ. Eosinophils and endomyocardial fibrosis: A review of clinical and experimental studies 1980–86. In: Kawai C, Abelmann WA, eds. *Pathogenesis of Myocarditis and Cardiomyopathy: Recent Clinical and Experimental Studies.* Cardiomyopathy Update. Vol 1. Tokyo, Japan: University of Tokyo Press; 1987:292–310.

52. Fauci AS, Harley JB, Roberts WC, et al. The idiopathic hypereosinophilic syndrome: Clinical, pathophysiological and therapeutic considerations. *Ann Intern Med.* 1982;97:78–86.

53. Lanham JG, Churg J. Churg-Strauss syndrome. In: Churg A, Churg J, eds. *Systemic Vasculitides.* New York, NY: Igaku-Shoin; 1991:101–120.

54. Lanham JG, Elkon KB, Pusey CD, et al. Systemic vasculitis with eosinophilia and asthma: A clinical approach to the Churg-Straus syndrome. *Medicine.* 1984;63:65–81.

55. Virella G, Virella I, Leman RB, et al. Anti-oxidized low-density lipoprotein antibodies in patients with CAD and normal healthy volunteers. *Int J Clin Lab Res.* 1993;23:95–101.

56. Yla-Herttuala S, Palinski W, Butler SW, et al. Human and rabbit atherosclerotic lesions contain IgG that recognize epitopes of oxidized LDL. *Arterioscler Thromb.* 1994;14:32–40

57. Bergmarf C, Wu R, de Faire U, et al. Patients with early-onset peripheral vascular disease have increased levels of autoantibodies against oxidized LDL. *Arterioscler Thromb Vasc Biol.* 1995;15:441–445.

58. Cominacini L, Garbin U, Pastorino AM, et al. Predisposition to LDL oxidation in patients with and without angiographically established CAD. *Arteriosclerosis.* 1993;99:63–70.

59. Bui MN, Sack MN, Mouissatsos G, et al. Autoantibody titers to oxidized low-density lipoprotein in patients with coronary atherosclerosis. *Am Heart J.* 1996;131:663–667.

60. Salonen JT, Yla-Herttuala S, Yamamoto R, et al. Autoantibody against oxidized LDL and progression of carotid atherosclerosis. *Lancet.* 1992;339:883–887.

61. Kabarov AE, Tertov VV. Saenko VA, et al. The atherogenic effect of lupus sera: Systemic lupus erythematosus-derived immune complexes stimulate the accumulation of cholesterol in cultured smooth muscle cells from human aorta. *Clin Immunol Immunopathol.* 1992;63:214–220.

62. Branch DW, Mitchell MD, Miller E, et al. Preeclampsia and serum antibodies to oxidized LDL. *Lancet.* 1994;343:645–646.

63. Maggi E, Bellazzi R, Gazo A, et al. Autoantibodies against oxidatively modified LDL in uremic patients undergoing dialysis. *Kidney Int.* 1994;46: 869–876.

64. Fogelman AM, Schechter I, Seager J, et al. Malondialdehyde alteration of LDL leads to cholesterol ester accumulation in human monocyte-macrophages. *Proc Natl Acad Sci U S A.* 1980;77:2214–2218.

65. Huang YH, Ronnelid J, Frostegard J. Oxidized LDL induces enhanced antibody formation and MHC class II dependent IFN-gamma production in lymphocytes from healthy individuals. *Arterioscler Thromb Vasc Biol.* 1995;15:1577–1583.

66. Cathcart MK, Morel DW, Chisolm GM. Monocytes and neutrophils oxidize LDL making it cytotoxic. *J Leukoc Biol.* 1985;38:341–350.

67. Witzum JL. Free radicals and antioxidants: The oxidation hypothesis of atherosclerosis. *Lancet.* 1994;344: 793–795.

69. O'Connell JB, Mason JW. Therapeutic implications of immune mechanisms in myocarditis. *Springer Semin Immunopathol.* 1989;11:43–49.

70. Dale JB, Chiang RY, Lederer JW. Recombinant tetravalent group A streptococcal M protein vaccine. *J Immunol.* 1993;151:2188–2194.

71. Medaglini D, Pozzi G, King TP, et al. Mucosal and systemic responses to a recombinant protein expressed on the surface of the oral commensal bacterium *Streptococcus gordonii* after oral colonization. *Proc Natl Acad Sci U S A.* 1995;92:6868–6872.

CHAPTER 26

Autoimmune Disorders of the Reproductive System

Francesco M. Fusi, MD, Richard A. Bronson, MD,
and S. Kenneth Tung, MD

Theoretically, it may be possible to raise an autoimmune response directed against gametes in both men and women. However, the only clinically relevant form of autoimmunity of the reproductive system is the production of antisperm antibodies (ASAs). Although the prevalence of such antibodies is negligible in the general population and relatively low in infertile men, the simple detection of ASAs is not enough to give a prognostic value to the chance of conceiving. This chapter first discusses the pathogenesis of ASAs and the most important tests for their diagnosis. However, because the detection of ASAs alone does not confirm a diagnosis of autoimmune infertility and is not directly related to reproductive prognosis, the other possible effects of antisperm antibodies on various sperm functions are discussed as well.

Antisperm Autoimmunity

Antisperm autoimmunity is a particular form of autoimmunity primarily directed against antigens that may not be recognized as "self" by the immune system. In fact, spermatozoa possess a variety of unique tissue-specific antigens not present in the individual during the fetal period, when immune self-recognition takes place and tolerance toward self occurs. Because spermatogenesis is not initiated until puberty, antigens unique to spermatozoa are not included in that recognition process. Their physiologic development must proceed in an environment that limits their exposure to the male immune system to avoid eliciting an immune response.

Several mechanisms of defense prevent the recognition of spermatozoa by the immune system. The first line of defense against the development of a sperm-specific autoimmune response is the blood-testis barrier. The tight junctions between Sertoli's cells divide the seminiferous tubules into adlumenal and basal compartments, excluding the passage of lymphocytes and high-molecular-weight proteins, such as immunoglobulins (Igs) and complement.[1,2] In addition, the Sertoli's cells form an immunologic barrier by actively phagocytosing and degrading sperm and residual products of spermatogenesis that would otherwise be a major source of antigenic stimulation. Only about one fifth of the sperm produced leave the testes, the remaining four fifths being resorbed.[3] Additionally, Sertoli's cells probably produce immunoregulatory factors by secreting transferrin, which has been shown to inhibit lymphocyte blastogenesis and complement-mediated cell lysis.[4] The barrier between the reproductive system and the immune system is less effective in the rete testis and the efferent ductules, so these sites are more accessible to cellular immune components. As has been demonstrated in mice, sperm-sensitized activated T lymphocytes transferred to recipient males exhibit the ability to react with autoantigens in this region, as well as in the vas deferens.[5] Conversely, dilution of sperm antigens in the rete testis[6] and its poor vascularization[7] may limit the interchange between intraluminal and intravascular compartments.

In addition to the barrier mechanisms that limit the contact of sperm antigens with the immune systems, an active semen-related immunosuppression appears to exist. Several lines of evidence have been presented for the existence of immunosuppressive factors within semen. Seminal plasma inhibits the ability of T and B lymphocytes to proliferate in response to mitogen or antigen challenge,[8,9] impairs antibody-dependent cell-mediated cytotoxicity,[10] and blocks the recognition of tumor cells or virally infected cells by natural killer and cytotoxic T lymphocytes.[11,12] In addition, it inhibits phagocytosis by macrophages and polymorphonuclear leukocytes[13] and the action of complement.[14] Soluble receptors for IgG (FcgRIII) have been detected within human seminal plasma,[15] raising the possibility that they play a role in blocking antibody-mediated sperm damage by binding to the Fc portion of the immunoglobulin molecule. Given that spermatozoa can induce the activation of complement by the alternative pathway,[16] it is possible that spermatozoa modulate the immune response via C3a, which suppresses antibody production by B lymphocytes in vitro.[17] Evidence also exists for active cellular immunosuppressive activity within the male reproductive system and in semen. Suppressor T lymphocytes have been detected in the interstitium of the testis and in the submucosal regions of the epididymis[18]; the ratio between suppressor and helper T lymphocytes in semen indicates the prevalence of suppression activity.[19]

Conditions that alter the balance between the exposure of the male immune system to sperm antigen and immunosuppressive factors may lead to antisperm antibody production. Vasectomy is associated with autoimmunity to spermatozoa in 60% to 70% of men,[20] perhaps mediated by absorption of an increased amount of sperm antigens that cannot be balanced by immunosuppressive factors. Unilateral obstruction of the vas deferens may also be responsible for ASA production.[21] Congenital obstruction of the vas deferens, seen in patients with cystic fibrosis, has been associated with the appearance of ASAs.[22] A correlation between the onset of puberty in boys with cystic fibrosis and the development of autoimmunity to sperm has been observed.[23]

Testicular trauma,[24] torsion,[25] biopsy,[26] and tumors[27] also have been associated with the production of ASAs. Witkin and Toth[28] have presented evidence that genital tract infections, which can act as adjuvants for immune activation, are related to ASA production. Nongonococcal urethritis (in particular, that resulting from *Chlamydia*) has been associated with antisperm antibodies.[29] Using an enzyme-linked immunosorbent assay (ELISA) with a recombinant *Chlamydia*-specific lipopolysaccharide fragment to detect antichlamydial antibodies and immunobead binding to detect ASAs, a strong correlation between antisperm IgG and IgA detected on motile spermatozoa and antichlamydial IgA in semen was found,[30] suggesting that an immune response to *Chlamydia* is associated with the development of an autoimmune response to spermatozoa.

Other possible causes of sperm antibody formation are related to the failure of immunosuppressive mechanisms. It has been postulated that a decrease in the number or activity of suppressor T cells in the male genital tract or in semen may play a role in the production of antisperm antibodies by B lymphocytes and plasma cells. In fact, men who have undergone a vasectomy and whose semen contains antibody-labeled spermatozoa have a predominance of helper T cells in their ejaculates.[19] In addition, the lack of immunosuppressive factors in the seminal plasma and/or the diminution of Fcg receptors or their inactivity may induce an immune response. It has been proposed that abnormal expression of antigens by spermatozoa or evidence of certain immunodominant antigens may cause lymphocyte activation.[31,32]

A different pathogenesis of autoimmunity to spermatozoa has been suggested for homosexual men. Under experimental conditions, the rectal insemination of spermatozoa in rabbits elicits a systemic immune response,[33] and gastric administration of homologous spermatozoa to rats results in ASA production associated with decreased fertility.[34] In humans, a higher prevalence of ASAs has been described in homosexual men than in heterosexual men from infertile couples.[35,36] Antisperm antibodies can be detected in serum in 40% to 50% of homosexual men.[37] Bronson et al[36] observed a higher prevalence of antisperm antibodies of the IgM class relative to IgG and IgA in sera from homosexual men when compared with autoimmune heterosexual men. The authors proposed that this might reflect differences in the etiology of autoimmunity to sperm between the 2 groups.

Antisperm autoimmunity is relevant in some forms of male reproductive failure. Unlike the established role of antibody-mediated infertility, the way in which cell-mediated immunity to spermatozoa induces reproductive failure is just beginning to be understood. Leukocytospermia can result in pathologic deficits via the production of cytokines by white blood cells.[38] A correlation between a positive leukocyte migration inhibition factor assay and asthenospermia has been described,[39] suggesting that a cell-mediated immune response might play a role in male infertility.

Most of the clinical and experimental evidence, however, is related to the effects of ASAs in the pathogenesis of sperm functional failure. Immunity to spermatozoa is not an all-or-nothing phenomenon: the effects of antibodies on fertility depend on their titer, the class of immunoglobulins produced, their affinity for specific epitopes displayed by spermatozoa, the nature of the antigens involved, and other associated phenomena such as the time between ejaculations. When approaching a case of supposed autoimmune infertility, a strict analysis of both clinical and laboratory data must be carried out. Although a simple, basal method to detect ASAs is the first step in an approach to the problem, the heterogeneity of sperm antigens involved and the different effects determined by immunoglobulin isotypes and titers make clinical interpretation of the data very difficult. A rational approach to the diagnosis and therapy of autoimmune infertility can be based on 2 different levels of analysis: (1) diagnosis of the presence of ASAs and (2) evaluation of the effects of such antibodies on sperm function.

Diagnosis of the Presence of Antisperm Antibodies

Several techniques have been described to detect antisperm antibodies on the surface of spermatozoa or in serum, but most of them have been abandoned because of poor correlation with clinical findings. These techniques include agglutination, immobilization, immunofluorescence, ELISA, and binding to immunoreactive beads.

Spermagglutination Techniques

These tests are based on the possibility of antibody-bound spermatozoa forming agglutinates. The first test described was the gelatin agglutination test,[40] in which spermatozoa are suspended in a gelatin medium and progressive dilutions of serum (previously heated to 56°C) are added. The evaluation of agglutinates is macroscopic in the tube. Shulman and Hekman[41] described a variant of this test in capillary tubes, but it was far less sensitive.

The tray agglutination test (TAT) is still used in some laboratories. It is based on the use of a microchamber filled with liquid paraffin, to which spermatozoa and different concentrations of serum are added. The evaluation is performed under an inverted microscope, and the presence of antibodies is suggested when agglutinations are present at dilutions greater than 1:32.

Both of these tests are able to detect only agglutinating antibodies present in serum. Agglutination depends on the number of antibody molecules bound and the class of immunoglobulins, because multivalent immunoglobulins, such as IgM and IgA, are more likely to induce agglutination. The low sensitivity of these tests precludes their usefulness as solitary screening tests to detect ASAs. Also, their specificity is not very high because bacteria, fungi, or steroids can induce non–antibody-dependent sperm agglutination. The TAT can be considered useful, but not essential, for routine use.

Sperm Immobilization Techniques

These tests can be useful for the detection of IgM and IgG antibodies; they are based on complement-dependent sperm immobilization. Complement-dependent damage to cell membrane integrity can be evaluated by scoring the sperm motility or through the use of viable staining. The best known of these tests, the sperm immobilization technique (SIT), was first described by Fjallbrant[42] and modified by Isojima et al.[43] Motile spermatozoa are placed in small test tubes with various dilutions of serum (previously heated to 56°C) and a complement source, such as AB human serum or guinea pig or rabbit complement. Hamerlink and Rumke[44] and De Almeida and Jouannet[45] proposed the use of eosin and trypan blue, respectively, to detect complement-mediated sperm killing, while Husted and Hjort[46] proposed the contemporaneous evaluation of immobilization and staining.

The methods based on sperm immobilization are sensitive in detecting complement-mediated sperm damage by antibodies and allow serum titration. However, they can be used only to detect serum antibodies and are not useful to study local or IgA-mediated immunity. The ability of complement-fixing antibodies to immobilize sperm is dependent on their location and the extent of binding on the spermatozoon surface.[47] The SIT is used in many laboratories and is useful for the diagnosis of ASAs, although it does not give complete information and must be used in conjunction with other tests.

Indirect Immunofluorescence

Indirect immunofluorescence microscopy, first described for the diagnosis of ASAs by Hjort and Hansen,[48] is based on the use of antihuman antibodies conjugated with fluorescein isothiocyanate (FITC). The original technique used spermatozoa fixed with methanol. This method allows the detection of antibodies bound directly to the sperm surface and of serum antibodies (via the exposure of antibody-free spermatozoa to the test serum). However, it presents some disadvantages. First, sperm fixation can destroy relevant antigens or expose internal antigens, whose reactivity with serum immunoglobulins is not relevant for infertility. Second, FITC-conjugated immunocomplexes can react nonspecifically with spermatozoa. Third, the scoring under fluorescent illumination is long, difficult, and very subjective and does not allow a precise localization of the binding site on the cell surface.

The use of nonfixed spermatozoa with a flow cytometric analysis of fluorescence is an interesting approach that may become one of the tests of choice in the future. Some preliminary studies[49] show that flow cytometric analysis may allow the detection of the proportion of antibody-bound spermatozoa, their titer in serum, and the quantity of antibodies bound to each cell surface.

Enzyme-Linked Immunosorbent Assays

Several ELISAs have been proposed to detect ASAs in serum. Some of them use sperm extract, others fixed spermatozoa. No correlation between the positive reactions obtained using an ELISA and other known tests have been found, suggesting that this test is not useful in the evaluation of antisperm antibodies.

Mixed Antiglobulin Reaction Test

Jager et al[50] in 1978 first presented the use of a mixed antiglobulin reaction in the detection of sperm surface–bound immunoglobulins. A drop of a suspension of Rh-positive red cells, previously coated with human anti-D IgGs, is placed on a slide with a drop of sperm suspension and rabbit antihuman IgG. In the presence of ASAs, mixed agglutinations form between spermatozoa and erythrocytes. The test can be performed directly or indirectly; that is, to detect directly sperm-bound antibodies or serum antibodies that bind antibody-free spermatozoa.

This test has the advantage of recognizing antibodies irrespective of their agglutinating or immobilizing activity. It also presents some disadvantages. First, motile spermatozoa are needed to evaluate the test. Second, the original test allows the evaluation of only antisperm IgG. Third, the mixed agglutination barely allows a specific localization of the portion of the cell that attracts antibodies. These disadvantages have been partially overcome by a recent improvement that uses smaller beads instead of red blood cells. The improved test is one of those most commonly used to detect ASAs and has good sensitivity as well as specificity (useful for clinical diagnosis).

Immunobead Binding

This test, first described by Bronson et al,[51] is based on the use of small polyacrylamide beads, covalently coated with rabbit antihuman immunoglobulins directed against human IgG, IgA, or IgM. A drop of sperm suspension and a drop of specific immunobeads are thoroughly mixed on a slide. After a few minutes, the spermatozoa covered with beads can be evaluated.

This is the principal test used today to detect ASAs because it presents several advantages:

- It allows evaluation of the proportion of antibody-bound motile spermatozoa.
- It allows evaluation of the class of immunoglobulins.
- It shows the exact localization of binding (head, midpiece, tail).

When at least 20% of spermatozoa are antibody bound, the test is considered positive. The major limit of the test is that it can be performed only when motile spermatozoa are available. Variants to the assay have been presented using other types of beads.[52] The test is essential for the detection of ASAs.

In the future, the detection of ASAs may be optimized with a combination of flow cytometric analysis (which might determine the exact proportion of sperm bound by antibodies, their class, and the amount of antibody bound to cells) and immunobead binding, which allows the exact localization of antibodies.

Evaluation of the Effects of Antisperm Antibodies on Sperm Function

The mere detection of ASAs does not confirm a diagnosis of autoimmune infertility and is not related to the reproductive prognosis. Antisperm antibodies can act in different ways to impair sperm functions. Semen parameters are more frequently altered when IgM is present in association with IgA.[53] In many cases (mostly when IgG is present), sperm parameters may appear normal. Antisperm antibodies can affect the transport mechanisms of spermatozoa within the female genital tract, alter sperm capacitation or the acrosome reaction, interfere with egg fertilization, or have postfertilization effects on the zygote and preimplantation embryo.

Sperm Transport

As a first step in the passage through the human female genital tract, spermatozoa must penetrate and progress through cervical mucus to gain entry into the uterus and fallopian tubes. The association between abnormal or inhibited mucus penetration and the presence of ASAs was first reported in 1969, when Fjallbrant[54] demonstrated that antisperm antibodies obtained from infertile patients or from immunized rabbits inhibited in vitro penetration of human cervical mucus by human spermatozoa. Sperm penetration through cervical mucus in situ is evaluated clinically by means of a postcoital test, which consists of the evaluation of the number and motility of spermatozoa present in the cervical mucus 8 to 12 hours after intercourse and during ovulation. The results of a postcoital test depend on mucus quality and particularly sialic acid biochemistry,[55] sperm concentration in semen,[56] the pattern of sperm motility,[57] and the proportion of spermatozoa labeled with antibodies.[51] Many studies have demonstrated that ASAs affect sperm penetration into and motility within cervical mucus.[51,58] The greater the proportion of antibody-bound sperm, the fewer sperm are able to enter and pass through cervical mucus, and when all spermatozoa are coated with antibodies, it is uncommon to see motile spermatozoa in the mucus.[51] Hence, men with a large proportion of antibody-bound sperm should be considered functionally oligospermic, despite normal sperm concentration in semen.

Both antisperm IgG and IgA have been found in cervical mucus following its liquefaction with bromelain.[59] Kremer and Jager[60] suggested that IgA antibodies were responsible for the shaking of antibody-labeled spermatozoa within cervical mucus. They postulated that locally secreted IgA was attached via the secretory component to glycoproteins of the cervical mucus. Later, Jager et al[61] showed that IgG also induces a shaking phenomenon, suggesting that other mechanisms are involved, and implicated the Fc region of the immunoglobulin molecule. It has been suggested that disulfide exchanges between sulfhydryl residues of sperm-bound immunoglobulins and glycoprotein molecules of mucin may lead to impairment of antibody-labeled sperm motion within cervical mucus.[51] In one study,[62] monoclonal antibodies raised against spermatozoa from several species, including man, directed against epitopes present on the surface of live sperm impaired human sperm penetration through a column of bovine cervical mucus, whereas monoclonal antibodies directed against subsurface epitopes in another study[63] did not.

The fact that monoclonal antibodies raised in mice[63] and polyclonal antibodies raised in rabbits[54] impair the ability of human spermatozoa to penetrate cervical mucus suggests that this is a non–species-specific effect. Studies performed using an IgA1 protease derived from *Neisseria gonorrhoeae* demonstrated that pretreatment of IgA-coated spermatozoa with this protease improved their mucus-penetrating ability.[64] This protease cleaves a single peptide bond of the heavy chain of IgA1, liberating the Fc portion of the molecule.[65] The fact that IgA-labeled (but not IgG-labeled) spermatozoa treated with this protease show an improved ability to penetrate into and sustain motility within cervical mucus, although they remain coated by IgA Fab,[66] suggests that penetration failure might not be due to the Fab portion of antibodies or to sperm surface antigens, but to the Fc portion. Alternatively, the effect may be due to a different activity of univalent versus multivalent IgA. However, these findings confirmed earlier data presented by Jager et al,[67] which demonstrated that spermatozoa exposed to Fab preparations of antisperm IgA are able to penetrate cervical mucus, in contrast to those exposed to intact immunoglobulins. It may be postulated that human cervical mucus possesses a receptor for the Fc portion of the immunoglobulin molecule.

A correlation between the regional specificity of ASAs to the spermatozoon surface and their ability to impair penetration of cervical mucus also has been observed. Binding of IgG and IgA immunoglobulins to the tails of spermatozoa is not associated with an alteration of their mucus-penetrating ability.[51] In contrast, sperm head–directed antibodies, mainly those of IgA class, and antibodies of both IgA and IgG classes directed against antigens on the principal piece of the sperm tail severely impair the ability of spermatozoa to penetrate mucus.[68]

Both the immunoglobulin class and the regional specificity of antibodies are important for the second mechanism of sperm transport impairment—complement-mediated immobilization. Immunoglobulins G and M can activate the complement cascade, which results in the target cell lysis. Whereas a single molecule of IgM is necessary to lyse a red blood cell, approximately 1,000 molecules of IgG are required.[69] Monomeric IgA does not activate the classical complement pathway. Complement proteins have been found in several secretions in the female genital tract, such as those of the cervix,[70] uterus,[71] fallopian tubes,[72] and ovarian follicle.[73–75] Price and Boettcher,[70] using hemolysis of red blood cells exposed to anti–red blood cell antibodies, showed that the complement activity in cervical mucus is much lower and was only 10% of the activity observed in serum. This observation may explain why complement-mediated sperm immobilization within cervical mucus does not take place immediately after sperm penetration into the mucus, but requires 4 to 8 hours.

The regional specificity of antibody binding to the spermatozoon surface is also an important factor in complement-mediated immobilization. Immunoglobulin G antibodies directed against the head, the middle piece, or the end piece were found to be ineffective in promoting complement-mediated loss of sperm motility, whereas a high degree of sperm immobilization was observed when IgG binding occurred on a majority of the sperm tail or when IgM labeled the end piece.[76] Hence, the amount of antibody, its location, and its isotype all play a role in sperm immobilization. An accessory mechanism that interferes with fertilization via ASAs may be via antibody-dependent cell-mediated cytotoxicity. Macrophages that populate the female genital tract may interact with the Fc portion of immunoglobulins or with C3 fixed by IgG and IgM antibodies, promoting phagocytosis as demonstrated by the lysis of indium In 111–labeled spermatozoa by peritoneal macrophages when spermatozoa are covered by specific antibodies.[77] The β_2 integrin CD11b/CD18 (CR3) appears to be involved in the adhesion events that take place in ASA- and complement-mediated immune destruction of spermatozoa by neutrophils; it promotes the adhesion of neutrophils to IgG- and C3-bound spermatozoa, potentiating the release of oxygen radicals at the site of membrane contact.[78]

Sperm Capacitation and Acrosome Reaction

Freshly ejaculated spermatozoa are unable to penetrate oocytes and must undergo a series of calcium-dependent biochemical and structural changes before they are capable of fusing with the egg plasma membrane. First, spermatozoa must undergo plasma membrane modifications (called capacitation), which enable them to undergo the acrosome reaction. This reaction consists of loss of the plasma membrane of the rostral portion of the spermatozoon head, the shedding of the acrosomal cap (a modified secretory granule situated over this region), and exposure of the inner acrosomal membrane.[79] Only acrosome-reacted sperm can penetrate the zona pellucida and fuse with the egg plasma membrane. The release of the acrosomal contents, which contain the enzymes acrosin (a trypsinlike protease) and hyaluronidase, plays a role in the spermatozoon's passage through the cumulus oophorus and the zona pellucida, allowing its contact with the egg plasma membrane. There is evidence that ASAs may induce a premature acrosome reaction,[80] which may alter the ability of the sperm to penetrate the zona and shorten their fertilizing life span.[81] Bronson et al[82] demonstrated that IgG ASAs directed against the rostral portion of the head in the presence of complement can increase the number of acrosome-reacted spermatozoa, as detected by ultrastructural studies. Other antibodies may have the opposite effect on the acrosome reaction; for example, a monoclonal antisperm antibody has been reported to block the calcium ionophore-induced acrosome reaction.[81] The presence of sperm immobilizing antibodies in sera appears to affect both the spontaneous and the calcium ionophore (A23187)–induced acrosome reaction of donor spermatozoa exposed to these sera.[83]

Sperm-Egg Interaction

Antisperm antibodies directed against antigens involved in the interaction between male and female gametes may alter fertilization by affecting the ability of spermatozoa to bind to the zona pellucida and to the egg plasma membrane. Several lines of evidence have indicated that ASAs may interfere with sperm recognition of the zona pellucida in humans and other mammals. During the process of fertilization, spermatozoa bind to species-specific receptors on the zona pellucida. In mice, several monoclonal antibodies can inhibit the binding of spermatozoa to zona pellucida.[84] In guinea pigs, autoantibodies induced by vasectomy block zona binding and in vitro fertilization.[85] The ability of specific antisera to block fertilization in the rabbit demonstrated that a specific autoantigen, RSA-1, was involved in zona recognition.[86]

In a series of experiments using donor spermatozoa exposed to sera containing ASAs, Bronson and coworkers[87] showed that the presence of these antibodies on the sperm surface interferes with their recognition of human zonae pellucidae of oocytes that had been removed surgically and stored in salt. When the ASA titer was lowered by absorption of these sera with spermatozoa before their exposure to test sperm, a partial recovery of zona binding ability was observed. These experiments suggested that the isotype of ASA bound to the head of the sperm may be important in determining the degree of impairment of zona binding; IgA was more inhibitory than IgG. In addition, the total immunoglobulin labeling of the sperm surface seemed to be an important prognostic factor, because when 100% of spermatozoa were labeled with antibody, the impairment of zona binding was more evident.

A similar experiment[88] using live oocytes obtained by follicular aspiration for in vitro fertilization confirmed these findings of the effect of ASAs. Further studies[89] performed with salt-stored human zonae pellucidae, bisected to allow each egg to act as its own internal control, demonstrated that antibodies directed against the sperm head can affect zona binding,[90] but not in every case. This suggests that the impairment depends on the antigens against which antibodies are directed; that is, whether they are the functional epitopes of a zona receptor ligand.

Many studies have addressed the effect of ASAs on sperm oolemmal fusion, using the ability of zona-free hamster oocytes to be penetrated by capacitated human spermatozoa. In 1976, Yanagimachi et al[91] reported that hamster eggs removed from their vestments (the cumulus oophorus and the zona pellucida) could be penetrated by the acrosome-reacted sperm of several species, including humans. A number of investigators have shown that homologous antibodies can affect the penetration of hamster oocytes by human spermatozoa.[58,92–95] In some studies, the inhibitory properties were found to be retained by IgG fractions of antisera,[58,96] and in one study the Fab fractions from three antisera were found to be inhibitory.[97] In apparent contrast with these findings, Bronson et al[98] found that some sera containing ASAs promote the penetration of zona-free hamster eggs by human spermatozoa after enhancing adhesion to the oolemma. These observations were confirmed by Aitken et al,[99] who showed that purified IgG from patient sera containing ASAs can promote human sperm penetration of zona-free hamster eggs, inhibit penetration, or be inactive.

Bronson and colleagues[100] observed that when ASAs promoted penetration, the number of oolemmal adherent antibody-labeled sperm was greatly increased. However, once these sperm adhered to the oolemma, their chance of penetrating the egg was the same as that for antibody-free spermatozoa from the same ejaculate. This finding suggests that the promotion of egg penetration by ASAs is solely due to their promotion of sperm-oolemma binding. Evidence has been presented that Fcγ receptors, present on the oolemma of both hamster[101] and human[102] oocytes, may account for the increased adherence of antibody-labeled sperm to eggs. Zona-free hamster eggs preincubated with IgG Fc to occupy oolemmal Fcγ receptors bound fewer IgG-labeled spermatozoa than did unexposed eggs. Using Fab preparations of monoclonal antibodies directed against FcγRI, FcγRII, and FcγRIII, all three receptors were found on the oolemma of unfertilized human eggs, and their ability to bind human and murine IgG-Fc also was shown.[102] The promotion of oolemmal binding of spermatozoa coated with ASAs via the interaction of oolemmal Fc receptors and the Fc portion of immunoglobulins could lead to a higher number of sperm penetrations. This mechanism could result in polyspermic fertilization of oocytes in vivo, diminishing the chances of reproductive success, because polyploid embryos exhibit diminished preimplantation growth potential and a higher rate of spontaneous abortion.[103]

Conversely, in those cases where the penetration of oocytes is inhibited by ASAs, the antibodies are probably directed against fertilization antigens that play a role in sperm–egg plasma membrane fusion. Antibodies directed against the rabbit antigens RSA-1, RSA-2, and RSA-3, which also cross-react with human spermatozoa, block penetration of zona-free hamster oocytes.[104] Naz et al[105] identified a 23-kd sperm membrane glycoprotein (FA-1) and demonstrated that a monoclonal antibody directed against FA-1 completely blocked the fertilization of zona-free hamster oocytes by human spermatozoa. Antisperm antibodies from immunoinfertile men also were studied for the presence of antibodies directed against FA-1. When anti–FA-1 antibodies were present, the penetration of hamster oocytes was reduced and was inversely related to monospecific anti–FA-1 absorbance.[52] The monoclonal antibody MH61—raised against human spermatozoa, reacting mainly with capacitated and acrosome-reacted sperm, and barely reactive with fresh sperm—was found to almost completely inhibit the penetration of hamster eggs by human spermatozoa.[106]

Retrospective and prospective analysis of fertilization data from programs performing in vitro fertilization provide another means of assessing the possible effects of ASAs on fertilization. Clarke and associates[107,108] showed that fertilization could be achieved at higher frequencies in women with humoral ASAs when culture medium was supplemented with nonimmune serum in place of patient serum. These data suggest that the presence of ASAs in the in vitro fertilization culture medium results in an impairment of fertilization. Immunoglobulins of the IgA class appeared to be more effective in impairing fertilization than those of the IgG class.

A more critical examination of the results of in vitro fertilization in women with immunities to sperm revealed both a diminished fertilization rate and a diminished embryonic cleavage rate, resulting ultimately in a diminished chance of pregnancy.[109] In this study, bovine serum albumin was used in the culture medium in lieu of patient serum if significant levels of serum ASAs were present. In women for whom patient sera was used, 44% of eggs were fertilized in 50 cycles versus 75% for the bovine serum albumin controls. The percentage of high-quality embryos was 49% in the immunologic infertile group versus 75% for the control subjects. Ten clinical pregnancies occurred in the former group versus 18 in the latter. Although they are promising because they illustrate that significant pregnancy rates can be achieved despite the presence of ASAs, these results suggest either that these antibodies cannot be eliminated from the egg by washing, hence impairing fertilization, or that the antibodies may be cytotoxic to the egg.

Other studies gave different conclusions. For example, in a small cohort of patients undergoing in vitro fertilization, where ASAs were present in the woman (group a), the man (group b), or neither (control), Pagidas et al[110] failed to find differences in egg fertilization, embryo development, or pregnancy rate.

Clarke et al[111] and De Almeida et al[112] studied the relationship between ASAs in the ejaculates of men with autoimmunity to sperm and human in vitro fertilization. Both groups found that when more than 80% of spermatozoa were labeled with head-directed IgA or a combination of IgA and IgG, there was a low fertilization rate of human oocytes. In another study, Junk et al[113] suggested that fertilization rates were adversely affected if the autoimmunity against spermatozoa was due to the presence of both IgG and IgA antibodies, whereas when only IgG or IgA was present, the impairment was less evident. They concluded that inhibition of fertilization may be caused by a synergistic effect of both classes of antibodies. Other authors, in in vitro fertilization trials, did not find any difference between antibody-positive and antibody-negative samples in the outcome of fertilization attempts.[114] Although the results of these studies are suggestive, it is difficult to analyze the effects of ASAs on in vitro fertilization. In effect, the small number of patients complicates serious statistical analysis, because the association of nonimmunologic factors related to egg quality and sperm penetrating ability may bias the results in a group. Yeh et al[115] correlated the class of ASAs with the outcome of in vitro fertilization. Using logistic regression, they did not find significant effects with IgG or IgA antibodies, but IgM antibodies were more effective. When more than 40% of spermatozoa were labeled with IgM and more than 60% with IgA, the fertilization rate dropped significantly. The most effective IgM antibodies were those directed against the head of the spermatozoa.

Another effect of ASAs in the outcome of in vitro fertilization can be exerted on early cleavage of fertilized ova. Naz[116] identified 2 glycoproteins of 14 + 3 and 18 + 3 kd in an extract from human spermatozoa and raised antibodies in rabbits. Extracted by affinity purification from human sera with ASAs, some antibodies were reactive against these bands. During in vitro fertilization in mice, ova fertilized by spermatozoa exposed to such antibodies failed to cleave. In the same patients from which the antibodies were obtained, in vitro fertilization presented the same problem of cleavage. Naz concluded that these sperm surface antigens may provide an extranuclear signal to oocytes to divide.

Summary

From all the data discussed, it appears that a wide range of effects can be determined by ASAs. Although the prevalence of these antibodies in the general population is 0% to 2% and in infertile men is 7% to 26%,[117] the detection of ASAs is not enough to give a prognostic value to the chance of conceiving. Although a number of indirect measures of sperm function can be performed in the presence of ASAs, including the postcoital test, induction of the acrosome reaction, and sperm penetration assay, only direct observation of human sperm with zona-intact human eggs at in vitro fertilization can document the actual effects of ASAs on fertilization. An important breakthrough, however, in the assessment of the reproductive prognosis of autoimmune sperm infertility will be made with the exact determination of the epitopes specifically involved in the binding of spermatozoa to the zona pellucida and sperm-oolemma interaction.

References

1. Hamilton DW. Structure and function of the epithelium lining the ductuli efferentes, ductus epididymis and ductus deferens. In: Greep RO, Astwood AB, eds. *Handbook of Physiology*. Washington, DC: American Physiological Society; 1975:259.
2. Gilula NB, Fawcett DW, Aoki A. The Sertoli cell occluding junctions and gap junctions in mature and developing mammalian testis. *Dev Biol*. 1976;50:142–148.
3. Johnson L, Petty CS, Neaves WB. Further quantification of human spermatogenesis: Germ cell loss during postprophase of meiosis and its relationship to daily sperm production. *Biol Reprod*. 1983;29:207–213.
4. Skinner MK, Cosand WL, Griswold MD. Purification and characterization of testicular transferrin secreted by rat Sertoli cells. *Biochem J*. 1984;218:313–320.
5. Tung KSK, Yule TD, Mahi-Brown CA, et al. Distribution of histopathology and Ia positive cells in actively induced and passively transferred experimental autoimmune orchitis. *J Immunol*. 1987;138:752–759.
6. Jones RC. The nature of the barrier to autoimmunity in the excurrent ducts of the mammalian testes. In: Boettcher B, ed. *Immunological Influences on Human Fertility*. New York, NY: Academic Press; 1977:67.

7. Kormana M, Reijonen K. Microvascular structure of the human epididymis. *Am J Anat*. 1976;145:23–41.

8. Lord EK, Senabaugh GF, Stites DP. Immunosuppressive activity of human seminal plasma, I: Inhibition of in vitro lymphocyte activation. *J Immunol*. 1977;118:1706–1711.

9. Marcus ZH, Freisheim JH, Houk JL. In vitro studies in reproductive immunology, I: Suppression of cell-mediated immune response by human spermatozoa and fractions isolated from human seminal plasma. *Clin Immunol Immunopathol*. 1978;9:318–323.

10. James K, Szymaniesc S. Human seminal plasma is a potent inhibitor of natural killer cell activity in vitro. *J Reprod Immunol*. 1985;8:61–76.

11. Marcus ZH, Misgav N, Zacut H. Inhibition of natural killer cell activity by a fraction of human seminal plasma. *IRCS J Med Sci*. 1984;12:897–903.

12. Witkin SS. Suppressor T lymphocytes and cross-reactive sperm antigens in human semen. *AIDS Res*. 1984;1:339–345.

13. Witkin SS. Selective activation of functional suppressor cells by human seminal fluid. *Clin Exp Immunol*. 1986;64:364–369.

14. Tarter TH, Alexander NJ. Complement-inhibiting activity of seminal plasma. *Am J Reprod Immunol*. 1984;6:28–31.

15. Thaler CJ, Faulk WP, McIntyre JA. Soluble antigens of IgG gamma receptors in human seminal plasma. *J Immunol*. 1989;143:1937–1939.

16. Witkin SS, Richards JM, Bedford JM. Influence of epididymal maturation on the capacity of hamster and rabbit spermatozoa for complement activation. *J Reprod Fertil*. 1983;69:517–521.

17. Morgan EL. The role of prostaglandin in C3a-mediated suppression of human in vitro polyclonal antibody responses. *Clin Immunol Immunopathol*. 1987;44:1–11.

18. El-Demiry M, James K. Lymphocyte subsets and macrophages in the male genital tract in health and disease. *Eur J Urol*. 1988;14:226–245.

19. Witkin SS. Mechanisms of active suppression of the immune response to spermatozoa. *Am J Reprod Immunol Microbiol*. 1988;17:61–64.

20. Alexander NJ, Anderson DJ. Vasectomy: Consequences of autoimmunity to sperm antigens. *Fertil Steril*. 1979;32:253.

21. Hendry WF, Parslow J, Stedronska J, et al. The diagnosis of unilateral testicular obstruction in subfertile males. *Br J Urol*. 1982;54:774–777.

22. D'Cruz OJ, Haas GG, de La Rocha R, et al. Occurrence of serum antisperm antibodies in patients with cystic fibrosis. *Fertil Steril*. 1991;56:519–527.

23. Bronson RA, O'Connor WJ, Wilson TA, et al. Correlation between puberty and the development of autoimmunity to spermatozoa in men with cystic fibrosis. *Fertil Steril*. 1992;58:1199–1204.

24. Haensch R. Spermatozoen-autoimmunphaenomene bei genitaltraumen und verschlubbazoospermie. *Andrologia*. 1973;5:147–151.

25. Mastrogiacomo I, Zanchetta R, Graziotti P, et al. Immunological and clinical study in patients after spermatic cord torsion. *Andrologia*. 1982;14:25–29.

26. Hjort T, Husted S, Linnet–Jepsen P. The effect of testis biopsy on autosensitization against spermatozoal antigens. *Clin Exp Immunol*. 1974;18:201–209.

27. Guazziero S, Lembo A, Ferro G, et al. Sperm antibodies and infertility in patients with testicular cancer. *Urology*. 1985;26:139–144.

28. Witkin SS, Toth A. Relationship between genital tract infections, sperm antibodies in seminal fluid, and infertility. *Fertil Steril*. 1983;40:805–808.

29. Shahmanesh M, Stedronska J, Hendry WF. Antispermatozoal antibodies in men with urethritis. *Fertil Steril*. 1986;46:308–311.

30. Witkin SS, Kligman I, Bongiovanni AM. Relationship between an asymptomatic male genital tract exposure to Chlamydia trachomatis and an autoimmune response to spermatozoa. *Hum Reprod*. 1995;10:2952–2955.

31. Mathur S, Williamson HO, Genco PV, et al. Sperm immunity in infertile couples: Antibody titers are higher against the husband's sperm than to sperm from controls. *Am J Reprod Immunol*. 1983;3:18–22.

32. Mathur S, Chao L, Goust J, et al. Special antigens on sperm from autoimmune infertile men. *Am J Reprod Immunol*. 1988;17:5–13.

33. Richards JM, Bedford JM, Witkin SS. Rectal insemination modifies immune responses in rabbits. *Science*. 1984;224:390–392.

34. Allardyce RA. Effect of ingested sperm on fecundity in the rat. *J Exp Med*. 1984;159:1548–1551.

35. Witkin SS, Sonnabend J. Immune response to spermatozoa in homosexual men. *Fertil Steril*. 1983;39:337–342.

36. Bronson RA, Cooper GW, Rosenfeld DW, et al. Comparison of antisperm antibodies in homosexual and infertile men with autoimmunity to spermatozoa. 30th Annual Meeting, Society for Gynecologic Investigation; March 17–20, 1983; Washington, DC.

37. Wolff H, Schill WB. Antisperm antibodies in infertile and homosexual men: Relationship to serologic and clinical findings. *Fertil Steril*. 1985;44:673–677.

38. Turek PJ, Lipshultz LI. Immunologic infertility. *Urol Clin North Am*. 1994;21:447–468.

39. Dimitrov DG, Urbanek V, Zverina J, et al. Correlation of asthenozoospermia with increased antisperm cell-mediated immunity in men from infertile couples. *J Reprod Immunol*. 1994;27:3–12.

40. Kibrik S, Belding DL, Merril B. Methods for the detection of antibodies against mammalian spermatozoa. *Fertil Steril*. 1952;3:430–438.

41. Shulman S, Hekman A. Antibodies to spermatozoa 1: A new macroscopic agglutination technique for their detection, using immotile sperm. *Clin Exp Immunol.* 1971;9:137–141.

42. Fjallbrant B. Interrelation between high levels of sperm antibodies, reduced penetration of cervical mucus by spermatozoa, and sterility in men. *Acta Obstet Gynecol Scand*. 1968;47:102–105.

43. Isojima S, Li TS, Ashitaka Y. Immunologic analysis of sperm-immobilizing factor found in sera of women with unexplained infertility. *Am J Obstet Gynecol.* 1968;101:677–682.

44. Hamerlink J, Rumke KB. A test for the detection of cytotoxic antibodies to spermatozoa in men. *J Reprod Fertil*. 1968;17:191–195.

45. De Almeida P, Jouannet P. Dexamethasone therapy of infertile men with sperm autoantibodies: Immunological and sperm follow-up. *Clin Exp Immunol.* 1981;44:567–575.

46. Husted S, Hjort T. Microtechniques for simultaneous determination of immobilizing and cytotoxic sperm antibodies. *Clin Exp Immunol*. 1975;22:256–263.

47. Bronson RA, Cooper GW, Rosenfeld DL. Autoimmunity to spermatozoa: Effect on sperm penetration of cervical mucus as reflected by postcoital testing. *Fertil Steril*. 1984;41:609–614.

48. Hjort T, Hansen KB. Immunofluorescent studies on human spermatozoa. *Clin Exp Immunol*. 1971;8:9–13.

49. Nikolaeva MA, Kulakov VI, Ter-Avanesov GV, et al. Detection of antisperm antibodies on the surface of living spermatozoa using flow cytometry: Preliminary study. *Fertil Steril*. 1994;59:639–644.

50. Jager S, Kremer J, Van Slochteren-Draaisma T. A simple method for antisperm antibodies detection in the human male: Detection of spermatozoal surface IgG with the direct mixed antiglobulin reaction carried out on untreated fresh human semen. *J Fertil.* 1978;23:1–12.

51. Bronson RA, Cooper GW, Rosenfeld DL. Sperm antibodies: Their role in infertility. *Fertil Steril.* 1984;42:171–183.

52. Hall JL, Engel D, Naz RK. Significance of antibodies against human sperm FA-1 antigen in immunoinfertility. *Arch Androl*. 1994;32:25–30.

53. Gonzales GF, Kortebani G, Mazzolli AB. Effect of isotypes of antisperm antibodies on semen quality. *Int J Androl*. 1992;15:220–228.

54. Fjallbrant B. Cervical mucus penetration by human spermatozoa treated with anti-spermatozoal antibodies from rabbit and man. *Acta Obstet Gynecol Scand.* 1969;48:71–77.

55. Lutjen PJ, McBain JC, Trounson AO. Biochemical aspects of spermatozoal cervical mucus interaction. *Proc Fertil Soc Aust*. 1984;3:26–34.

56. Jette NT, Glass RH. Prognostic value of the post-coital test. *Fertil Steril*. 1972;23:29–36.

57. Mortimer D, Pandya IJ, Sawers RS. Relationship between sperm motility characteristics and sperm penetration into cervical mucus in vitro. *J Reprod Fertil*. 1986;78:93–102.

58. Alexander NJ. Antibodies to human spermatozoa impede sperm penetration of cervical mucus or hamster eggs. *Fertil Steril*. 1984;41:433–439.

59. Clarke GN, Stojanoff A, Cauchi MN, et al. Detection of antispermatozoal antibodies of IgA class in cervical mucus. *Am J Reprod Immunol*. 1984;5:61–65.

60. Kremer J, Jager S. Characteristics of anti-spermatozoal antibodies responsible for the shaking phenomena with special regard to immunoglobulin class and antigen-reactive sites. *Int J Androl*. 1980;3:143–152.

61. Jager S, Kremer J, Kuiken J, et al. The significance of the Fc part of antispermatozoal antibodies for the shaking phenomenon in the sperm-cervical mucus contact. *Fertil Steril*. 1981;36:792–797.

62. Anderson DJ, Johnson PM, Alexander NJ, et al. Monoclonal antibodies to human trophoblast and sperm antigens: Report of two WHO-sponsored workshops, June 30, 1986, Toronto, Canada. *J Reprod Immunol*. 1987;10:231–257.

63. Bronson RA, Cooper GW. Effect of sperm-reactive monoclonal antibodies on the cervical mucus penetrating ability of human spermatozoa. *Am J Reprod Immunol Microbiol*. 1987;14:59–61.

64. Bronson RA, Cooper GW. Documentation of IgA1 and IgA2 antisperm antibodies within seminal fluid. *Am J Reprod Immunol*. 1988;18:7–10.

65. Plaut AG. The IgA1 proteases of bacteria. *Ann Rev Microbiol*. 1983;37:603–665.

66. Bronson RA, Cooper GW, Rosenfeld DL, et al. The effect of an IgA1 protease on immunoglobulins bound to the sperm surface and sperm cervical mucus penetrating ability. *Fertil Steril*. 1987;47:985–991.

67. Jager S, Kremer J, Kuiken J, et al. Induction of the shaking phenomenon by pretreatment of spermatozoa with sera containing antispermatozoal antibodies. *Fertil Steril*. 1981;36:784–791.

68. Wang C, Gordon Baker HW, Jennings MG, et al. Interaction between human cervical mucus and sperm surface antibodies. *Fertil Steril*. 1985;44:484–488.

69. Humphrey JH, Dourmashkin RR. Electron microscopic studies on immune cell lysis. In: *CIBA Foundation Symposium on Complement*. Boston, MA: Little, Brown & Co; 1965:175.

70. Price RJ, Boettcher B. The presence of complement in human cervical mucus and its possible relevance to infertility in women with complement-dependent sperm immobilizing antibodies. *Fertil Steril*. 1979;36:61.

71. Dhindsa DS, Schumacher GFB, eds. *Immunological Aspects of Infertility and Fertility Regulation*. New York, NY: Elsevier/North–Holland; 1980:13.

72. Yang SL, Schumacher GFB, Broer KA, et al. Specific antibodies and immunoglobulins in the oviductal fluid of the rhesus monkey. *Fertil Steril*. 1983;39: 359–369.

73. Schumacher GFB. Humoral immune factors in the female reproductive tract and their changes during the cycle. In: Dhindsa DS, Schumacher GFB, eds. *Immunological Aspects of Infertility and Fertility Regulation*. New York, NY: Elsevier/North-Holland; 1980:93.

74. Clarke GN, Hsieh C, Koh SH, et al. Sperm antibodies, immunoglobulins and complement in human follicular fluid. *Am J Reprod Immunol*. 1984;5:179.

75. D'Cruz OJ, Haas GG, Lambert H. Evaluation of antisperm complement-dependent immune mediators in human ovarian follicular fluid. *J Immunol*. 1990;144: 3841–3848.

76. Bronson RA, Cooper GW, Rosenfeld DL. Correlation between regional specificity of antisperm antibodies to the spermatozoan surface and complement-mediated sperm immobilization. *Am J Reprod Immunol*. 1982;2:222–225.

77. London SN, Haney AF, Weinberg JB. Macrophages and infertility: Enhancement of human macrophage-mediated sperm killing by antisperm antibodies. *Fertil Steril*. 1985;43:274–278.

78. D'Cruz OJ, Haas GG Jr. Beta 2 integrin (CD11b/CD18) is the primary adhesive glycoprotein complex involved in neutrophil-mediated immune injury to human sperm. *Biol Reprod*. 1995;53:1118–1130.

79. Yanagimachi R. Sperm-egg fusion. In: Bronner F, ed. *Current Topics in Membranes and Transport*. Orlando, FL: Academic Press; 1988:3–43.

80. Lansford B, Haas GG, DeBault LE, et al. Effect of antisperm antibodies on the acrosomal reactivity of human sperm. In: *The American Fertility Society Program and Abstracts*. 44th Annual Meeting; October 10-13, 1988; Atlanta, GA.

81. Wolf DP. Acrosomal status quantitation in human sperm. *Am J Reprod Immunol*. 1989;20:106–113.

82. Bronson RA, Cooper GW, Phillips DM. Effects of sperm-reactive antibodies and complement on the ultrastructure of human spermatozoa. *Ann N Y Acad Sci*. 1987;513:574–576.

83. Tasdemir I, Tasdemir M, Fukuda J, et al. Effects of sperm-immobilizing antibodies on the spontaneous and calcium-ionophore (A23187)-induced acrosome reaction. *Int J Fertil Menopausal Stud*. 1995;40:192–195.

84. Saling PM, Lakoski KA. Mouse sperm antigens that participate in fertilization, II: Inhibition of sperm penetration through the zona pellucida using monoclonal antibodies. *Biol Reprod*. 1985;33:527–536.

85. Huang TTF, Tung KSK, Yanagimachi R. Autoantibodies from vasectomized guinea pigs inhibit fertilization in vitro. *Science*. 1981;213:1267–1269.

86. O'Rand MG. Inhibition of fertility and sperm-zona binding by antiserum to the rabbit sperm membrane auto-antigen RSA-1. *Biol Reprod*. 1981;25:621–628.

87. Bronson RA, Cooper GW, Rosenfeld DL. Sperm-specific isoantibodies and autoantibodies inhibit the binding of human sperm to the human zona pellucida. *Fertil Steril*. 1982;38:724–729.

88. Tsukui S, Noda Y, Yano J, et al. Inhibition of sperm penetration through human zona pellucida by antisperm antibodies. *Fertil Steril*. 1986;46:92–96.

89. Yanagimachi R, Lopata A, Odom CB, et al. Retention of biologic characteristics of zona pellucida in highly concentrated salt solution: The use of salt stored eggs for assessing the fertilizing capacity of spermatozoa. *Fertil Steril*. 1979;31:562–574.

90. Mahoney MC, Blackmore PF, Bronson RA, et al. Inhibition of human sperm-zona pellucida tight binding in the presence of antisperm antibody positive polyclonal patient sera. *J Reprod Immunol*. 1991;19:287–301.

91. Yanagimachi R, Yanagimachi H, Rogers BJ. The use of zona-free animal ova as a test-system for the assessment of the fertilizing capacity of human spermatozoa. *Biol Reprod*. 1976;15:471–476.

92. Dor J, Rudak E, Aitken RJ. Antisperm antibodies: Their effect on the process of fertilization studied in vitro. *Fertil Steril*. 1981;35:535–541.

93. Requeda E, Charron J, Roberts KD, et al. Fertilizing capacity and sperm antibodies in vasostomized men. *Fertil Steril*. 1983;39:197–203.

94. Haas GG, Ausmanas M, Culp L, et al. The effect of immunoglobulin occurring on human sperm in vivo on the human sperm/hamster ova penetration assay. *Am J Reprod Immunol Microbiol*. 1985;7:109–112.

95. Abdel-Latif A, Mathur S, Rust PF, et al. Cytotoxic sperm antibodies inhibit sperm penetration of zona-free hamster eggs. *Fertil Steril*. 1986;45:542–549.

96. Haas GG, Sokoloski JE, Wolf DP. The interfering effect of human IgG antisperm antibodies on human sperm penetration of zona-free hamster eggs. *Am J Reprod Immunol Microbiol*. 1980;1:40–43.

97. Menge AC, Mangione CM, Dietrich JW, et al. Effect of antisperm antibodies in serum and cervical mucus on the capacity of human sperm to penetrate zona-free hamster ova. *Arch Androl*. 1984;12:83–88.

98. Bronson RA, Cooper GW, Rosenfeld DL. Ability of antibody-bound sperm to penetrate zona-free hamster eggs. *Fertil Steril*. 1981;36:778–783.

99. Aitken RJ, Hulme MJ, Henderson CT, et al. Analysis of the surface labelling characteristics of human spermatozoa and the interaction with anti-sperm antibodies. *J Reprod Fertil*. 1987;80:473–485.

100. Bronson RA, Fusi F, Cooper GW, et al. Antisperm antibodies induce polyspermy by promoting adherence of human sperm to zona-free hamster eggs. *Hum Reprod*. 1990;5:690–696.

101. Bronson RA, Fleit HB, Fusi F. Identification of an oolemmal Fc receptor: Its role in promoting binding of antibody-labelled human sperm to zona-free hamster eggs. *Am J Reprod Immunol*. 1990;23:87–92.

102. Bronson RA, Fusi FM, Fleit HB. Monoclonal antibodies identify Fcγ receptors on unfertilized human oocytes but not spermatozoa. *J Reprod Immunol.* 1992;21:293–307.

103. Hassold TJ, Chan N, Funkhauser S, et al. A cytogenetic study of 1000 human abortions. *Ann Hum Genet.* 1980;44:151–178.

104. O'Rand MG, Irons GP. Monoclonal antibodies to rabbit sperm autoantigens, II: Inhibition of human sperm penetration of zona-free hamster eggs. *Biol Reprod.* 1984;30:731–736.

105. Naz RK, Alexander NJ, Isahakie M, et al. Monoclonal antibody to a human germ cell membrane glycoprotein that inhibits fertilization. *Science.* 1984;225:342–344.

106. Okabe M, Nagira M, Kawai Y, et al. A human sperm antigen possibly involved in binding and/or fusion with zona-free hamster eggs. *Fertil Steril.* 1990;54:1121–1126.

107. Clarke GN, McBain JC, Lopata A, et al. In vitro fertilization results for women with sperm antibodies in plasma and follicular fluid. *Am J Reprod Immunol Microbiol.* 1985;8:130–131.

108. Clarke GN, Lopata A, Johnston WIH. Effect of sperm antibodies in females on human in vitro fertilization. *Fertil Steril.* 1986;46:435–441.

109. Vasquez-Levin M, Kaplan P, Guzman I, et al. The effect of female antisperm antibodies on in vitro fertilization, early embryonic development and pregnancy outcome. *Fertil Steril.* 1991;56:84–90.

110. Pagidas K, Hemmings R, Falcone T, et al. The effect of antisperm autoantibodies in male or female partners undergoing in vitro fertilization-embryo transfer. *Fertil Steril.* 1994;62:363–368.

111. Clarke GN, Lopata A, McBain JC, et al. Effect of sperm antibodies in males in human in vitro fertilization (IVF). *Am J Reprod Immunol Microbiol.* 1985;8:62–66.

112. De Almeida M, Gazagne I, Jeulin C, et al. In vitro processing of sperm with autoantibodies and in vitro fertilization results. *Hum Reprod.* 1989;4:49–53.

113. Junk SM, Matson PL, Yovich YM, et al. The fertilization of human oocytes by spermatozoa from men with antispermatozoal antibodies in semen. *J In Vitro Fert Embryo Transf.* 1986;3:350–352.

114. Sukcharoen N, Keith J. The effect of the antisperm auto-antibody-bound sperm on in vitro fertilization outcome. *Andrologia.* 1995;27:281–289.

115. Yeh WR, Acosta AA, Seltman HJ, et al. Impact of immunoglobulin isotype and sperm surface location of antisperm antibodies on fertilization in vitro in the human. *Fertil Steril.* 1995;63:1287–1292.

116. Naz RK. Effects of antisperm antibodies on early cleavage of fertilized ova. *Biol Reprod.* 1992;46:130–139.

117. Heidenreich A, Bonfig R, Wilbert DM, et al. Risk factors for antisperm antibodies in infertile men. *Am J Reprod Immunol.* 1994;31:69–76.

SECTION IV

General Guidelines for the Introduction of New Tests and Standardization of Laboratory Tests

CHAPTER 27

General Immunologic Methods for the Evaluation of Autoimmune Diseases

James T. Wu, PhD

Autoantibodies against various organelles, enzymes, proteins, and nuclear DNA have been found in sera from patients with various autoimmune diseases. Detection of these autoantibodies relies on their specific affinity binding to the antigens in various preparations on tissue sections (immunohistologically) or in solution (immunochemically). The affinity, or equilibrium dissociation constant, between the autoantibody and the antigen determines the specificity and sensitivity of the test. Because there is usually more than one type of autoantibody present in patient serum, purity of the antigen preparation conceivably affects the specificity of the autoantibody detection.[1] Less-sensitive methods based on a secondary antigen-antibody reaction, such as those leading to precipitation or agglutination, are not covered here.

Selection of a method for autoantibody detection also is affected by whether the antigen is soluble or not, and whether identification of autoantibodies against a specific protein or an entire organelle is desired. Autoantibodies against cellular components such as DNA, DNA protein complexes, histone proteins, and nonhistone nuclear proteins can be detected in systemic lupus erythematosus (SLE) and related diseases. Autoantibodies against cellular organelles can be detected immunohistologically using a slice of frozen tissue or fixed cells; this method is advantageous in that it does not require solubilization or purification of the antigen. The immunohistochemical technique also gives the pattern of antigen distribution within a specific type of tissue. However, it is less sensitive and specific and is not suitable for large-scale screening.

When soluble pure antigen is available, enzyme-linked immunosorbent assay (ELISA) becomes the method of choice.[2] It provides superior specificity and sensitivity when the antigen is highly purified. This technique also allows simultaneous screening of a large number of specimens. Recently, the use of recombinant protein as antigen has become increasingly popular for the detection of autoantibodies following the ELISA procedure. Recombinant mitochondria proteins, peptides coded for the 74-kd and the 52-kd mitochondria autoantigens, were used to establish ELISA.[3] The synthetic portion of the protein molecule (eg, N- and C-terminal peptides of glutamic acid decarboxylase [GAD]) or specific epitope on an oxidized low-density lipoprotein molecule also have been used as antigens for the identification of autoantibodies.[4] Using the synthetic portion of the protein molecule may avoid problems associated with antigen isolation, such as alteration of the antigen during purification.

Another procedure that has been used to avoid antigen isolation and purification is immunoblot. This is the method frequently used to detect autoantibodies against certain antigens in a specific type of cell or tissue extract. High-resolution electrophoresis is usually employed to separate the proteins of the extract, followed by transferring the separated protein onto a membrane and then staining with patient serum containing autoantibodies. This technique is highly sensitive and specific. All the methods mentioned here complement each other. If required, they can be used simultaneously for a complete identification of autoantibodies.

Autoantibodies are immunoglobulins (Igs), but not necessarily IgG; occasionally, they appear as IgA and IgM. Therefore, antihuman IgG alone should not be used as the secondary antibody for visualization. Antihuman IgA and antihuman IgM also should be tested during the initial screening.

This chapter describes various methods of identifying autoantibodies, from simple diffusion in agarose gel to the sophisticated immunoblot procedure. The selection of an appropriate method is dependent on the instrumentation available, the sensitivity and specificity required, and the type of specimen to be used. Even the simplest double gel diffusion, if used properly, can be very sensitive and capable of providing important information.

Gel Immunodiffusion

Gel immunodiffusion is performed mainly using agarose gel as the supporting medium. Cellulose acetate membrane, formerly a popular supporting medium, is seldom used. The high water content and large pore size of the agarose gel allow the antigens and antibodies to migrate through the gel by diffusion, driven either by the concentration gradient or by an electric field as in counterimmunoelectrophoresis (CIE). When antigen and antibody diffuse toward each other in the gel, a precipitin line is formed when the concentrations of both antigen and antibody reach an equivalence. The purity of the agarose gel makes the precipitin lines clear and easy to distinguish. Procedures of gel immunodiffusion are mostly qualitative but provide semiquantitative information based on the concentrations of antigen used and the position of the precipitin lines.

Both double diffusion and CIE procedures require wells in the gel plates. Antigen and antibody solutions are placed in separate wells. Depending on the size and shape of the antigen molecule, immunoprecipitates are formed at the point of equivalence for each antigen-antibody pair after several hours of diffusion. Typically, double diffusion requires overnight incubation in a humidified chamber, whereas only 1 or 2 hours are needed to perform CIE. A longer incubation time and electrophoresis (for double diffusion and CIE, respectively) may be required depending on the shape and size of the antigen molecule.

Agarose gels with different degrees of purity are available. In general, the higher the purity of the gel, the better it performs in terms of sensitivity and clarity. However, in CIE, it is important to use agarose gel with a high electroendosmosis (EEO) for the antibody to travel in an opposing direction to that of the antigen. If pure agarose is used for preparing the gel film in CIE, both antigen and antibody travel toward the anode and would never meet to form a precipitin line.

In the past, agarose gel was cast on a glass plate, which has largely been replaced by Gelbound (FMC Bioproducts, Rockland, ME), a specially treated flexible polyester film that allows easier handling and storage as well as retention of the plates as a permanent record. For most gel film, gels of 0.8% to 1% wt/vol are prepared in phosphate-buffered saline (PBS). The thickness of the agarose gel is usually maintained at about 1 mm. A puncher is needed to make uniform circular holes in the gel for filling the specimens. Each well holds about 8 µL of liquid. At the end of immunodiffusion, precipitin lines in wet untreated agarose gel can be viewed under indirect light against a black background when the concentration of antigen is at or above 10 to 50 µg/mL. However, at lower concentrations, the gel plate is washed overnight in PBS to remove soluble proteins, pressed dry, and then subjected to dye or silver staining.

When the precipitin lines are stained with dye, this can greatly increase the sensitivity of detection. Amido black and Coomassie brilliant blue R-250 are the most frequently used dyes for this purpose. Amido black is less sensitive, but gives a cleaner background. Coomassie brilliant blue R-250 is approximately 3 times more sensitive, but it takes much longer to reduce the background staining. Before reacting with the dye, the gel plate is soaked in PBS to remove all soluble proteins left in the gel, dried, and then soaked in the dye solution. If the soluble proteins are not removed or the plate is not dried prior to the dye reaction, very high background staining results. The most sensitive staining is by silver reagent. Because silver reagent is designed for polyacrylamide gel, it may not be applicable to agarose gel and a special silver reagent must be used. Silver staining is about 10 times more sensitive than Coomassie blue for protein visualization; nanogram concentrations of protein are visible with silver staining.[5] Proteins in agarose gel, not visible by Coomassie blue, can be restained using silver reagent, even after the dried film has been stored for months. Commercial silver stain kits for agarose gel, such as the Titan gel silver stain kit from Helena Laboratories (Beaumont, TX), are available.

Double Diffusion

Double diffusion (Ouchterlony technique) is the simplest technique available for identifying autoantibodies. This method does not require any sophisticated instrumentation. Although it is basically a qualitative method, it also can provide some semiquantitative data. At the present time, the method has largely been replaced by ELISA. However, when used properly, it provides information no other methods can. For example, the specificity of certain autoantibodies can be identified by comparing the precipitin line to a pure antigen preparation placed in the well next to the sample well. It is also possible to confirm that a positive result from an ELISA is not due to interferences. The technique should remain largely as a research tool and occasionally as an adjunct test for other procedures.

Essentially, in double diffusion, antigen-antibody solutions are placed in separate wells within the agarose gel. Many different well arrangements can be made, a few of which are shown in **Figure 27-1**. The most frequently used arrangement (Figure 27-1A) is one in which the antigen solution is placed in the center well and various dilutions of the patient specimen are placed in the surrounding wells. Commercial templates for this arrangement are available. The distance between the central well and the surrounding wells is usually 1 cm, but one template has a distance of 0.5 cm. In the latter arrangement, neither the antigen nor autoantibody has very far to travel in the agarose gel and they remain at relatively higher concentrations when they meet to form a precipitin line. The appearance of a heavy precipitin line at the position closer to the antigen well indicates that a high concentration of autoantibody is present in the specimen. As the sample is diluted further, the precipitin line becomes

Double immunodiffusion (Ouchterlony technique)

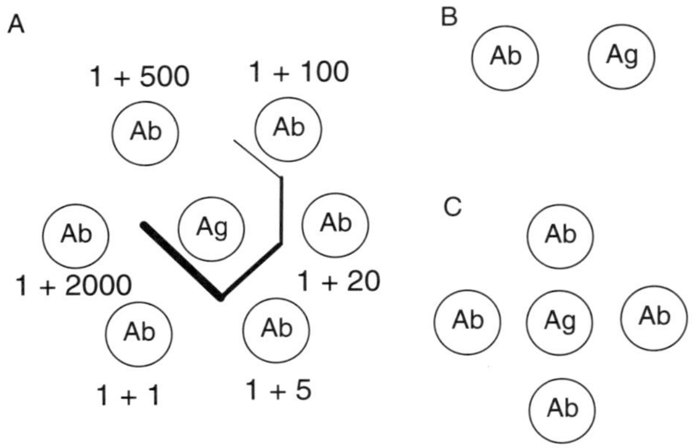

Figure 27-1. Various arrangements of sample wells for double diffusion. The distance between the antigen (Ag) and antibody (Ab) wells may vary from 1 to 0.5 cm. Each well has a diameter of about 0.25 cm and can hold approximately 8 μL when the gel film is 1 mm thick.

lighter and moves closer to the autoantibody well. No precipitin line is visible for the wells containing sample at 1:500 and 1:2,000 dilutions. In these wells, the concentration of the antigen exceeds that of the autoantibody when the specimen is highly diluted, so no precipitation forms. Conceivably, the position of the precipitin line gives a semiquantitative impression of the concentration of autoantibody in the specimen when a known amount of antigen is used for detection.

Double diffusion can be used to detect two different autoantibodies. The sensitivity of the method can be adjusted depending on the well arrangement and staining method used. A short distance between wells means that both the antigen and the autoantibody are maintained at higher concentrations, thus improving the sensitivity of autoantibody detection. If the 0.5-cm template is used with the silver reagent for staining, sensitivity can be improved to the high nanogram level.

The major steps of double diffusion are

- Diffusion
- Washing in PBS to remove soluble proteins
- Press drying the gel film
- Staining

Although the method is simple, it has the disadvantage of being time-consuming. The whole procedure can take several days to complete if the antigen molecule is large. Compared with other techniques, double diffusion is considered the least sensitive.

Example

Jaskowski et al[6] compared double diffusion with enzyme immunoassay for screening autoantibodies to extractable nuclear antigens. They pointed out that double diffusion was the traditional method for identifying specific autoantibodies but was time-consuming and expensive when testing large numbers of clinical specimens because large amounts of expensive antigen were required. The kit used in their study can be obtained from INOVA Diagnostics (San Diego, CA).

Counterimmunoelectrophoresis

In double diffusion, both antigen and antibody solutions are allowed to diffuse in all directions (360°) from the well. Only a portion of the entire antigen and antibody meet and form a precipitin line. Consequently, the majority of the antigen and antibody are wasted in double diffusion. In CIE, the application of the electric field not only accelerates the diffusion process, but forces the antigen and antibody to move in opposite directions. Therefore, all the antigen and antibody are involved in the formation of the precipitin line. The time required for the diffusion is shortened greatly and the sensitivity of autoantibody detection is improved. The time required to complete CIE depends on the well arrangement, the type of antigen molecule, and the voltage applied.

To perform CIE, a double row of wells is punched in the agarose gel (**Figure 27-2**) for which a commercial template is available. The distance between the antigen and antibody wells can be fixed at 0.5 or 1 cm. Using a 0.5-cm template in combination with silver reagent allows the detection of antibody concentrations of less than 100 ng. In this technique, the antigen is placed in the cathodic wells and the specimens to be tested are placed in the opposite anodal wells. It is important to ensure that the agarose used to make the film contains high EEO, such as in Seakem HE and Seakem ME from FMC Corporation, Bio Products, Rockland, ME. The agarose gel also should be dissolved in the electrophoresis buffer rather than PBS, as in double diffusion. Impure agarose is used to prepare gel for CIE because during electrophoresis the electroendosmotic flow created by the high EEO agarose makes the antibody migrate toward the anode and meet the antigen, which usually moves toward the cathode under alkaline conditions.

Counterimmunoelectrophoresis was used in the past in the routine identification of hepatitis-associated antibodies.[7] Using agarose gel film, only 8 μL of liquid

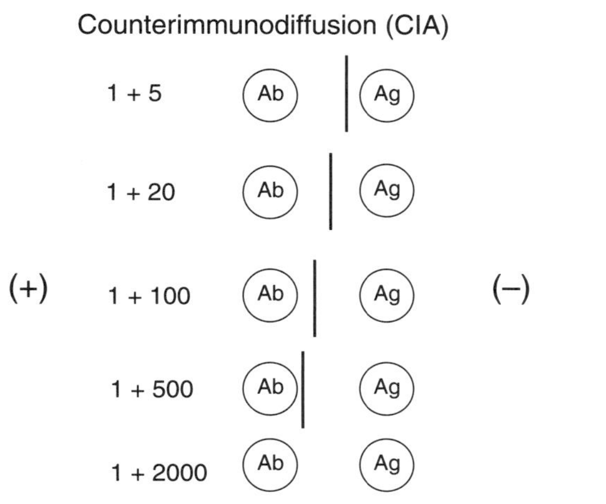

Figure 27-2. Arrangement of wells commonly used for counterimmunoelectrophoresis. The distance between the antigen and antibody wells may vary from 1 to 0.5 cm (see Figure 27-1).

is required to fill each well. For the detection of hepatitis-associated antibodies, electrophoresis is carried out at 40 mA for 30 minutes. To perform CIE, a power supply and an electrophoresis chamber are needed in addition to the agarose gel. Precipitin lines are visualized using the same procedure as in double diffusion.

Example

Even though cellulose acetate paper currently is seldom used as a solid support for electrophoresis, it was used by Delpech et al[8] to detect specific autoantibodies in sera from patients with SLE. The researchers placed 25 µL of 5 mg/mL protein antigen on the cathodic side and 15 µL of undiluted sera on the anodal side. Counterimmunoelectrophoresis was carried out at 80 V for 2 hours in tris-glycine buffer (pH 9). Precipitin lines were fixed and stained with Coomassie brilliant blue. A much smaller sample volume is required with greater test sensitivity if agarose film is used instead of cellulose acetate, especially if silver reagent is used for staining.

Indirect Immunofluorescence

Immunofluorescence is a powerful technique for detecting autoantibodies against intra- and extracellular components in both histologic sections and cultured cells. In indirect immunofluorescence (**Figure 27-3**), a fluorochrome is linked to the secondary antihuman immunoglobulin antibodies, usually rabbit or goat, which are used to bind to the antigen-bound human autoantibodies for visualization by fluorescence microscope. This technique usually uses frozen tissue sections or tissue culture cell monolayers from human organs as the source of antigen for the identification of autoantibodies in patient serum. Unfixed, frozen, and paraffin-embedded sections of human tissues also may be used. HeLa cell preparation is used for the detection of antinuclear antibodies.

Indirect immunofluorescence can be used to detect antibodies against cytoskeletal system, fibroblasts, and special cells fixed with methanol. Autoantibodies against chromatin, kinetochores, nucleoli, nuclear matrix, nuclear bodies, mitochondria, ribosomes, and (occasionally) Golgi apparatus are commonly identified with this technique. Isolation and purification of specific soluble antigens are not necessary. Another advantage associated with indirect immunofluorescence is its ability to provide an immunoreactivity pattern, showing the location and pattern of distribution of antigens in a specific type of tissue and cell. Multicolor immunofluorescence also can be used in this way when identification of antibodies against more than one antigen is required; it is possible to find multiple autoantibodies against different antigens in the same serum. This technique is particularly useful for the detection of "anticellular antibodies," or autoantibodies against antigens associated with specific tissue (**Table 27-1**).

Because protein A, a cell wall protein of *Staphylococcus aureus*, binds with high affinity to the Fc region of immunoglobulin molecules, especially of the IgG class, fluorescently conjugated protein A has been used to replace the secondary antibody to reduce background labeling in indirect immunofluorescence. However, the amplification is low and is limited by

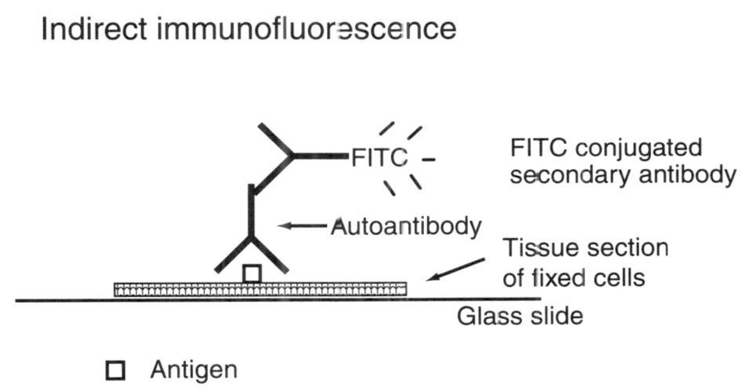

Figure 27-3. Schematic of test format for indirect immunofluorescence.

Table 27-1. Excitation and Emission Maxima of Common Fluorochromes

Fluorochrome	Absolute Maximum (nm)	Emission Maximum (nm)	Color of Fluorescence
Texas red	596	615	Deep red
Lissamine-rhodamine-B	570	590	Red
Rhodamine isothiocyanate	554	573	Red
Fluorescein isothiocyanate	492	515	Green
Aminomethyl coumarin acetic acid	350	450	Blue

the protein's lower affinity for immunoglobulins of some species, particularly sheep, goat, and rat, and for some IgG subclasses in other species.

In general, the major steps involved in indirect immunofluorescence are

- Specimen preparation, such as fixing cells in cold acetone, fixing tissue in periodate-lysine-paraformaldehyde, preparation of Bouin's fluid-fixed paraffin-embedded sections of tissue, and fixing all types of cells isolated from tissues or cultured cells with methanol
- Incubation with an appropriately diluted specimen
- Incubation with appropriately diluted fluorescein isothiocyanate (FITC)–conjugated $F(ab')_2$ fragments of goat antihuman immunoglobulins (IgG + IgM + IgA)
- Mounting of the slides in phosphate-buffered glycerol after washing in PBS
- Examination by incident fluorescence microscopy using an excitation wavelength of 495 nm

Controls are fixed cells incubated with FITC-conjugated antibody alone. Background staining is assessed by using monoclonal IgG or IgM antibodies that do not react with human tissues. Both frozen sections or formaldehyde-fixed organ tissue can be used for immunostain. Visualization of autoantibodies can be made by fluorescence microscopy.[9]

Because each cell type contains thousands of different antigens, human autoantibodies to DNA show cross-reactivity with synthetic polynucleotides, cardiolipin, and other phospholipids. It is possible for autoantibodies to react either with the same molecule in several different tissues, with common antigenic determinants on different molecules in multiple organs, or with both. Immunofluorescence is not as specific and sensitive as ELISA. For example, autoantibodies to mitochondria detected in human sera contain multiple specificities and also may be present in the sera of healthy individuals.

The fixatives used have an impact on the intensity of immunostaining. Takino et al[10] used the immunoperoxidase method to study the location of antigens that react with islet cell cytoplasmic antibodies within the human pancreatic beta cells. They found that the most intense staining was observed in islets of those tissue sections fixed in periodate-lysine-paraformaldehyde, and weak staining was observed in those fixed in cold ethanol, 4% paraformaldehyde, or cold acetone. No positive staining was seen in sections fixed in 3% glutaraldehyde.

Examples

Solimena et al[11] employed indirect immunofluorescence using frozen sections of formaldehyde-fixed rat brain to incubate (immunostain) both serum and cerebrospinal fluid from patients with stiff-man syndrome. They found autoantibodies staining all gray-matter regions. These autoantibodies were identical to those against glutamic acid decarboxylase.

Using cryostat sections of normal human and rabbit renal tissue, Konishi et al[12] were able to identify autoantibodies against renal tubular cells in a patient with Graves' disease and distal renal tubular acidosis. The immunofluorescence technique revealed that positive cells extending from the cortex to the outer medulla appeared to be collecting duct cells. The researchers' use of 2 different fluorescence labels—the tetramethylrhodamine isothiocyanate–conjugated peanut lectin and FITC-conjugated goat antihuman IgG—allowed them to determine that the patient's autoantibodies were reactive with 2 types of intercalated cells.

Dobersen et al[13] used immunofluorescence to study sera from 36 patients with type 1 diabetes for the capacity of lysing beta cells. The study revealed an islet cell cytoplasmic autoantibody in 20 patients with diabetes and an islet cell surface antibody in 23 patients. The islet cell cytoplasmic autoantibodies were detected by standard indirect immunofluorescence on sections of Bouin's fixed human pancreas. Islet cell surface antibodies were detected by indirect immunofluorescence with viable rat islet cells. For antigen preparation, the cells were plated at a density of 2×10^4 cells per well in 96-well tissue culture trays. Test serum (50 µL) was diluted in PBS at a ratio of 1:2 and added to the wells, incubated at 37°C for 30 minutes with 50 µL of FITC-conjugated goat antihuman IgG (heavy and light chains), and then examined under a fluorescence microscope.

Enzyme Immunoassays

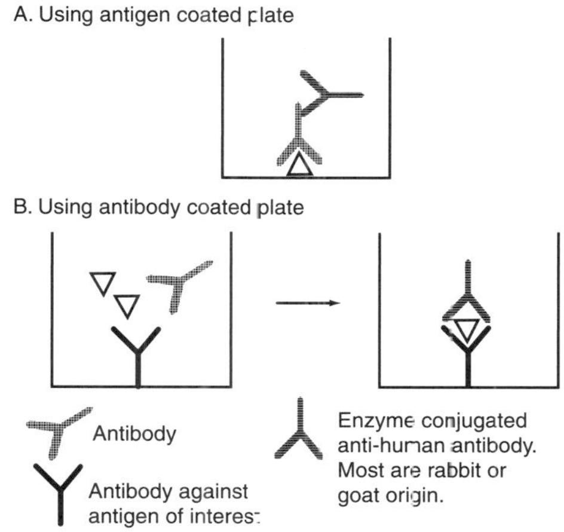

Figure 27-4. The 2 main test formats for enzyme-linked immunosorbent assay to detect autoantibodies. (**A**) An antigen-coated solid phase is used. (**B**) An antibody-coated microplate is used.

Enzyme-Linked Immunosorbent Assays

Enzyme-linked immunosorbent assay is the most sensitive, specific, and quantitative type of assay. This technique can handle large numbers of specimens simultaneously, making it suitable for screening. A soluble pure antigen preparation is preferred. Essentially, 2 major test formats are used for the detection of autoantibodies: an antigen-coated solid phase and an antibody-coated solid phase.

Antigen-Coated Solid Phase

In the first format, a soluble pure antigen is coated on the solid phase (**Figure 27-4A**). A polystyrene microplate is usually used as the solid phase (a polystyrene tube or bead also can be used). A microplate is recommended because it requires less reagent and is generally easier to operate. The test specimen is then added and captured by the antigen coated on the solid phase. After the removal of unbound antibody by washing, labeled anti-immunoglobulin is added. If the label is an enzyme, the enzyme substrate is added after unbound conjugate has been washed away. The intensity of the color developed by the bound enzyme conjugate is used to measure the amount of antibody present in the specimen. Recent advances in recombinant technology have made it possible to use well-defined and pure antigens in this test format. The type of autoantibody detected depends on the type of antigen(s) used to coat the solid phase.

Examples

Van de Water et al[3] coated microtiter plates with 100 µL of purified recombinant fusion proteins at 2 mg/L in carbonate coating buffer (pH 9.6). After blocking, serum samples were diluted 1:1,000 in blocking buffer, and 100 µL of the diluted serum was added to the plates in duplicate wells. After washing, a peroxidase-conjugated secondary antibody histidine-rich protein antihuman immunoglobulin (polyvalent) (1:4,000) was added for final quantification.

To detect antibody to cardiolipin (phospholipid antigen), researchers[14] placed 200 µL of a solution of cardiolipin (Avanti Polar Lipids, Alabaster, AL) in ethanol-chloroform (90 mg/L) in microtiter wells, evaporated by air jet. After washing, 200 µL of a 1:10 dilution of test serum was added and incubated in duplicate specimens for 7 hours in a humid chamber at room temperature. Following washing, autoantibody was measured by ELISA using alkaline phosphatase–conjugated antipolyvalent human immunoglobulin and developed with *p*-nitrophenyl phosphate in diethanolamine buffer. Color intensity was read at 405 nm (a single positive serum sample was used as the calibrator). Specific, rapid, and sensitive detection of 2 distinct mitochondrial autoantibodies in sera from patients with primary biliary cirrhosis was made possible by using the recombinant 74- and 52-kd mitochondrial proteins.[3] The autoantigens were prepared with a full-length human clone encoding the 74-kd mitochondrial autoantigen and a human cDNA clone for the 52-kd autoantigen. For the ELISA, round-bottom polystyrene microtiter plates (Immulon I, Dynatech Labs, Alexandria, VA) were coated with 100 μL of the purified recombinant fusion proteins (2 μg/mL). One hundred microliters of diluted serum (1:1,000 in blocking buffer) was added to the wells. After incubation for 1 hour at 37°C, a peroxidase-conjugated secondary antihuman immunoglobulin (1:4,000) was used for qualification.

Ohta and colleagues[4] used synthetic peptides for the characterization of autoantibodies. Synthetic N-terminal peptides ($GAD_{65}N$ and $GAD_{67}N$) and a C-terminal peptide ($GAD_{67}C$) of human GAD isoforms were used to identify isoforms of glutamic acid decarboxylase.

Antibody-Coated Solid Phase

Pure antigen is not always available, and loss or denaturation of antigen frequently occurs during the isolation and purification process. An antigen coating, especially on a microplate where the available surface area is limited, cannot tolerate too many impurities. The alternative is to coat the solid phase with monoclonal or polyclonal antibody, from either humans or animals, such as rabbits or goats. The coating antibody should react with the same epitopes as those reacting with the autoantibodies so that a competitive format can be established. The antibody-coated solid phase is then incubated with both the specimen containing autoantibodies and the semipurified antigen preparation in a microtiter well. In this test format, the coating antibody and the specimen autoantibodies compete for the soluble antigen, and the antigen does not have to be purified. Consequently, the amount of antigen captured by the solid phase is inversely related to the amount of autoantibody contained in the specimen. The amount of captured antigen is quantified by the addition of an enzyme-labeled secondary antibody.

Example

Gruber et al[2] carried out an ELISA using this format to detect liver-kidney microsomal autoantibodies, soluble liver antigen autoantibodies, and mitochondria antigen autoantibodies based on inhibition of the binding of the detecting (coating) antibody by sera containing the autoantibodies. Purified gamma-globulin fractions from positive patient sera were used to coat the microplates, which were used to capture the antigen (mitochondrial fraction or microsomal fraction) after blocking and washing. The microplates were incubated with patient sera of unknown specificity. Subsequently, the plates were washed and incubated first with diluted biotinylated gamma-globulin fraction of the corresponding specificity and then with avidin-peroxidase.

Particle Concentration Fluoroimmunoassays

Microplate is generally recognized as a convenient solid phase for ELISAs. Many instruments are available to facilitate the pipetting, washing, incubation, and absorbency reading. Conceivably, the entire microplate assay can be semiautomated.

Because of the limited surface area for protein binding in microwells, microwell assays can only accommodate concentrations in the nanogram range. One way to overcome this problem is to use antigen or antibody to coat a microsphere (fine polystyrene particle), which has a much larger surface area (**Figure 27-5**). A solid phase with a large surface area tolerates impurities in the antigen coating preparation. Pure antigen may not be required for autoantibody detection when a microsphere is selected as the solid phase for ELISA.

Example

Karjalainen et al[15] were able to use this technique to detect autoantibodies against bovine serum albumin (BSA) in patients with type 1 diabetes. The researchers coated microspheres with a large quantity of BSA. First, 20 μL of serum (1:100 to 1:1,000 dilution) was added to 96-well unidirectional-flow vacuum filtration plates (IDEXX, Portland, ME), each containing 20 μL microspheres (0.125% wt/vol) covalently

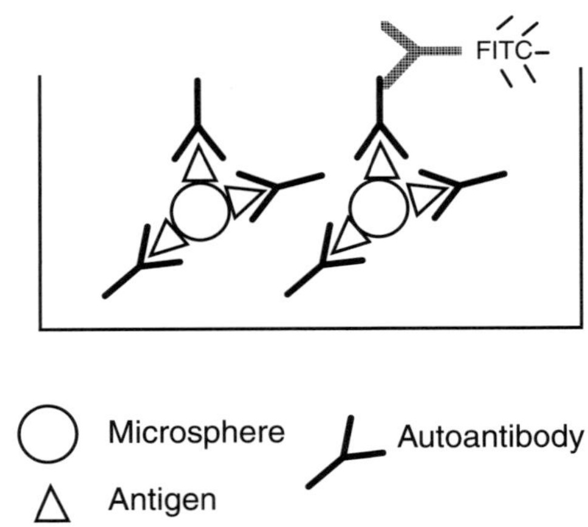

Figure 27-5. Schematic of a microsphere being used for the detection of autoantibodies.

conjugated with BSA. Ovalbumin (0.1% wt/vol) in PBS containing 1% Tween-20 was used to prevent nonspecific binding. After 1 to 3 minutes of incubation and washing, unbound proteins were removed by vacuum filtration, and 100 μg of affinity-purified fluorescein-conjugated goat antihuman IgG, IgA, IgM, or IgD was added to each well. Bound fluorescence was read and transmitted to personal computers for automated data processing. The assay had a sensitivity of 1 ng of IgG or IgA per mL of sample and 10 ng of IgM per mL of sample; the intra-assay and interassay coefficient of variation ranged from 8% to 10%.

Immunoblotting

Immunoblotting (or Western blot) is a technique used mainly for identification of an antigen in a solution containing a mixture of proteins. Because the last step of antigen visualization uses an antibody specific for a certain antigen for immunostaining, the technique also should be useful for identifying the presence or absence of autoantibody if the known antigen fixed on the membrane is overlayered with human serum. Immunoblotting has the advantage of combining the resolution of gel electrophoresis with the specificity of antibody staining. This technique does not require a pure antigen for autoantibody detection because gel electrophoresis—either sodium dodecyl sulfate (SDS) gel electrophoresis or agarose gel electrophoresis—separates antigens from other proteins before reacting with specimens containing autoantibodies.

Immunoblotting also provides information about some of the characteristics of antigens that bind to the autoantibody. For example, the relative molecular weight of the monomer protein (the antigen) can be determined at the same time the protein itself is identified. To its detriment, immunoblotting is labor-intensive and requires both a skillful technologist and more sophisticated laboratory equipment. The procedure can only process a few specimens at a time and is unsuitable for a large number of specimens.

The procedure can be divided into 6 major steps: antigen preparation, gel electrophoresis, transfer of the separated proteins to a membrane support, blocking of nonspecific binding sites on the membrane, application of specimens, and visualization.

Cells or tissues containing the antigen of interest are first subjected to extraction with an appropriate buffer. In most cases, a crude extract can be run directly on a gel without further purification. However, if the antigen is one of the minor proteins at very low concentration, semipurification may be needed first to remove some of the major contaminant proteins from the extract. Before electrophoresis, the extract or concentrated extract should be dialyzed against the sample buffer designed for the particular electrophoresis system.

Agarose gel electrophoresis, polyacrylamide gel electrophoresis (PAGE), and isoelectrofocusing on agarose gel can be employed for the separation of an antigen from other proteins. It is well known that transferring proteins from agarose gel to a nitrocellulose membrane is easier and more quantitative because of the large pore size of the agarose gel. The SDS-PAGE system has been used frequently because of the superior resolution achieved. However, the resolution obtained with isoelectrofocusing is even better. Because all blotting techniques require a successful transfer of proteins from the gel, it is helpful to consider the pore size of the gel to be used. Usually, the lower the percentage of the acrylamide and crosslinker, the easier the transfer.

Nitrocellulose is the most commonly used membrane. Proteins can be transferred onto a nitrocellulose membrane either by a simple diffusion, vacuum-assisted solvent flow or by electrophoretic elution. Electrophoretic transfer is the most commonly used method and is highly recommended. The major advantage is its speed and the completeness of transfer.

Before sample application, it is essential to block the membrane to prevent nonspecific binding of autoantibody. Blocking can be achieved with a variety of protein or detergent solutions. Two blocking solutions that are compatible with nearly all detection systems are nonfat dried milk and BSA. The sample to be tested should be diluted with PBS containing protein (such as 3% BSA) at various concentrations.

Detection of the antigen-bound autoantibody band with enzyme-labeled antihuman antibodies from animals is the most popular method of visualization. Again, the autoantibody may not be IgG. Initially, both enzyme-conjugated antihuman IgG, IgM, and IgA should be tested.

Examples

Solimena et al,[11] using immunoblotting, were able to determine that the autoantibodies found in serum and cerebrospinal fluid from patients with stiff-man syndrome were against glutamic acid decarboxylase.

Gruber et al[2] also performed SDS-PAGE and immunoblotting for the detection of autoantibodies against mitochondria and microsomes.

Protein fractions of antigen preparations of mitochondria, microsomes, and "100,000 g" supernatant or cell lysates of HT-29 cells were separated by SDS-PAGE under reducing conditions, according to Laemmli et al.[16] The resolved proteins were blotted onto nitrocellulose paper, which was then incubated for 30 minutes at room temperature with patient sera (diluted 1:50 in PBS with 1% BSA). The paper was incubated with labeled rabbit antihuman IgG antiserum. Some blots were developed using enhanced chemiluminescence.

Summary

In this chapter, various methods for the detection of human autoantibodies have been described, including gel immunodiffusion, indirect immunofluorescence, enzyme immunoassay, and immunoblotting. In addition to describing the principles and characteristics of individual methods, the advantages, disadvantages, and sensitivity to various methods have also been discussed in detail. More than one example for each method is cited from the literature to illustrate how these methods were actually being applied clinically.

References

1. Nichols WS, Nakamura RM. Antibody patterns in autoimmune disease. *Lab Man*. 1984;9:39–47.
2. Gruber R, Felber E, Pape GR, et al. Detection of autoantibodies against M2, LKM-1, and SLA in liver diseases by standardized uniform ELISA-techniques. *J Clin Lab Anal*. 1994;8:284–292.
3. Van de Water J, Cooper A, Surh CD, et al. Detection of autoantibodies to recombinant mitochondrial proteins in patients with primary biliary cirrhosis. *N Engl J Med*. 1989;320:1377–1380.
4. Ohta M, Obayashi H, Ichimura T, et al. Immunological characterization of antibodies against synthetic peptides of glutamic acid decarboxylase. *Clin Chim Acta*. 1996;251:81–89.
5. Willoughby EW, Lambert A. A sensitive silver stain for proteins in agarose gels. *Anal Biochem*. 1983;130: 353–358.
6. Jaskowski TD, Schroder C, Martins TB, et al. Comparison of three commercially available enzyme immunoassays for the screening of autoantibodies to extractable nuclear antigens. *J Clin Lab Anal*. 1995;9: 166–172.
7. Gocke DJ, Howe C. Rapid detection of Australia antigen by counterimmunoelectrophoresis. *J Immunol*. 1970;104:1031–1032.
8. Delpech A, Gilbert D, Daliphard S, et al. Antibodies to Sm, RNP and SSB detected by solid-phase ELISAs using recombinant antigens: A comparison study with counter immunoelectrophoresis and immunoblotting. *J Clin Lab Anal*. 1993;7:197–202.
9. Satoh J, Prabhakar BS, Haspel MV, et al. Human monoclonal autoantibodies that react with multiple endocrine organs. *N Engl J Med*. 1983;309:217–220.
10. Takino H, Yoshimura T, Kawasaki E, et al. Immunoelectron microscopic localization of antigens which react with islet cell cytoplasmic antibodies within human pancreatic beta cells. *J Clin Lab Anal*. 1992;6:410–416.
11. Solimena M, Folli F, Denis-Donini S, et al. Autoantibodies to glutamic acid decarboxylase in a patient with stiff-man syndrome, epilepsy, and type I diabetes mellitus. *N Engl J Med*. 1988;318:1012–1020.
12. Konishi K, Hayashi M, Saruta T. Renal tubular acidosis with autoantibody directed to renal collecting-duct cells. *N Engl J Med*. 1994;331:1593–1594.
13. Dobersen MJ, Scharff JE, Ginsberg-Fellner F, et al. Cytotoxic autoantibodies to beta cells in the serum of patients with insulin-dependent diabetes mellitus. *N Engl J Med*. 1980;303:1493–1498.
14. Barbi G, Keil LB, Gaito AD, et al. Spectrotype distributions of circulating IgG from patients with systemic lupus erythematosus. *Clin Chem*. 1992;38: 1988-1994.
15. Karjalainen J, Martin JM, Knip M, et al. A bovine albumin peptide as a possible trigger of insulin-dependent diabetes mellitus. *N Engl J Med*. 1992;327: 302–307.
16. Laemmli UK. Cleavage of structural proteins during the assembly of the head of bacteriophage T4. *Nature*. 1970;227:680–684.

CHAPTER 28

The Introduction of New Tests to the Clinical Laboratory

Helene M.A. Paxton, PhD, MS, MT

The introduction of a "new" clinical test by the laboratory is determined by how the test is to be used and by its current regulatory status and device classification. A new test can be (1) a totally different analyte, (2) a modification of a previous test, (3) a change in the type of specimen required, (4) a change from a manual test to an automated one, or (5) a new method.[1] The intended use of the test or how it is to be employed in the management of patients largely regulates the amount of validation to which it must be subjected before use (eg, the inherent risk to the patient of reporting the test result).

The laboratory ultimately controls how a test is used and marketed to its physician base. Therefore, the laws governing the laboratory are the determinants by which a new test is introduced. The Department of Health and Human Services, Health Care Financing Administration Public Health Service regulation called the Clinical Laboratory Improvement Amendments of 1988; Final Rule (CLIA), 42 CFR Part 405[2] is the latest set of regulations affecting the laboratory.

Test of Moderate Complexity

If a new test is of moderate complexity as defined by CLIA and is cleared by the Food and Drug Administration (FDA) for in vitro diagnostic use, the laboratory only needs to meet the quality control and quality assurance parameters designated in the manufacturer's package insert and the requirements for a test of moderate complexity as defined by CLIA. One of the CLIA requirements is that the laboratory needs to participate in an external proficiency testing program deemed by CLIA as acceptable for the analyte in question. If a proficiency test is unavailable, the laboratory must split samples with another laboratory to ensure comparability. Laboratories may need to take specific action on other aspects of the quality assurance rules and are urged to review the appropriate specialty checklist for compliance.

A particularly difficult parameter, even in moderate complexity tests, is the establishment of normal ranges and the validation of analyte ranges. This requirement is the most problematic, because it is cumbersome and costly for many small laboratories. Many laboratories ask whether they may use published normal reference ranges found in the package insert or in peer-reviewed journals for their normal range if they cannot perform a normal range study to satisfy the statistical requirements. The answer is complex.

By strict standards, a laboratory needs to establish its own normal ranges and validate its analyte ranges based on its ethnic population base; therefore, it should run the test on a normal set of sera defined by a set of currently healthy blood donors. The sera should include the entire adult age range as well as pediatric populations (not found in blood donors). Autoimmune tests are especially sensitive to age-related normal ranges because some analytes occur with increasing frequency in older individuals. It is suggested that normal range studies be subdivided by decades and include an approximately equal number of men and women as appropriate for the test in question. Ethnic diversity becomes problematic for laboratories doing studies that extend across state lines. Therefore, it is suggested that such laboratories arrange for the appropriate collection of "normal samples" across their service areas with their participating clients. In all cases, the normal range studies performed by individual laboratories must contain enough samples to be statistically significant, and findings should be compared with published normal ranges for the analyte whenever possible.

Issues of prevalence (number of patients per 100,000 who have the disease at the time of the study) and incidence of disease (number of cases in a given year per 100,000) may need to be considered. Prevalence equals incidence multiplied by duration of disease. When considering autoimmune diseases, there is generally a high prevalence rate even though the incidence in the general population is low because such diseases are chronic and last each patient's lifetime.

Age groups may be critically important to setting appropriate analyte ranges. Furthermore, when comparing ranges between 2 tests measuring the same analyte, the methodologies should be similar because different methods often yield different values and have different thresholds of sensitivity. Other quality control issues of precision, accuracy, and test performance criteria are well defined in the regulations and are not discussed here.

Test of High Complexity or "Home Brews"

Many of the assays discussed in this book are not likely to be FDA approved or to have a defined FDA classification status. The 1976 Medical Device Amendment[3] placed most analytes in 3 regulatory classifications that are based on their inherent safety and effectiveness and perceived risk. "New analytes" are unclassified and by definition class III (high risk) until classified otherwise by the FDA. These analytes generally fall in the "home brew" category. Furthermore, such analytes are considered high-complexity tests by CLIA and are often marketed by diagnostic companies, if available commercially, as "research use only" (RUO) tests.

Limits are being placed on these RUOs by the new compliance document being generated by the FDA. This Compliance Policy Guide (CPG) will affect both RUO and investigational-use-only devices.[4] High-complexity tests that have not been cleared by the FDA or cleared moderate- or high-complexity tests that have been modified by the user (another type of home brew) must follow the CLIA Subpart K rule.[2]

A new FDA category of reagents, known as analyte specific reagents (ASRs), are now available and by definition are considered home brews.[5] The ASRs include under a single regulation those pre-1976 devices that were not classified previously and post-1976 devices, many of which were home brews. The regulation was finalized and became effective November 23, 1998; it is expected to simplify requirements for most low-risk products. The drawback is that the FDA will now have jurisdiction over home brews and thus will be involved in the regulation of laboratories, especially those involved in interstate commerce. However, the risk of such inspections is minimal due to the staff shortage at the FDA. Laboratories should be careful in their advertising claims for such test offerings because the FDA will inspect false claims, which are viewed as a risk to patients.

The positive side of the ASR rule is that it should allow more consistency in the quality of manufacturing of the components of home brew tests due to manufacturers' adherence to good manufacturing practices and certain labeling requirements. Manufacturers cannot give laboratories "intended use" or clinical information with regard to these reagents, and laboratories must include a disclaimer in patient reports when using an ASR in a home brew test.

Things to Consider Before Starting

Before test validation can begin, it must be determined whether the new test will be qualitative (positive/negative readout) or quantitative, and whether it is a screening test or a monitoring test, because the stringency standards for performance vary by type. The laboratory and clinicians using the test must clearly understand the differences between these types of assays.

They also must have some idea as to the pretest probability (prevalence in the population); that is, tests with good sensitivity (80%) and specificity (90%) where there is only a 1% chance of disease in the population—those with a positive assay will still have only a 7.5% probability of having the disease. Disease prevalence is frequently not taken into account when a new test is introduced. This failure has sometimes led to inappropriate and unnecessary testing.

In a screening test, the sensitivity must be high and the specificity can be lower, although these parameters must be adjusted based on the clinical impact and medical risk of false positives and false negatives (ie, how many false positives or false negatives are acceptable to those using the tests). These can be costly as well as controversial decisions, as in screening tests for prostate specific antigen or breast cancer. If a test is used for monitoring (pretest probability of disease is high), the test must have high specificity and high precision and thus have high predictive value (posttest probability). The test sensitivity can be lower because the patient population is well defined.[6,7]

If a test is designated for screening purposes, it is presumed that a confirmatory test is available. Customarily, only those patients who are positive on a screening test are retested by the confirmatory test and are not considered true positives unless the initial test is confirmed. It should be obvious that some false-positive samples are acceptable in a screening test, but false negatives are not; false positives will be confirmed, whereas false negatives will not be retested and will be missed—resulting in an incorrect diagnosis.

Sensitivity and specificity generally are not changeable in a qualitative test except by between-run variability by the user, but the manufacturer may change the threshold value, affecting the sensitivity and specificity of the test. In a quantitative test, the threshold of a test's positivity can be changed by the user. This again affects the sensitivity and specificity and is critical in defining analytic and significant ranges for patient management.

The Laboratory's Responsibility

When introducing a new high-complexity test, the laboratory must define the test's intended use and the analyte being measured; the patient sample requirements, sample collection, storage, and preservation; reportable ranges for patients; and a step-by-step protocol. This protocol should include, as appropriate:

- Test performance or instrument operation instructions
- Test system maintenance procedures
- Preparation and storage of reagents
- Calibrators, controls, and other materials used in testing
- Control procedures, including the type of materials and frequency of assay
- Calibration procedures, including the type of materials (reference preparations) and frequency of assay
- A definition of acceptable reporting units
- Actions to be taken if calibration or control results do not meet the acceptable range of values
- The correct interpretation of test end points
- The course of action when the test becomes inoperable
- The course of action when the test end point cannot be determined (eg, it is beyond linearity, or below the lowest threshold)[8]
- Confidence limits, tolerance limits, coefficients of variation, standard deviations, and precision parameters that must be determined and recorded

Method accuracy studies should illustrate that the test system is not affected by systematic error when using the following:

- Reference materials assayed by several study participants generating data that prove there is no statistically significant difference between the test results and the value of the reference material
- Patient samples instead of reference materials, proving that there is no statistically significant difference between test results obtained on patient reference material due to the effects of sample matrix
- Patient samples containing common interfering substances, proving there is no introduction of error in the presence of these substances

Statistical treatment of data must reflect the intended use of the test and take into consideration the type of data generated. Questions to be asked include

- Do the data reflect a "normal distribution" (parametric) or are the data nonparametric?
- What is the best comparison between the 2 tests (do the tests have the same median) if there are 2 tests to compare, as in modifications, changes in sample, or automation?

The appropriate sensitivity and specificity values must be generated and compared with previous analytes or gold standards.[6]

Introducing the New Test

It is clear from this discussion that bringing a new test to the laboratory is no longer a simple task and is fraught with regulatory and validation pitfalls. The laboratory has to further consider the marketing and cost of the test both as a basis for revenue and cost for the patient (whether the test is reimbursable). If it is considered a home brew or a research test, reimbursement by Medicare may be impossible. Is the test safe and effective? Is it acceptable in the medical community? It is important for the laboratory to remember there may not be agreement between or even within state and federal agencies. The laboratory as the provider must challenge its own state agencies and be prepared to defend the test's clinical utility with good prevalence data, the diagnostic power of the test result, and the relevance of results to patient management in order to get payment. In an age of contained medical costs and health care management, this is a most difficult task.

References

1. National Committee for Clinical Laboratory Standards. *Glossary and Guidelines for Procedures, Reagents and Reference Materials*. Approved Guidelines, NCCLS publication DL1-A. Villanova, PA: NCCLS; 1986.
2. Health Care Financing Administration. Medicare, Medicaid and CLIA Programs: Clinical Laboratory Improvement Amendments of 1988; Final Rule (42 CFR Part 405). *Federal Register*. February 2, 1992;57:7002–7186.
3. Department of Health and Human Services. Medical Device Amendments of 1976, 21 USC 360c(a)(1); 21 CFR Parts 809 and 864. *Federal Register*. March 14, 1996;61:10484–14489.
4. US Food and Drug Administration. *FDA Compliance Policy Guide on Commercialization of Research and Investigational Use In Vitro Diagnostic Devices*. Washington, DC: FDA; January 5, 1998.
5. Medical Devices; Classification/Reclassification; Restricted Devices; Analyte Specific Reagents, 21 CFR Parts 809 and 864. *Federal Register*. November 21, 1997;62:62243–62260.
6. Galen RS, Gambino SR. Sensitivity, specificity, prevalence and incidence. In: *Beyond Normality. The Predictive Value and Efficiency of Medical Diagnoses*. New York, NY: John Wiley & Sons; 1975:9–14.
7. Riegelman RK, Hirsh RP. Diagnostic discrimination of tests. In: *Studying a Study and Testing a Test*. 2nd ed. Boston, MA: Little Brown & Company; 1989:151–163.
8. Public Health Service. Letter concerning moratorium of classifying laboratory testing devices as waived tests. Guidelines for requesting waivers. December 19, 1994.

CHAPTER 29

Current Status of Standards and Control Materials for Laboratory Tests

Robert M. Nakamura, MD

Several organizations are involved in standards and reference preparations for use in clinical diagnostics. Those in the United States include the National Committee for Clinical Laboratory Standards (NCCLS), College of American Pathologists (CAP), Centers for Disease Control and Prevention (CDC), Arthritis Foundation (AF), American Association of Clinical Chemists, and Biological Response Modifier's Program of the National Cancer Institute. International organizations involved in reference preparations are the World Health Organization (WHO); National Institute of Biological Standards and Control of the United Kingdom; International Union of Immunological Societies (IUIS); United Kingdom External Quality Assessment Schemes for Autoimmune Serology and Special Immunochemistry; International Laboratory for Biological Standards of the Netherlands; Community Bureau of Reference (BCR), Belgium; and International Federation of Clinical Chemistry (IFCC).

Few written source materials are available on this subject. The CAP prepared a document titled *Standards, Reference Materials and Method—A Practical Guide to the Medical Laboratory*, the last edition of which was published in 1984. In January 1994, the NCCLS, in cooperation with CAP and its National Reference System for Clinical Laboratory (NRSCL) Council, produced a sourcebook that compiled information on methods and materials useful to the general clinical laboratory: *Sourcebook of Reference Methods, Materials, and Related Information for the Clinical Laboratory; Proposed Guideline* (NCCLS Document NRSCL 12-P Vol. 14 No. 1).

This chapter discusses some of the available reference materials that may be useful to the clinical diagnostic laboratory. Other useful reference materials and calibrators are highlighted in chapters that discuss specific assays.

Definitions and Nomenclature

Before examining the reference materials, it is necessary to establish the universal terminology used in association with these materials.[1–3] Important terms include the following:

- WHO international standards. An international unit has been assigned to each of these standards for biologic substances. Member states have agreed to subject such substances to national quality control measures and to express the potency of the substances in international units or their equivalents.
- WHO international reference preparations. International units may or may not be assigned to these preparations, which are biologic substances provided as a service but for which national quality control measures have not been agreed on as obligatory.
- WHO international reference reagents. High-specificity reagents for qualitative use in identification.
- National standards. These standards have designated unitage calibrated in terms of WHO international standards or international reference preparations.
- WHO reference laboratories working standards (international or national). These materials are often the same as the WHO international standards or the national standards, with unitage directly related to these.

Other standards (eg, manufacturers' standards, research laboratory standards) may have provisional units designated by the source laboratory if no units exist.

The International Standards Organization has the following additional definitions:

- Reference material (RM). A material or substance, one or more properties of which are sufficiently well established to be used for the calibration of an apparatus or for the verification of a measurement method. A reference material is intended to transfer the value of measured quantity (physical, chemical, biologic, technologic) between one place and another. It may be in the form of a pure or mixed gas, liquid, or solid, or even a simple manufactured object.
- Certified reference material. An RM accompanied by, or traceable to, a certificate stating the property value(s) concerned, issued by an organization that is generally accepted as technically competent.

Once specifications for a standard or reference material have been established, a pool of sufficient material should be collected. The minimum number of ampoules in the pool should be 4,000 for an international standard or reference preparation.[4] It is generally agreed that for worldwide use and ease of transportation, a standard should be lyophilized.

Four principal criteria should be satisfied before a preparation can be defined as a biologic reference material[5]:

- The preparation should be as pure as possible.
- The preparation should be stable.

- The preparation should have specific activity.
- Specific activity should be definable in units, where possible.

Units of Measurement

The assignment of international units (IU) as applied to biologic materials is completely arbitrary. For any given substance, an IU is continuous and represents the same amount of activity with each succeeding standard. This is ensured by comparing the new standard with the old in an international collaborative assay and by assigning unitage to the new standard. By expressing the activity of a new standard in terms of that of the old standard, the activity of one unit of the material remains the same even though the weight of dried material that contains this activity in the new standard is likely to be different.[6]

International units have been assigned to initial reference preparations for immunoglobulins (Igs). The IU of IgG has, by definition, the same activity as 0.8147 mg of the dry powder present in an ampoule of the international research standard for human serum Igs G, M, and A. Of course, no one would try to weigh out this amount, but the total contents of the ampoule would be reconstituted in a suitable volume of diluent with the knowledge that this volume contains 100 IU of IgG. An IU of IgE, on the other hand, has the same activity as is present in 0.006562 mg of the dry powder in an ampoule of the international reference preparation of human serum IgE. Accepting the arbitrary nature of units, it also must be accepted that—just as there is no relationship between units of length and mass—there is no relationship between the unit of a specific antigen or antibody and the unit of a second different antigen or antibody.[6]

Reference Preparations for Autoantibodies to Nuclear and Intracellular Antigens

ANA (Homogeneous WHO 66/33)

In 1971, Anderson et al[7] reported on a collaborative international study of a proposed research standard for antinuclear factor 66/33 (homogeneous). This material was adopted by the WHO and the IUIS as an international reference preparation. Each ampoule was defined to contain 100 IU. After dilution of the contents in 1 mL of liquid, a concentration of 100 IU/mL is obtained. **Table 29-1** indicates where this and other standards and reference materials may be obtained.

Several groups of researchers[3,7,13] have recommended the use of WHO 66/33 as follows: If the determined end point of the WHO standard 66/33 is 1:160 in a particular laboratory, the end point dilution contains 1/160 × 100 IU/mL = 0.625 IU/mL. (The undiluted 66/33 contains 100 IU/mL.)

For another laboratory with another system, the end point might represent fewer or more IU/mL of antinuclear antibody (ANA) activity. The differences among laboratories and systems may be nullified by expressing results of test sera in IU/mL calculated by multiplying the reciprocals of their dilutions at their titration end points by the number of units of activity present in the reference preparation at its titration end point in the particular laboratory.

The WHO 66/33 standard has been available since 1970, but its use is not widespread. There are several reasons:

- WHO 66/33 is probably an inappropriate reference for speckled or other patterns of nuclear fluorescence.
- The ANA titer is dependent on total antibody content and antibody avidity. Sera with similar total amounts of antibody but varying avidity may give different end points.
- WHO 66/33 contains mostly IgG ANA and is thus best used in comparing test sera containing ANA activity of the IgG class.
- Many laboratories use the immunofluorescence antinuclear antibody (IFM-ANA) screening test for ANA. Quantitative results often are obtained by testing one or two serum dilutions, such as 1:20 and 1:160, indicating the intensity of fluorescence.[3]

Feltkamp et al[14] did a collaborative laboratory study with the use of WHO 66/33. The study showed an improvement of interlaboratory comparability for the homogeneous fluorescence pattern when the common reference standard was used. Molden et al[15] showed that IFM-ANA tests can be monitored with the use of AF/CDC reference sera of defined antibody specificities.

WHO/IUIS IgM Class ANA

The IUIS immunofluorescence committee, established in 1971, was instrumental in developing a reference serum containing ANA of the IgM class

Table 29-1. Places to Obtain Standards, Reference Preparations, and Source Materials

Materials	Source
WHO (antinuclear factor 66/233 [homogeneous])	Central Laboratory of the Netherlands Red Cross Blood Transfusion Service, Plesmanlaan, 125, Amsterdam, the Netherlands
FITC-labeled sheep antihuman Ig (480010), FITC-labeled sheep antihuman IgM (anti-mu chain), and IgM class ANA (HL)	WHO Immunology Unit, Unit 1211, Geneva 28, Switzerland[8, 9]
WHO/IUIS 480010 conjugate	WHO Immunology Unit, Unit 1211, Geneva 28, Switzerland[3]
Wo/80 and other WHO standards	Central Laboratory of the Netherlands, Red Cross Blood Transfusion Service, Plesmanlaan, 125 Amsterdam, the Netherlands[8] or Department of Reagents CLB, PO Box 9190, 1006 AD Amsterdam, the Netherlands[10]
CAP reference preparation (lot #C103BG) for anti-SS-A/Ro	College of American Pathologists, 325 Waukegan Road, Northfield, IL 60093-2750
RPPHS (CAP/BCR/IFCC)	College of American Pathologists, 325 Waukegan Road, Northfield, IL 60093-2750 or Community Bureau of Reference, Commission of the European Community, 200, Rue de la Loi, 1049 Bruxelles, Belgium
Antiphospholipid antibody standards	E. Nigel Harris, M. Phil., M.D., Division of Rheumatology, Department of Medicine, University of Louisville, KY 40292; (current address) Morehouse School of Medicine, 720 Westview Drive Southwest, Atlanta, GA 30310-1495[11,12]
Primary standard calibrators for IgG anti–β_2-GPI	Vincent A. De Bari, M.D., St. Joseph's Hospital and Medical Center, 703 Main Street, Paterson, NJ 0750
Standards NIBS 66/387 (antithyroid microsome serum) and WHO ECBS 1979 (antithyroglobulin reference standard)	National Institute for Biological Standards and Control, Holly Hill, Hampstead, London, NW3 6RB, United Kingdom
Standards to various human cytokines (information and materials)	National Institute of Biological Standards and Control, PO Box 1193, Potters Bar EN6 3QH, United Kingdom
Reference reagents for murine and human cytokines	Dr Craig W. Reynolds, Biological Response Modifiers Program, NCI-FCRDC, Building 1052, Room 253, Frederick, MD 21702-1201
WHO standard for C-reactive protein 1986 (85/506); WHO 106 international reference human serum for smooth muscle (antiactin) antibody; WHO 1066 human rheumatoid arthritis serum (rheumatoid factor)	International Laboratory for Biological Standards, Central Laboratory, Netherlands Red Cross Blood Transfusion Service, Plesmanlaan 125, Amsterdam, the Netherlands[8,10]
Autoantibodies 64/2 (first British standard for rheumatoid serum, human); 64/93 (antithyroglobulin serum, human); 66/387 (antithyroid microsome serum, human); 67183 (primary biliary cirrhosis serum, human); 90/656 (cardiolipin antibody)	National Institute of Biological Standards and Control, Blanche Lane, South Mimms, Potters Bar EN6 30G, United Kingdom[10]

Abbreviations: WHO = World Health Organization; FITC = fluorescein isothiocyanate; IUIS = International Union of Immunological Societies; CAP = College of American Pathologists; RPPHS = reference preparations for protein in human serum; BCR = Community Bureau of Reference (Belgium); IFCC = International Federation of Clinical Chemistry; Ig = immunoglobulin; β_2-GPI = β_2-glycoprotein I; ECBS = Expert Committee on Biological Standardization.

(HL, containing heavy and light chains). A freeze-dried batch of ANA-positive serum was pooled from six patients with systemic lupus erythematosus.[8,9] The ampoule contained 100 arbitrary units of ANA activity as lyophilized serum. The end point was the highest dilution showing the minimal nuclear staining distinguishable from a negative reaction.

WHO/IUIS 480010

The IUIS committee also helped to develop two WHO/IUIS international fluorescein isothiocyanate (FITC)–conjugated antibody preparations, which are used in IFM-ANA test methods. The quality of the conjugate is extremely important for accurate diagnostic results. The Medical Research Council of the United Kingdom assembled a working party to define the specifications of the preparation, conjugation, and characterization of fluorescent conjugates.[16] Subsequently, the IUIS standardization committee encouraged development of the sheep antihuman Ig conjugate 480010 and helped conduct an international collaborative study with the WHO reference standard 66/33.

The 480010 conjugate was submitted to the WHO Expert Advisory Panel on Biological Standardization as an international standard and was accepted as such by WHO and IUIS. Each 0.5-mL ampoule of 480010 is defined as containing 100 IU/500 µL (or 200 IU/mL).

The quality of the conjugate is based on its specificity and potency performance. The conjugate 480010 was prepared from an antiserum raised by immunization with human IgG and human $F(ab')_2$, which resulted in strong anti-IgG and good reactivity with IgM and IgA. The conjugate reacts with heavy and light chains of IgG and with the light chains of IgM and IgA.

The potency of the conjugate is assessed by the presence of dilutions of conjugates against dilutions of the same middle layers of serum in a chessboard titration on a tissue substrate. A good conjugate should give a constant titer for the middle layer serum over a wide range of conjugate dilutions. The constant end point dilution of the middle layer is the plateau titer and the highest conjugate dilution at which the plateau titer is maintained is the plateau end point of the conjugate.[17] The working dilution of a conjugate is at least twice the concentration at the plateau end point.

Standard preparations of FITC-conjugated anti-IgM and anti-IgG also have been prepared and accepted by WHO and IUIS. Both standards contain 100 IU/ampoule.

WHO Standard for Antibodies to Double-Stranded DNA

In 1988, Feltkamp and coworkers[18] developed the first international standard for antibodies to double-stranded DNA (dsDNA) antibodies, coded Wo/80. The Wo/80 sera were obtained after recalcification of plasma taken from a patient with systemic lupus erythematosus. Vials were filled with 500 µL of serum and lyophilized. The specimens contained no other autoantibodies in measurable quantities.

The Wo/80 serum vials were tested in 8 laboratories by the immunofluorescence technique for *Crithidia lucidiae*. The titers varied between 1:20 and 1:640 (mean, 1:160). In 7 laboratories, the Farr assay for DNA antibodies with the Amersham kit also was performed on the Wo/80 specimens. At a dilution of 1:40, a mean binding percentage of about 50% was observed. After reconstitution with 500 µL of distilled water, the vials were labeled to contain 100 IU/500 µL or 200 IU/mL.

AF/CDC Reference Sera for Autoantibodies to Nuclear and Intracellular Antigens

In 1980, the AF, in collaboration with the CDC, established the Committee on Antinuclear Antibody Serology.[19–21] The committee was to establish a repository of ANA reference sera to be made available to researchers and clinical laboratories in the United States and other countries. The ANA reference reagents were intended to serve as primary reference standards defining ANA specificities and be used by clinical laboratories to define their own secondary reference reagents.

In 1982, the committee AF/CDC prepared and assayed reference preparations using the methods listed in **Table 29-2**. The 5 reference sera provided reference reagents for ANAs defined in the following terms:

- Three patterns of fluorescent antinuclear antibodies: homogeneous/rim pattern and 2 different speckled nucleoplasmic patterns
- Four different antinuclear antibodies identified by immunodiffusion analysis: antibodies to native DNA, SS-B/La, nuclear ribonucleoprotein (nRNP), and Sm

The bank of reference reagents at the AF/CDC laboratory was expanded to include 5 more reference

Table 29-2. ANA Reference Sera Established by the AF/CDC[19,20]*

Analytes	Assay Method	Assay Readout	Specificities of Reference Sera				
			CDC1 FANA and Anti-nDNA	CDC2 FANA and Anti–SS-B/La	CDC3 FANA Only	CDC4 Anti-nRNP Only	CDC5 Anti-Sm Only
ANA	Immuno-fluorescence microscopy	Pattern titer	H/R 1:5:512 (1:160-1:640)	Sp 1:160 (1:80-1:320)	Sp 1:320 (1:180-1:640)		
Anti-nDNA	Millipore filter Farr assay *Crithidia lucidiae*	%DNA-bound DNA-bound Titer	74% (64%-82%) 85% (75%-95%) 1:90 (1:180-1:320)				
ANA-SS-B/La	Immunodiffusion	Titer		1:40 (1:16-1:80)			
ANA-nRNP	Immunodiffusion	Titer				1:64 (1:32-1:80)	
Anti-Sm	Immunodiffusion	Titer					1:64 (1:32-1:64)

Abbreviations: ANA = antinuclear antibodies; AF/CDC = Arthritis Foundation/Centers for Disease Control and Prevention; FANA = fluorescence ANA; nDNA = nuclear DNA; nRNP = nuclear ribonucleoprotein; H/R = homogeneous/rim; Sp = speckled pattern.
**Results show the median value with range of values.*

ANAs,[20,21] which were processed and analyzed in the same way as the first 5 reagents. The reference reagents were made available in 1988 and are described in **Table 29-3**.

As of June 1994, a total of 1,598 laboratories from 58 different countries had received AF/CDC ANA reference sera (Byrd MG, personal communication, 1994). These preparations have been of great value to researchers and clinical laboratories in the standardization of IFM-ANA. Those with defined specificities for dsDNA, SS-B/La, nRNP, and Sm were compared with the commonly used IFM-ANA substrates, including mouse kidney sections and human epithelial (HEp-2) tissue culture cells. Use of the reference sera was recommended for IFM-ANA testing.[15,22,23]

In October 1992, the AF/CDC committee was reorganized and is now called the IUIS-ANA subcommittee. Participating organizations include the CDC, AF, WHO, Internal League Against Rheumatism, and the European League Against Rheumatism.[8,24,25]

Table 29-3. Reference Antinuclear Antibodies Available From the AF/CDC ANA Reference Laboratory[20,21]

Reagent	Immunologic Features
AF/CDC1	Homogeneous pattern ANA (doubles as antinative DNA)
AF/CDC2	Anti-La (SS-B)
AF/CDC3	Speckled pattern ANA
AF/CDC4	Anti-U_1RNP (U_1 small nuclear RNP)
AF/CDC5	Anti-Sm (U_1, U_2, U_5, $U_{4/6}$, small nuclear RNP)
AF/CDC6	Nucleolar pattern ANA
AF/CDC7	Anti–SS-A/Ro
AF/CDC8	Centromere-pattern ANA
AF/CDC9	Anti–Scl-70 (DNA topoisomerase 1)
AF/CDC10	Anti–Jo-1 (histidyl-transfer RNA synthetase)

Abbreviations: ANA = antinuclear antibodies; U_1RNP = uridine-rich ribonucleoprotein.

College of American Pathologists Reference Serum for Anti–SS-A/Ro Antibodies

In 1991, the College of American Pathologists' Standards Committee and Immunology Resource Committee prepared a monospecific reference serum containing only anti–SS-A/Ro nuclear antibody.[26] This reference preparation (lot #C103BG) has an assigned value of positive immunodiffusion precipitin antibody to SS-A/Ro and a positive range of titer of 1:4 to 1:32. This reference serum should be used to test IFM-ANA substrate cell lots for the presence of the SS-A/Ro antigen. In addition, the monospecific anti–SS-A/Ro reference serum can be used for specific identification of unknown anti–SS-A/Ro by immunodiffusion analyses.

Reference Preparations for Serum Proteins

The WHO, with various collaborating organizations, has developed reference preparations for IgG, IgA, IgM, and IgE,[27,28] which were initially expressed in international units.[6] In the late 1970s, Reimer et al[28] prepared a reference material for human serum proteins. This material was lyophilized in vaccine vials and became first the CDC/USNRP (US National Reference Preparation) and then the WHO Reference Preparation for Six Human Serum Proteins (WHO 6HSP).[29] International units were arbitrarily assigned to WHO 6HSP for 6 proteins (albumin, α_1-antitrypsin, ceruloplasmin, α_2-macroglobulin, transferrin, and C3 component of complement).

In collaboration with the CDC, the CAP produced a series of reference preparations for serum proteins (RPSP-1 to RPSP-4) and assigned mass units to them.[30] During the process of preparing RPSP-1 to RPSP-3, a "drift of values" was assigned by consensus against the preceding reference material. RPSP-4 was assigned values similar to the final and currently accepted reference preparations for protein in human serum (RPPHS). This project was a collaborative effort of the BCR, IFCC, and CAP.

The RPPHS was prepared from pooled human serum (obtained from 364 healthy donors), which had been clarified to eliminate lipoprotein.[31,32] It contained sodium azide (1.0 g/L), benzamidine chloride (0.157 g/L), and aprotinin (80,000 IU/L) as preservatives. After microfiltration and filling, the material was freeze-dried, resulting in a mean weight of 71.8 mg lyophilizate per vial with a mean residual moisture of 0.57%. The intended use of the product was for standardization of the 14 serum proteins listed in **Table 29-4**.

The concentrations of the 14 proteins contained in this material were assigned using existing international and national reference preparations and purified

Table 29-4. Human Serum Proteins[31,32]

Analyte	Assigned Value (g/L)	95% CI (g/L)	International Units (IU/ML)	95% CI (IU/ML)
Immunoglobulin A	1.96	1.92-2.00	125	(122.4-127.6)*
Immunoglobulin G	9.68	9.58-9.78	117	(115.8-118.2)
Immunoglobulin M	0.797	0.774-0.820	105	(102-108)
Complement C3	1.091	1.064-1.118	89	79-99
Complement C4	0.151	0.146-0.156	60	(58-62)
Albumin	39.7	38.9-40.5	97	93-101
α_1-Antitrypsin	1.206	1.195-1.217	91	87-95
α_1-Acid glycoprotein	0.656	0.651-0.661	NA	
α_2-Macroglobulin	1.64	1.59-1.69	79	75-83
Haptoglobin	0.893	0.884-0.902	NA	
Transferrin	2.45	2.39-2.51	100	96-104
Ceruloplasmin	0.205	0.194-0.216	67	57-77
Prealbumin	0.243	0.225-0.261	NA	
C-reactive protein	0.0392	0.0373-0.0411	0.0392	0.0373-0.0411

Abbreviations: CI = confidence interval NA = not applicable (no WHO reference available).
**Values in parentheses are calculated using the uncertainty for g/L. Separate standards of deviation were not done for international units.*

proteins.[31,32] The mass/volume values for IgA, IgG, IgM, C3, C4, albumin, α_2-macroglobulin, haptoglobin, and ceruloplasmin were assigned from the CDC's US National Reference Preparation for Human Serum Proteins (USNRP—120575/C); those for C-reactive protein were from the WHO's First International Standard for Human C-Reactive Protein (85/506); and those for prealbumin (transthyretin), α_1-antitrypsin, α_1-acid glycoprotein (orosomucoid), and transferrin were from highly purified proteins. For α_1-antitrypsin, α_1-acid glycoprotein (orosomucoid), and transferrin, values based on the USNRP were also given for comparison purposes.

International units for IgA, IgG, and IgM were assigned from the WHO International Reference Preparation for Human Serum Immunoglobulins (67/86); those for C3, albumin, α_2-macroglobulin, and ceruloplasmin came from the WHO International Reference Preparation for six Human Serum Proteins (4/2); and those for C4 came from the WHO First Reference Preparation for Complement Components (5/4).

The values for prealbumin (transthyretin), α_1-antitrypsin, α_2-acid glycoprotein (orosomucoid), and transferrin were assigned from purified proteins because the values in the USNRP are now different from those currently accepted by the scientific community or, in the case of prealbumin, were never established.

Value transfer is based on the linear relationship of several dilutions of the reference material in which the overall regression is used to determine the ratio of concentrations. The slope of regression is then used to assign the values for the proteins. The value assignment was undertaken by collaborating laboratories in Europe, Japan, and the United States. The methods employed were nephelometry and turbidimetry, using a variety of instruments.[31,32]

Antiphospholipid Antibodies

The detection of autoantibodies to cardiolipin is an established method for assessing the risk of thrombosis in antiphospholipid antibody syndrome. Data have indicated that anticardiolipin antibodies in patients with this syndrome are directed against epitopes on the phospholipid binding plasma protein β_2-glycoprotein I (β_2-GPI).[33–36] The conventional anticardiolipin enzyme assays thus detect antibodies to 2 specificities: autoantibodies directed against β_2-GPI, and β_2-GPI independent anticardiolipin.[37–39] Tincani et al[40] have shown that anti–β_2-GPI autoantibodies in human antiphospholipid syndrome sera are directed to epitopes located on native β_2-glycoprotein and preserved during species evolution.

Assays are being developed to detect specific autoantibodies to β_2-GPI in patients suspected of thrombosis with the antiphospholipid syndrome. Erickson et al[41] described a reference calibrator for IgG antibodies to β_2-GPI.

Autoantibodies to Thyroperoxidase and Thyroglobulin

At the 1995 National Association of Clinical Biochemists Symposium, Feldt-Rasmussen[42] reported on the analytic and clinical performance goals for testing autoantibodies to thyroperoxidase, thyroglobulin, and thyrotropin receptor. According to that report, thyroperoxidase antibody results in quantitative international units; she employed a standard from the Medical Research Council 66/387, a serum containing thyroid microsomal antibody, with each vial containing 3,000 IU.

In a previous study, Groves et al[43] reported on primary standardization for the enzyme-linked immunosorbent assay (ELISA) of serum thyroperoxidase and thyroglobulin antibodies.

The standards NIBS 66/387 "antithyroid microsome serum," and WHO Expert Committee on Biological Standardization (ECBS) 1979 "antithyroglobulin reference standard" were obtained from the National Institute for Biological Standards and Control (see Table 29-1).

Antineutrophilic Cytoplasmic Antibodies

In 1989, Wiik[44] outlined a standard indirect immunofluorescence procedure for the detection of antineutrophilic cytoplasmic antibodies (ANCAs). There have been 2 international cooperative studies to evaluate the value of indirect immunofluorescence and solid phase techniques for ANCA detection. The first study[45] concluded that the indirect immunofluorescence procedure showed comparable results using strongly positive sera, even though the studies were performed with different methods.

The second study was conducted to help standardize solid phase enzyme types of assays for ANCAs. It was concluded that purified proteinase-3 and purified myeloperoxidase can be used in standardized ELISAs for ANCA detection.[46] The study used 3 purified preparations of proteinase-3 and 1 preparation of purified myeloperoxidase. It showed that ELISAs using purified proteinase-3 and myeloperoxidase can be standardized to a coefficient of variation of approximately 20% and 34%, respectively, between different testing laboratories.[46] The indirect immunofluorescence test results were comparable in terms of positivity and negativity and staining patterns, but not in respect to quantitative titers.

Islet Cell Antibody Assays

An international workshop was begun in 1985 to standardize the islet cell antibody (ICA) assay.[47] In this first workshop, analyses of coded serum samples from diabetic patients revealed that the detection limits and titer levels varied markedly between laboratories for identical serum samples. One sample of a high-titer serum, which was read as positive by all the participating laboratories, was selected to serve as an international reference serum.[48] In a second workshop, the use of a standard serum improved standardization and precision in the ICA assay.[49] In this workshop, arbitrary values of 5, 10, 20, 40, and 80 JDF units were assigned to 1:16, 1:8, 1:4, and 1:2 dilutions and a neat sample of the standard serum. A standard curve was used to correct reported results to JDF units.[49] The third[50] and fourth[51] workshops demonstrated that the use of a JDF unit standard improved the ICA assay quantitation and precision. The results from the fourth workshop also demonstrated excellent specificity, good concordance, and an ability to separate control sera from defined type 1 diabetes–related subjects.[51] Workshop serum samples were lyophilized at the University of Florida at Gainesville, coded, and sent to 47 participating laboratories worldwide.

There are many different methods, substrates, and procedure variations in indirect immunofluorescence tests for islet cell antibodies. Landin-Olsson[52] presented evidence that the precision of the islet cell antibody assay depends on the individual tissue pancreas.

Reference Reagents for Human Cytokines

The WHO ECBS has given considerable effort to developing international standards for various cytokines through an evaluation process in international collaborative studies. Standards have been developed for interleukin-1α and interleukin-1β,[53] macrophage colony-stimulating factor,[54] interleukin-3,[55] interleukin-4,[56] interleukin-6,[57] tumor necrosis factor,[58] and other cytokines.

The Biological Response Modifiers Program (National Cancer Institute) and the Division of Microbiology and Infectious Diseases (National Institute of Allergy and Infectious Diseases) in collaboration with the National Institute for Biological Standards and Control (United Kingdom) have made available reference reagents for murine and human cytokines. The reagents are available in small amounts (approximately 1 µg/sample) for use in the calibration of in vitro bioassays and in-house standards only and are not to be used for experimental purposes. Several of the human reference reagents currently available are

- Interferon α, β, and γ
- Interleukin-1α, -1β, and 2 through 10
- Leukemia inhibitory factor
- Granulocyte colony-stimulating factor
- Granulocyte-macrophage colony-stimulating factor
- Macrophage colony-stimulating factor
- Transforming growth factor–α and transforming growth factor–β

Whiteside[59] wrote an excellent review of cytokine measurements and interpretation of cytokine measurements in human disease.

Other Available Reference Preparations

Table 29-1 lists additional reference preparations and autoantibodies, as well as where to find them.

Summary and Recommendations

There has been considerable progress in the standardization of procedures and available reference preparations. Of course, standards and reference preparations comprise only a part of any quality assurance and improvement program. The ultimate goal of standardization is for various clinical laboratory test results to be interchangeable and for an exchange of data to be made with confidence.

With the development of more rapid and sensitive assays, there is a need for the continuous development of new reference preparations that are adaptable to the new methods. For example, there is a need for a future generation of reference preparations and standards that will demonstrate specific antibody reactivity on sensitive assays, such as ELISAs. These types of reference preparations are currently being developed by the Standards Committee of the Association of Medical Laboratory Immunologists. In addition, efforts should be made toward the characterization and standardization of specific antigen preparations that may be natural or of recombinant technologic origin. New reference preparations also will be needed to address the new nucleotide molecular assays in the clinical laboratory.

References

1. Batty I. Standards and quality control in clinical immunology. In: Thompson RA, ed. *Techniques in Clinical Chemistry*. 2nd ed. Oxford, England: Blackwell Scientific; 1981:306–324.
2. Holborow EJ, Johnson GD, Chantler S. Use of international reference preparations for immunofluorescence. In: Wick G, Traill KN, Schwanenstein K, eds. *Immunofluorescence Technology: Selected Theoretical and Clinical Aspect*. New York, NY: Elsevier Biomedical; 1982:1–10.
3. Holborow EJ, ed. *Standardization in Immunofluorescence*. Oxford, England: Blackwell Scientific; 1970.
4. Outschoorn AS, Bangham DR, Evans DG, et al. Guidelines for the preparation and establishment of reference materials and reference reagents for biological substances. *WHO Expert Committee on Biological Standardization Twenty-Ninth Report*, Geneva, Switzerland: World Health Organization; 1978.
5. Perkins FT. The establishment and use of biological standards. In: Dumonde DC, Steward MW, eds. *Laboratory Tests in Rheumatic Diseases: Standardization in Laboratory and Clinical Practice*. Baltimore, MD: University Park Press; 1979:73–79.
6. Batty I. Standardization of immunological reagents. In: Dumonde DC, Steward MW, eds. *Laboratory Tests in Rheumatic Diseases: Standardization in Laboratory and Clinical Practice*. Baltimore, MD: University Park Press; 1979:81–91.
7. Anderson SE, Addison IE, Dixon HG. Antinuclear factor serum (homogeneous): An international collaborative study of the proposed research standard 66/233. *Ann N Y Acad Sci*. 1971;177:337–345.
8. Feltkamp TEW. Standards and reference preparations. In: van Venrooij WJ, Maini RN, eds. *Manual of Biological Markers of Diseases*. Norwell, MA: Kluwer Academic Publishers; 1993;A11:1-12.
9. Feltkamp TEW. Standards for ANA and anti-DNA. *Clin Rheumatol*. 1990;9(suppl):74–81.
10. Ward AM. *United Kingdom External Quality Assessment Scheme for Autoimmune Serology and Special Chemistry*. Sheffield, UK: Department of Immunology; 1996.
11. Harris EH. The second international anti-cardiolipin standardization workshop/the Kingston antiphospholipid antibody study (KAPS) group. *Am J Clin Pathol*. 1990;94:476–484.
12. Harris EH. Anticardiolipin wet workshop report: Fifth international symposium on antiphospholipid antibodies. *Am J Clin Pathol*. 1994;101:616–624.
13. Johnson GD, Chantler S, Batty I, et al. Use and abuse of international reference preparations in immunofluorescence. In: Dumonde DC, Steward MW, eds. *Laboratory Tests in Rheumatic Diseases: Standardization in Laboratory and Clinical Practice*. Baltimore, MD: University Park Press; 1979:93–100.
14. Feltkamp TEW, Klein F, Janssens MBJA. Standardization of the quantitative determination of antinuclear antibodies (ANA's) with a homogeneous pattern. *Ann Rheum Dis*. 1988;47:906–909.
15. Molden DP, Nakamura RM, Tan EM. Standardization of the immunofluorescence test for autoantibody to nuclear antigens (ANA): Use of reference sera of defined antibody specificity. *Am J Clin Pathol*. 1984;82:57–66.
16. Working party recommendations on the characterization of antisera as reagents. *Immunology*. 1971;20:1.
17. Beutner EH, Kumar V, Krasny SA, et al. Defined immunofluorescence in immunodermatology. In: Beutner, EH, Chorzelski TP, Kumar V, eds. *Immunopathology of the Skin*. 3rd ed. New York, NY: John Wiley & Sons; 1987:3–40.
18. Feltkamp TEW, Kirkwood TBL, Maini RN, et al. The first international standard for antibodies to double-stranded DNA. *Ann Rheum Dis*. 1988;47:740–746.
19. Tan EM, Fritzler MJ, McDougal JS, et al. Reference sera for antinuclear antibodies, I: Antibodies to native DNA, Sm, nuclear RNP, and SS-B/La. *Arthritis Rheum*. 1982;25:1003–1005.
20. McDougal JS, Kennedy S, McDuffie FC. Standards and quality assurance for immunologic tests: Standards and reference materials for autoantibodies to nuclear antigens. In: Rippey JH, Nakamura RM, eds. *Diagnostic Immunology: Technology Assessment and Quality Assurance*. Skokie, IL: College of American Pathologists; 1983:147–155.
21. Tan EM, Feltkamp TEW, Alarcón-Segovia D, et al. Reference reagents for antinuclear antibodies. *Arthritis Rheum*. 1988;31:1331. [Letter]
22. Nakamura RM, Bylund DJ, Tan EM. Current status of available standards for quality improvement of assays for detection of autoantibodies to nuclear and intracellular antigens. *J Clin Lab Anal*. 1994;8:360–368.
23. Charles PJ, van Venrooij WJ, Maini RN. The consensus workshops for the detection of autoantibodies to intracellular antigens in rheumatic diseases: 1989–1992. *Clin Exp Rheumatol*. 1992;10:507–511.

24. Tan EM. International cooperative activities in standardization of antinuclear antibodies. In: van Venrooij WJ, Maini RN, eds. *Manual of Biological Markers of Diseases*. Norwell, MA: Kluwer Academic Publishers; 1993;A1:1–5.

25. Kalden JR. WHO/IUIS standardization programme. *Clin Exp Rheumatol*. 1992;10:513–514.

26. Bylund DJ, Nakamura RM. Importance of detection of SS-A/Ro autoantibody in screening immunofluorescence tests for autoantibodies to nuclear antigens. *J Clin Lab Anal*. 1991;5:212–218.

27. Taylor RN, Huong AY, Fulford KM, et al. Quality Control for Immunologic Tests. HEW Publication No. 79-8376. Atlanta, GA: Centers for Disease Control and Prevention; 1979.

28. Reimer CB, Smith SJ, Hannon WH, et al. Progress towards international reference standards for human serum proteins. *J Biol Stand*. 1978;6:133–138.

29. WHO Expert Committee on Biological Standardization. *Twenty-ninth Report*. Technical Report Series 626. Geneva, Switzerland: World Health Organization; 1978:19.

30. Reimer CB, Smith SJ, Wells TW, et al. Collaborative calibration of the U.S. National and the College of American Pathologists reference preparations for specific serum proteins. *Am J Clin Pathol*. 1982;77: 12–19.

31. Johnson AM. A new international reference preparation for proteins in human serum. *Arch Pathol Lab Med*. 1993;117:29–31.

32. Whicher JT, Ritchie RF, Johnson AM, et al. New international reference preparation for proteins in human serum (RPPHS). *Clin Chem*. 1994;40:934–938.

33. Matsuura E, Igarashi Y, Yasuda T, et al. Anticardiolipin antibodies recognize β_2-glycoprotein I structure altered by interacting with an oxygen modified solid phase surface. *J Exp Med*. 1994;179:457–462.

34. Roubey RAS, Eisenberg RA, Harper MF, et al. "Anticardiolipin" autoantibodies recognize β_2-glycoprotein I in the absence of phospholipid: importance of antigen density and bivalent binding. *J Immunol*. 1995;154:954–960.

35. Roubey RAS. Review: Immunology of the antiphospholipid antibody syndrome. *Arthritis Rheum*. 1996;39:1444–1454.

36. Emlen W. Antiphospholipid antibodies: new complexities and new assays. *Arthritis Rheum*. 1996;39:1441–1443. [Editorial]

37. Roubey RAS, Maldonado MA, Byrd SN. Comparison of an enzyme-linked immunosorbent assay for antibodies to β_2-glycoprotein I and a conventional anticardiolipin immunoassay. *Arthritis Rheum*. 1996;39:1606–1607. [Concise communication]

38. Matsuura E, Igarashi Y, Fujimoto M, et al. Heterogeneity of anticardiolipin antibodies defined by the anticardiolipin cofactor. *J Immunol*. 1992;148:3885–3891.

39. Roubey RAS, Pratt CW, Buyon JP, et al. Lupus anticoagulant activity of autoimmune antiphospholipid antibodies is dependent upon β_2-glycoprotein I. *J Clin Invest*. 1992;90:1100–1104.

40. Tincani A, Spatola L, Prati E, et al. The anti-β_2-glycoprotein I activity in human anti-phospholipid syndrome sera is due to monoreactive low-affinity autoantibodies directed to epitopes located on native β_2-glycoprotein I and preserved during species' evolution. *J Immunol*. 1996;157:5732–5738.

41. Erickson EN Jr, Najmey SS, Keil LB, et al. Reference calibrators for IgG antibodies to β_2-glycoprotein I: Preparation, properties, and availability to investigators. *Clin Chem*. 1996;42:1116–1117.

42. Feldt-Rasmussen U. Analytical and clinical performance goals for testing autoantibodies to thyroperoxidase, thyroglobulin, and thyrotropin receptor. *Clin Chem*. 1996;42:160–163.

43. Groves CJ, Howells RD, Williams S, et al. Primary standardization for the ELISA of serum thyroperoxidase and thyroglobulin antibodies and their prevalence in a normal Welsh population. *J Clin Lab Immunol*. 1990;32:147–151.

44. Wiik A. Delineation of a standard procedure for indirect immunofluorescence detection of ANCA. *Acta Pathol Microbiol Immunol Scand*. 1989;97(suppl 6):12–13.

45. Hagen EC, Andrassy K, Csernok E, et al. Immunological standardization: Development and standardization of solid phase assays for the detection of anti-neutrophil cytoplasmic antibodies (ANCA): A report on the second phase of an international cooperative study on the standardization of ANCA assays. *J Immunol Methods*. 1996;196:1–15.

46. Hagen EC, Andrassy K, Chernok E, et al. Immunological standardization: The value of indirect immunofluorescence and solid phase techniques for ANCA detection: A report on the first phase of an international cooperative study on the standardization of ANCA assays. *J Immunol Methods*. 1993;159:1–16.

47. Bottazzo GF, Gleichmann H. Report of the first international workshop on the standardisation of cytoplasmic islet cell antibodies. *Diabetologia*. 1986;29: 125–126.

48. Gleichmann H, Bottazzo GF. Progress toward standardization of cytoplasmic islet cell-antibody assay. *Diabetes*. 1987;36:578–584.

49. Bonifacio E, Lernmark A, Dawkins RL, et al. Serum exchange and use of dilutions have improved precision of measurement of islet cell antibodies. *J Immunol Methods*. 1988;106:83–88.

50. Bonifacio E, Boitard C, Gleichmann H, et al. Assessment of precision, concordance, specificity, and sensitivity of islet cell antibody measurement in 41 assays. *Diabetologia*. 1990;33:731–736.

51. Greenbaum CJ, Palmer JP, Nagataki S, et al. Improved specificity of ICA assays in the Fourth International Immunology of Diabetes Serum Exchange Workshop. *Diabetes*. 1992;41:1570–1574.

52. Landin-Olsson M. Precision of the islet-cell antibody assay depends on the pancreas. *J Clin Lab Anal*. 1990;4:289–294.

53. Poole S, Gaines Das RE. Immunological standardization: The international standards for interleukin-1α and interleukin-1β: Evaluation in an international collaborative study. *J Immunol Methods*. 1991;142:1–13.

54. Mire-Sluis AR, Gaines Das RE, Thorpe R, et al. Immunological standardization: The international standard for macrophage colony stimulating factor (M-CSF): Evaluation in an international collaborative study. *J Immunol Methods*. 1995;179:141–151.

55. Mire-Sluis AR, Gaines Das RE, Thorpe R, et al. Immunological standardization: Implications for the assay and biological properties of interleukin-3: Results of a WHO international collaborative study. *J Immunol Methods*. 1996;194:1–12.

56. Mire-Sluis AR, Gaines Das RE, Thorpe R, et al. Immunological standardization: Implications for the assay and biological activity of interleukin-4: Results of a WHO international collaborative study. *J Immunol Methods*. 1996;194:13–25.

57. Gaines Das RE, Poole S. Immunological standardization: The international standard for interleukin-6: Evaluation in an international collaborative study. *J Immunol Methods*. 1993;160:147–153.

58. de Kossodo S, Houba V, Grau GE, et al. Assaying tumor necrosis factor concentrations in human serum: A WHO international collaborative study. *J Immunol Methods*. 1995;182:107–114.

59. Whiteside T. Cytokine measurements and interpretation of cytokine assays in human disease. *J Clin Immunol*. 1994;14:327–339.

INDEX

Numbers in **boldface** refer to pages on which images, figures, and tables appear.

A

B

C

D

E

F

G

H

I

M

N

O

P

Q

R

S

T

U

V

W

X

Y

Z